Diagnostic Patient Studies
in Surgery

Diagnostic Patient Studies in Surgery

Bernard Sigel, M.D.

Professor and Chairman
Department of Surgery
Medical College of Pennsylvania
Philadelphia, Pennsylvania

Lea & Febiger 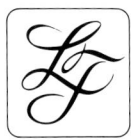 *Philadelphia 1986*

Lea & Febiger
600 Washington Square
Philadelphia, PA 19106-4198
U.S.A.
(215) 922-1330

Library of Congress Cataloging-in-Publication Data
Main entry under title:

Diagnostic patient studies in surgery.

  Includes bibliographies and index.
  1. Diagnosis, Surgical. I. Sigel, Bernard, 1930–
[DNLM: 1. Endoscopy. 2. Physical Examination.
3. Radiography. 4. Radionuclide Imaging. 5. Surgery,
Operative. 6. Ultrasonic Diagnosis. WB 200 D536]
RD35.D45   1986   616.07′5   85-23999
ISBN 0-8121-0996-1

Copyright © 1986 by Lea & Febiger. Copyright under the International Copyright Union. All rights reserved. This book is protected by copyright. *No part of it may be reproduced in any manner or by any means without written permission from the publishers.*

PRINTED IN THE UNITED STATES OF AMERICA

Print No.   4   3   2   1

Preface

How we make a diagnosis in surgical practice has changed radically in recent years. The basic history and physical examination have remained essentially the same, but newer methods of assessment that complement the history and physical examination have transformed the practice of medicine. These methods are patient and laboratory studies. Although such studies have increased our ability to detect and to diagnose disease, they also present problems characteristic of other technologic advances. Such problems relate to the appropriate uses of new technology. Appropriate uses can only follow an understanding of the basics and application of diagnostic procedures employed in surgery.

The term "patient studies" refers to one of the two major types of diagnostic techniques. Patient studies are diagnostic procedures that require the presence of the patient. These studies are different from laboratory studies, which are performed on specimens, such as blood, urine, or tissue, obtained from patients and processed later in a laboratory prepared to do chemical, immunologic, microbiologic, morphometric, or some other type of analysis. Some diagnoses require a combined use of patient and laboratory studies. For example, imaging or endoscopy, both of which are patient studies, may be used to guide placement of a biopsy needle to obtain a specimen for tissue analysis. Basically, three types of patient studies are performed. All have evolved since the nineteenth century, although many may be traced to antiquity. The three types of patient studies are imaging procedures, endoscopy, and function analyses.

Much of the growth and development of modern medical science and technology can be attributed to advances in patient studies. The use of these studies in surgical practice has had a significant impact on the management of patients. Patient studies have become an indispensable aspect of the management of many conditions treated by surgical means; however, they have also become numerous and sometimes risky, complex, and expensive. This book is intended to help surgeons to understand the commoner patient studies available to them in the management of their patients. This help is provided as a short reference about patient studies and a guide to their use.

A number of technologic advances, occurring mostly since World War II, have given rise to the many patient studies available today. These advances are largely related to rapid developments in science and technology as a whole and include such developments as new energy sources for imaging (ultrasound, nuclear products, magnetic resonance), new materials (fiber optics), and new computational abilities brought about by integrated circuits. Many patient studies have recently undergone rapid change. A means of evaluating this progress is to consider the many branches of medicine and the types of physicians active in the performance of each major type of patient studies.

The field of medical imaging has grown extensively and has given rise to the specialty of diagnostic radiology, which provides physicians skilled in the performance and interpretation of radiographic images. This field has been enriched by advances in nuclear medicine, ultrasound, computer tomography, magnetic resonance imaging, and specialized procedures employing the injection of contrast material. Although some specialists perform their own imaging procedures, the specialists in diagnostic radiology have largely become the main providers of imaging expertise.

The situation is different wtih endoscopy. Endoscopic procedures are performed by physicians and surgeons specializing in diseases of certain systems, such as the genitourinary, gastrointestinal, and respiratory tracts. Not all specialists perform endoscopic studies, however, and many rely on colleagues to perform requisite endoscopic examinations.

Function analyses do not provide an image or an endoscopic view, but rather information about physiologic processes and how they may be deranged. Many function tests began as physiologic investigation. Function analyses are as diverse as the organs and systems that they evaluate. Consequently, these tests are usually supervised and interpreted by physicians in a variety of medical specialties. Function analyses range from the commonplace electrocardiogram to the less-common 24-hour monitoring of esophageal hydrogen ion concentration.

The point about patient studies in surgery is the extensive number and wide assortment of tests that usually require the involvement of other physicians in a variety of specialties. Surgeons who request patient studies have increasing difficulty in deciding which procedures to order and how to respond to their results. Indeed, the errors that may occur in the diagnostic workup of a patient are often related to which tests to perform and when. Although much is now known about patient studies used in surgical diagnosis, this knowledge is available in a multiplicity of sources such as separate textbooks on the various forms of imaging, endoscopy, and function analysis. These sources are usually directed to physicians within a specialty such as radiology or gastrointestinal endoscopy. On the other hand, the standard textbooks of surgery can devote little space to patient studies. This book attempts to follow a middle course by providing information about diverse types of patient studies for surgeons. We have tried to bring together a number of topics related to the surgical applications of the three types of patient studies into a single volume that can be used by the general and subspecialty surgeon as a reference and guide. Because of limits relating to the nature and quantity of material that may be presented in a reasonable manner, much selectivity was necessary in defining the scope and content of this book. This can be best expressed in terms of what we emphasized and what we restricted.

Our approach has been to present topics that relate to general as well as some specialty applications of patient studies. These topics include all major imaging modes in use today, the commoner endoscopic procedures, and function analyses applicable to most workups of the cardiac, genitourinary, respiratory, gastrointestinal, and neurologic systems. Space has prevented us from including other topics such as otolaryngologic and ophthalmologic procedures. We feel justified in excluding these examinations because a surgeon undertaking a diagnostic workup seldom requests specific otolaryngologic or ophthalmologic procedures, but rather seeks a consultant who, in turn, obtains specific tests. The situation is different for most of the patient studies described in this book because we have selected procedures that a surgeon is more likely to request directly. Such procedures may be new or well established. This book aims to acquaint the surgeon with some new procedures and to summarize the current status of other tests that might be required during the management of a surgical patient.

Diagnostic Patient Studies in Surgery is limited because less emphasis is placed on technique and interpretation than on short explanatory descriptions of the studies, their strengths and weaknesses, and the main indications for their use. Our primary aim in preparing the book was not to teach the surgeon how to perform or to interpret patient studies, but rather to teach an understanding of how the tests are best used during the diagnostic process. The emphasis is on the surgeon as decision maker regarding which tests to order, the timing of these tests, and the meaning of test results.

This book is further limited by not providing specific approaches or algorithms for performing diagnostic workups of individual problems. The book describes many types of patient studies that the surgeon may consider, but it does not initiate the problem-solving search. The surgeon must have already started the diagnostic process and must have some idea of which studies should be performed. Questions about the possible use of a particular study should prompt the reader to refer to a section or chapter dealing with that study. This book need not be read sequentially because each chapter is independent, except the chapter on general principles of radiation, which is background reading for other topics in radiographic imaging. For those wishing further information, each chapter contains references to the literature or suggestions for general reading in the subject. For common patient studies, however, this book should provide adequate background information. I hope that this book will promote a more informed and cost-effective use of patient studies in surgical practice.

Philadelphia, PA   Bernard Sigel, M.D.

Contributors

HERAND ABCARIAN, MD, FACS
Professor of Surgery
University of Illinois College of Medicine at Chicago
Chairman, Section of Colon Rectal Surgery
Cook County Hospital
Chicago, Illinois

ELENA ADLER, MD
Assistant Professor of Anesthesia and Pediatrics
Children's Hospital Medical Center
Cincinnati, Ohio

JOHN A. BARRETT, MD
Assistant Professor of Surgery
University of Illinois at Chicago
Director, Trauma Unit
Cook County Hospital
Chicago, Illinois

JOHN M. BECKER, MD
Clinical Assistant Professor of Medicine
University of Pennsylvania
School of Medicine
Radiologist, Presbyterian-University of Pennsylvania Medical Center
Philadelphia, Pennsylvania

GEORGE BERCI, MD, FACS
Clinical Professor of Surgery
UCLA School of Medicine-Los Angeles
Associate Director, Dept. of Surgery
Director, Division of Surgical Endoscopy
Cedars-Sinai Medical Center
Los Angeles, California

C. THOMAS BOMBECK, MD
Professor of Surgery
Chief, Section of Surgical Gastroenterology
University of Illinois
Chicago, Illinois

LUIGI BONAVINA, MD
Research Associate
Creighton University
Dept. of Surgery
Omaha, Nebraska

GRAEME M. BYDDER
Senior Lecturer
Royal Postgraduate Medical School
Hammersmith Hospital
London, England

GERALD W. CHODAK
Associate Professor of Surgery
Pritzger School of Medicine
The University of Chicago Medical Center
Chicago, Illinois

ROBERT H. CHOPLIN, MD
Associate Professor of Radiology
Bowman-Gray School of Medicine
Radiologist, North Carolina Baptist Hospital
Winston Salem, North Carolina

PETER L. COOPERBERG, MD
Professor of Radiology
University of British Columbia
Chief, Section of Ultrasound
Dept. of Radiology
Vancouver General Hospital
Vancouver, BC Canada

MICHAEL C. DALSING, MD
Conrad Jobst Fellow in Peripheral Vascular Surgery
Northwestern University Medical School
Chicago, Illinois

TOM R. DeMEESTER, MD
Chairman, Dept. of Surgery
Professor of Thoracic and Cardiovascular Surgery
Creighton University
Omaha, Nebraska

FREDERICK J. DOHERTY
Assistant Professor of Radiology
Director, Diagnostic Ultrasound
Tufts University New England Medical Center
Boston, Massachusetts

CONTRIBUTORS

DANIEL H. DUNN, MD
Assistant Professor of Surgery
SUNY Downstate Medical Center
Associate Director of Surgery
Long Island College Hospital
Brooklyn, New York

M. MICHAEL EISENBERG, MD
Professor of Surgery
Vice-Chairman, Dept. of Surgery
SUNY Downstate Medical Center
Director of Surgery
Long Island College Hospital
Brooklyn, New York

WILLIAM S. FRANKL, MD, MS
Professor of Medicine
Co-Director, Likoff Cardiovascular Institute of Hahnemann University
Philadelphia, Pennsylvania

EDWARD G. GRANT, MD
Associate Professor of Radiology
Associate Professor and Director of Ultrasound
Georgetown University Hospital
Washington, D.C.

GWENDOLYN B. GRAYBAR, MD
Professor of Anesthesiology
Attending Anesthesiologist
University Hospital
Birmingham, Alabama

JOHN R. HAAGA, MD
Professor of Radiology
Director of Diagnostic Radiology
Head, Section of Body Computed Tomography
University Hospital of Cleveland
Cleveland, Ohio

GERALD M. KLEIN, MD
Attending Radiologist
Metropolitan Hospital
Springfield, Pennsylvania

GREGORY P. LEWIS, MD
Mason Clinic in Seattle
Seattle, Washington

WELLS MARTIN, III, MD
Clinical Assistant Professor of Radiology
Department of Radiology
High Point Regional Hospital
High Point, North Carolina

GARY J. MERLOTTI, MD
Assistant Professor of Surgery
University of Illinois at Chicago
Associate Director
Trauma Unit
Cook County Hospital, Chicago, Illinois

DAVID J. OTT, MD
Associate Professor of Radiology
Bowman Gray School of Medicine
Wake Forest University
Winston-Salem, North Carolina

HENRY W. SCHOENBERG, MD
Professor and Chairman
Section of Urology
The University of Chicago
Chicago, Illinois

CARL L. SCHULTZ
Assistant Professor of Radiology
Case Western Reserve University
University Hospitals of Cleveland
Cleveland, Ohio

BERNARD SHAPIRO, MD
Chairman, Division of Nuclear Medicine
Dept. of Radiology
Albert Einstein Medical Center
Philadelphia, Pennsylvania

DIMITRIOS G. SPIGOS, MD
Professor of Radiology
Chief, Special Procedures
University of Illinois College of Medicine at Chicago
Chicago, Illinois

GEORGE N. STEIN, MD
Professor of Radiology
University of Pennsylvania School of Medicine
Radiologist, Presbyterian-University of Pennsylvania Medical Center
Philadelphia, Pennsylvania

PAUL A. THOMAS, MD
Professor of Surgery, University of Illinois
Chief, Surgical Service, Veterans Administration Medical Center
Attending Staff, Division Cardio-Thoracic Surgery at both University of Illinois Hospital and Cook County Hospital
Chicago, Illinois

JOHN V. WHITE, MD
Fellow in Peripheral Vascular Surgery
Northwestern University Medical School
Chicago, Illinois

ANDREW C. WILBUR, MD
Assistant Professor of Radiology
University of Illinois
College of Medicine at Chicago
Chicago, Illinois

DONALD K. WOOD, MD
Associate Professor of Clinical Surgery
University of Illinois at Chicago
Assistant Chief, Surgical Service
Veterans Westside Medical Center
Staff Surgeon, at both University of Illinois Hospital and Cook County Hospital, Chicago, Illinois

JAMES S.T. YAO, MD, PhD
Professor of Surgery
Director, Blood Flow Laboratory
Northwestern University Medical School
Chicago, Illinois

Contents

Part I: Imaging

Chapter 1. Radiologic Physics, Technique, and Radiobiology 3
Robert H. Choplin
Wells Martin, III

Chapter 2. Plain Film Radiography of the Skeleton 13
Robert H. Choplin
Wells Martin, III

Chapter 3. Plain Film Radiography of the Chest and Abdomen 43
Robert H. Choplin

Chapter 4. Ultrasound Imaging 59
Edward G. Grant
Frederick J. Doherty

Chapter 5. Radionuclide Scanning 97
Bernard Shapiro

Chapter 6. Computed Tomography 127
Carl L. Schultz
John R. Haaga

Chapter 7. Angiography 153
Andrew C. Wilbur
Dimitrios G. Spigos

Chapter 8. Luminal Contrast Studies of the Bile and Pancreatic Ducts .. 183
Section 1. Oral Cholecystography and Intravenous Cholangiography
Joseph M. Becker
George N. Stein

Section 2. Percutaneous Transhepatic Cholangiography and Endoscopic Retrograde Cholangiopancreatography
Gerald M. Klein
George N. Stein

Chapter 9. Luminal Contrast Studies of the Gastrointestinal Tract 213
David J. Ott

Part II: Endoscopy, Function Studies, and Magnetic Resonance Imaging

Chapter 10. Studies of the Urinary Tract 243
Gerald W. Chodak
Harry W. Schoenberg

CONTENTS

Chapter 11.	Rationale and Selection of Diagnostic Procedures for Airway and Chest Diseases .... Paul A. Thomas Donald K. Wood	255
Chapter 12.	Upper Gastrointestinal Endoscopy .... C. Thomas Bombeck	263
Chapter 13.	Lower Gastrointestinal Endoscopy .... Herand Abcarian	275
Chapter 14.	Diagnostic Laparoscopy .... George Berci	283
Chapter 15.	Abdominal Paracentesis and Lavage for Trauma .... John A. Barrett Gary J. Merlotti	293
Chapter 16.	Diagnostic Pulmonary Function Tests .... Gwendolyn Graybar Elena Adler	299
Chapter 17.	Cardiac Function Studies .... William S. Frankl	311
Section 1.	Electrocardiography	
Section 2.	Cardiac Catheterization	
Section 3.	Bedside Hemodynamic Monitoring	
Chapter 18.	Prolonged Esophageal pH Monitoring .... Luigi Bonavina Tom R. DeMeester	353
Chapter 19.	Esophageal Motility Studies .... C. Thomas Bombeck	365
Chapter 20.	Gastroduodenal Function Studies .... Daniel H. Dunn M. Michael Eisenberg	369
Chapter 21.	Vascular Laboratory Tests in Peripheral Vascular Disease .. Michael C. Dalsing John V. White James S. T. Yao	379
Chapter 22.	Fine-Needle Abdominal Aspiration .... Gregory P. Lewis Peter L. Cooperberg	401
Chapter 23.	Clinical Magnetic Resonance Imaging .... G. M. Bydder	413
Index	....	429

Part I

IMAGING

1

Radiologic Physics, Technique, and Radiobiology

Robert H. Choplin ■ Wells Martin, III

Although detailed knowledge of the physics and technique of radiology is unnecessary for clinical practice, an overview of these processes may be helpful in understanding some of the limitations of x-ray equipment and the reasons for the appearance of x-ray films. It may also be useful as background information for discussing potential technical problems with a radiologist or technologist. For readers with greater interest in this subject, several excellent texts are available.[1-3]

A developed radiograph is the product of a complex process that includes generation of an x-ray beam, passage of that beam through an object with which it interacts to create spatial differences in intensity, and the capture of those spatial inequalities on a receptor. It is possible to alter each of these processes, with differences in the resulting image. Although radiologists attempt to alter the processes to enhance an area of interest, the final product always reflects a compromise between enhancement and suppression of desired and undesired variables. When viewing a radiograph, it is sometimes possible to tell which variables have been altered, but often it is not.

GENERATION OF AN X-RAY BEAM

X rays are electromagnetic radiations with properties of both waves and particles. They travel at the speed of light, have wavelengths of 0.1 to 1 angstrom (for diagnostic x-ray studies) and energy levels of 10 to 300 kiloelectron volts (keV). X rays are produced by bombardment of a target by a stream of electrons in a vacuum tube (Fig. 1–1). When the electrons hit the target, they may interact with the nuclei of target atoms to produce *bremsstrahlung* (general radiation), which emerges as a beam with a peak and a spectrum of lesser-energy x rays (Fig. 1–2). Electrons may also interact with a target-atom electron to produce characteristic radiation, which has a single energy level. Charac-

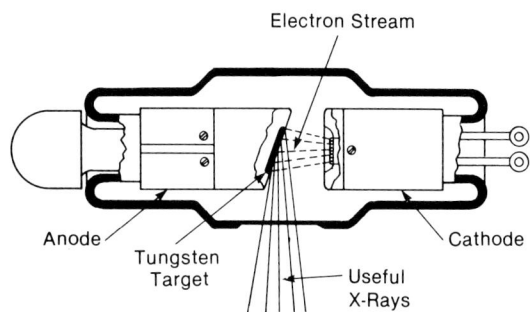

FIG. 1–1. Cross-sectional view of an x-ray tube. A stream of electrons is accelerated across a vacuum tube in such a way that they collide with a target, which is usually made of tungsten. Interaction between these electrons and the tungsten atoms produces x-rays. Because the tube is shielded, x-rays may only leave through a small window.

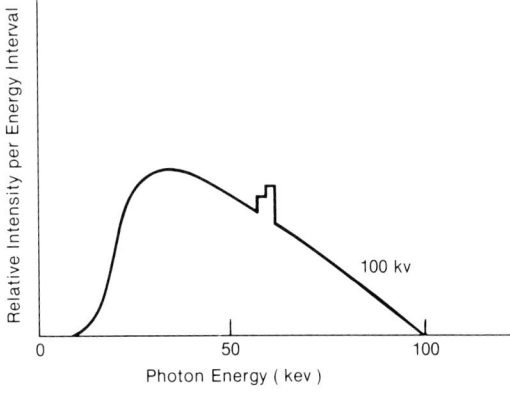

FIG. 1–2. Photon energies in an x-ray beam produced by *bremsstrahlung*. The beam is composed of x-ray photons of energies ranging from about 10 to 100 keV, with the majority of photons occurring at lower energy levels. The step up at 62 keV results from the characteristic radiation of tungsten.

3

teristic radiation contributes 0 to 30% of the total energy of an x-ray beam, depending on how it is produced. Both the peak energy and the total amount of x rays in the beam may be controlled by an operator. X-ray equipment is usually constructed to suit desired needs and ranges from simple machines useful for imaging the chest and the extremities to more complex and powerful units suitable for angiography.

INTERACTION OF X RAYS WITH MATTER

Such interaction occurs at the atomic level, as well as with the object under radiographic study.

Interactions at the Atomic Level

As an x-ray beam traverses an object, interactions take place at the level of the atom. Although an x-ray photon may interact with matter in five basic ways, only the photoelectric effect and Compton scattering are important in diagnostic radiology. Photoelectric reactions are more likely to take place when the average energy level of the x-ray photons is low and when the tissues under study are composed of higher-atomic-number atoms, such as bones.

A photoelectric reaction takes place when an x-ray photon collides with a tightly bound electron from an atom's *inner* shell and ejects it from its orbit. When this reaction happens, the photon is completely absorbed, and spatial differences in beam intensity (shadows) are created as other x-ray photons completely traverse the object. The photoelectric effect therefore plays a major role in creating the contrast differences between tissues and allows their visualization. Unfortunately, films exposed using low-photon-energy beams result in a high radiation dose to the patient. Because of this high absorbed radiation dose, one attempts to obtain films at low enough photon energy levels to provide some photoelectric effect and therefore crisp images, but at high enough energy levels to maintain minimum radiation exposure.

Compton scattering is the other important interaction between x-ray photons and atoms. When a high-energy x-ray photon strikes a free electron in the *outer* shell of an atom, it ejects the electron from its shell and is itself deflected in a new direction. The distribution of scattered photons varies with the energy of the incident beam in such a way that photons are scattered in an increasingly forward direction as the average energy of the beam increases (Fig. 1–3). Because scattered radiation is deflected randomly, it adds to overall film blackening and decreases the difference in intensity between black and white regions of a film. This decrease in contrast may degrade the imaged because scattered radiation may account for 50 to 90% of the photons emerging from a patient. As with the photoelectric effect, a compromise must be made in selecting the energy level used in taking a radiograph. Decreasing beam energy lessens Compton scatter, but increases the radiation dose to the patient. Increasing beam energy lessens the radiation dose, but increases the amount of scatter and therefore degrades the image.

Interaction with the Object to be Radiographed

An x-ray beam is characterized by a quality variable, which is the average energy of the photons, and by a quantity variable, which is the number of photons. Beam intensity is the product of these two variables. Attenuation is the reduction in intensity of the x-ray beam by either absorption or deflection of photons as it traverses an object. Attenuation across an absorber occurs in an exponential fashion, so the intensity of a beam emerging from a patient may be as little as 1% of the intensity at entrance. Attenuation is influenced by the energy of the incident beam, the density of the absorber, the atomic number of the absorber, and the electrons per gram of tissue. The first two factors are of primary importance in diagnostic radiology. Most radiographs must be taken with a beam energy of 60 to 120 keV, an energy level at which Compon reactions predominate and at which differential attenuation almost entirely depends on tissue density.

Scatter Reduction

The x-ray beam exiting from a patient consists of both primary and scattered radiation and has as-

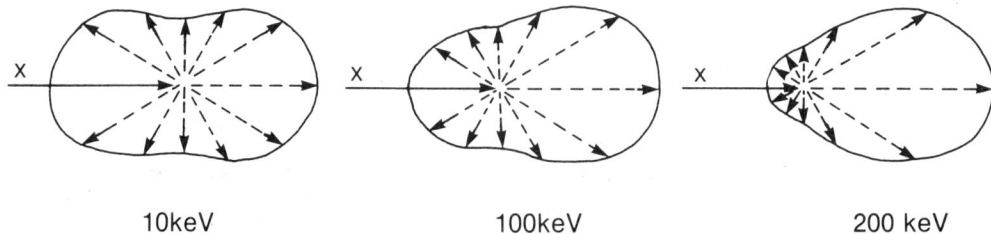

FIG. 1–3. The distribution patterns from Compton scattering occurring with beams of three different energy levels. As the average energy of the beam increases, the deflected (scattered) photon is more likely to continue in a forward direction.

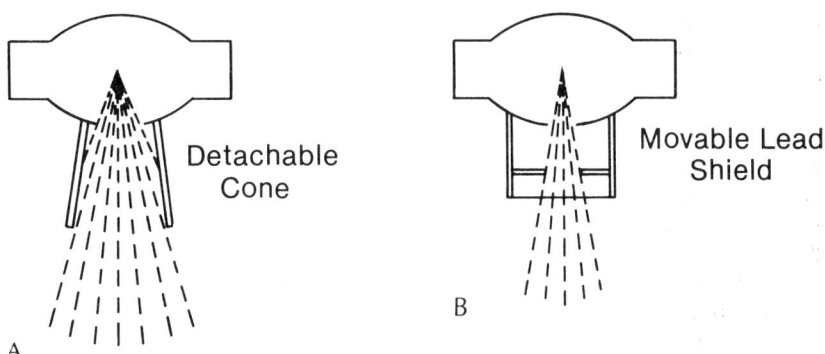

FIG. 1-4. Radiation beam restrictors. X-ray beams are restricted to a size appropriate to examine a body part by using detachable cones *(A)* of various sizes or a collimator. *B,* The collimator has movable lead shields that can be adjusted to limit the x-ray field.

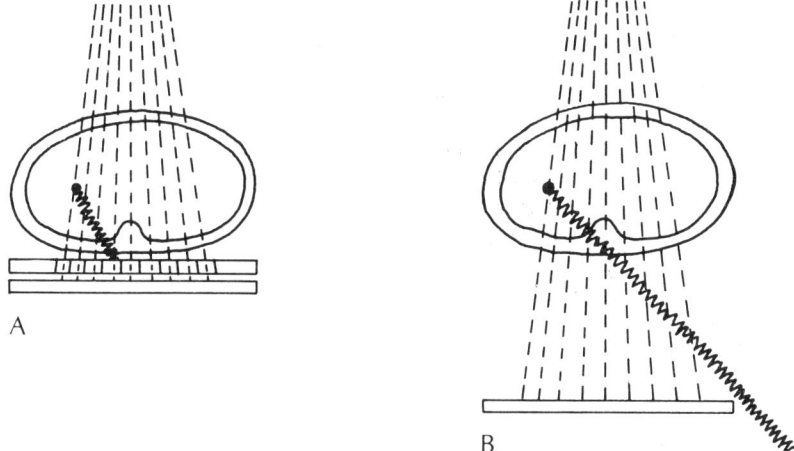

FIG. 1-5. Reduction of scattered radiation; two methods. *A,* A grid consisting of lead foil strips and aluminum has been placed between the patient and the film. Because the scattered radiation (zig-zag line) is not parallel to the lead strips, it cannot reach the film to degrade the image. *B,* An air gap of about 20 cm has been placed between the patient and the film. Because of this gap, a scattered photon (zig-zag line) may not hit the film.

sumed spatial differences in intensity because of interactions with various anatomic structures. The amount of scattered radiation increases not only with increasing beam energy, but also with the size of the x-ray field and the part examined. For example, an x-ray beam in an abdominal study has more scatter radiation than an x-ray beam in the radiographic study of a finger. The amount of scattered radiation may be minimized by decreasing field size or part thickness and by the use of grids or an air gap when the beam has left the patient. Field size is decreased by using cones or a collimator to restrict the beam as it comes from the x-ray tube (Fig. 1-4). Scattered radiation in the beam exiting from a patient may be reduced by use of either a grid or an air gap (Fig. 1-5). A grid is constructed of parallel strips of lead foil interposed between strips of radiolucent material, usually aluminum or an organic compound. A grid allows passage of primary radiation, but only minimal amounts of scattered radiation pass through because they are not parallel to the lead foil. An air gap between the patient and the receptor decreases scattered radiation because the majority of the scattered photons do not hit the film. Use of either an air gap or a grid requires a slight increase in radiation dose to the patient.

IMAGE RECEPTORS

To study the information carried by the x-ray beam, the beam must be captured on an appropriate receptor. This capture may be accomplished by exposure of film, by a film-screen system, by a xeroradiographic system, or by a fluoroscopic screen. Information capture with processing before display, as in computed tomography or some digital imaging system, is beyond the scope of this chapter and is discussed in the chapters devoted to computed tomography (CT) and angiography.

Although film may be directly exposed by x rays, this method is insensitive, and the radiation doses are too high for routine use, except for radiographs of extremities. To keep radiation doses low, almost all films are taken using intensifying screens. These film-screen systems are plastic screens in which an inorganic salt, called a phosphor, has been imbedded. When exposed to x rays, the phosphor emits a large amount of light per x-ray photon, and this light exposes the film. A number of phosphors are available, each of which is usually matched to a particular film; the result is a film-screen combination with a defined speed (sensitivity to x rays) and resolving power. In general, as the speed of a system increases, its ability to resolve detail decreases. One must therefore make a compromise between radiation dose and film quality. Systems must be selected according to the requirements of the anatomic part to be imaged.

A fluoroscopic screen uses either zinc cadmium sulfide or cesium iodide as the phosphor because these compounds emit light in the blue-to-green area of the visible spectrum, the region of maximum sensitivity of the retina. The image on a fluoroscopic screen may be viewed directly, through a system of mirrors, or by a television system. Image intensifiers, devices that magnify the light output from the fluoroscopic screen, are used with almost all modern fluoroscopic equipment.

Xeroradiography is a means of capturing the x-ray image by use of an electrostatically charged selenium plate. The plate is partially discharged when exposed to x rays, and a powder of charged particles is used to develop the electrostatic image, which is then transferred to paper. Because the radiation dose required for exposure of a xeroradiographic plate is higher than that required for film-screen systems, the technique is unsuitable for general radiography. Xeroradiography has an advantage over film in imaging soft tissue detail, however. This advantage has made xeroradiography popular for mammography. When the technique was first used for this purpose, xeroradiographic mammograms could be performed at a radiation dose lower than that required for film mammograms. Since that time, modifications in both film-screen systems and mammographic x-ray units have made it possible to produce high-quality film mammograms at a lower radiation dose than needed for xeroradiography. Both forms of breast imaging are in widespread use and are considered acceptable.

BODY-SECTION RADIOGRAPHY

Body-section imaging has used conventional tomography for many years. The development of CT scanning, gray-scale ultrasonography, and magnetic resonance imaging have made body section imaging one of the most rapidly evolving areas in medical diagnosis. Each technique is discussed in a separate chapter of this book. The principle underlying all these methods is to view a section of the body unencumbered by confusing overlapping anatomic structures.

Conventional tomography is body-section radiography that uses movements of the radiographic tube and x-ray film to blur unwanted information while keeping the region of interest in focus.[4] The simplest form of tomography is a linear movement of both the radiographic tube and the film, but in opposite directions with respect to the patient (Fig. 1–6). The focal plane is at the level of the axis of rotation of the beam. Theoretically, only a single plane is in sharp focus, and defocusing is progressive as one moves above or below that plane. In practice, however, a section appears to have "thickness;" the objects in that region are in focus, and objects outside that plane are out of focus. Because the effectiveness of blurring depends on the total length of tube travel, equipment has been developed to move the tube and film in long, complex motions, as illustrated in Figure 1–7. This equipment is more expensive than simple linear units. One disadvantage of linear tomography, however, is its inability to blur linear structures that are parallel to the line of tube motion. This phenomenon happens because the

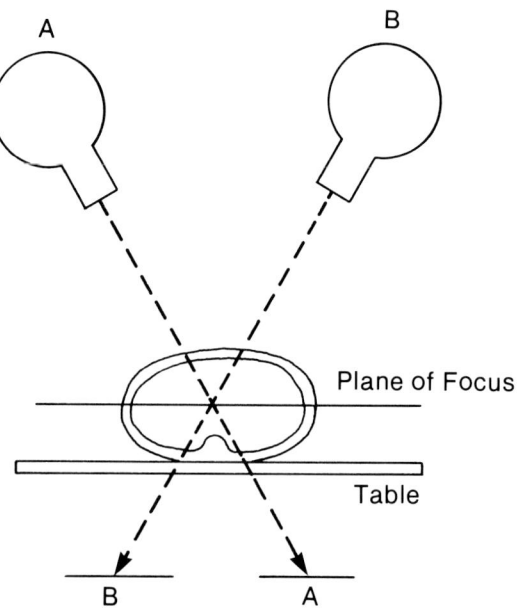

FIG. 1–6. Tomography. The radiograph is performed while the x-ray tube and film move from A to B, resulting in a plane of focus. To obtain images at other levels, the patient is moved up or down with respect to the plane of focus.

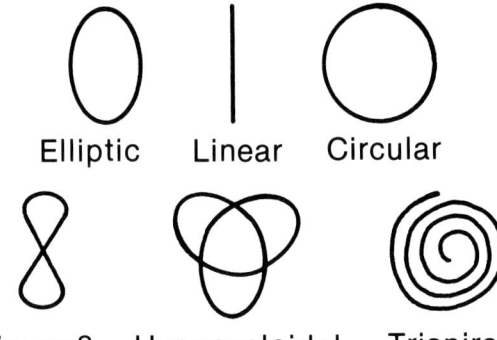

FIG. 1–7. Pathways of movement for tomography. The tube and film are moved in opposite directions along one of these pathways. The complex pathways have more effective blurring, but they are expensive. Each pathway results in its own artifacts.

projected image of the linear structure moves so little. As such, linear tomography may not be beneficial in evaluating some structures, such as bones, which are linear and cannot be oriented perpendicular to tube travel to avoid this artifact (Fig. 1–8).

PERCEPTION OF THE RADIOGRAPHIC IMAGE

Perception of the radiographic image is a complex process involving acquisition of visual information, psychophysiologic processing of the information into a recognizable pattern, and assignment of an appropriate meaning to that pattern.[5] Although much of this process takes place unconsciously and is poorly understood, several factors can be used to optimize one's ability to make a diagnosis.

Perception of any light signal depends on the state of foveal adaptation, which becomes less sensitive as the ambient lighting becomes brighter. Therefore, extraneous lighting should be excluded as much as possible, to lower the threshold for signal detection. In addition, perception depends on the difference between the signal and the background. Elimination of possible sources of reflected light is therefore important in maximizing the signal-to-noise ratio.

The visual system is much more sensitive to contrast than to brightness. Although contrast is often thought of as the difference in illumination between two points, it may also be considered as the rate of change of illumination with respect to distance across the retina. The greater the rate of change, the greater the contrast and the more apparent an "edge" becomes. The lower the rate of change, the more difficult it is to detect an abnormality. Some radiologic diagnosis depends on detection of abnormal opacity, but to a lesser extent than on margin detection. The posteroanterior and lateral images and CT scan of a patient with a ganglioneuroma clearly demonstrate this principle; one sees the reason that this lesion is obvious on the posteroanterior film and invisible on the lateral film (Fig. 1–9). Finally, one's ability to detect subtle margins changes with viewing distance. It has been suggested that films should always be viewed not only from a normal distance of about 30 inches, but from an increased viewing distance or through minifying lenses, both of which have the effect of sharpening contrast differences.

RADIATION PROTECTION

Protection from radiation involves measurement and restriction of doses, as well as an understanding both of the effects of radiation and of permissible limits.

Measurement of Radiation

Radiation measurements may be expressed in terms of exposure, absorbed dose, or biologic effectiveness.[1] The original unit of exposure, the roentgen, is that amount of radiation that ionizes air under standard conditions releasing electrons equal to a charge of 2.58×10^{-4} coulombs/kg air. The roentgen is limited in that it applies only to x or gamma rays and cannot be accurately measured at beam energy levels higher than 3 million electron volts (3 MeV), a level above which most modern radiotherapy equipment operates. The biologic consequences of radiation are related more closely to the portion of the x-ray beam that is absorbed by the patient than to the exposure itself. Although the absorbed dose is proportional to exposure, the relationship is complex, and the number of units of absorbed dose varies with the energy of the beam and the composition of the absorber. The unit of absorbed dose, the rad, is equal to an energy transfer of 100 ergs/g irradiated material from any form of ionizing radiation. The rem, a unit of dose equivalent, measures biologic effectiveness and is required for a comparison of the effects of different types of ionizing radiation. For x and gamma rays in the diagnostic energy range, all these units of measure are close enough to be considered equal. Dosages from x-ray or nuclear medicine examinations of patients are preferably expressed in rad or mrad (1/1000 rad). The International System of Units (SI) has suggested changing the name of the unit of absorbed dose from rad to Gray and the unit of biologic effectiveness from rem to Sievert. A Gray equals 100 rad, and a Sievert equals 100 rem. The method of calculation of these quantities is unchanged.[6]

Effects of Ionizing Radiation

Ionizing radiation used in diagnostic imaging includes x rays and gamma rays. Gamma rays are qualitatively similar to x rays, but they are a product

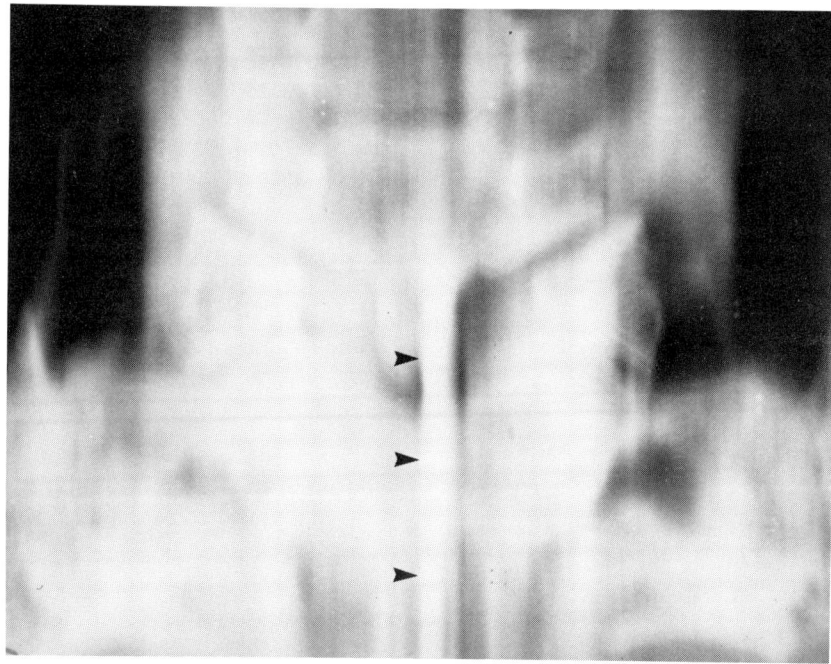

FIG. 1–8. Linear tomogram of the atlas and axis; tube travel is along the craniocaudad axis. Note tha bones perpendicular to tube travel (cortical margins of C1 and C2 lateral masses) are demonstrated in detail. Bones parallel to tube travel are not well detailed, and the nasal septum produces a parasite line (arrowheads).

of radioactive decay and are most widely used in nuclear medicine studies. Ionizing radiation exerts its biologic effects through the transfer of energy to one or more atoms by ejecting electrons from stable electron orbits. When an electron is ejected, an ion pair is formed, an unstable high-energy state develops, and the ions may enter into chemical reactions that could not occur in the atom's stable state. Through these chemical reactions, the biologic effect ultimately takes place.[7-10]

The consequences of radiation may be expressed at either the cellular or tissue level (somatic effect) or at the level of the population as a whole (genetic effects). The somatic effects occur in an individual who has been irradiated, whereas the genetic effects occur in the progeny of such an individual. Most often, the cellular effect of radiation is a deletion in the base sequence of a nucleotide. Because these molecules exert a major effect over all cellular functions, one or more of these functions may be lost because of the deletion. Whether or not this loss is of consequence depends on the exact function lost, on the existence of alternate functions, and on the capacity for the function to be repaired or replaced. The effect on a tissue or organ depends on the amount and type of radiation, the speed with which it is delivered, the age of the organism at the time of radiation, and the kind of tissue irradiated. The most rapidly proliferating tissues are the most radiosensitive, and vice versa.

The most important somatic effect of radiation is the production of solid tumors and leukemia; however, these effects have only been demonstrated at dose levels well above those delivered in diagnostic radiology. Estimates extrapolated from data on patients receiving higher doses suggest that the increased incidence of fatal cancer in the population receiving low doses ($<$ 100 rad) of radiation would be about 4 cases per million per rad per year. Because the background incidence is 160,000 cases of fatal cancer per million persons per year, massive population studies would be needed to detect this effect. In view of this requirement, it is not actually known whether low-dose radiation exposure causes cancer or leukemia.

Radiation is also known to produce gene mutations and chromosomal aberrations. As with the somatic effects, the estimated increased incidence of abnormalities due to genetic effect is small and is overshadowed by the background incidence of more than 10 genetic defects per 100 pregnancies. To date, no study has clearly demonstrated any genetic effect of radiation in man.

Irradiation of pregnant experimental animals has

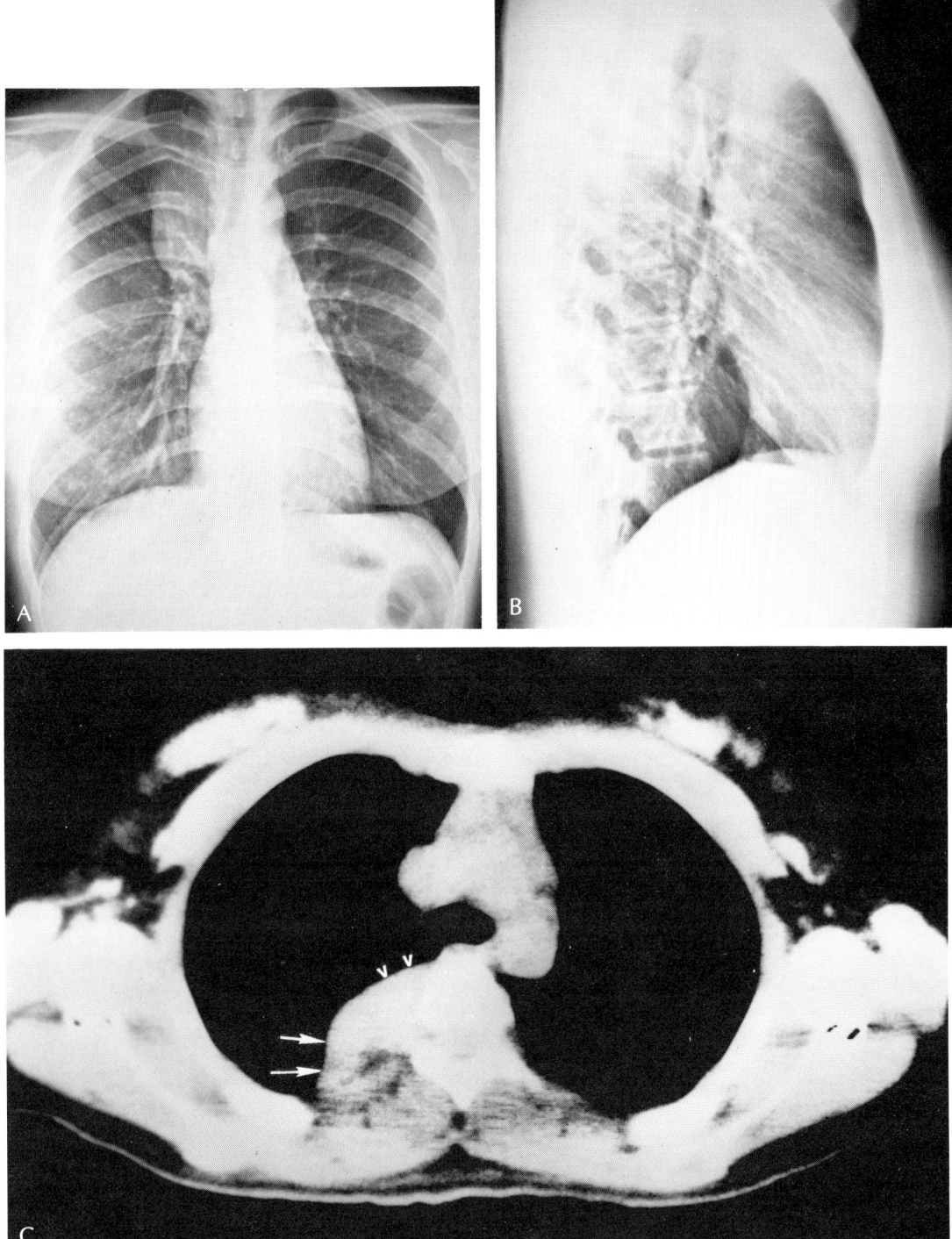

FIG. 1-9. Edge perception in radiology. A mediastinal mass is clearly visible in the posteroanterior (PA) view *(A)* and is virtually invisible on the lateral view *(B)*. *C,* The CT scan shows the lateral margin of the tumor (arrows) to be nearly parallel to the x-ray beam in a PA projection; the anterior margin (arrowheads) is less parallel to the laterally projected beam and does not generate an edge. Moreover, the tumor is posteriorly located, so its increased radiopacity is not detectable on the lateral view because of the "normal" increased radiopacity of the shoulders.

Table 1–1. Maximum Permissible Radiation Exposure Limits (REM)

Occupational Exposure	Quarterly	Annually
Whole body	3	5
Hands	25	75
Other organs	5	15
Fetus	—	0.5
General Population		
Genetic	—	0.17
Somatic	—	0.17

(Adapted from National Council on Radiation Protection and Measurements: Basic Radiation Protection Criteria. NCRP Report No. 39. Washington, DC, NCRP, 1971.)

Table 1–2. Estimated Radiation Doses for Selected Examinations (RAD)

Radiographic study	Mean skin dose per film	Mean gonadal dose per examination	
		Men	Women
Chest	0.05	—	—
Abdomen	0.77	0.1	0.22
Upper gastrointestinal tract	0.8	—	—
Lower gastrointestinal tract	0.63	0.3	1.7
Oral cholecystogram	0.77	—	—
Cervical spine	0.25	—	—
Lumbar spine	2.5	0.22	0.72
Pelvis	0.5	0.36	0.21
Hip	1.0	0.6	0.12
Arm	0.13	—	—
Leg	0.11	—	—
Mammogram	0.4	—	—

(From Pizzarello, D.J., and Witcofski, R.L.: Medical Radiation Biology. 2nd Ed. Philadelphia, Lea & Febiger, 1982.)

caused many fetal malformations, depending on the stage of embryonic development at the time of irradiation; however, such effects have not been clearly demonstrated in man, either in patients receiving medical radiation during pregnancy or in survivors of nuclear explosions. In light of this data and the high background incidence of congenital abnormalities, the National Council on Radiation Protection and Measurements (NCRP) has provided guidelines for the management of women found to be pregnant after medical radiation exposure. At radiation doses to the pelvis of under 5 rad, the additional risk of fetal abnormality from the radiation is thought to be small, and the pregnancy should be continued. Therapeutic abortion performed solely because of radiation exposure should not be considered until the radiation dose approaches 15 rad. Because a radiation dose approaching that level would require multiple radiographic studies involving the pelvic area within a short time, the health of the mother would probably be the overriding consideration in assessment of the situation.

Permissible Exposure Limits

Although it is wise to adhere to the concept that ionizing radiation is harmful and exposure should be held to a minimum, man has always lived in an environment of naturally occurring radiation. The average person in the United States receives 102 mrem radiation exposure per year in the form of cosmic x rays, ultraviolet light, and gamma rays from naturally occurring radionuclides.

Permissible exposure limits are recommended by the NCRP, a private organization of scientists expert in radiation. The limits are recommended in light of available knowledge concerning the known effects of radiation.[11-12] Since the first recommendations in 1931, the limits have been progressively reduced. An attempt is made to set the limits at a level below which no biologic effect is detectable. Maximum permissible limits deal primarily with occupational exposure. No recommendations exist with regard to diagnostic or therapeutic x-ray exposure because the overriding concern is the health of the patient. Physicians taking radiographs should strive to obtain examinations at the minimum radiation dose to the patient consistent with diagnostic-quality films. Maximum permissible radiation exposure limits and the average dose to patients for a variety of examinations are provided in Tables 1–1 and 1–2.

REFERENCES

1. Christensen, E.E., Curry, T.S., III, and Dowdey, J.E.: An Introduction to the Physics of Diagnostic Radiology. 2nd Ed. Philadelphia, Lea & Febiger, 1978.

2. Johns, H.E., and Cunningham, J.R.: The Physics of Radiology. 3rd Ed. Springfield, IL, Charles C Thomas, 1974.
3. Hendee, W.R.: Medical Radiation Physics. 2nd Ed. Chicago, Yearbook Medical Publishers, 1979.
4. Littleton, J.T. (ed.): Tomography: Physical Principles and Clinical Applications. Golden's Diagnostic Radiology, Section 17. Baltimore, Williams & Wilkins, 1976.
5. Tuddenham, W.J.: The visual physiology of roentgen diagnosis. A. Basic concepts. AJR, 78:116, 1957.
6. International Commission on Radiation Units and Measurements (ICRU): Radiation Quantities and Units. ICRU Report 33. Washington, DC, ICRU, 1980.
7. Little, J.B.: Cellular effects of ionizing radiation. N. Engl. J. Med., 278:308, 369, 1968.
8. Pizzarello, D.J., and Witcofski, R.L.: Medical Radiation Biology. 2nd Ed. Philadelphia, Lea & Febiger, 1982, p. 5.
9. Witcofski, R.L.: The effects of radiation exposure from radiopharmaceuticals used in diagnostic studies. *In* Third International Radiopharmaceutical Dosimetry Symposium. Edited by E.E. Watson, T. Schlafke-Stelson, and J.L. Coffey. Oak Ridge, TN, Bureau of Radiological Health, 1980, p. 45.
10. National Council on Radiation Protection and Measurements: Medical Radiation Exposure of Pregnant and Potentially Pregnant Women. NCRP Report No. 54. Washington, DC, NCRP, 1977.
11. Wagner, H.N., Jr.: Radiation: The risks and benefits. *In* Symposium on the perception of the risk of radiation. AJR, 140:595, 1983.
12. National Council on Radiation Protection and Measurements: Basic Radiation Protection Criteria. NCRP Report No. 39. Washington, DC, NCRP, 1971.

2

Plain Film Radiography of the Skeleton

Wells Martin, III ■ Robert H. Choplin

Plain film radiography of the head, back, and extremities includes simple projection radiography and tomography of these areas without the use of contrast materials. Although findings on plain films may require clarification or definition of the extent of disease by more sophisticated radiologic examinations such as computed tomography, myelography, or arthrography, many such findings are sufficient for definitive therapeutic decisions. The number of films obtained during a "routine" examination varies from institution to institution, but one should include enough studies to be able to evaluate the important anatomic structures in at least two projections. Although desired information may not be present on films from a routine examination, it may often be obtained with a simple radiograph performed in a different projection. For these reasons, the surgeon should have some understanding of the anatomic features visible on common radiographic projections, of the way in which radiographic studies may be limited by the patient's clinical status or regional anatomic features, and of the appropriate studies for answering specific clinical questions. Because it is not possible to review this subject in great detail, the reader in need of more information should consult the references cited.

HEAD

Common plain film examinations of the head include the skull, facial bones, paranasal sinuses, and mandible. Because of the anatomic complexity of this area and because of the superimposition of structures, numerous projections are required to isolate specific structures, for optimal visualization. To evaluate symmetry accurately, frontal views must be nonrotated, and oblique views must be comparable but opposite in projection. Although these studies can be obtained with any simple radiography unit, units designed to visualize cranial and facial structures (dedicated head units) allow consistently reproducible, high-quality examinations. These units move around the patient's head at any desired angle and allow the entire examination to be accomplished with a minimum of motion or discomfort to the patient. Finally, a co-operative patient who voluntarily remains immobile during the study is required. Because obtaining high-quality studies requires meticulous radiographic technique and precise positioning of the patient, only well-trained, dedicated personnel should perform these examinations.

Technique

SKULL. A routine skull series includes the following projections: frontal, which may be either posteroanterior (PA) or anteroposterior (AP), an inclined PA (Caldwell), a half-axial AP (Towne), a right or left lateral, and an axial (base). The films may be obtained with the patient in either the erect or the supine position. The frontal films are obtained with the x-ray beam directed at various angles in relation to the orbitomeatal line (Fig. 2–1A). The lateral view is obtained with the x-ray beam directed either perpendicular or horizontal to the x-ray table, depending on the patient's position (Fig. 2–1B and C). Additions to this series include oblique or tangential views, to demonstrate whether lesions occur in the diploic space and the degree to which such lesions involve one of the tables of the skull (Fig. 2–2).

FACE. Radiography of the face most commonly includes one or a combination of the following series: facial bones, paranasal sinuses, and mandible. Although the facial bone and paranasal sinus series usually constitute different examinations, they include almost exactly the same projections. The major difference is technical; the films from the paranasal sinus series are confined (coned down) to a smaller area, to allow a more optimal examination.

The facial bone series almost always includes PA, lateral, and steeply inclined PA (Waters') views. Other films frequently included are inclined PA (Caldwell), axial (base), and half-axial (Towne) views. The paranasal sinus series generally includes all the foregoing projections. Ideally, both examinations should be performed with the patient in an upright position, but if that is not possible, at least one projection, usually the lateral, should be performed with a horizontal beam, to allow visual-

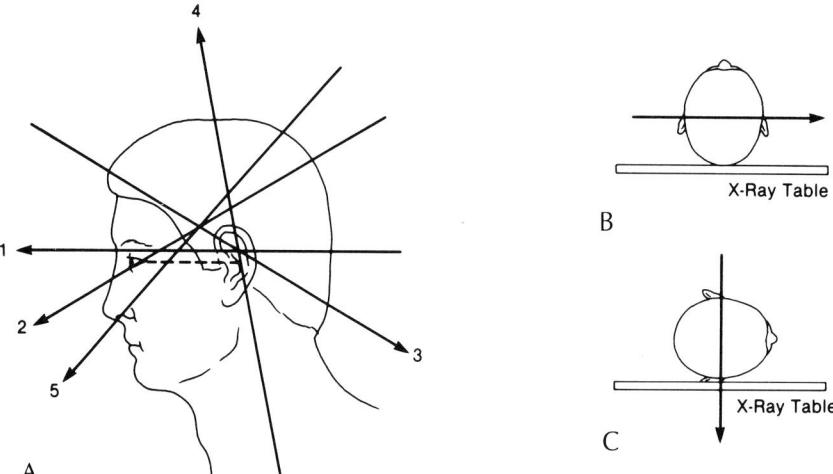

FIG. 2–1. Radiographic projections for skull, facial bone, and paranasal sinus series. *A,* Posteroanterior or anteroposterior view (1), with the x-ray beam parallel to the orbital-meatal (OM) line (dashed); (2) inclined posteroanterior (Caldwell) view), with the x-ray beam angled 15° caudal to the OM line; (3) half-axial anteroposterior (Towne) view, with the x-ray beam angled 30° caudal to the OM line; (4) axial (base) view, with the x-ray beam angled 100° cephalad to the OM line; and (5) steeply inclined posteroanterior (Waters') view, with the x-ray beam angled 37° caudal to the OM line. *B,* Horizontal-beam (cross-table) lateral view, with the x-ray beam parallel to the examination table and perpendicular to the x-ray film; the patient's head is not turned. *C,* Standard lateral view, with the x-ray beam perpendicular to the examination table and the x-ray film; the patient's head is turned to one side.

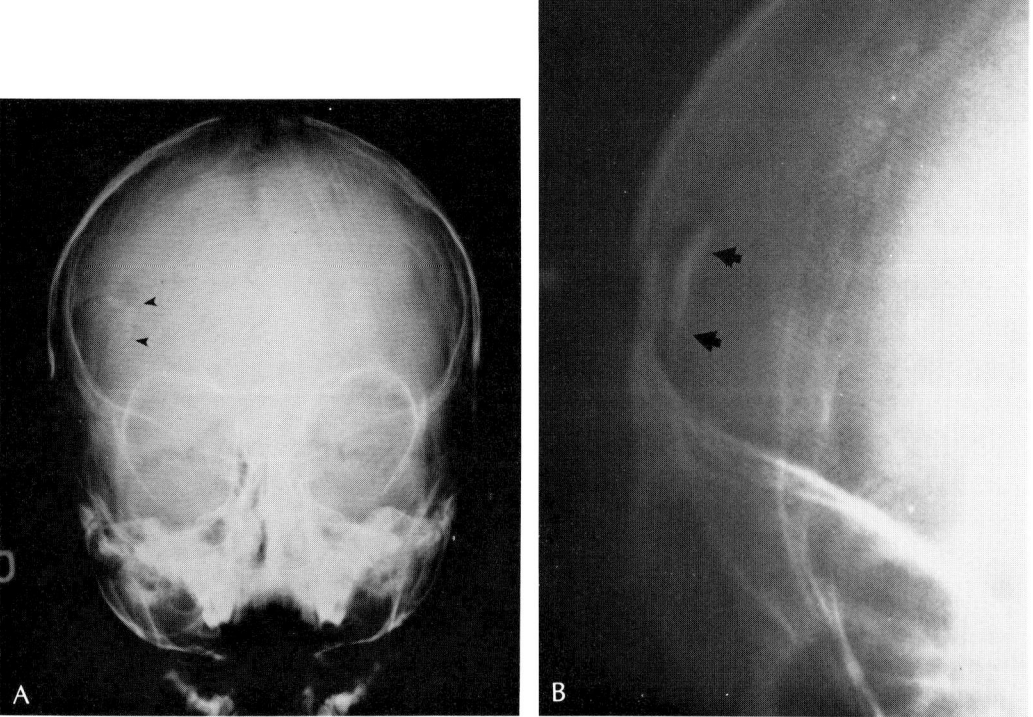

FIG. 2–2. Tangential view of the skull; depressed skull fracture. *A,* Anteroposterior view shows a fracture (arrowheads) of the right frontal bone. *B,* Tangential view shows the degree of depression of the bone fragment (arrows).

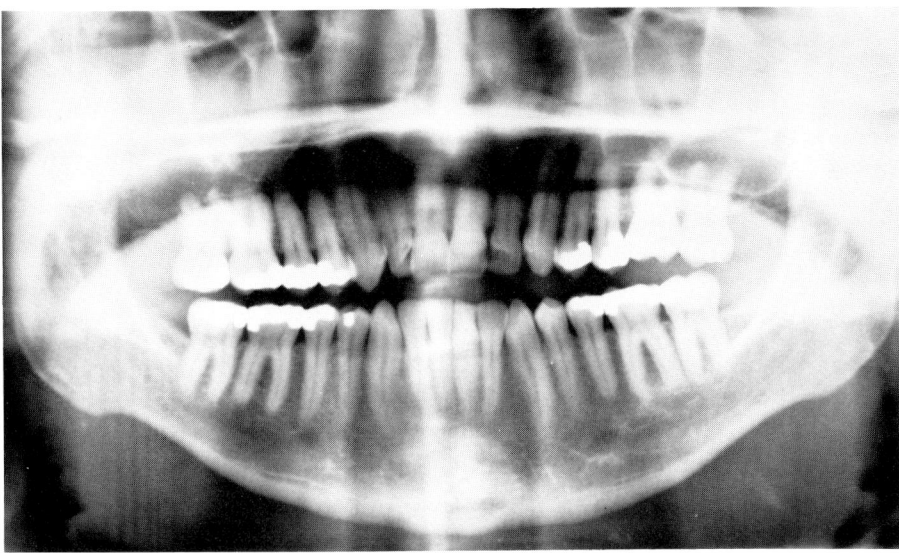

FIG. 2–3. Panoramic radiograph in which the mandible alone is in focus while superimposed facial structures and the cervical spine are blurred.

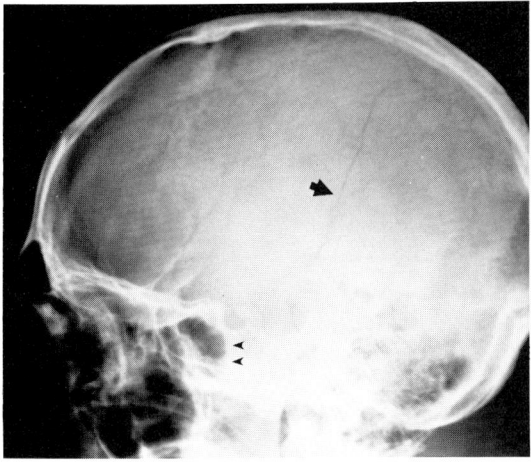

FIG. 2–4. Horizontal-beam (cross-table) lateral view of the skull. The air-fluid level present in the sphenoid sinus (arrowheads) indicates a basilar skull fracture. The patient also has a linear skull fracture of the parietal bone (arrow).

ization of air-fluid levels. Despite technically optimal examinations, tomography is often required to detect or to define the extent of disease in this anatomically complex area.

The mandible may be examined by a series of views, the composite of which allows for visualization of the entire bone, or, alternately, by a single panoramic radiograph. The mandible series usually includes AP, both right and left oblique, and Towne views of the temporomandibular joints. The panoramic radiograph is obtained with a specialized unit in which the x-ray tube and the film cassette rotate about the patient's head in an elliptic path, resulting in a plane of focus along the arch of the mandible (Fig. 2–3).

Indications and Limitations

TRAUMA. Head injuries are common indications for radiologic studies.

Skull. Skull radiography is often performed routinely for any type of head trauma, although, in recent years, avoidance of its overuse has been stressed.[1] A number of efficacy studies have shown a high correlation between certain high-yield clinical criteria and the presence of skull fractures. For example, Phillips has suggested the following criteria:[2]

1. Unconsciousness, including unarousable alcoholic unconsciousness, at the time of presentation to an emergency facility.
2. Documented decreasing level of consciousness or progressive mental deterioration.
3. A history of previous craniotomy, with a shunting tube in place.
4. Skull depression or a subcutaneous foreign body palpable or identified by probe through a laceration or puncture wound.
5. Hemotympanum or fluid discharge from the ear.
6. Cerebral spinal fluid discharge from the nose.
7. Mastoid ecchymosis (Battle's sign).
8. Bilateral orbital ecchymosis (raccoon eyes).
9. Unexplained focal neurologic signs.

When these high-yield guidelines are followed, the use of skull radiography may be reduced by 30 to 50%.[2,3] Other important factors in determining whether a skull series is indicated include the cli-

16   *IMAGING*

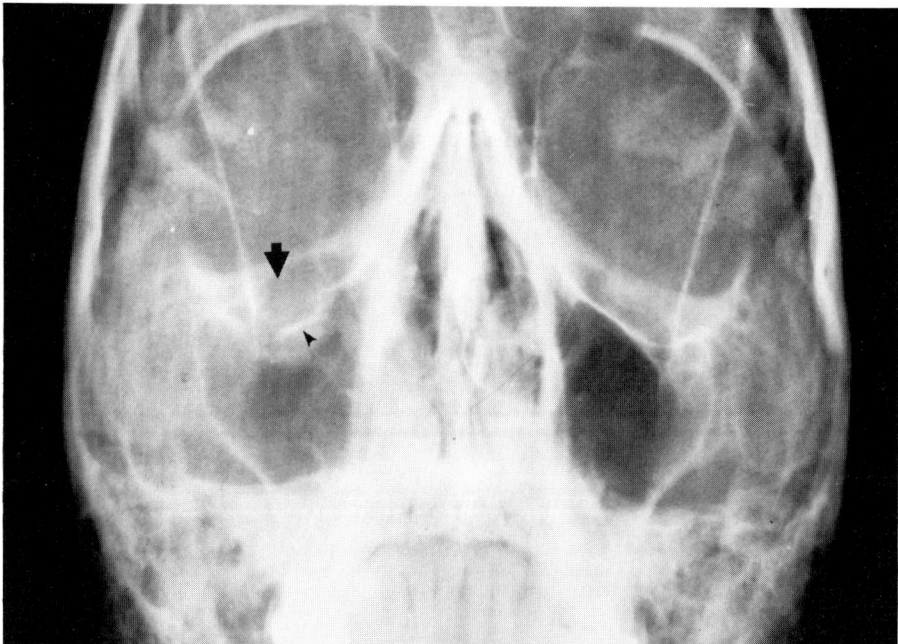

FIG. 2–5. Asymmetry of facial structures; blow-out fracture of the right orbit. Soft tissue density in the maxillary antrum (arrow) is asymmetric in appearance, when compared to the normal left side. Note the depressed bone fragment from the orbital floor (arrowhead).

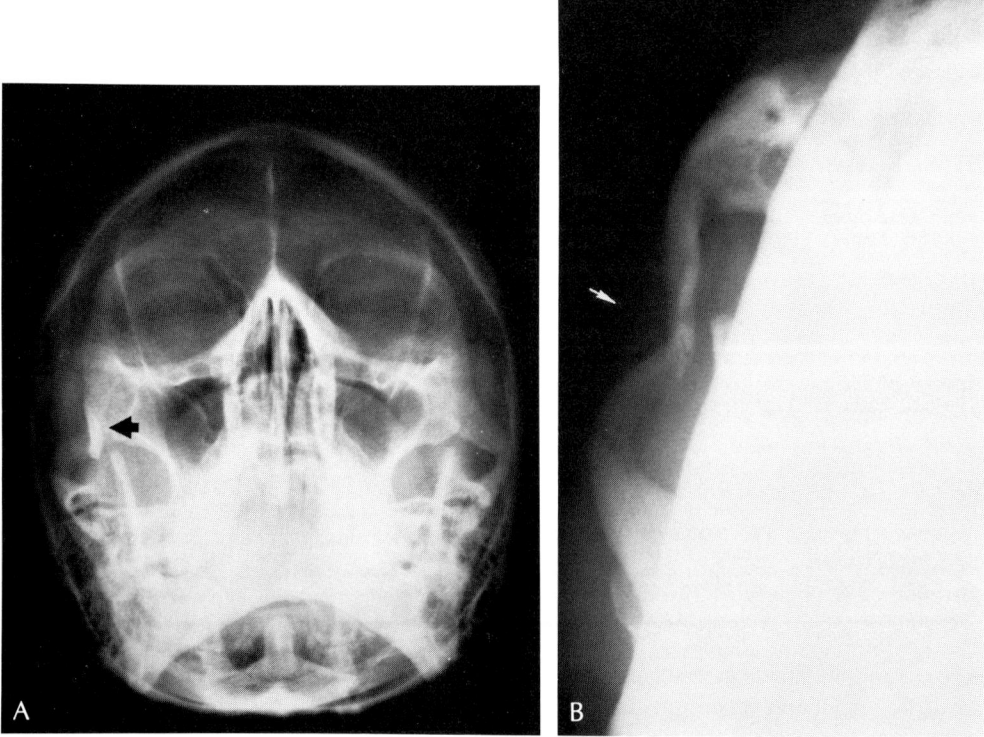

FIG. 2–6. Special view of the facial bones; right zygomatic arch fracture. *A,* A Waters view demonstrates an ovoid opacity projecting over the right zygomatic arch that is not present on the left (arrow). *B,* A special zygomatic arch view (tangential axial view) better shows this opacity to be a depressed fracture of the arch (arrow).

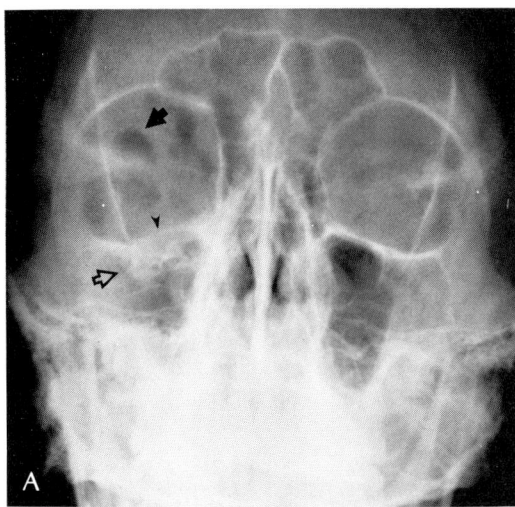

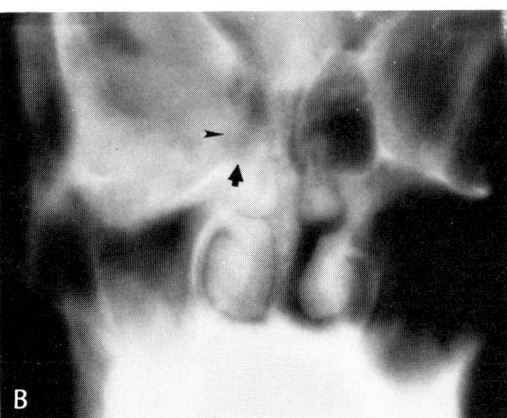

FIG. 2–7. Conventional tomography in facial fractures; blow-out fracture of the right orbit. *A,* A Waters view shows orbital air (arrow), interruption of the inferior orbital rim (arrowhead), and soft tissue density in the maxillary antrum (open arrow). *B,* A facial tomogram shows opacification of the right ethmoid sinus (arrow) and loss of visualization of the lateral wall of the ethmoid sinus (arrowhead); these findings were not clearly identified on the plain film.

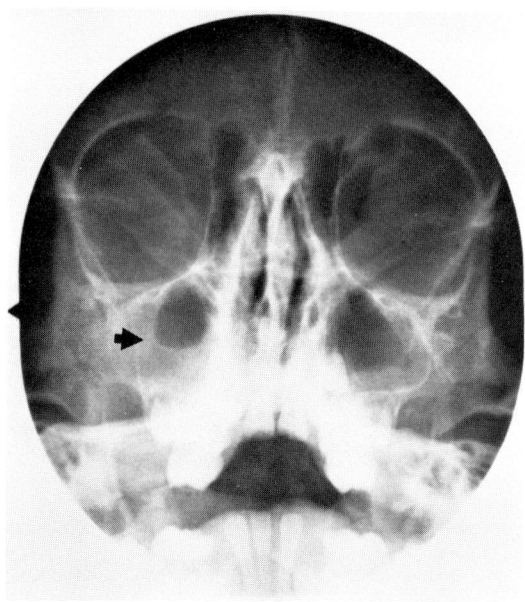

FIG. 2–8. An upright Waters view in paranasal sinus examination. The upright view shows an air-fluid level (arrow) in the right maxillary sinus in this patient with acute sinusitis.

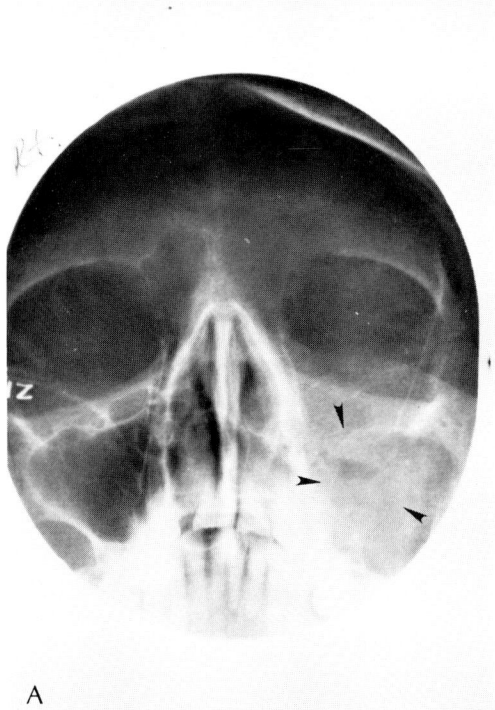
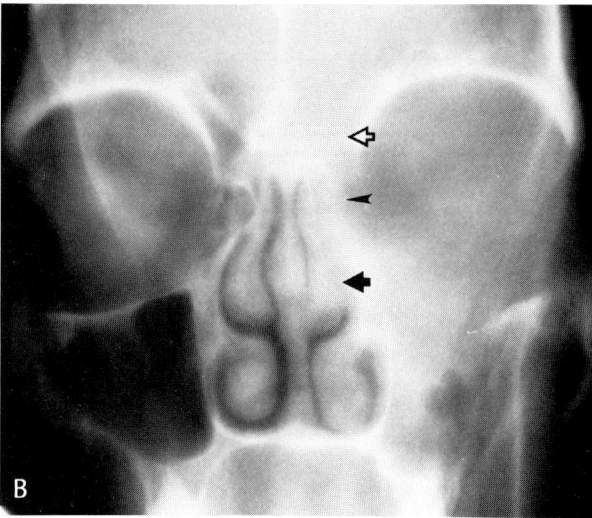

FIG. 2-9. Conventional tomography of the paranasal sinuses; carcinoma of the maxillary antrum. *A,* A Waters view shows opacification of the left maxillary antrum and destruction of the walls of the maxillary antrum (arrowheads). *B,* A facial tomogram shows tumor extension into the nasal cavity (arrow), the ethmoid sinus (arrowhead), and the frontal sinus (open arrow); such extension was not clearly visible on the plain films.

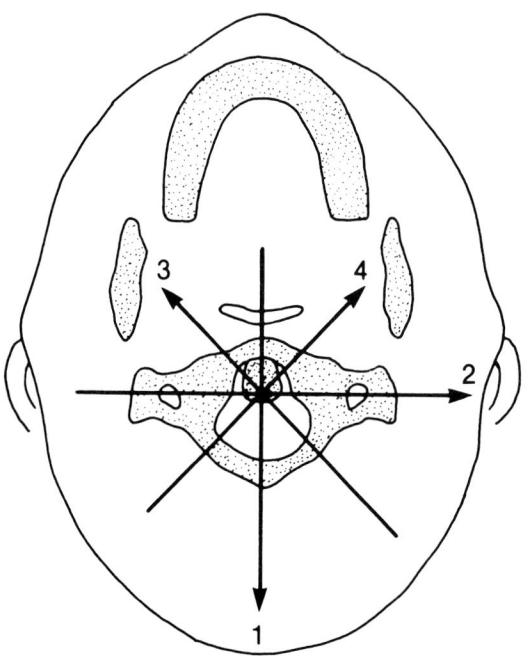

FIG. 2-10. Radiographic projections of the cervical spine. Anteroposterior (1), lateral (2), obliques (3 and 4) views. The open-mouth odontoid view is obtained as an anteroposterior view.

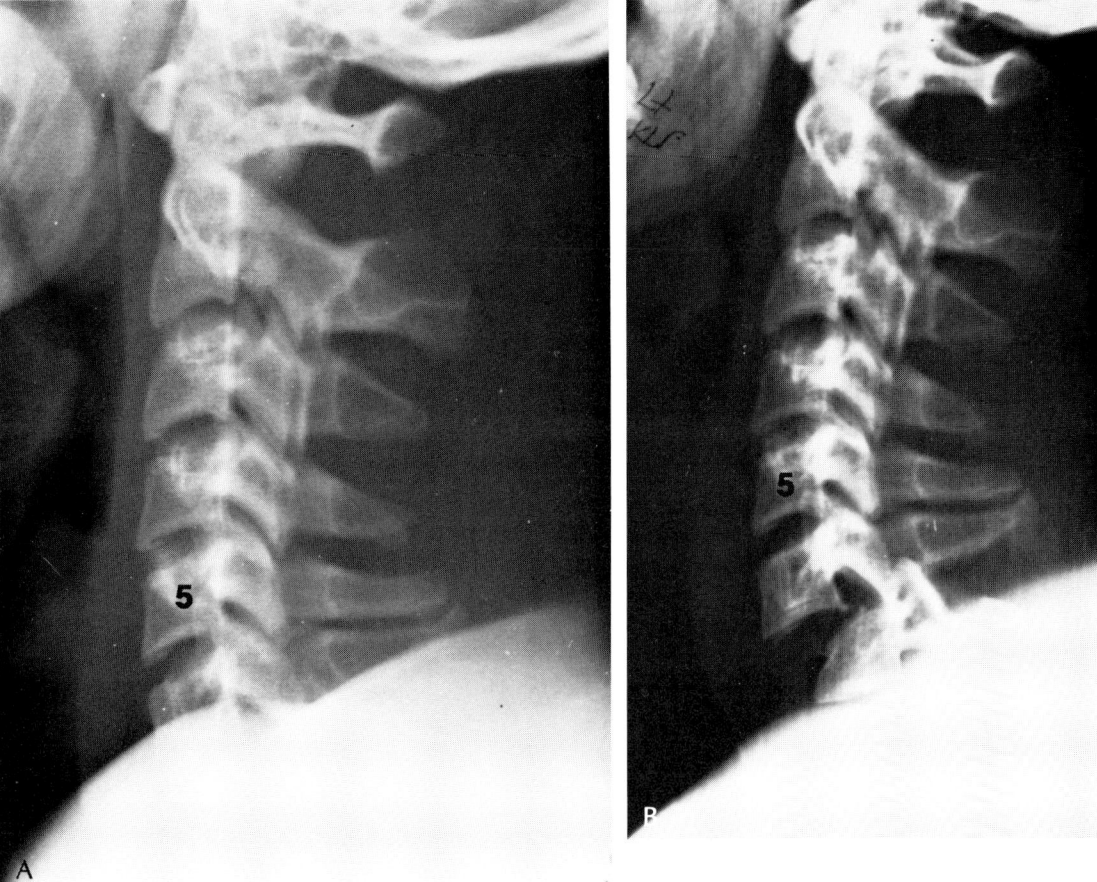

FIG. 2-11. Traction for visualization of the cervicothoracic spine; C6, C7 subluxation. A, An inadequate lateral view of the cervical spine showing only C1 through C6 vertebral bodies. B, A repeat view of the same patient with traction on the patient's arms now shows C7 and the obvious subluxation.

nician's past experience, the patient and associated family pressures, and medicolegal concerns, however.[4] Moreover, because the neurologic sequelae of head trauma are more closely related to the intracranial disorder than to the presence or absence of skull fracture, some authors consider computed tomography to be the procedure of choice in evaluating these patients.[5]

If one decides to obtain skull films, one must determine whether the examination may be done in the hospital x-ray department or whether it must be done using mobile equipment. Radiographic examinations are of higher quality and have fewer limitations when performed in a hospital x-ray suite. Although the standard skull series is easily performed in a conscious and co-operative patient, the inability to immobilize unco-operative patients completely makes diagnostic-quality examinations difficult to obtain. Thus, the examination must often be deferred or limited in scope.

In patients who are unconscious or who have suspected spinal injuries, the entire examination must be performed in a supine position. All views will thus be in an AP projection, except the horizontal-beam lateral film, which is important for evaluating air-fluid levels in the paranasal sinuses (Fig. 2-4). In addition to the skull series in an unconscious patient, a horizontal-beam (cross-table) lateral radiograph of the cervical spine should be obtained, to exclude an unstable cervical spinal fracture. If possible, this radiograph should be obtained prior to the passage of endotracheal tubes, to prevent further injury from neck manipulation. Because of the need to extend the neck in obtaining an axial view of the skull, such a radiograph should be obtained only when a cervical spinal evaluation has been completed.[6] A summary of recommended procedures for radiography of the skull in unconscious patients is as follows:

1. Examinations should be performed when the patient's condition is clinically stable.
2. Whether to perform a portable or a conventional examination depends on the patient's condition.

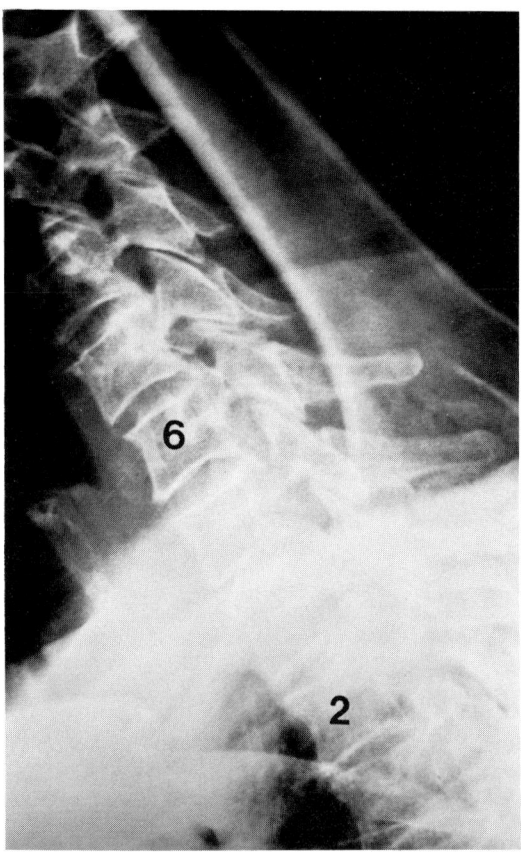

FIG. 2–12. Swimmer's view. By elevating one arm and rotating both shoulders slightly, the cervicothoracic junction can often be seen well. This view is generally obtained when traction on the patient's arms does not allow for adequate visualization of the cervicothoracic area.

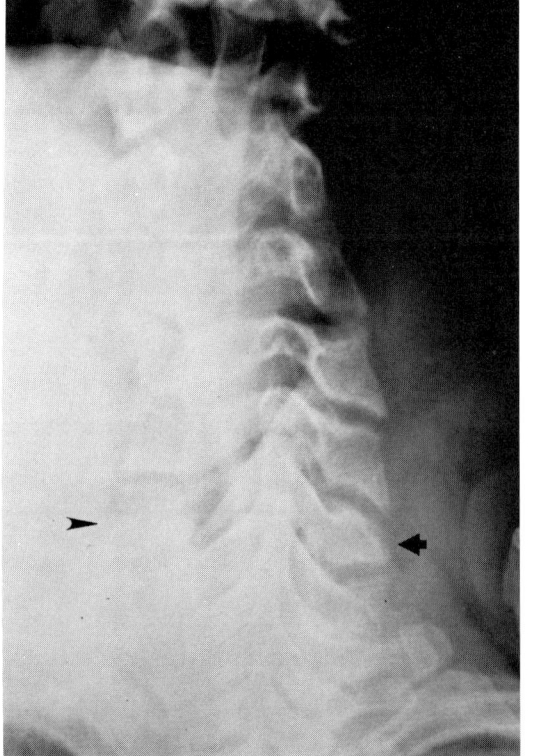

FIG. 2–13. Special view of the posterior arches of the cervical spine (Pillar view). The x-ray beam is angled caudally with the patient's head rotated to each side for each exposure. A compression fracture of the left articular mass of C6 is identified (arrow). Note the normally shaped articular mass on the opposite side at the same level (arrowhead).

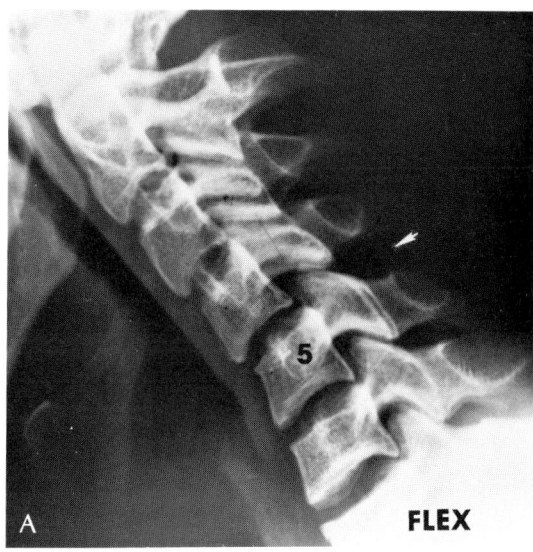
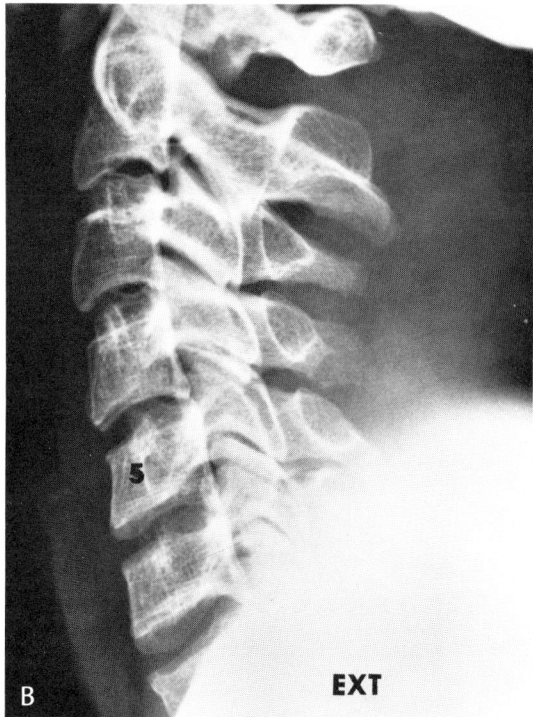

FIG. 2–14. Flexion and extension views of the cervical spine. *A,* the flexion (FLEX) view shows anterior subluxation of C4 on C5, as well as widening of the interspinous space at the same level (arrow). *B,* Compare *A* with the normal relationship when patient is in extension (EXT).

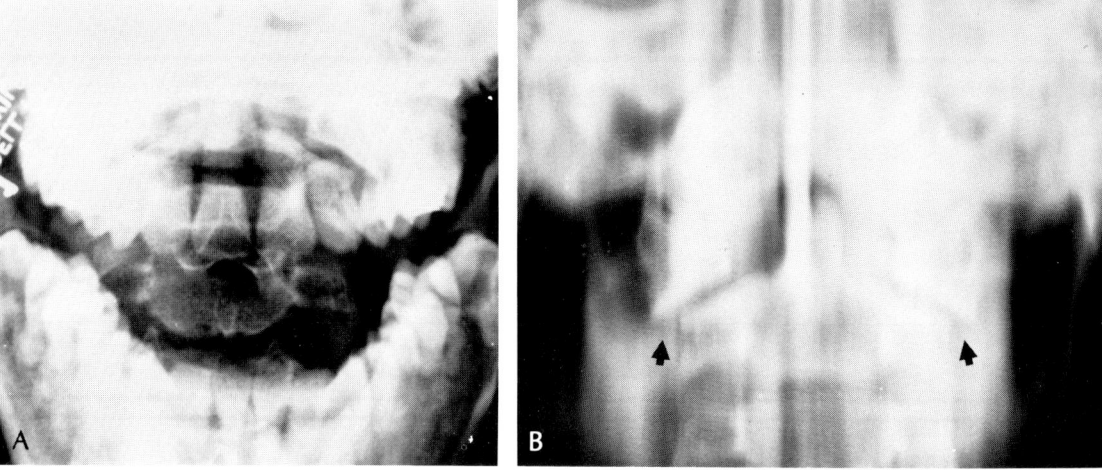

FIG. 2–15. Conventional tomography in fractures; Jefferson burst fracture. *A,* Open-mouth odontoid view is suboptimal and is unable to show the relationship of C1 to C2. *B,* Conventional tomogram shows the lateral offset of both lateral masses of C1 on C2 (arrows) indicative of a fracture of C1.

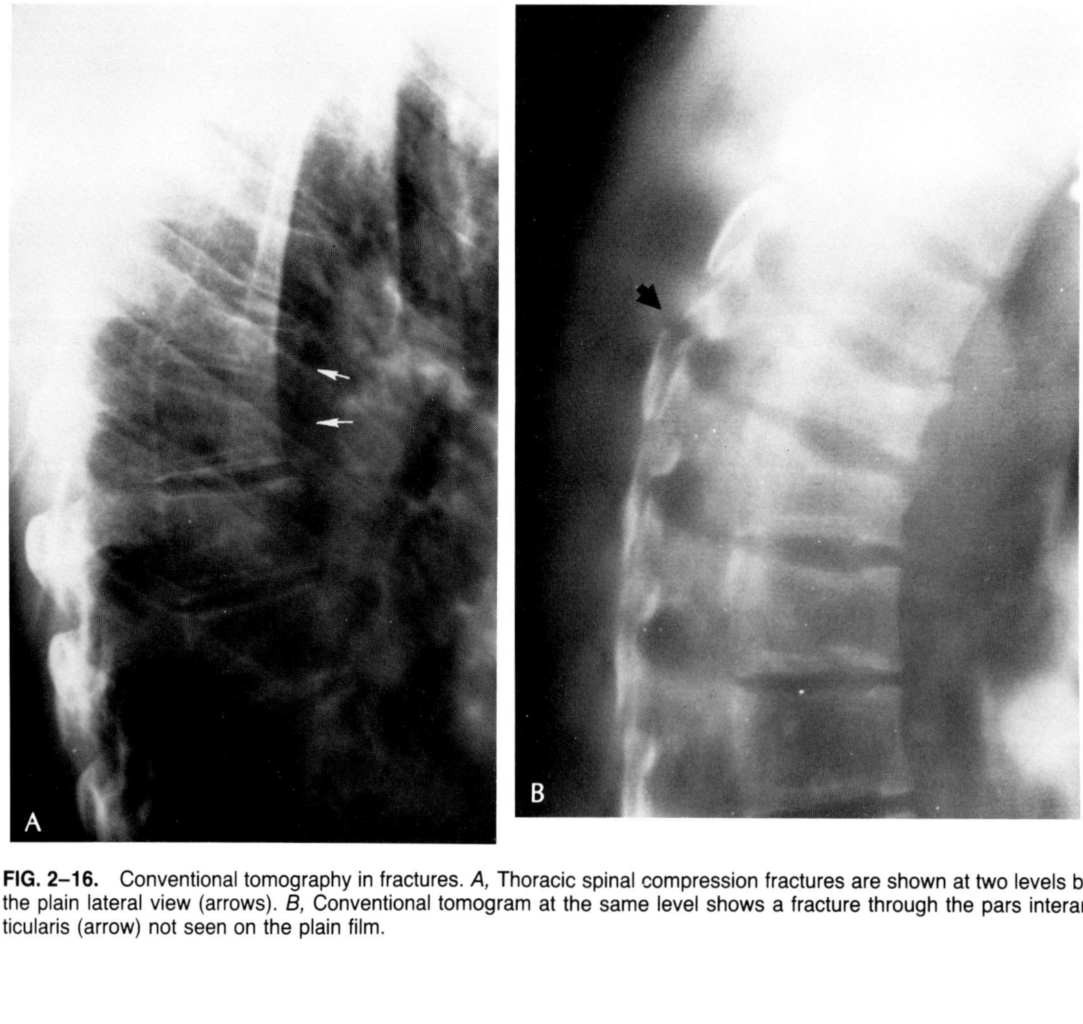

FIG. 2–16. Conventional tomography in fractures. *A,* Thoracic spinal compression fractures are shown at two levels by the plain lateral view (arrows). *B,* Conventional tomogram at the same level shows a fracture through the pars interarticularis (arrow) not seen on the plain film.

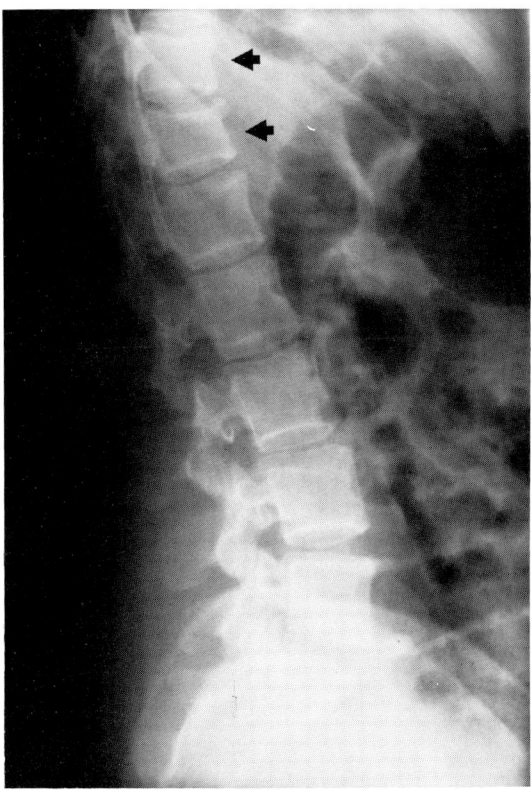

FIG. 2–17. Inclusion of the lower thoracic spine in a lumbar spine series. Thoracic spinal compression fractures of T11 and T12 (arrows) are identified on the lumbar spinal examination. These fractures would have been missed if only the lumbar spine had been imaged.

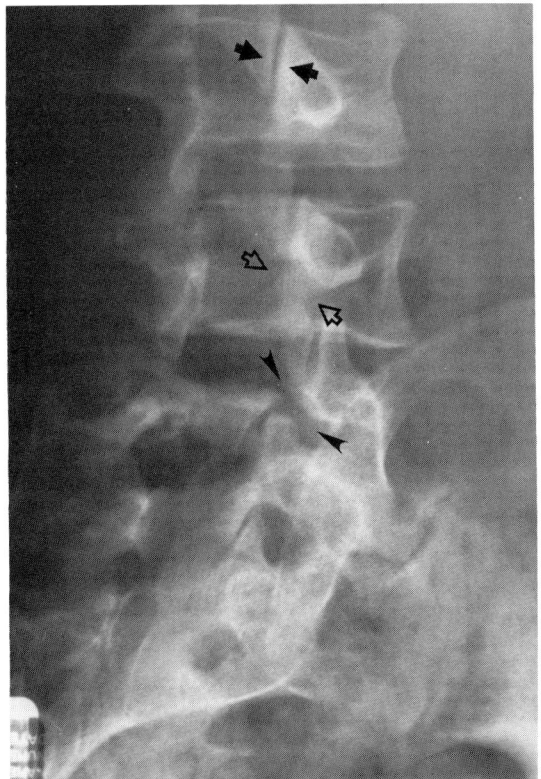

FIG. 2–18. Oblique lumbar spinal view. Normal apophyseal joint (arrows) is well outlined. A pars interarticularis defect (spondylolysis) (arrowheads) is demonstrated. A normal intact pars interarticularis allows for comparison (open arrows).

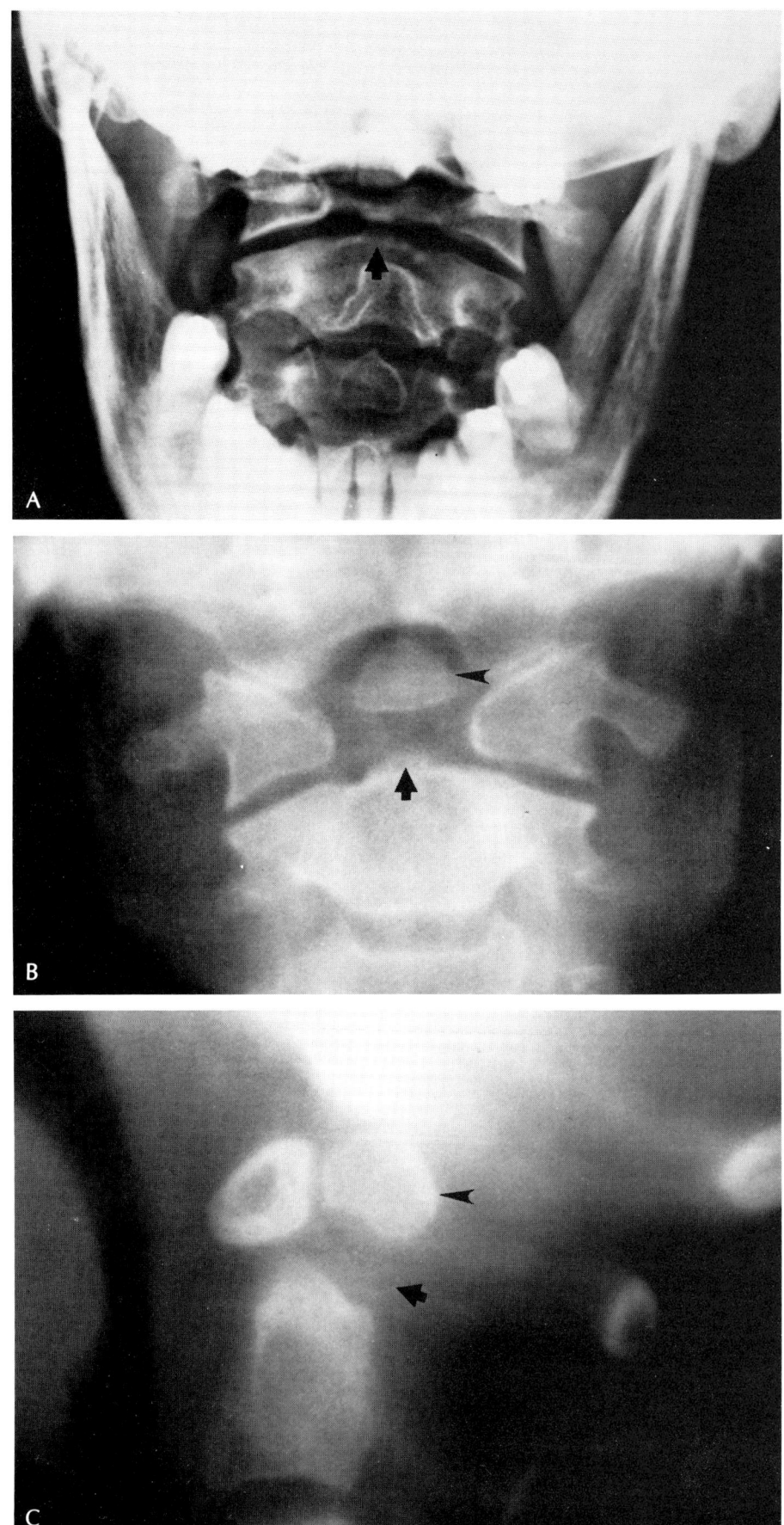

FIG. 2–19. (Legend on facing page.)

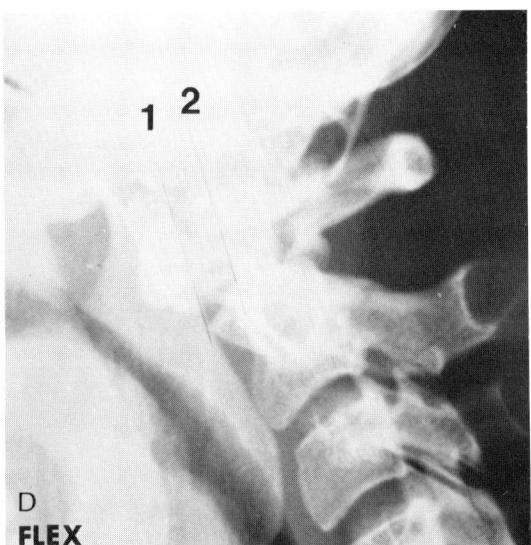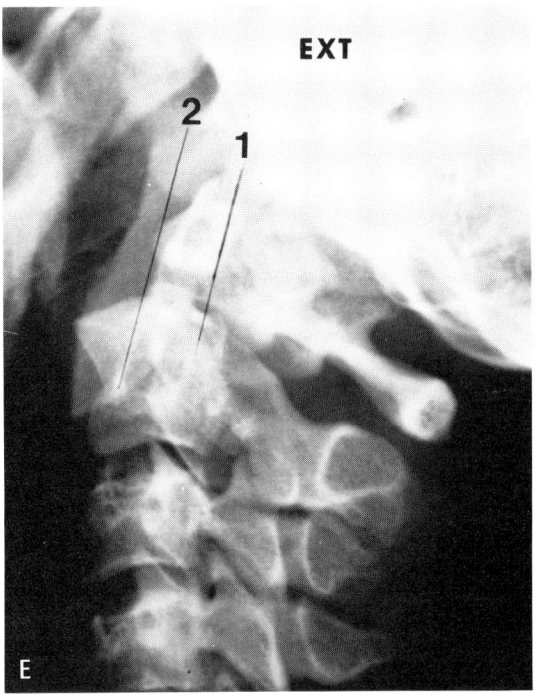

FIG. 2–19. Conventional tomography and special views in congenital cervical spine abnormality; hypoplasia of the odontoid process with the presence of an os odontoideum. A, Open-mouth odontoid view shows a defect at the base of the odontoid process (arrow). B and C, Anteroposterior and lateral tomograms confirm the defect at the base of the odontoid process (arrow) and show the presence of the os odontoideum (arrowhead). D and E, Flexion (FLEX) and extension (EXT) views show marked hypermobility at the atlantoaxial joint. Note the reversal of the lines marking the anterior arch of C1 (1) and the body of C2 (2). Cervical spinal fusion was performed at this level.

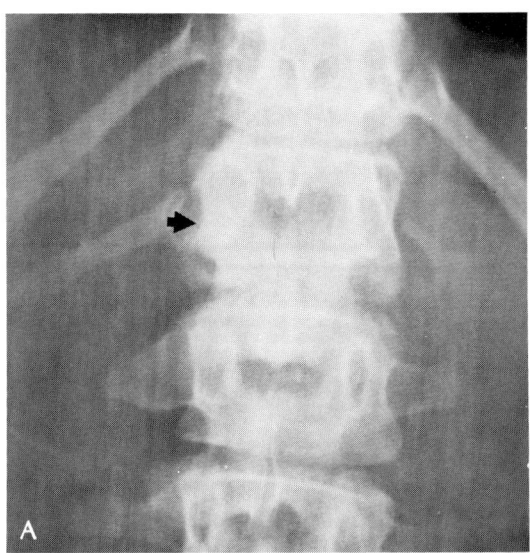
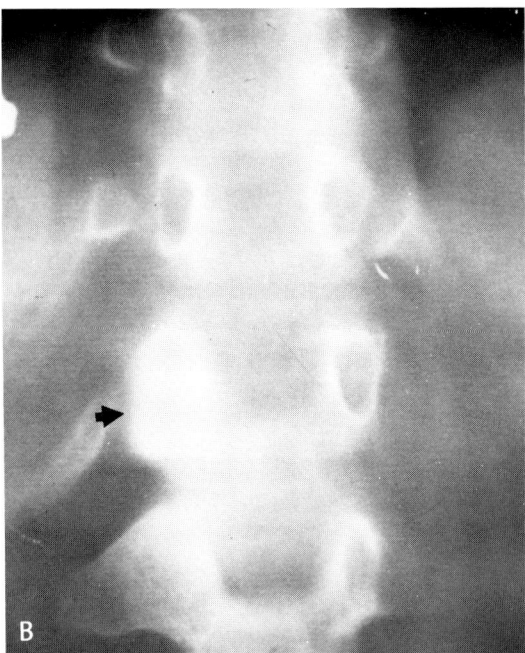

FIG. 2–20. Conventional tomography of the spine; osteoid osteoma. *A,* Plain anteroposterior film of T12 shows slight increased density of the right pedicle (arrow). *B,* Conventional tomogram shows a sclerotic pedicle (arrow) confirming the suspicious plain film findings.

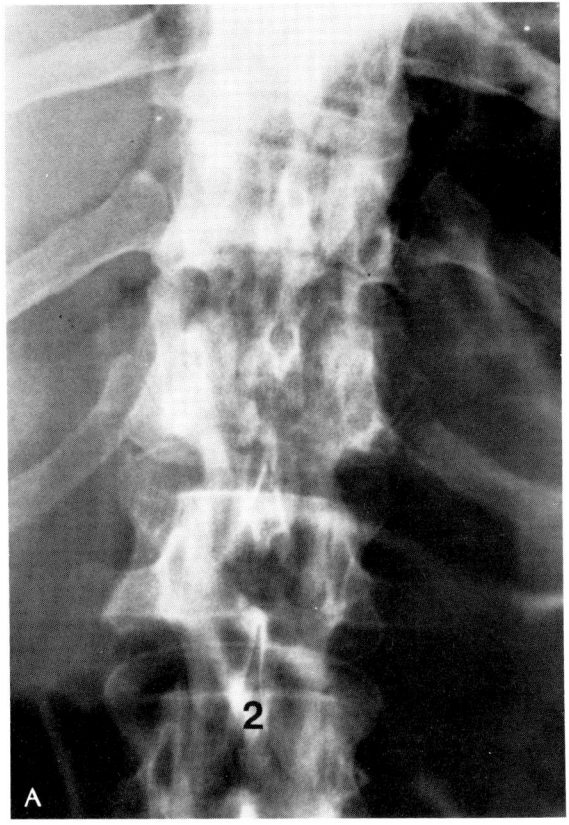 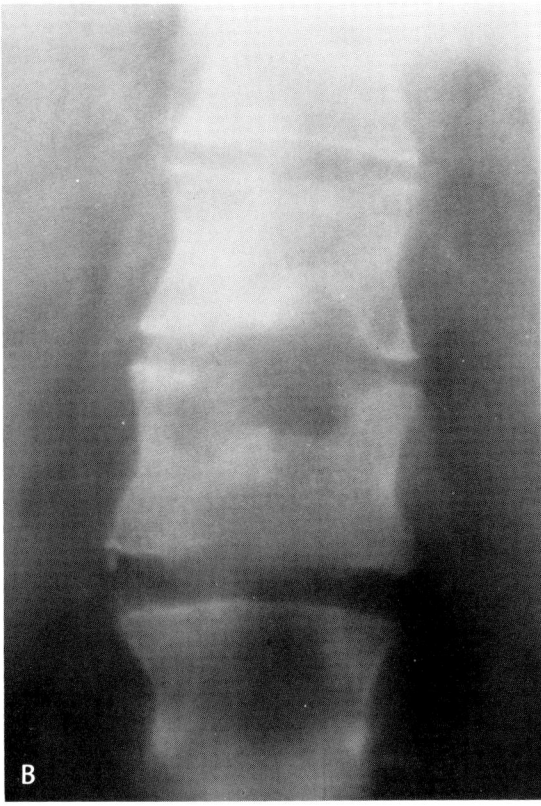

FIG. 2–21. Conventional tomography of the spine in inflammatory disease; osteomyelitis. A, Plain anteroposterior film of the lower thoracic spine shows a poorly defined superior end plate of the T12 vertebral body; compare it with the superior end plate of L2. B, Conventional tomogram clearly shows the destruction of the inferior end plate of T11 vertebral body and the superior end plate of T12 vertebral body.

3. A horizontal-beam (cross-table) lateral view of the cervical spine should be obtained prior to intubation, to exclude an unstable cervical spinal injury.
4. Anteroposterior, horizontal-beam lateral, and Towne views of the skull are indicated.

If the patient's condition is clinically unstable, a portable skull series may have to be obtained, usually including only the AP, Towne, and horizontal-beam lateral views. The Towne view should be included because up to 25% of skull fractures are detectable on this projection only.[7]

FACIAL TRAUMA. Trauma is one of the most common indications for facial bone radiography. Nonrotated frontal projections are mandatory to evaluate symmetry. Any asymmetry requires an explanation and may be due to either bone or soft tissue abnormality (Fig. 2–5). None of the views previously described in a standard facial bone series enable one to see the zygomatic arch optimally, and gross fractures may appear subtle or may be missed entirely. When the results of the clinical examination suggest a fracture in this area, specific zygomatic arch views (Fig. 2–6), or facial tomography, should be performed. Tomography, including pantomography, is often beneficial in determining the presence of fractures when plain film findings are equivocal or in defining the extent of such fractures when their presence has been noted (Fig. 2–7).

NONTRAUMATIC CONDITIONS. Despite the clear advantages of tomographic imaging in many such situations, plain radiography has a place in the evaluation of nontraumatic conditions of the head.

Skull. Almost all nontraumatic processes involving the skull can be imaged on a standard radiographic skull series. In conditions such as osteomyelitis and metastasis, radionuclide bone scanning may detect abnormalities before any bone destruction is visible on plain films. Nonetheless, plain films are helpful in evaluating progression or resolution of disease once destruction has been identified. For evaluation of the sella turcica, AP and lateral coned-down views may suffice, although tomography is often needed for adequate visualization. For evaluation of intracranial processes of any type, computed tomography is the current method of choice.

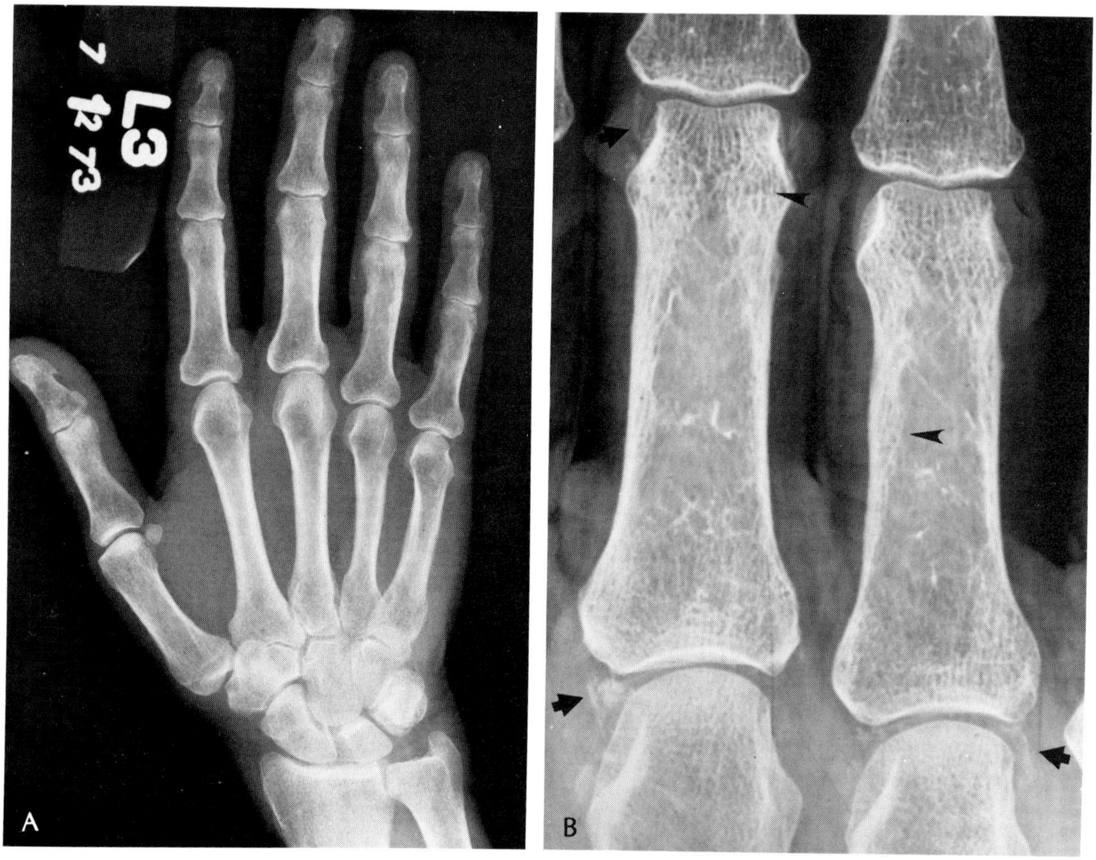

FIG. 2-22. Magnification radiography. *A,* Normal hand. *B,* Magnification view of a different patient shows soft tissue calcification (arrows) clearly located within the synovium; the magnification also provides better definition of the fine trabecular structure of bone (arrowheads).

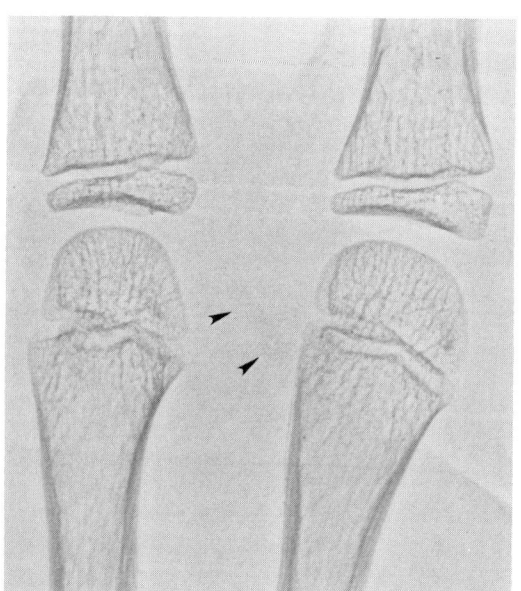

FIG. 2-23. Xeroradiography. Xeroradiograph of the soft tissues of the hand shows a density (arrowheads) not seen on a plain radiograph. This feature represented a wooden foreign body.

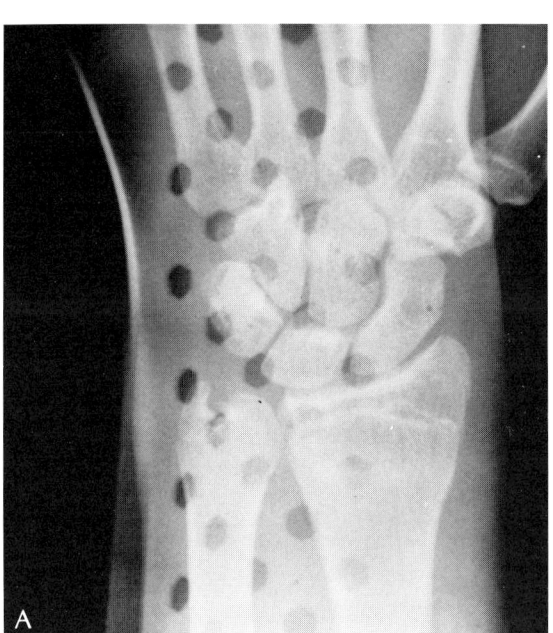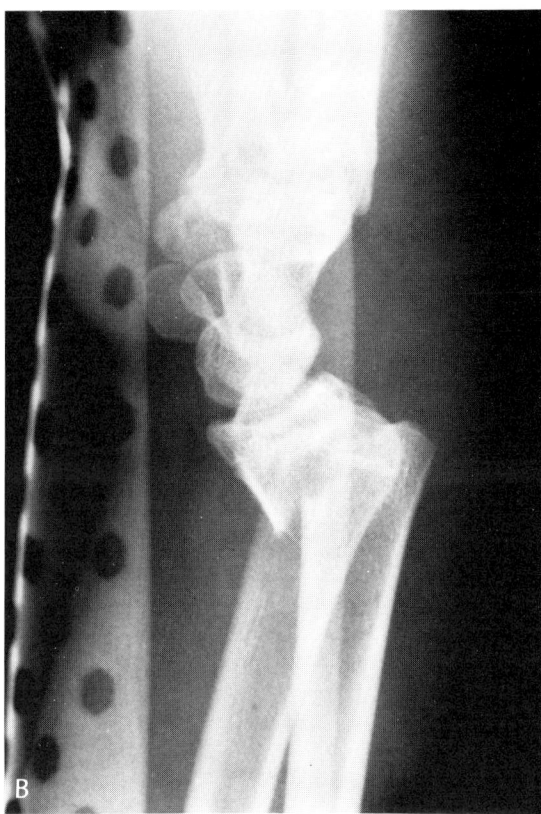

FIG. 2–24. Necessity for two views in radiography of the extremities. *A,* An anteroposterior view shows apparent anatomic alignment of fracture fragments. *B,* The lateral view shows marked apex dorsal angulation.

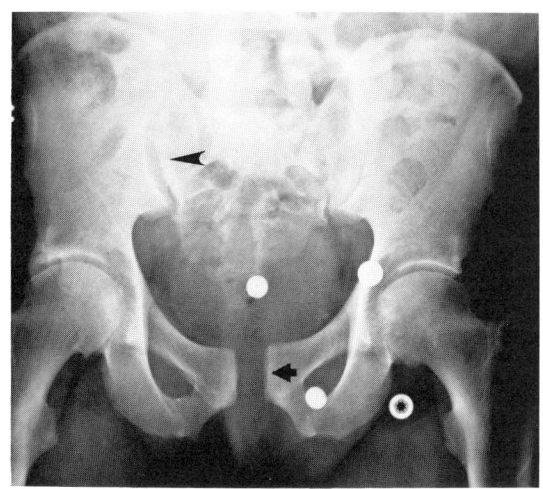

FIG. 2–25. Fractures of ring or ring-like structures; pelvic fractures. Diastatic fractures through the symphysis pubis (arrow) and the right sacroiliac joint (arrowhead) are present. Compare the right sacroiliac joint with the normal left sacroiliac joint.

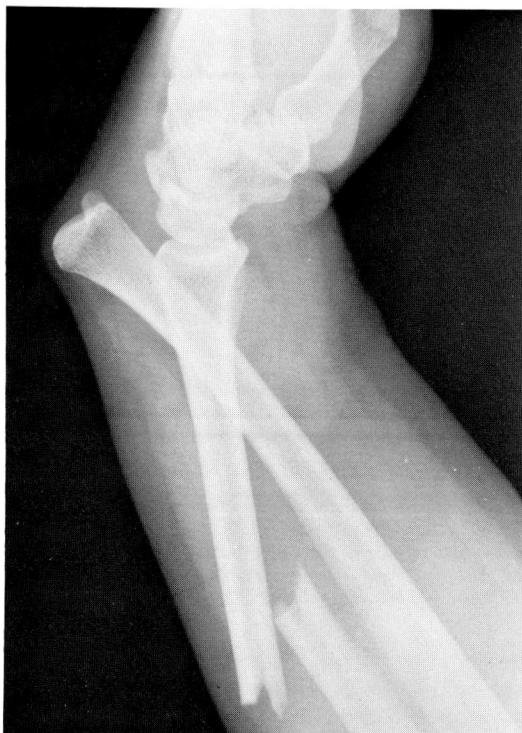

FIG. 2-26. Fracture-dislocation of paired bones. An angulated fracture of the distal radius with an associated distal radioulnar dislocation is present (Galeazzi fracture). The patient's proximal forearm is normal.

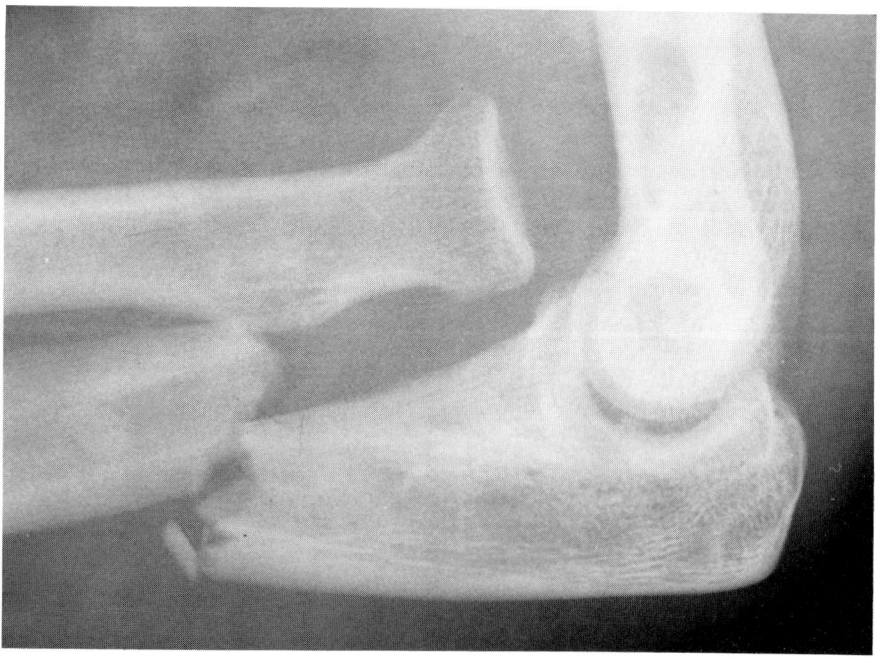

FIG. 2-27. Fracture-dislocation of paired bones. A fracture of the proximal ulna with volar angulation is associated with a volar dislocation of the radial head (Monteggia fracture). The distal forearm is normal.

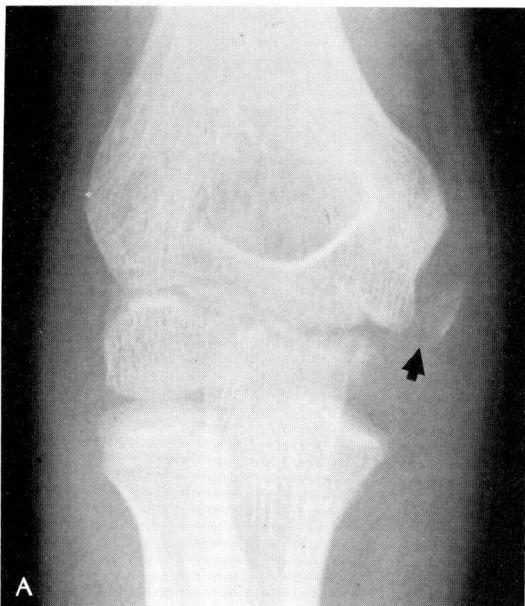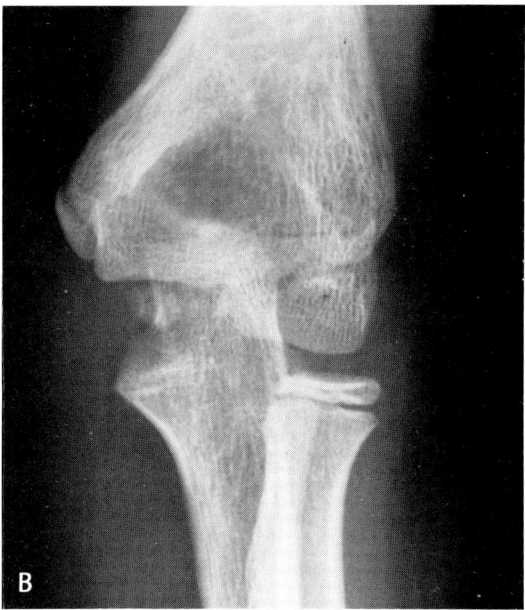

FIG. 2-28. Comparative views in children. A, An avulsion fracture of the medial epicondylar apophysis (arrow) is suspected on this anteroposterior view of the elbow. B, A normal anteroposterior view for comparison confirms the separation of the apophysis.

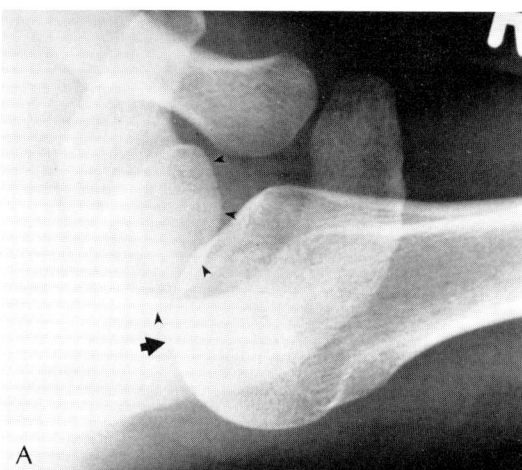
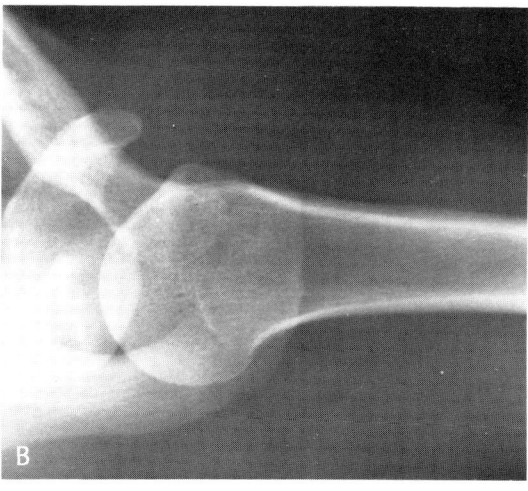

FIG. 2-29. Axillary projection of the shoulder. A, The humeral head (arrow) is dislocated posteriorly in relation to the glenoid (arrowheads). B, A postreduction axillary projection of the shoulder shows the normal glenohumeral relationship.

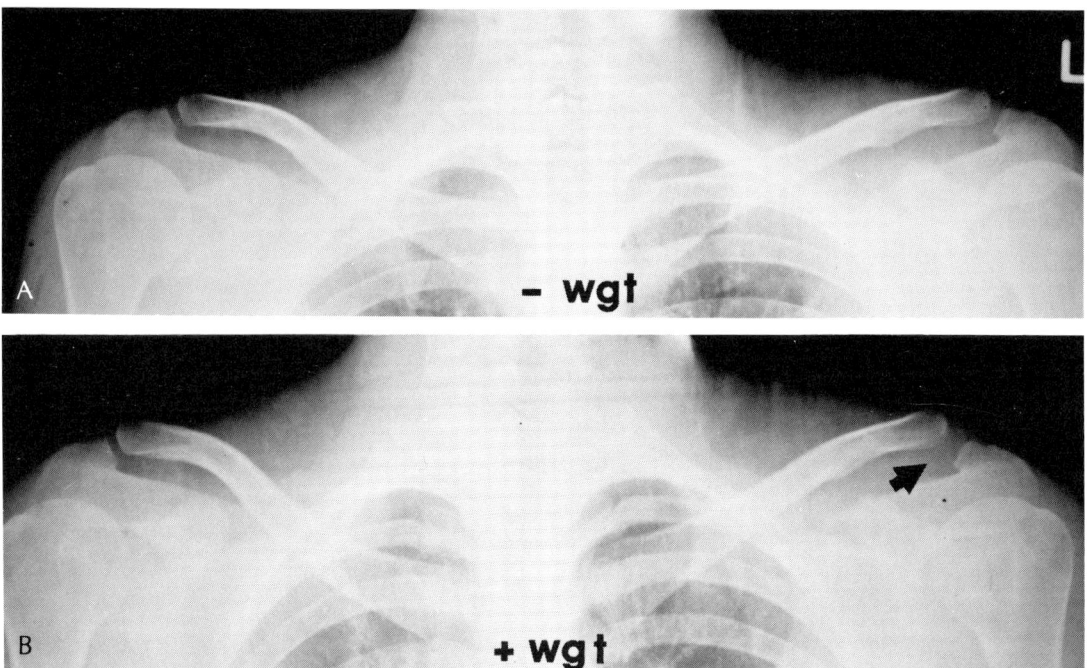

FIG. 2–30. Acromioclavicular joint views. *A*, Non-weight-bearing (− wgt) view of both acromioclavicular joints appears symmetric. *B*, Weight-bearing (+ wgt) view of both acromioclavicular joints shows a separation of the left acromioclavicular joint (arrow).

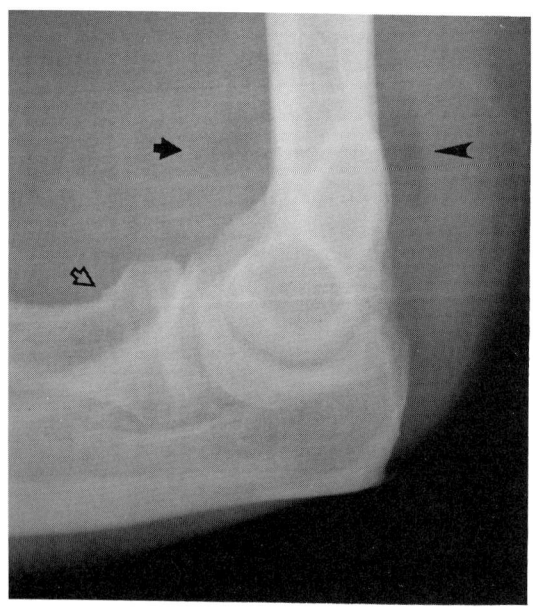

FIG. 2–31. Lateral projection of elbow and effusions. The anterior fat pad (arrow) is displaced, and the posterior fat pad (arrowhead) is visualized. The presence of these signs should make one suspicious of a fracture in a patient with trauma. A small, nondisplaced radial head fracture is present (open arrow).

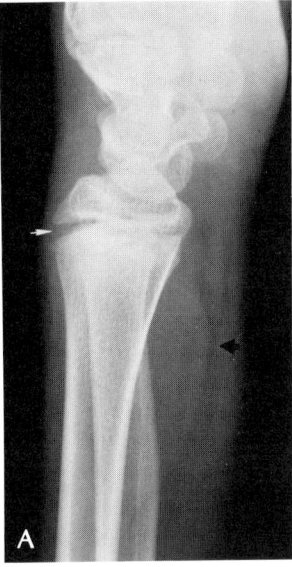
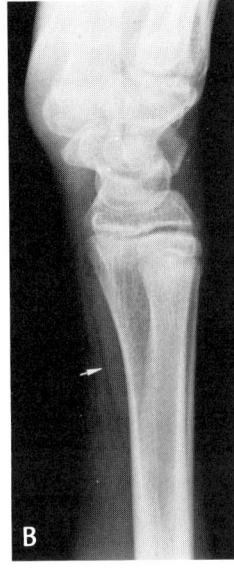

FIG. 2-32. Carpal soft tissue planes and fractures. *A,* A lateral projection of the wrist shows displacement of the pronator quadratus fat plane (black arrow). The presence of such displacement suggests a fracture in the region of the wrist or the distal radius. The question of epiphyseal separation of the distal radial epiphysis is raised (white arrow). *B,* Comparative view of the normal contralateral wrist confirms the suspicion of epiphyseal separation (Salter-Harris I fracture). Note also the normal appearance of the pronator quadratus fat plane (arrow).

Face. Radiographs of the facial bones and paranasal sinuses are often obtained in the evaluation of inflammatory or neoplastic disease (Fig. 2-8). Although the soft tissue components of disease may be readily identified on plain films, minimal areas of bone destruction or the extent of bone destruction may not be optimally imaged. In such instances, plain film facial tomography can be performed (Fig. 2-9).

BACK

Plain film radiography of the back includes examinations of the cervical, thoracic, and lumbosacral spine. As in radiography of the head, multiple projections are required to isolate various anatomic structures for optimal visualization. Each of the three basic examinations has routine projections, with variations if needed.

Technique

CERVICAL SPINE. A routine cervical spinal series includes AP, lateral, open-mouth odontoid, and both oblique views (Fig. 2-10). These views may be obtained in either an erect or a supine position, depending on the condition of the patient.

THORACIC SPINE. A routine thoracic spinal series includes AP and lateral views. The upper thoracic spine may not be visualized because of superimposition of the shoulders. A slight oblique (Fletcher) view, in which the shoulders are rotated away from the upper portion of the thoracic spine, is often obtained.

LUMBOSACRAL SPINE. The lumbosacral spine is routinely examined with full-length AP, full-length lateral, and coned-down lateral views of the lumbosacral junction. Because scatter radiation with subsequent image degradation is such a problem in the abdomen, optimal film quality can only be obtained when the radiographic beam is just large enough to visualize the spine. If a structure is not visualized to its greatest advantage by this routine set of films, additional projections, such as oblique views, may be obtained.

Indications and Limitations

TRAUMA. Spinal injuries are common indications for radiologic evaluation.

Cervical Spine. Approximately 10% of patients with unstable cervical spine fractures sustain further spinal cord injury after the initial trauma because of improper immobilization of the cervical spine or inadequate radiologic examinations.[8] Because these injuries are theoretically preventable, patients must be properly immobilized before the radiologic examination is performed. This end is often accomplished by using sandbags, although a variety of cervical collars are also available. In addition, radiographic technique must be meticulous to ensure a proper examination. No corners can be cut in the management of these patients.

Plain films of patients with suspected cervical spinal trauma usually include preliminary and final series, either of which may require tomography for clarification. The first series of films includes AP, lateral, and open-mouth odontoid views. In patients with severe head and neck trauma, the initial and most important view is the horizontal-beam lateral projection. If obvious fracture or subluxation is present, the patient should be placed in cervical traction before further views are obtained.

Because the percentage of injuries of the lower cervical spine is high, the cervicothoracic junction must always be visualized. Steady pulling of the patient's arms toward his feet often allows adequate visualization of this area without superimposition of the shoulder onto the radiograph (Fig. 2-11). If this region is not visualized with such traction, and if the patient is co-operative and has no neurologic injuries, a swimmer's view can be obtained (Fig. 2-12). If the patient is not co-operative or is neurologically impaired, tomography should be performed. In addition to the lateral projection in acute trauma, AP and open-mouth odontoid views should be obtained.

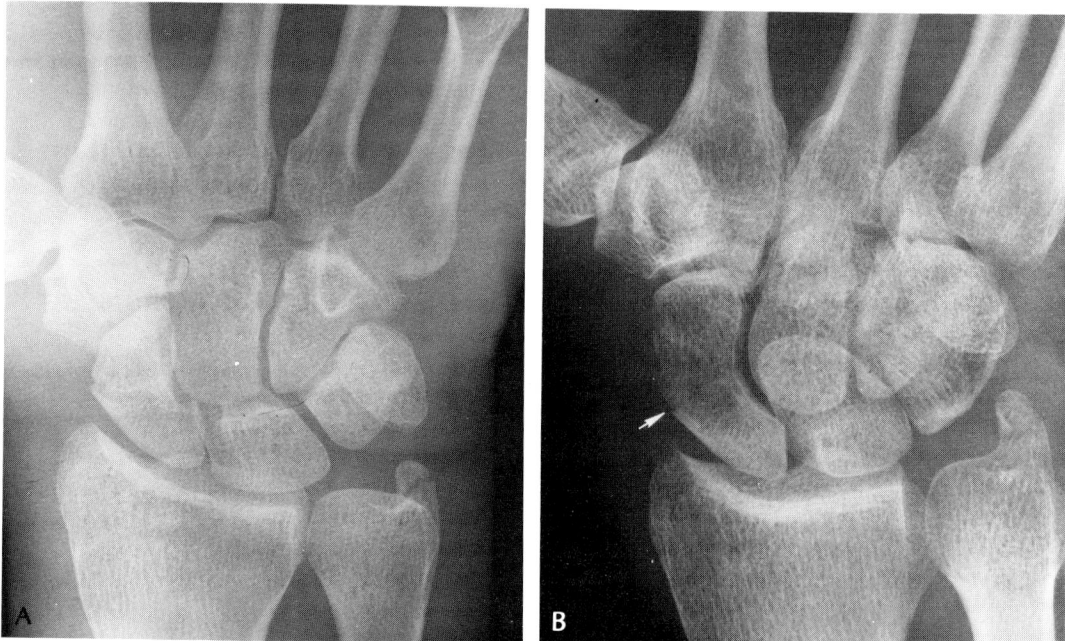

FIG. 2–33. Navicular view. *A,* Routine anteroposterior view of the wrist in a patient with a suspected navicular fracture shows only a fracture of the ulnar styloid. *B,* Special navicular view that elongates the navicular bone shows the suspected fracture (arrow).

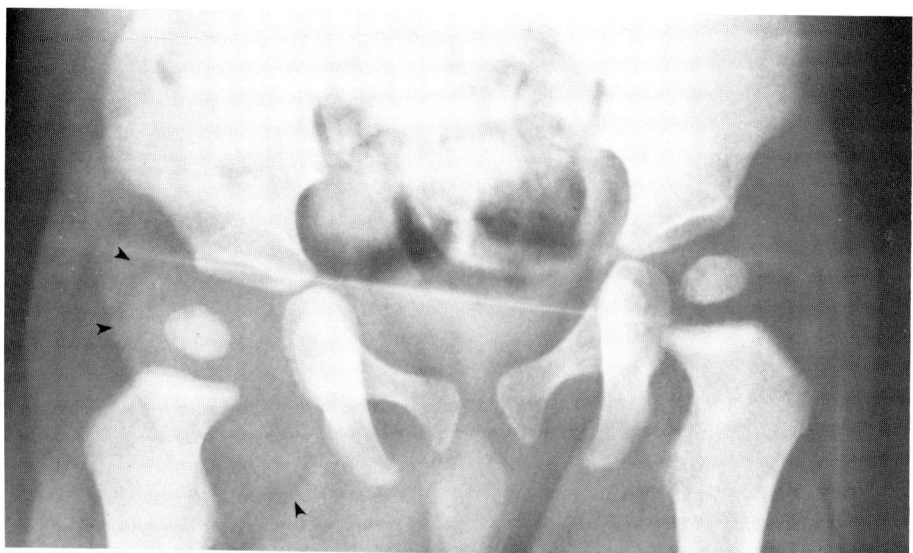

FIG. 2–34. Hip-joint effusion. Widening of the joint space and bowing of the fat planes around the right hip (arrowheads) are seen in a patient immediately after reduction of a dislocated hip. Compare with the normal left hip.

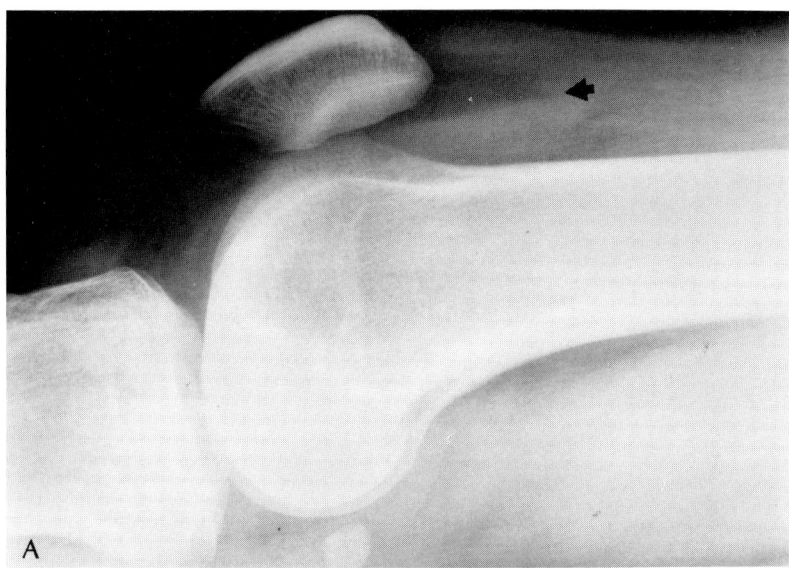
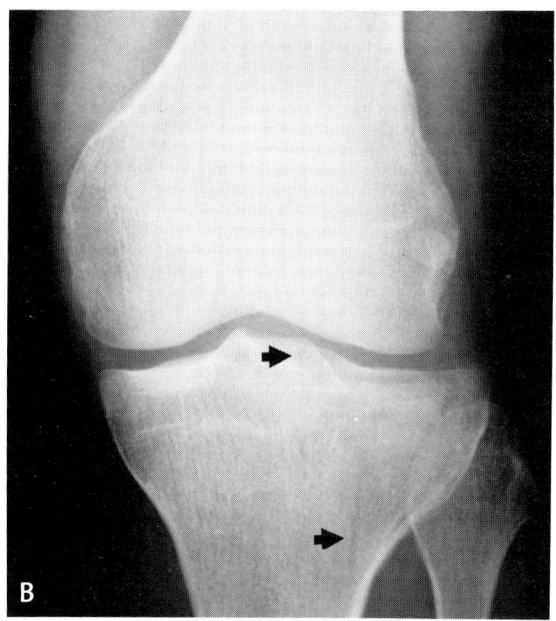

FIG. 2–35. Fat-fluid level in a knee indicating fracture. *A*, A horizontal-beam lateral view of the knee reveals a fat-fluid level (arrow) indicative of fracture. *B*, A nondisplaced linear fracture of the proximal tibia is present (arrows).

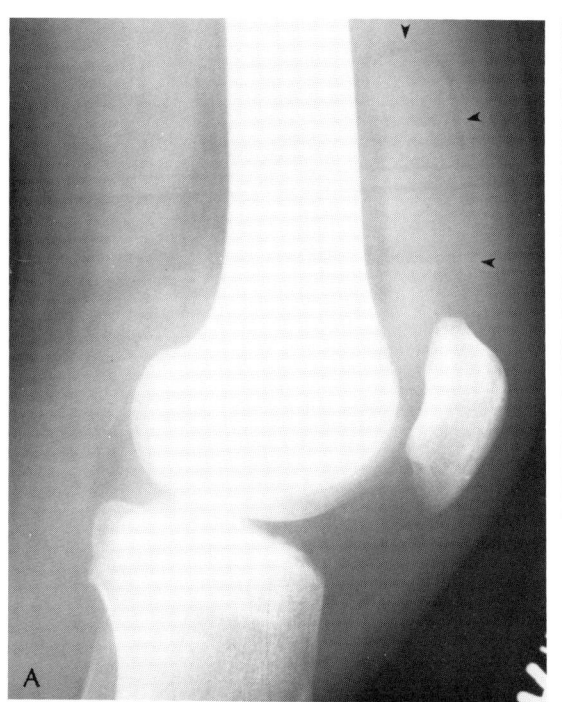
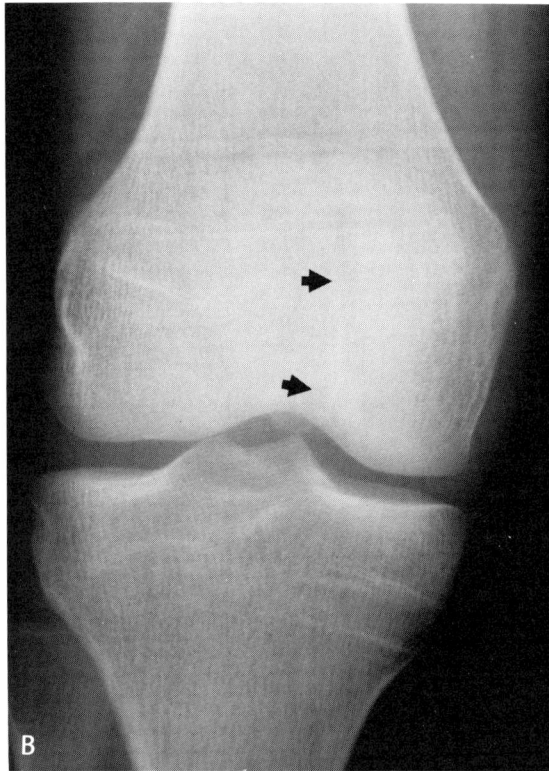
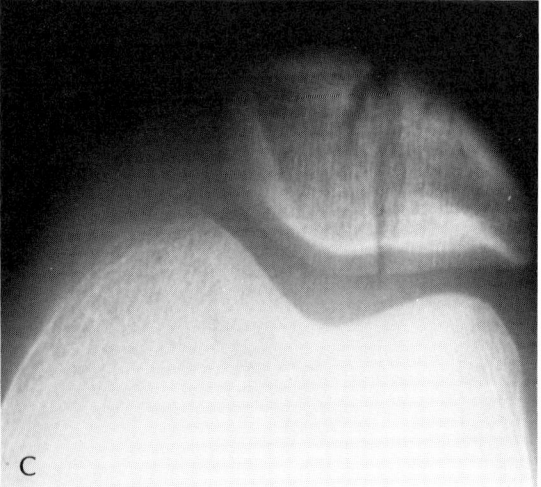

FIG. 2–36. Special view of the knee; sunrise view of the patella. *A,* A joint effusion is present (arrowheads). *B,* A lucency is suspected to overlie the distal femur and patella in the anteroposterior view (arrows). *C,* The sunrise view confirms the presence of a vertical fracture through the patella.

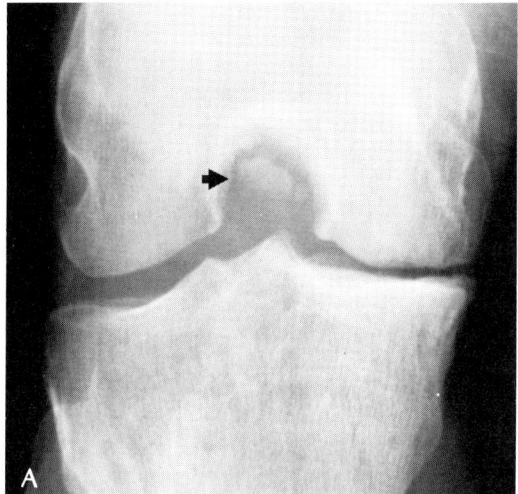

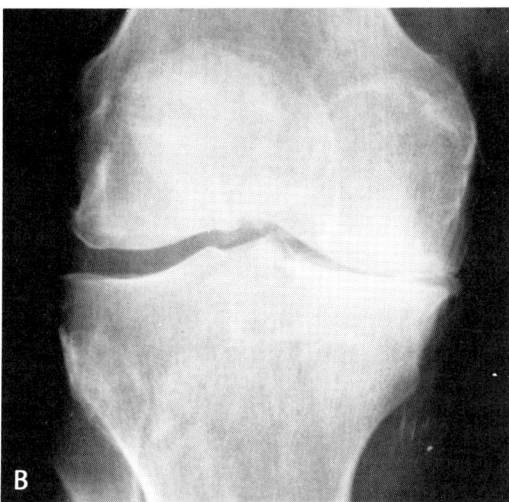

FIG. 2–37. Tunnel view of the knee. A, The intercondylar view shows a calcified loose body (arrow) in the intercondylar notch of the distal femur. B, The straight anteroposterior view of the knee does not allow for visualization of this loose body.

These projections may be obtained without moving the patient's head or neck.

The second series of films should be obtained only when the first series has excluded unstable fractures. This series includes some optional and erect lateral views. If the initial series has suggested an abnormality or if clinical findings warrant further evaluation, then additional films may be obtained, for optimal visualization of the pedicles, facet alignment, intervertebral foramina, or articular masses (Fig. 2–13). If no abnormalities are detected on the routine or subsequent special views, then erect lateral views in flexion and extension should be obtained before the patient is discharged from the hospital. These last views are helpful in evaluating

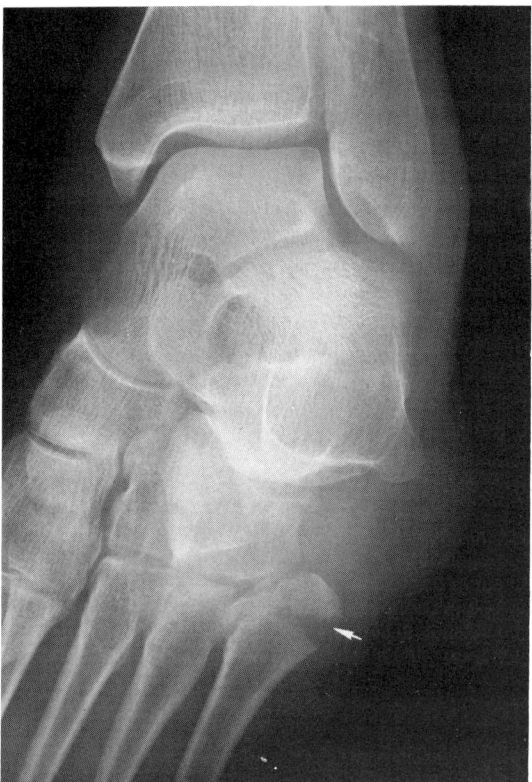

FIG. 2–38. Inclusion of the base of the fifth metatarsal bone in an examination of the ankle. A fracture of the base of the fifth metatarsal bone (arrow) is identified on the oblique view of the ankle. If only tarsal bones are imaged, this common fracture will be missed.

widening of the interspinous spaces, widening of the atlantoaxial joint space, and anterior subluxation of vertebral bodies, all of which may indicate ligamentous injury (Fig. 2–14). Flexion and extension views are potentially hazardous and should only be performed under the direct supervision of a physician in co-operative and neurologically intact patients in whom either no fracture or a stable fracture has been identified. The patient voluntarily flexes and extends the neck to the point of pain and no further. Forced flexion and extension are contraindicated.

Conventional tomographic examination of the cervical spine is common and is useful in patients with trauma. Indications include delineation of the extent of known fractures, high clinical suspicion of fracture in the face of a normal preliminary radiographic examination, and radiographic findings suggestive of fracture, such as subluxation, prevertebral soft tissue swelling, vertebral body compression of undetermined age, and abnormal alignment of the spinous processes on the AP view.[9] An example of a fracture of the first cervical vertebra

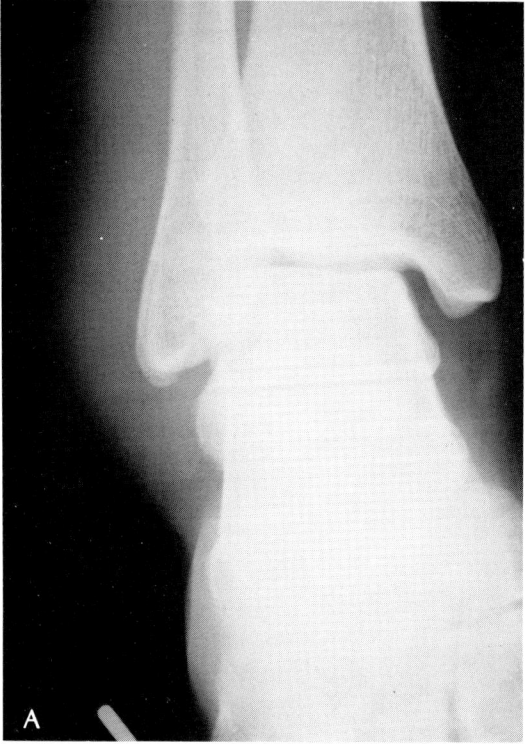

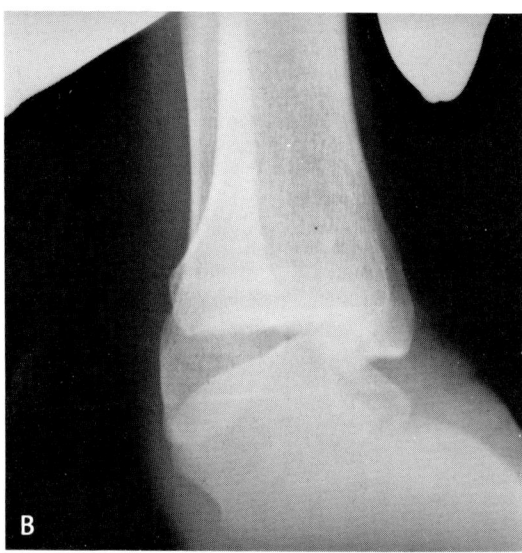

FIG. 2-39. Comparative views of the ankle. A, Non-stressed anteroposterior view of ankle shows soft tissue swelling laterally. B, Stress view in slight obliquity shows marked widening of the ankle mortise laterally, indicating ligamentous tear.

missed by an open-mouth odontoid view but detected by tomography is shown in Figure 2-15.

Recommended procedures for the radiographic examination of the cervical spine in the patient with suspected injury are as follows:

1. The examination should be performed when the patient's condition is clinically stable.
2. The physician should properly immobilize the patient's cervical spine.
3. One should perform a conventional or portable examination, depending on the patient's condition.
4. One should obtain horizontal-beam (cross-table) lateral, anteroposterior, and open-mouth odontoid views, with the patient in the supine position.
5. Tomograms should be ordered if suspicious or equivocal x-ray findings are present.
6. Flexion and extension views should be obtained if the roentgenograms are negative for fracture and if the patient is co-operative and has had no neurologic injuries.

Thoracic Spine. The routine spinal series of radiographs is usually adequate for detection of fractures and subluxations. In patients with major trauma and neurologic symptoms referrable to the thoracic spine, a horizontal-beam lateral view should be obtained before the patient is moved from the stretcher. If a potentially unstable fracture is present, the patient must be properly immobilized or placed in traction before further radiographs are obtained. Tomography of the thoracic spine is performed for indications similar to those for the cervical spine and improves diagnostic accuracy (Fig. 2-16).

Lumbar Spine. The routine examination of the lumbosacral spine is often adequate for evaluating trauma patients. The area examined should extend from T10 through the sacrum because pain from a fracture in this region is often poorly localized (Fig. 2-17). Oblique views of the lumbosacral spine are not routinely performed because, in one large series, they contributed to the interpretation only 2% of the time.[10] If abnormalities are suggested by the routine examination, or if the patient has persistent clinical symptoms, however, oblique views may be indicated. Anatomic structures visualized to best advantage on the oblique views include the pars interarticularis and apophyseal joints (Fig. 2-18). The role of conventional tomography in the examination of the lumbar spine is similar to that in examination of the cervical and thoracic spine.

NONTRAUMATIC CONDITIONS. Radiographic examination of the spine is indicated in many disorders, including degenerative diseases, neoplasia, congenital anomalies, and infectious processes. The initial examination for nontraumatic lesions

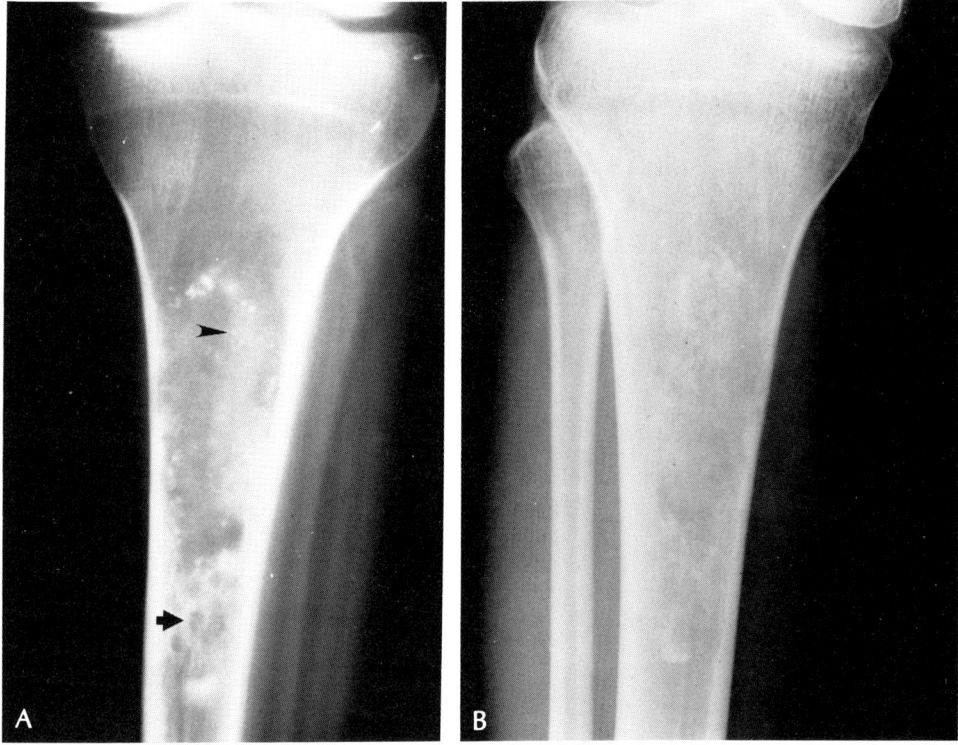

FIG. 2-40. Conventional tomography in neoplasms. *A,* A tomogram of a proximal tibial lesion demonstrates rings (arrow) and stipples (arrowhead) of calcification characteristic of a cartilaginous lesion such as this enchondroma. *B,* A plain anteroposterior film of the same area does not show the characteristics of this calcification in such detail.

should include the routine views as described. When further evaluation is necessary, either additional views or conventional tomography may help one to arrive at a diagnosis (Figs. 2-19 to 2-21). The radiographic examination of the spine has not proved helpful in pre-employment screening.[11,12]

EXTREMITIES

Primary radiography of the extremities uses a greater variety of techniques than radiography of the head or spine. In addition to plain films, simple tomography, fluoroscopy, magnification radiography, and xeroradiography may all be useful. Although computed tomography and ultrasonography may be helpful, they continue to be secondary techniques for imaging the extremities.

Techniques

Examinations of the long bones must include at least an AP and a lateral view. Pathologic processes cannot always be accurately localized with a single view, and the differential diagnosis is predicated on accurate localization. All examinations of joints should include at least one oblique view in addition to the AP and lateral views. Patients with certain types of trauma should have additional projections of specific regions, as discussed later in this chapter.

As in all areas of plain film radiography, conventional tomography should be performed if the routine examination is normal in the presence of a strong clinical suspicion of disease or if one needs to clarify the extent of disease. In addition, fluoroscopy and fluoroscopically positioned spot filming of the extremities and joint spaces are probably underused. Under fluoroscopic control, the radiologist may position the patient in such a way that a disease process is best seen. Fluoroscopically positioned spot films may be useful for detecting fractures when the routine examination is normal or equivocal, for locating or determining the extent of a fracture, for evaluating fibrous union within fractures, and for ascertaining the presence of osteochondritis dissecans.[13]

Special microfucus radiographic tubes built in the past several years have allowed the development of high-resolution magnification radiography. Although this technique allows earlier detection of abnormalities than is possible with conventional radiography, the equipment is expensive and the radiation dose to the patient is higher. Nonetheless, this technique can be applied to all general indica-

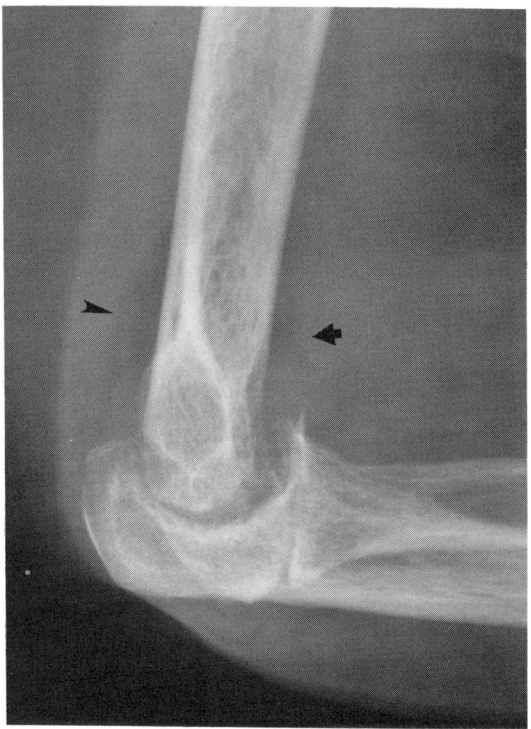

FIG. 2–41. Lateral projection of elbow and joint effusion. The anterior fat pad (arrow) is displaced, and the posterior fat pad (arrowhead) is visualized; these findings indicate an effusion. Erosions of the olecranon fossa are present. The effusion is secondary to rheumatoid arthritis, rather than to fracture, as in Figure 2–31.

tions for plain film radiography. It is useful particularly in the early detection of periosteal reaction in osteomyelitis, in the detection of fractures of the carpal navicular and metaphyseal avulsion fractures in abused children, in the detection and localization of soft tissue calcification (Fig. 2–22), and in the detection of subperiosteal resorptive changes and cortical tunneling in metabolic disorders such as osteomalacia.[14,15]

Xeroradiography may be helpful in specific instances. The unique physical properties of this technique allow for imaging of objects with low intrinsic contrast and objects with sharp edges. In selected cases, xeroradiography may be useful for detection and localization of soft tissue foreign bodies that cannot be seen with conventional radiography[16] (Fig. 2–23).

Indications and Limitations

TRAUMA. Several principles should be followed in evaluating patients with trauma. Two views of both pre- and postreduction examinations are necessary when evaluating fractures (Fig. 2–24). When a fracture is identified on routine views of a long bone, the joint closest to the fracture should also be radiographed because of the high incidence of associated injury. Identification of one fracture in a ring or ring-like structure should lead to a search for a second disruption. This disruption may occur as another bone fracture or by dislocaiton at a joint. Although this principle is classically demonstrated in the pelvis (Fig. 2–25), the paired bones of the leg and forearm should be thought of as functional rings (Figs. 2–26 and 2–27). If an examination detects an angulated fracture or dislocation of either of the paired long bones, the entire length of both bones as well as the opposite joint should be imaged to detect possible associated fractures or dislocations. Finally, in children and adolescents with unfused growth centers, comparative views of the normal side may be indicated. These views should not be obtained in all patients because of the increased radiation dose, but such studies are helpful when findings are equivocal (Fig. 2–28).

Efficacy studies analogous to those in skull radiography have reported criteria with a high yield of fracture detection in trauma to the extremities. For example, Brand and colleagues have outlined the following criteria[17]:

1. Gross signs of fracture, such as bone deformity, bone instability, and crepitation.
2. Point tenderness.
3. Ecchymosis or severe swelling in an upper extremity.
4. Moderate-to-severe pain during weight bearing in the hip or thigh.
5. Positive clinical examination of the knee.

Strict use of these criteria would have reduced x-ray use by 12% for upper extremities and 19% for lower extremities in a large study, but because of demands by patients, the actual reductions were 5 and 16%, respectively. Acknowledging medicolegal factors, the expectations of patients, and the possibility that this list of criteria may not be all inclusive, these criteria are still useful in determining which patients are most likely to benefit from a radiographic examination of an extremity. Reported factors with a low yield of fracture detection included pain at rest, generalized tenderness, limitation of motion, moderate swelling, and pain during weight bearing for injuries distal to the knee.[17]

Shoulder. In trauma to the shoulder, the internal and external rotational AP films should be accompanied by a film clearly depicting the relationship between the humeral head and the glenoid. This relationship may be demonstrated on a transthoracic lateral view, an axillary projection (Fig. 2–29), or a 45° posterior oblique film. When acromioclavicular joint injury is suspected, films showing both acromioclavicular joints should be obtained, with and without weight bearing (Fig. 2–30). The weights should be tied to the patient's arms, and the patient should be instructed to relax as much as possible. Both these studies are done in an attempt to avoid false-negative examinations in muscular patients.

Elbow. A properly centered, true lateral projection is important for adequate evaluation of the soft tissues of the elbow. Because fractures of the distal humerus and radial head are often nondisplaced and subtle, attention is often called to their presence by the associated joint effusion and consequent fat-pad displacement (Fig. 2–31). Improperly obtained radiographs make recognition of these signs almost impossible. In addition, if a true lateral examination is not obtained, fracture alignment may be incorrectly shown.

Wrist and Hand. A properly centered, true lateral projection of the wrist is important for evaluating carpal bone alignment and soft tissue abnormalities. If the pronator quadratus fat plane is displaced or obscured, subtle distal radial and ulnar fractures should be suspected, and additional views or tomography should be obtained for confirmation (Fig. 2–32). When fractures of the carpal navicular bone are suspected but are not identified, a special view that projects the bone in its longest axis (navicular view) should be obtained (Fig. 2–33).

Pelvis and Hips. The plain film examination of the pelvis in patients with trauma includes an AP projection as well as an examination of the hips. The hip is examined in a true lateral projection or in a frog-leg lateral projection, which is actually an oblique projection of the proximal portion of the femur. Examination of the soft tissues in the region of the hip is important. Displacement of fat planes or asymmetry in the joint spaces may indicate a joint effusion secondary to trauma (Fig. 2–34).

Knee. In all instances of trauma to the knee, a lateral examination using a horizontal beam should be performed. A fat-fluid level in the suprapatellar pouch, which can only be visualized with this projection, is a reliable indicator of a fracture (Fig. 2–35). Additional films obtained at different projections (Fig. 2–36), fluoroscopy, or tomography may be required to show fractures not clearly identified on the routine knee series. In the knee, the intercondylar (tunnel) view aids in determining the presence of loose bodies (Fig. 2–37), as well as in detecting entities such as osteonecrosis and osteochondritis dissecans.

Ankle. In addition to the ankle joint itself, the lateral and oblique views should show the base of the fifth metatarsal bone. Fractures in this region are often thus detected and may cause ankle edema and "ankle" pain (Fig. 2–38). When soft tissue swelling is considerable, ligamentous injury should be suspected and may be confirmed by stress views (Fig. 2–39).

Foot. Patients who have fractured the calcaneus secondary to an axial compression force should have radiographs of the lumbar spine if any clinical symptoms are referrable to the area because of the increased incidence of associated vertebral body compression fractures.

NONTRAUMATIC CONDITIONS. Routine views of the extremities and joints are generally adequate as the initial plain film radiographic examination for nontraumatic conditions such as infection, neoplasm, metabolic and degenerative disorders, and congenital anomalies. Many of the principles described in relation to trauma also apply to patients with nontraumatic indications for plain film radiography (Fig. 2–40). Two views are required, to localize abnormalities and to formulate an accurate differential diagnosis. Careful examination of soft tissue fat planes and fat pads about the wrists, elbow, and hip are also necessary in patients with nontraumatic indications. Obscuration or displacement of these fat planes and fat pads may be seen in osteomyelitis, joint infections, and effusions secondary to inflammatory diseases (Fig. 2–41).

REFERENCES

1. Bell, R.S., and Loop, J.W.: The utility and futility of radiographic skull examination for trauma. N. Engl. J. Med., *284*:236, 1971.
2. Phillips, L.A.: Comparative evaluation of the effect of a high yield criteria list upon skull radiography. J. Am. Coll. Emerg. Physicians, *8*:106, 1979.
3. Cummins, R.O., et al.: High-yield referral criteria for posttraumatic skull roentgenography. JAMA, *244*:673, 1980.
4. Cummins, R.O.: Clinician's reasons for overuse of skull radiographs. AJR, *135*:549, 1980.
5. Federle, M.P., and Brant-Zawadski, M.B.: Computed Tomography in the Evaluation of Trauma. Baltimore, Williams & Wilkins, 1982, p. 1.
6. Harris, J.H., and Harris, W.H.: The Radiology of Emergency Medicine. Baltimore, Williams & Wilkins, 1981, p. 3.
7. Shaffer, M.A., and Doris, P.E.: Increasing the diagnostic yield of portable skull films. Ann. Emerg. Med., *11*:33, 1982.
8. Wales, L.R., Knapp, R.K., and Morishima, M.S.: Recommendations for evaluation of the acutely injured cervical spine: a clinical radiologic algorithm. Ann. Emerg. Med., *9*:49, 1980.
9. Maravilla, K.R., Cooper, R.P., and Sklar, F.H.: The influence of thin-section tomography in the treatment of cervical spine injuries. Radiology, *127*:131, 1978.
10. Rhea, J.T., et al.: The oblique view: an unnecessary component of the initial adult lumbar spine examination. Radiology, *134*:45, 1980.
11. Gibson, E.S., Martin, R.H., and Terry, C.W.: Incidence of low back pain and pre-employment x-ray screening. J. Occup. Med., *8*:515, 1980.
12. Foote, G.A.: Pre-employment radiography of the lumbosacral spine. The Nisbet Symposium, 1980: Radiology in Health Screening. Australas. Radiol., *26*:25, 1982.

13. Choplin, R.H., Gilula, L.A., and Murphy, W.A.: Fluoroscopic evaluation of skeletal problems. Skeletal Radiol., 7:191, 1981.
14. Sundaram, M., et al.: The clinical value of direct magnification radiography in orthopedics. Skeletal Radiol., 3:85, 1978.
15. Genant, H.K., et al.: Direct radiographic magnification for skeletal radiology. Radiology, 123:45, 1977.
16. Wolfe, J.N.: Xeroradiography of the bones, joints, and soft tissues. Radiology, 93:583, 1969.
17. Brand, D.A., et al.: A protocol for selecting patients with injured extremities who need x-rays. N. Engl. J. Med., 306:333, 1982.

3

Plain Film Radiography of the Chest and Abdomen

Robert H. Choplin

CHEST

Plain film examination of the chest is the most common of all radiographic studies; between 60 and 70 million examinations are performed each year in the United States.[1] Although this simple examination does have limitations, few other tests have its capacity for showing the presence and extent of disease while remaining inexpensive and causing virtually no discomfort to the patient.

Basic Radiographic Examination

The simplest chest examination is performed in the frontal projection; the lateral projection and other views are obtained by the dictates of the clinical situation or the initial radiographic findings. The frontal chest film may be taken in either the anteroposterior (AP) or the posteroanterior (PA) projection, although the PA view is thought to reflect heart size more accurately because of decreased magnification (Fig. 3–1). The study should be performed with the patient in the erect position in full inspiration, unless the patient's condition does not permit it. The majority of physicians today prefer films taken using 120 to 140 kVp and a wide-latitude film-screen combination. These studies have the best quality when antiscatter measures and phototiming are used. An optimally positioned study, as in Figure 3–2, includes the entire thorax, with the patient aligned to superimpose the sternoclavicular joints just on either side of the spine. When the film is properly exposed, the lower spine is visible through the heart, but its detail is obscured. The pulmonary vessels should be easily visible at least to the junction of the inner two-thirds and outer third of the lung. The films should be labeled with the patient's name or identification number, the date, a right or left marker, and the name or number of the technician. One may obtain chest radiographs with these features using simple equipment in outpatient settings as well as in hospitals.

Indications for and Efficacy of Chest Radiographs

The chest radiograph supplements the patient's medical history and physical examination by defining the anatomic location of disease more precisely. Because of the many disease processes that may affect the thorax, the indications for obtaining a chest radiograph are broad. Physicians have used these studies for diagnostic or screening purposes. Diagnostic radiographs identify or clarify abnormalities suspected because of specific symptoms or findings referable to the patient. Screening examinations are performed in a population of patients, most of whom are asymptomatic, to identify a specific disease process.

Most physicians consider chest radiography to be appropriate in the initial evaluation of patients with signs or symptoms referable to the thorax or of patients who have a disease with a high likelihood of cardiac or pulmonary involvement. Despite the long history of chest radiography, however, the exact contribution of the chest radiograph to the management of patients with new thoracic symptoms or established cardiopulmonary disease is not always clear. Several studies conducted in the last several years have attempted to clarify the point at which the chest radiograph is most useful. In a study of patients with acute chest complaints, the radiograph was avoidable during the initial evaluation in 96% of patients under 40 years of age if they had a normal physical examination and no hemoptysis.[2] Pneumonia was the most frequent abnormality missed. The chest radiograph can probably be safely deleted in the initial evaluation of this group of patients, although it should be obtained if symptoms persist. Similar studies have been conducted to develop guidelines for the proper use of chest radiography in the management of asthma and tuberculosis.[3,4] As greater emphasis is placed on cost containment, we shall need further studies that better define the

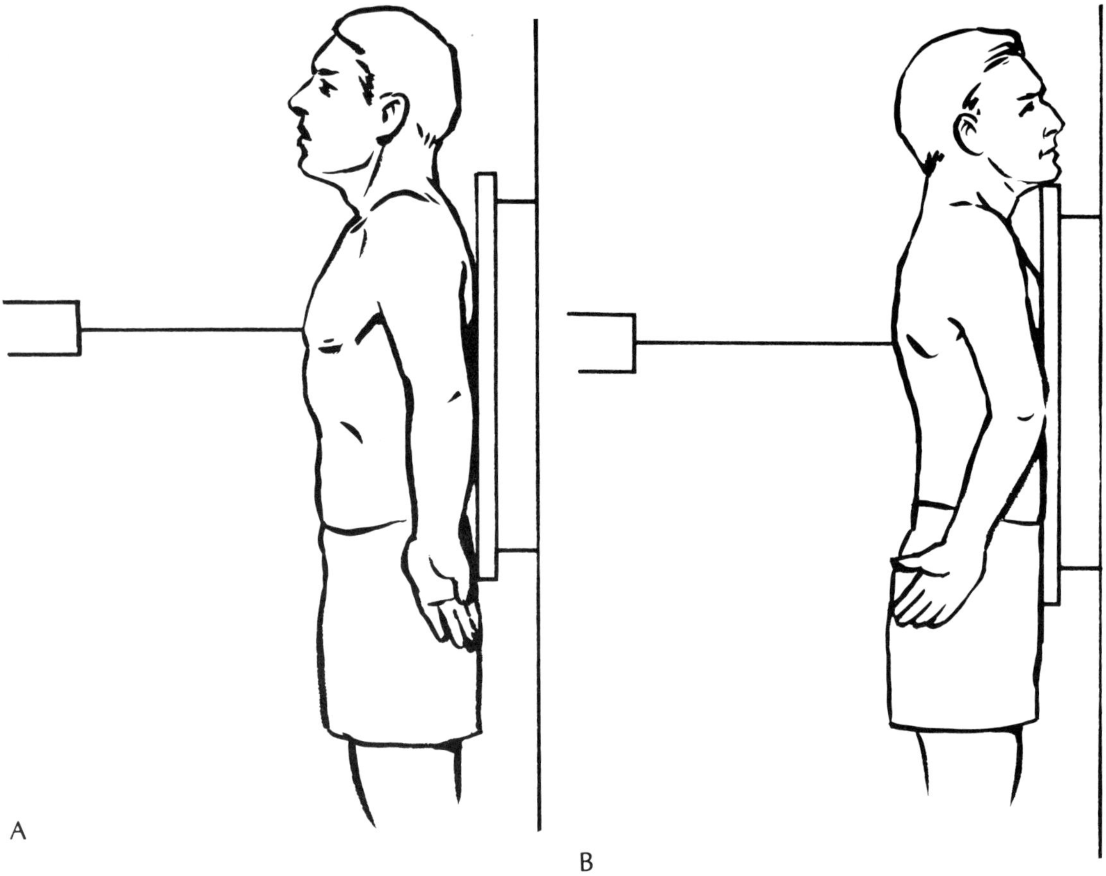

FIG. 3–1. Projections for frontal chest radiograph. The x-ray beam traverses the patient from anterior to posterior *(A)* or from posterior to anterior *(B)*. Structures closer to the film holder have less magnification than structures farther away.

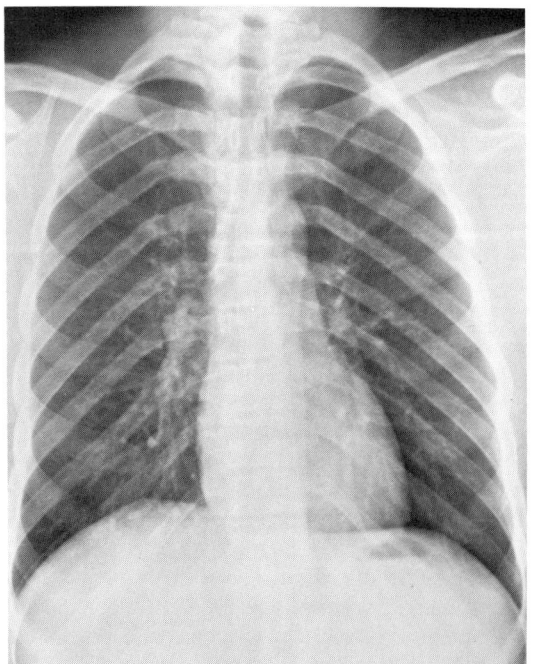

FIG. 3–2. Posteroanterior chest radiograph. Both sides of the inferior ribs and the top of the first rib should be visible, although the amount of external soft tissue depends on the patient's size. In full inspiration, the right hemidiaphragm is between the ninth and tenth posterior ribs.

effective use of these radiologic tests in many settings.

The presence of disease in asymptomatic patients is not always obvious on the chest radiograph. The reasons relate to the incidence of disease in the population, as well as to the limited ability of chest radiography to show early disease in the airways, lung interstitium, and mediastinum. Because of these limitations, guidelines for the use of chest radiographs to screen for disease have been developed by the United States government's Center for Devices and Radiological Health.[5] These guidelines have been reviewed and endorsed by many medical organizations, including the American College of Radiology, American College of Physicians, and the American College of Surgeons. The guidelines are as follows[5]:

1. Routine screening examinations of unselected populations performed by administrative mandate should be discontinued unless a significant yield of disease can be shown.
2. Routine prenatal chest radiographs should be discontinued.
3. A chest radiograph should not be required solely because of admission to a hospital.
4. Repeated chest radiographs have not been shown to be productive in most instances in regard to detection and control of tuberculosis. Chest radiographs should be performed whenever a specific medical indication exists, such as in initial evaluation of a tuberculosis skin-test convertor, symptomatic patients during treatment, and others.
5. Chest radiographs related to occupation should be obtained selectively, based on an individual's previous occupational and medical history, the clinical examination, and proposed job assignment. Follow-up examinations should take place at intervals consistent with the current understanding of the pathophysiologic features of the disease and its rate of progression.

In addition to the foregoing clinical situations, annotated bibliographies from the government report address screening for lung cancer and cardiovascular disease.[5] In neither of these situations has screening been of clear-cut benefit.

The need for chest radiography as a preliminary to nonthoracic surgical procedures is a controversial subject of great interest to surgeons. The practice is widespread, despite a lack of studies that clearly delineate the instances in which it is beneficial. One report has suggested that the yield of preoperative radiography can be increased by examining only patients with a clinical history of or findings suggesting cardiopulmonary disease, as follows[6]:

1. Previous cardiac or pulmonary disease.
2. History of smoking.
3. Occupational exposure to asbestos, dust, or fumes.
4. Serious systemic disease.
5. Previous or current cancer.
6. Symptoms suggestive of cardiac, pulmonary, or systemic disease.
7. Abnormal physical findings in the chest or abdomen.

By following the foregoing criteria, 41% of the preoperative chest radiographs in this study could have been avoided without deleterious effects on the patients.

Additional Radiographic Projections

Other projections that are helpful in detecting abnormalities or in fully assessing an observation from the frontal film include the erect lateral, lateral decubitus, apical lordotic, and oblique views. These projections are obtained as shown in Figure 3–3.

The erect lateral view is an integral part of radiographic evaluation in patients with cardiopulmonary disease and disorders with a high likelihood of involving the thorax, such as carcinoma. The examination is usually performed in the left lateral projection, to obtain a more accurate reflection of heart size. Although the lungs are superimposed on the lateral view, one may best obtain certain information about the heart, the pulmonary hila, other mediastinal structures, and the thoracic spine with this view. In an optimally positioned patient (Fig. 3–4), the central ray of the radiographic beam traverses the patient just inferior to the pulmonary arteries. The posterior ribs are almost superimposed, and the posterior cortex of the sternum is easily visualized. The patient's arms should be raised as much as possible to prevent obscuration of the upper mediastinum and lungs. The exposure should allow visualization of pulmonary vessels in the retrosternal air space.

When the chest radiograph is used for screening purposes, the lateral examination may be used selectively.[7] In patients aged 40 years or over, it should be included because it may contribute information up to 16% of the time. In patients between ages 20 and 39 years, however, it contributes to diagnosis in only 3% and should be performed selectively as needed.

The lateral decubitus examination is really a frontal projection using a horizontal beam and taken with the patient lying on his side. This projection helps one to assess gravitational influences on disease processes or to define the anatomic location of an abnormality (Figs. 3–5 and 3–6). Indications for this examination are as follows:

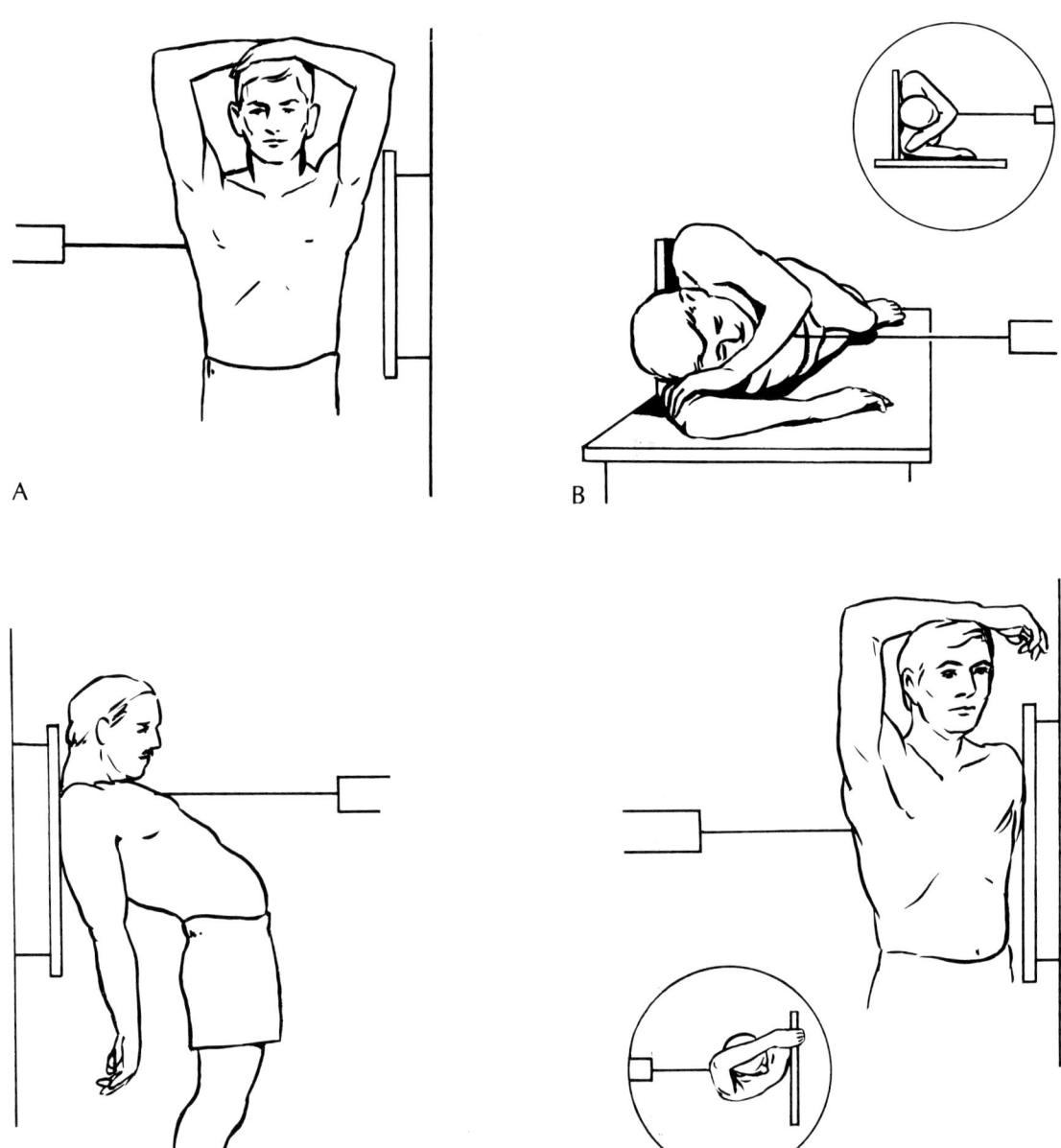

FIG. 3–3. Accessory Projections for Chest Radiography. *A,* Erect lateral view: the x-ray beam traverses the patient from side to side; the patient is standing, but he could be seated. *B,* Lateral decubitus view: the x-ray beam usually traverses the patient from anterior to posterior, but the direction could be reversed; the patient lies on the right side for a right lateral decubitus view and on the left side for a left lateral decubitus view; the x-ray beam is horizontal. *C,* Apical lordotic view: the x-ray beam traverses the patient from anterior to posterior; the patient leans back against the film holder. *D,* Oblique view: either an anteroposterior or a posteroanterior position is possible; unless the degree of obliquity is specified, a 45° posteroanterior projection is usually obtained; protocols vary widely for this projection; the patient is usually standing.

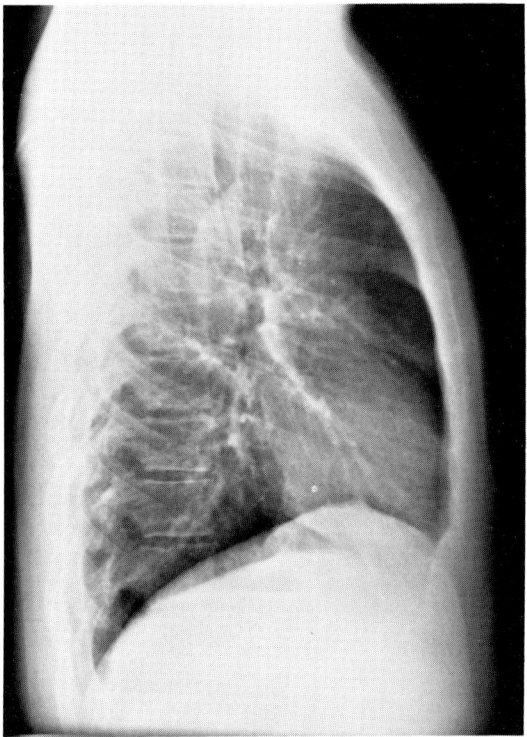

FIG. 3–4. Erect lateral chest radiograph. The posterior costophrenic angle must be visible, to detect small amounts of pleural fluid. The patient's arms must be raised sufficiently to show the retrosternal mediastinum clearly.

1. Demonstration of the free-flowing nature of the pleural fluid.
2. Aid in differentiation of pleural space from parenchymal lung disease.
3. Demonstration of the mobile nature of masses within cavities.
4. Confirmation of a pneumothorax when a supine radiograph suggests its presence and the patient cannot assume an erect position.
5. Demonstration of gravitational effects on pulmonary opacities (pulmonary edema and subsegmental microatelectasis shift to dependent lung while most other processes remain unchanged; most useful to distinguish pulmonary edema from pneumonia).

The apical lordotic and oblique views are usually obtained in an attempt to visualize portions of the lung or thorax by diminishing confusing opacities of the skeleton. These examinations are often unsatisfactory, however, because patients have difficulty assuming the necessary posture, or the optimal degree of obliquity has not been obtained by the technician. Clinician-ordered studies, therefore, may not resolve a problem, and the patient may be required to return to the hospital x-ray department for an

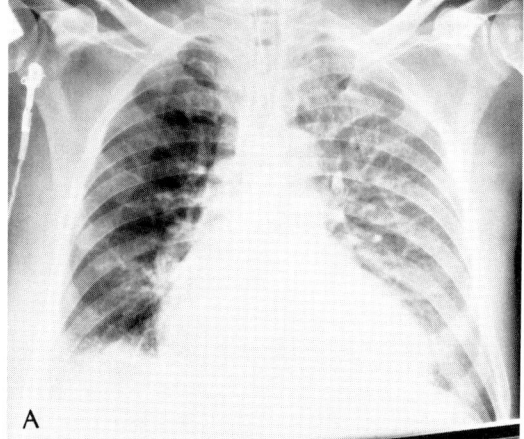

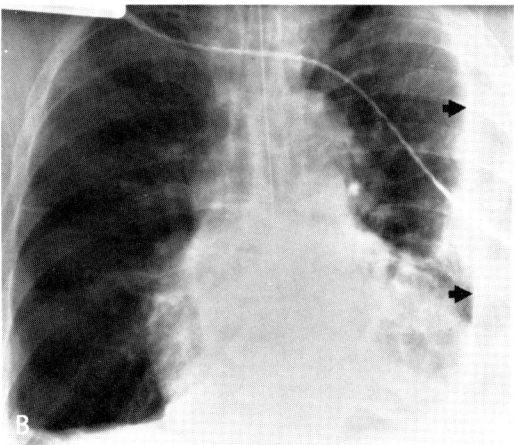

FIG. 3–5. Lateral decubitus projection: pleural fluid. A supine anteroposterior radiograph (A) demonstrates diffuse opacity of the left hemithorax without mediastinal shift; this finding suggests a pleural effusion. A left lateral decubitus view (B) confirms the presence of a moderate-sized, free-flowing pleural effusion (arrows).

additional study. Two alternatives to clinician-ordered studies are spot films obtained at the direction of the radiologist or fluoroscopically positioned spot films. Films from these studies are obtained in a position and degree of inspiration that best show any abnormalities present (Figs. 3–7 and 3–8). Indications for these studies are as follows:

1. Confirmation of the presence and anatomic location of a suspected abnormality, such as a possible pulmonary nodule.
2. Demonstration of calcification within a pulmonary nodule or pleural plaque.
3. Optimal demonstration of an abnormality for sequential measurement.
4. Demonstration of the vascular nature of some thoracic masses, such as azygos vein distention versus azygos lymph node enlargement.

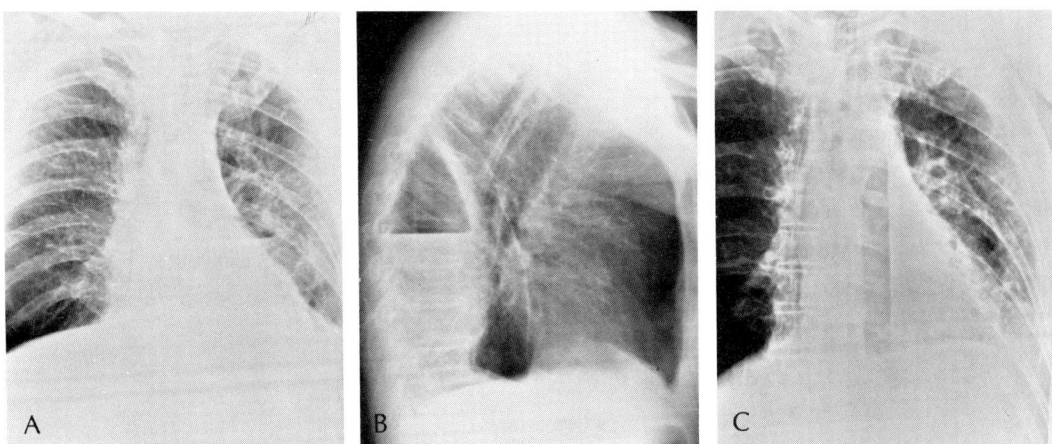

FIG. 3–6. Lateral decubitus projection: pleural space versus parenchymal lung disease. Anteroposterior (A) and lateral (B) radiographs demonstrate a large space in the posterior left hemithorax with air-fluid levels of similar length on both projections. The left lateral decubitus view (C) shows an air-fluid level longer than that seen on the erect views, confirming the location of the fluid in the pleural space.

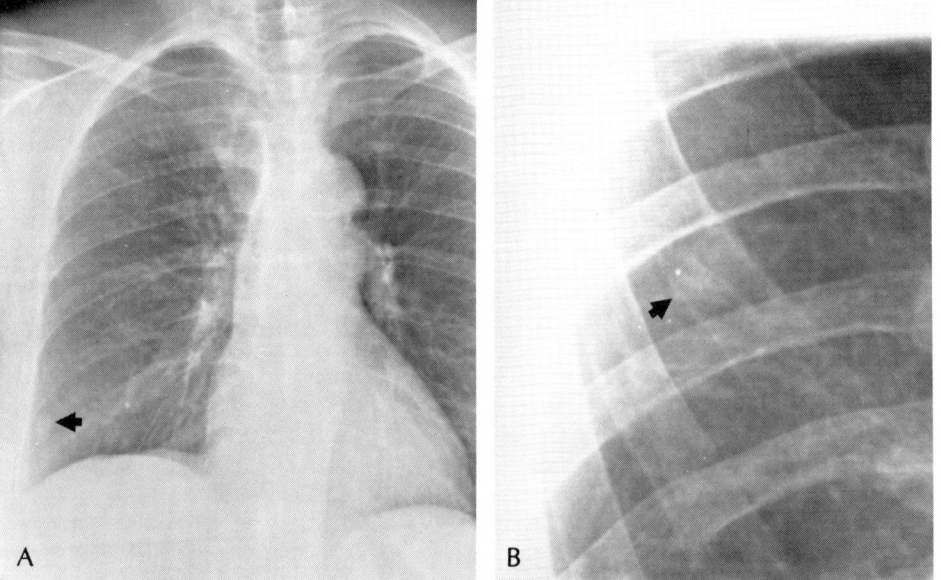

FIG. 3–7. Fluoroscopically positioned spot film. The posteroanterior chest radiograph (A) demonstrates a possible lung nodule (arrow) that could not be identified on the lateral projection and was not present a year earlier. The spot film (B) shows that the opacity relates to a healing rib fracture (arrow), which had presumably occurred when the patient had minor trauma 3 months earlier.

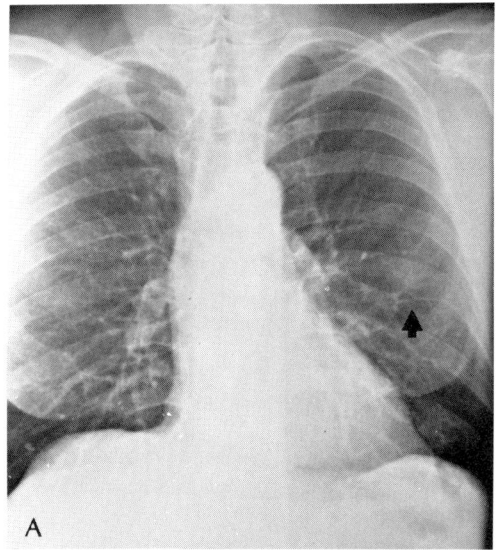

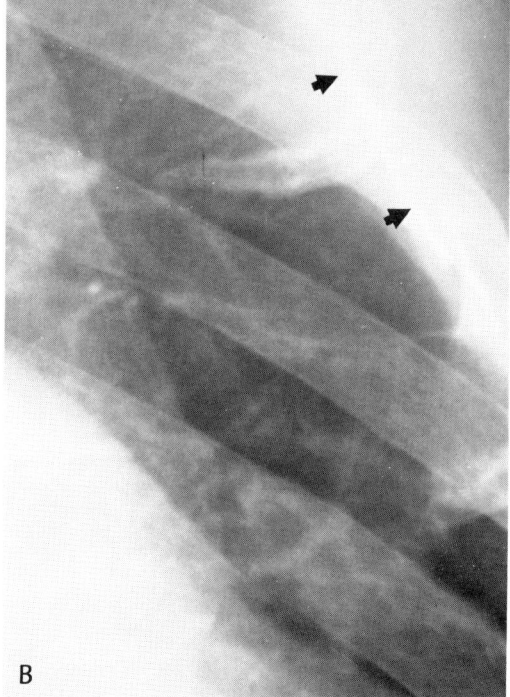

FIG. 3-8. Fluoroscopically positioned spot film. The posteroanterior chest radiograph (A) shows vague opacity over the left hemithorax (arrow). The spot film (B) shows a calcified pleural plaque (arrows) of asbestosis.

If conventional tomography is indicated, it usually can be accomplished without the need for another appointment.

Plain Film Tomography

The principles of conventional tomography are described in Chapter 1. The exact technique depends on the equipment available and the problem

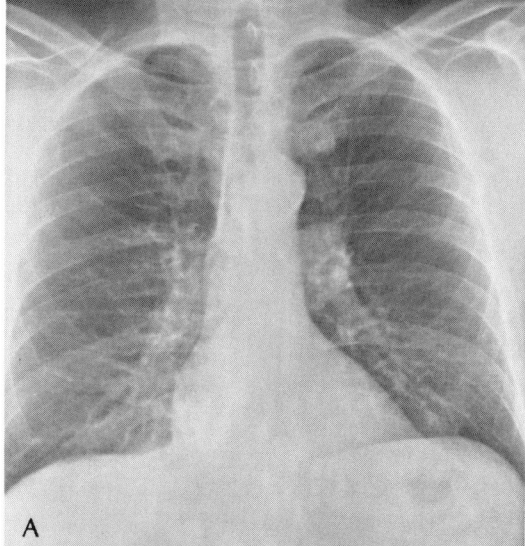

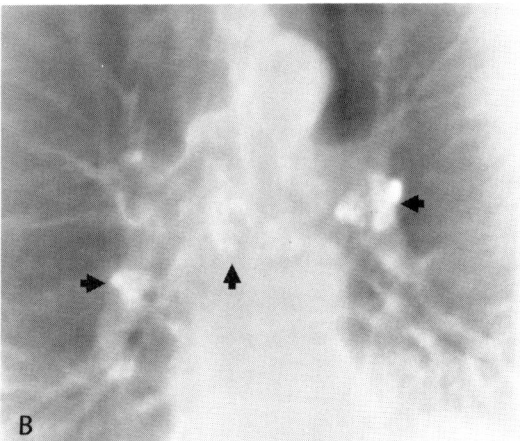

FIG. 3-9. Conventional tomography. The posteroanterior chest radiograph (A) suggests a left hilar mass. Conventional tomography (B) demonstrates calcified lymph nodes in both hila and the subcarinal region (arrows).

to be solved. Conventional tomography has been supplanted, in part, by computed tomography, but it continues to be a widely available, superb technique for resolving a number of diagnostic problems in the lungs, pulmonary hilus, or airways (Fig. 3-9). The indications for conventional tomography of the chest are as follows:

1. Confirmation of the presence and anatomic location of a suspected abnormality.
2. Demonstration of calcification within a pulmonary nodule.
3. Demonstration of cavitation within a pulmonary lesion.
4. Determination of the patency of the trachea and bronchi.

5. Demonstration of the walls of the trachea and bronchi.
6. Demonstration of calcified lymph nodes adjacent to the bronchi.
7. Demonstration of hilar lymph node enlargement.
8. Demonstration of pulmonary vascular abnormalities, such as arteriovenous malformation, anomalous venous drainage, and pulmonary venous varix.
9. Demonstration of the branching nature of masses, such as bronchoceles.
10. Demonstration of lung disease not identified on plain films, such as metastases and arteriovenous malformations.

Although cost and availability were formerly major considerations in deciding between conventional and computed tomography, often little difference exists today, and local conditions should dictate the decision if both techniques can answer the problem satisfactorily.

The tomographic sections should include enough films to bracket a questioned abnormality. The field of view should encompass the abnormality, as well as likely sites of secondary involvement. The intervals between tomographic sections should depend on the size of the structure to be defined.

In the search for previously unidentified disease, films should include sections from the posterior to the anterior ribs. With films taken at 1-cm intervals, one may reliably identify small nodules in the midzones of the lungs. Small nodules adjacent to the ribs or in the anterior or posterior costophrenic sulci are difficult to see and may be better detected by computed tomography.[8]

Mobile Unit Radiography

Mobile or portable unit radiography refers to radiographs taken with transportable equipment ranging from small, lightweight machines with simple generators and radiographic tubes to larger, heavier apparatus with considerable flexibility in the selection of factors for exposure. These units are in widespread use, but they are primarily located in hospitals and are used in intensive care units, surgical suites, and emergency departments, as well as for patients who cannot easily be moved. Maintaining a consistently high level of film quality is difficult because the tube-to-film distance may vary, because patients are frequently unable to co-operate during film positioning or are unable to achieve a certain degree of inspiration, and because medical devices such as orthopedic traction or special beds may create physical obstructions. Nonetheless, for proper interpretation, a technically adequate film should be properly labeled, with the patient's name

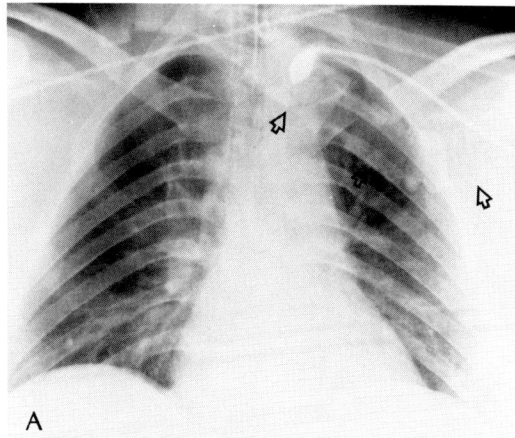

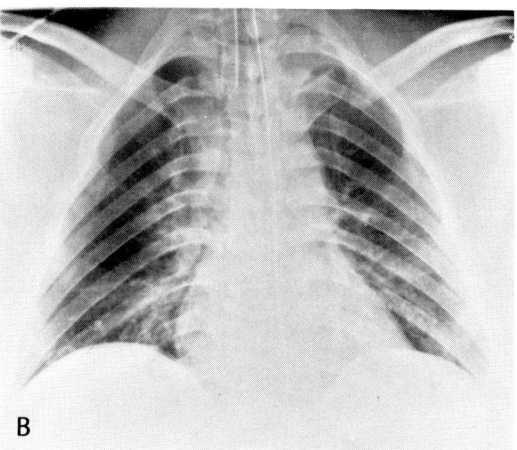

FIG. 3–10. Mobile unit radiography. The initial anteroposterior chest radiograph (A) shows the upper mediastinum and left hemithorax obscured by ventilator tubing (arrows). A repeat film (B) shows a widened mediastinum and left apical cap, which suggest the possibility of aortic rupture.

or identification number, the date and time, the position of the patient, and ventilator settings if appropriate. As far as practical, medical devices should be removed from the field of view because they may obscure significant pathologic features (Fig. 3–10).

Proper interpretation of mobile unit films is difficult at best, and the fewest mistakes are made when all appropriate personnel are informed of the patient's status and the therapeutic interventions performed. The most difficult films to interpret are those of patients in hospital intensive care units. For several years, daily interpretation sessions with intensive care unit physicians have been held at our hospital when each morning's films are obtained. These sessions maximize each group's awareness of a patient's problems. If sessions of this type cannot be held, then the radiologist should be told the specific reason for ordering the examination and the diagnostic question to be answered.

The decision to use mobile unit radiography may be based on the erroneous assumption that it can provide more rapid service with an acceptable-quality film. In a study of ordering patterns for mobile unit examinations at my institution, the only reason for obtaining a portable examination was an anticipated delay in the radiology department in one-third of these cases. Most hospital radiology departments can grant requests that patients not have to wait in the department. Because many radiology departments have a surcharge for mobile unit examinations, appropriate use of these requests could save these patients money.

Interpretation of Chest Radiographs

Proper interpretation of chest radiographs is difficult because of the myriad differences in film density, positioning of patients, level of inspiration, biologic variations of normal, and regions of anatomic complexity.[9,10] Although anyone with sufficient interest can develop skill in interpretation, errors continue to be a major problem in radiology. Errors by observers account for the majority of mistakes, although they may also occur because of suboptimal technical quality of a film or because the disease process cannot be demonstrated on plain radiographs. Performance errors may be either failures to make observations or improper assessments of the significance of a particular finding. Studies of eye movement patterns during radiographic interpretation suggest that abnormalities are often viewed, but are not reported. Presumably, these abnormalities are thought to represent errors of radiographic technique or to have a benign cause (Fig. 3–11). Alternately, errors of radiographic technique may be misinterpreted as real pathologic features (Fig. 3–12).

Strategies to decrease error rates in radiology have incorporated the technique of double interpretation, a method developed when it was realized that a single observer viewing a film once finds only 59 to 68% of the lesions actually present. A second viewing by the same observer or a single viewing by another observer increases the detection rate to 68 to 82%. The anatomic location of an abnormality has a significant influence on its detection rate. Most missed abnormalities are positioned in the lung apex (Fig. 3–13), adjacent to or superimposed over the hilum (Fig. 3–14), located in the posterior costophrenic sulcus, or obscured by bone. Lesions under 5 mm in diameter usually remain undetected until many are present. Provision of an appropriate medical history by the clinician, with notations on the patient's symptoms, physical signs, known diagnoses, treatment, and diagnostic questions, is helpful to the radiologist in the proper interpretation of films. At the same time, clinical physicians should become familiar with the radiographic signs of the diseases they commonly treat and should routinely view radiographs of their patients, to ensure double reading of these films. Through this type of co-operative effort, mistakes should be held to a minimum, and the patient will receive maximum benefit from the examination.

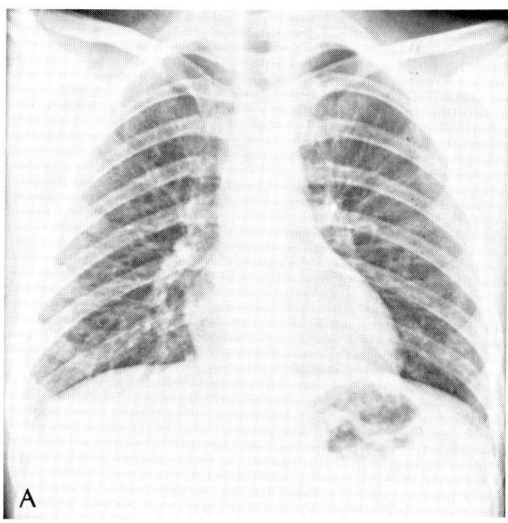

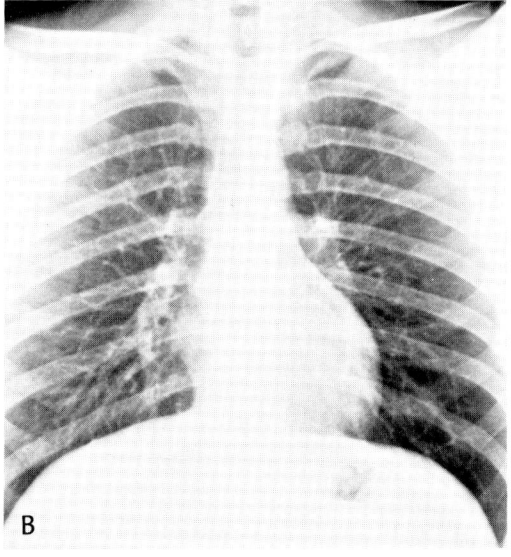

FIG. 3–11. Interpretation error: incorrect assessment. The posteroanterior chest radiograph (A) of a 19-year-old man who was treated with bleomycin for seminoma showed vague infiltrates and restricted lung volume (note the high diaphragm). The film was initially interpreted as a suboptimal examination because of the lack of inspiratory effort. The patient subsequently developed symptoms, and the bleomycin was stopped. The chest radiograph then returned to normal (B).

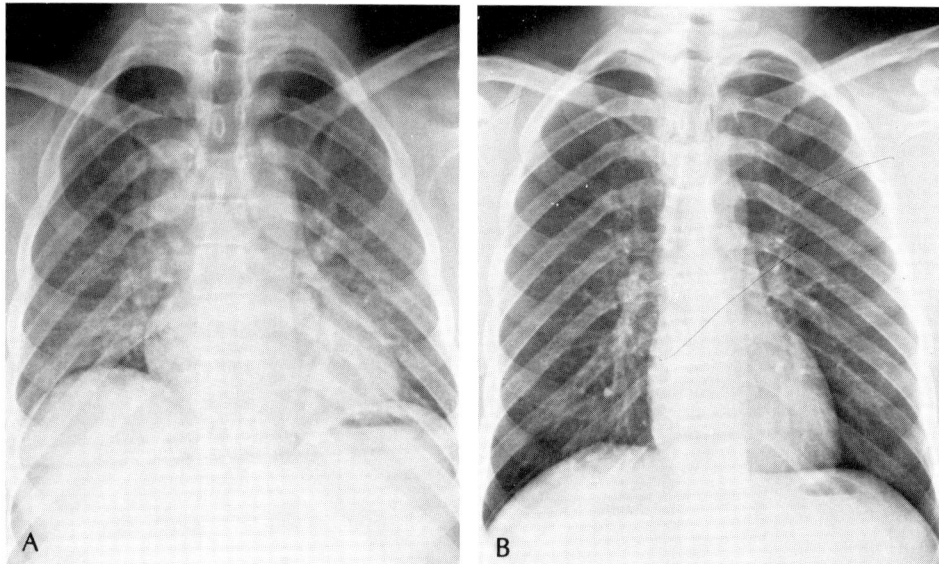

FIG. 3–12. Interpretation error: incorrect assessment. Posteroanterior chest radiograph *(A)* of an 18-year-old man with hand trauma initially interpreted as congestive heart failure because of lower lobe opacities and azygos vein enlargement. Because of the absence of symptoms, the radiograph was immediately repeated, with emphasis on full inspiration *(B)*. Note the normal appearance with the diaphragm positioned just inferior to the tenth posterior rib.

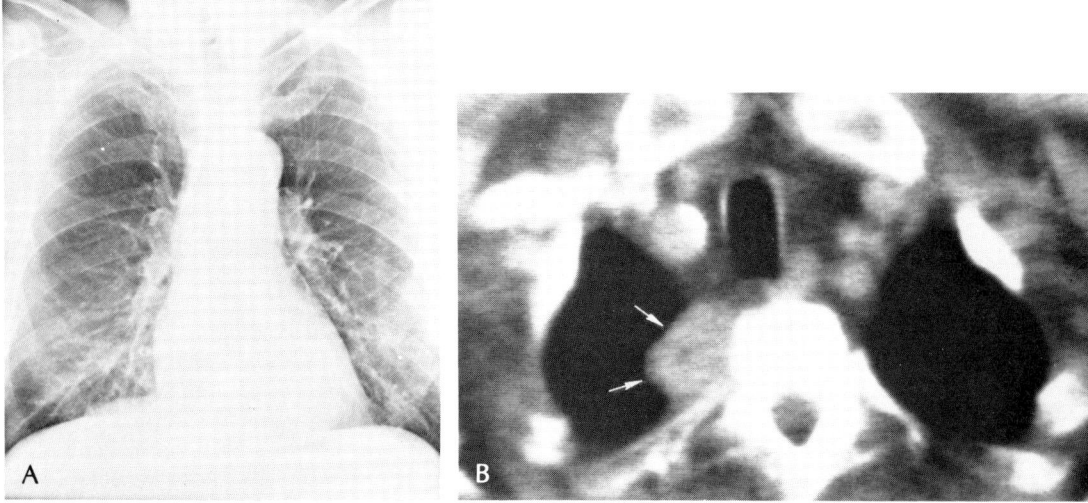

FIG. 3–13. Interpretation error: missed abnormality. The posteroanterior chest radiograph *(A)* of a 60-year-old man with a history of smoking and symptoms of Pancoast's tumor. This radiograph was initially interpreted as normal, although the right apex is asymmetrically dense, when compared to the left apex. A computed tomograph *(B)* through the lung apices shows carcinoma of the right upper lobe (arrows).

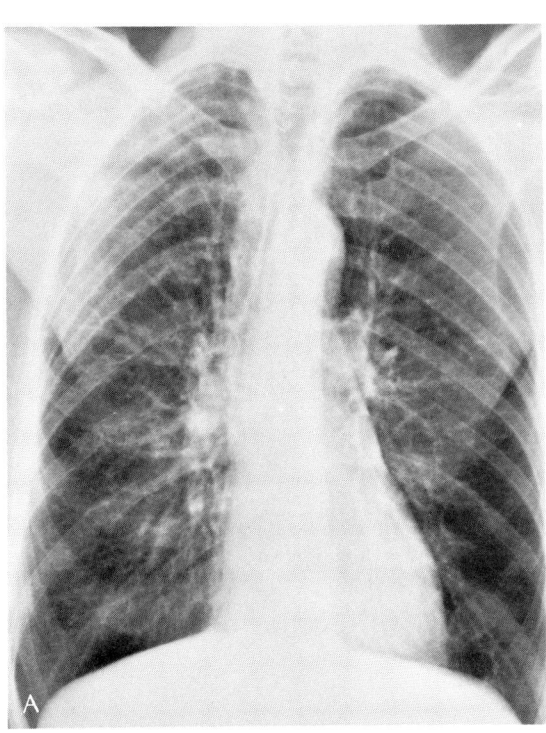
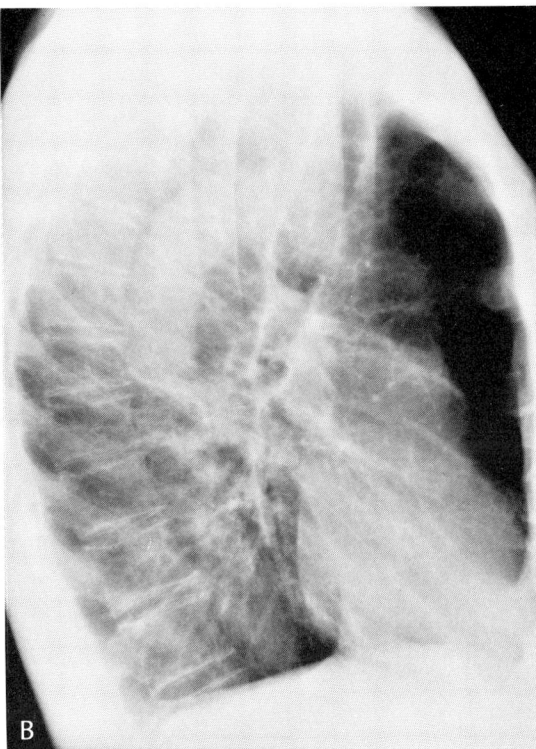
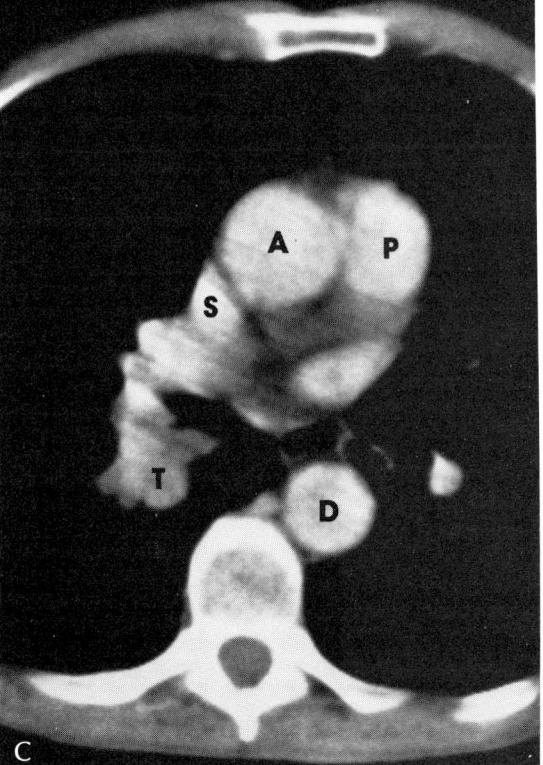

FIG. 3–14. Interpretation error: missed abnormality. Posteroanterior (A) and lateral (B) chest radiographs of a 60-year-old man with a history of smoking and cough. These radiographs were initially interpreted as evidence of obstructive airway disease. A computed tomograph (C) at 3.0 cm inferior to the carina shows the carcinomatous mass adjacent to the right interlobar pulmonary artery. A, Ascending aorta; D, descending aorta; P, main pulmonary artery; S, superior vena cava; T, tumor.

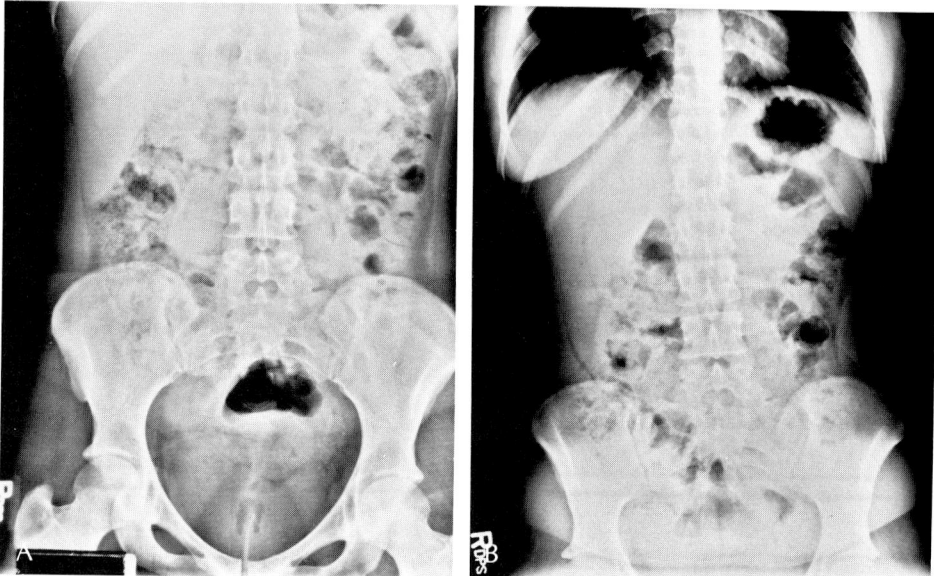

FIG. 3–15. Abdominal series: Positioning. The supine film *(A)* is centered so the symphysis pubis is visible, whereas the erect film *(B)* is centered higher, to ensure inclusion of the diaphragm. When a chest film is included, the erect film may be centered similar to the supine radiograph.

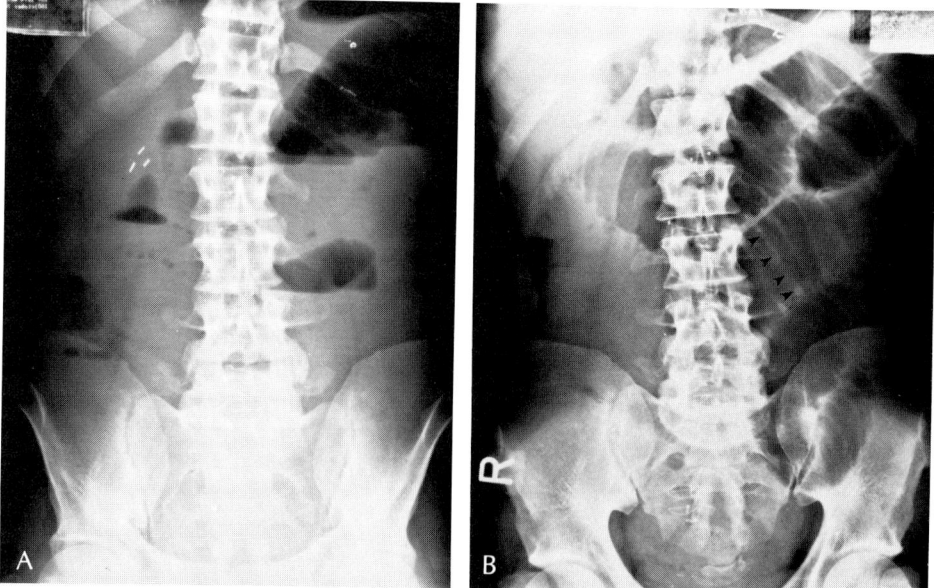

FIG. 3–16. Abdominal series: bowel gas patterns. Erect *(A)* and supine *(B)* views of the abdomen show dilated bowel in the superior abdomen. Although the small bowel could be mistaken for the colon on the erect film, the supine view clearly shows plicae conniventes (arrowheads), identifying it as small bowel.

ABDOMEN

Plain film radiography of the abdomen is a common examination; about 8 million studies are done each year in the United States.[1] Although abdominal radiographs are often dramatic and may be diagnostic of some processes, findings on many studies are nonspecific, and subsequent evaluation of specific organs or organ systems must be performed. The advent of computed tomography and gray-scale ultrasonography has had a real impact on the diagnosis of intra-abdominal disease. These newer techniques have led to a decline in the use of abdominal plain films, but ordinary radiographs still provide a low-cost, simple way of evaluating many intra-abdominal processes.

Radiographic Technique

Plain abdominal films are ordered either as a series that includes multiple projections or as a single film used to evaluate specific regions.[11,12] The exact positioning of the patient depends on the organ system of greatest interest. The films are usually obtained in the AP projection, although the PA projection may be used if necessary. To obtain adequate contrast, the films are taken at 60 to 75 kVp, and a grid should be used to decrease scattered radiation. The examination requires simple radiographic equipment and can be performed in either the inpatient or outpatient setting.

The abdominal radiographic series is designed primarily to evaluate the gastrointestinal tract and peritoneum (Fig. 3–15). It consists of a supine film and one taken with a horizontal beam. Most often, this horizontal-beam film is of an erect abdomen, but a left lateral decubitus view may be substituted. The abdominal films should be centered to include the symphysis pubis and the diaphragm. Large patients may require two films in each projection for an evaluation of the entire abdomen. Because the symptoms resulting from basilar pulmonary processes may suggest abdominal disease, a chest radiograph is usually considered part of an "acute abdomen series." This chest radiograph may be deleted in the follow-up of patients with known intra-abdominal processes, unless it is indicated on other grounds.

The erect or lateral decubitus films are important in evaluating air-fluid levels, in determining patterns of bowel distention (Fig. 3–16), and in recognizing small amounts of free intraperitoneal air (Fig. 3–17). The lateral decubitus film should be obtained with the patient's left side down, to catch any free air against the liver's edge or between the liver and the abdominal wall. Studies relating to pneumoperitoneum have shown that as little as 1 or 2 ml air can be detected. Small amounts of air are most easily

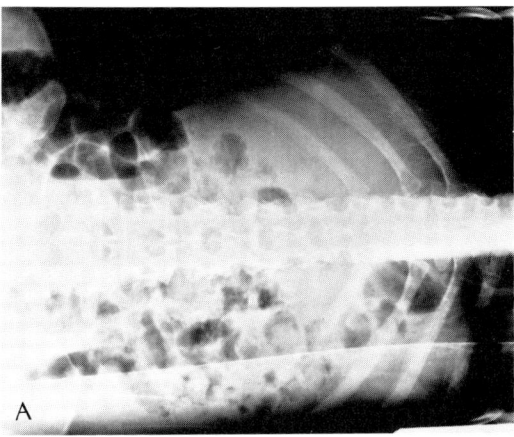
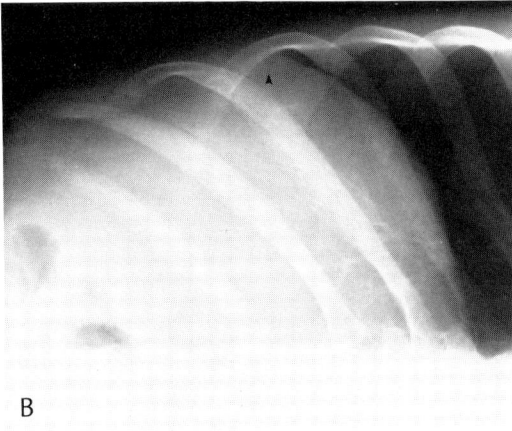

FIG. 3–17. Abdominal series: Pneumoperitoneum. The full film (A) and close-up view (B) of a left lateral decubitus abdominal radiograph show a small pneumoperitoneum collected between the liver and abdominal wall (B, arrowhead).

detected on a midinspiration, erect chest radiograph or a left lateral decubitus abdominal radiograph obtained during exhalation. Because it may take some time for the air to rise within the abdomen, the patient should be either erect for 15 to 20 min, for the chest radiograph, or in the lateral decubitus position for at least 5 min, for the left lateral decubitus film. Although a pneumoperitoneum may be recognized on a right lateral decubitus or supine lateral view, the amount of gas necessary is greater, and distention of adjacent bowel loops may result in confusing lucencies. At some institutions, the abdominal series includes the supine and erect films and both decubitus views, to allow for assessment of movement of gas within the bowel or peritoneum.

A plain film centered for the urinary tract, sometimes called a KUB (kidney-ureters-bladder) study, is positioned 2 to 4 cm inferior to the area of the previously described supine plain film, to ensure that the inferior margins of a distended bladder or stones

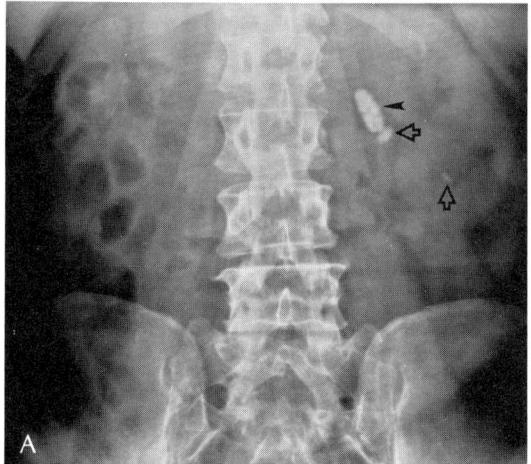
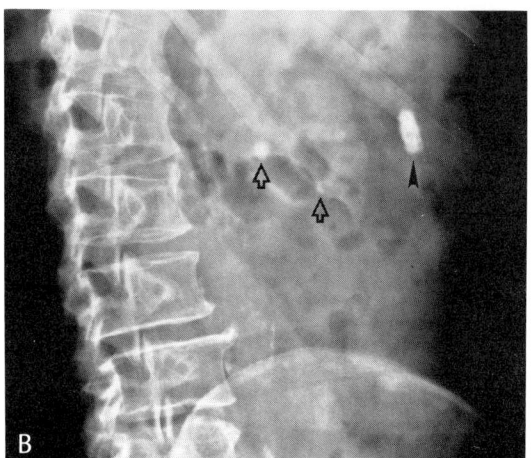
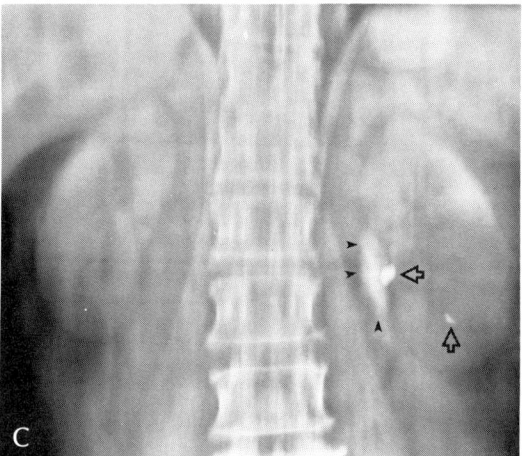
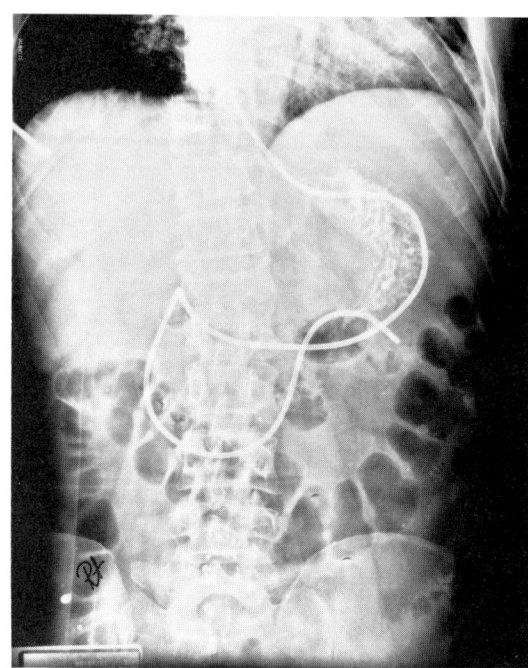

FIG. 3-19. Above. Abdomen: Location of medical devices on plain film. This supine anteroposterior radiograph is centered to the superior abdomen and inferior chest, to evaluate the position of a Frederick-Miller tube placed for enteral feeding.

FIG. 3-18. Left. Abdomen: plain film, oblique view, conventional tomography. The supine anteroposterior radiograph *(A)* shows three calcifications (arrows, arrowhead), only two of which project over the kidney on a left posterior oblique view *(B)*. A plain film tomogram *(C)* shows the two renal calcifications (arrows), as well as a blur artifact from the more anterior calcified mesenteric lymph node (arrowheads).

lying inferior to it are imaged. If opacities that may represent stones project over the urinary tract, oblique views may be obtained or plain film tomography may be done to confirm their location (Fig. 3–18). Plain film tomography may also be helpful in showing nephrolithiasis when findings on the plain films are equivocal or negative.

Plain films obtained to evaluate the size of an organ, to characterize masses, or to detect and localize foreign bodies are centered appropriately to the clinical question (Fig. 3–19). It is therefore important to advise the technician and radiologist of the reason for the examination.

Indications for and Efficacy of Abdominal Radiographs

Plain abdominal films have been obtained as part of the medical evaluation of a number of disorders that can be broadly grouped according to anatomic system. Indications for plain film radiography of the abdomen are as follows:

1. Assessment of solid organ (liver, spleen, kidney) size, position, and contour.
2. Determination of bowel-gas patterns that could indicate obstruction, nonobstructive distention, ischemia, or inflammation.
3. Determination of the presence of pneumoperitoneum, ascites, or intra-abdominal abscess.
4. Determination of the presence of urolithiasis, cholelithiasis, or appendicolithiasis.
5. Determination of the characteristics of palpable masses.
6. Determination of the presence of foreign bodies or medical devices.

The foregoing categories are meant to serve as guidelines. More accurate means of assessing many of these entities have developed in the past several years; for example, peritoneal abscess search with computed tomographic or radionuclide scanning.

In general, the plain film is not useful in evaluating patients with chronic abdominal complaints. Imaging of these patients should be directed to the organ system thought most likely to be involved, with examinations of those organs, such as upper or lower gastrointestinal series, intravenous urography, or pancreatic computed tomography. On the other hand, plain film examinations may prove useful in patients with acute abdominal symptoms. Because many such patients have negative radiographic examinations, high-yield criteria for ordering these studies have been developed, as follows[13]:

1. High clinical suspicion of bowel obstruction, renal-ureteral calculi, or intestinal ischemia.
2. High clinical suspicion of gallstones, if ultrasound is unavailable.
3. Trauma.
4. Moderate to severe abdominal tenderness.

The foregoing criteria apply to patients who are not hospitalized and may not be applicable to inpatient populations.

REFERENCES

1. Johnson, J.L., and Abernathy, D.L.: Diagnostic imaging procedure volume in the United States. Radiology, 146:851, 1983.
2. Benacerraf, B.R., et al.: An assessment of the contribution of chest radiography in outpatients with acute chest complaints: a prospective study. Radiology, 138:293, 1981.
3. Zieverink, S.E., et al.: Emergency room radiography of asthma: an efficacy study. Radiology, 145:27, 1982.
4. Albert, R.K., et al.: Monitoring patients with tuberculosis for failure during and after treatment. Am. Rev. Respir. Dis., 114:1051, 1976.
5. Center for Devices and Radiological Health: The selection of patients for x-ray examinations: chest x-ray screening examinations. Rockville, MD, United States Department of Health and Human Services, Food and Drug Administration, Government Printing Office Publication No. 017-015-00210-1, 1984.
6. Rucker, L., Frye, E.B., and Staten, M.A.: Usefulness of screening chest roentgenograms in preoperative patients. JAMA, 250:3209, 1983.
7. Sagel, S.S., et al.: Efficacy of routine screening and lateral chest radiogrpahs in a hospital-based population. N. Engl. J. Med., 291:1001, 1974.
8. Muhm, J.R., et al.: Comparison of whole lung tomography and computed tomography for detecting pulmonary nodules. AJR, 131:981, 1978.
9. Tuddenham, W.J. (Ed.): Symposium on perception of the roentgen image. Radiol. Clin. North Am., 7, 1969.
10. Stitik, F.P., and Tockman, M.S.: Radiographic screening in the early detection of lung cancer. Radiol. Clin. North Am., 16:347, 1978.
11. McCort, J.J. (Ed.): Abdominal Radiology. Baltimore, Williams & Wilkins, 1981.
12. Miller, R.E., Becker, G.J., and Slabaugh, R.D.: Detection of pneumoperitoneum: optimum body position and respiratory phase. AJR, 135:487, 1980.
13. Eisenberg, R.L., et al.: Evaluation of plain abdominal radiographs in the diagnosis of abdominal pain. Ann. Intern. Med., 97:257, 1982.

4

Ultrasound Imaging

Edward G. Grant ■ Frederick J. Doherty

Diagnostic ultrasound was used as early as 1950 in attempts to detect malignant tumors within the human breast and brain.[1] In the years following, however, little attention was paid to this method of imaging by the radiologic community. Extensive work with this technique was not begun until the 1960s, when bistable ultrasound enabled sonographers to display organ outlines for the first time. Prior to the development of bistable ultrasound, sonographic images were limited to A-mode displays, which were merely a series of amplitude spikes on a graph. Over the past 20 or so years, major advances in ultrasound technology have gradually taken us from the simple graphic A-mode display, through bistable organ outlines, to gray-scale images with excellent parenchymal detail, and finally to real-time ultrasound.

MECHANISM OF ACTION

Because ultrasound is so different from conventional radiography, a brief introduction about how it works and, probably equally as important, when it does not work should aid the clinician in the optimal use of this versatile imaging technique. Ultrasound is the most operator-dependent of all widely used methods of imaging. The sonographer physician is therefore essential during almost every examination and should be present to aid clinicians in interpreting the resultant images. Moreover, many of the images obtained for documentation during a real-time examination are freeze-frame pictures, or "stop-action shots" of a whole imaging procedure. They are much like the spot films obtained fluoroscopically, and for this reason, a close working relationship must exist between the ultrasound technician, the sonographer physician, and the referring clinician to gain the maximum benefit for the patient. The results can be gratifying to all.

Although human beings have made pictures with ultrasound for only 20 years or so, animals such as porpoises, manatees, and bats have been "imaging" with it for centuries. Like their animal counterparts, sonographers, through their transducers, produce a short burst of sound, lasting approximately one-thousandth of a second, and then listen to the returning echoes. This return of echoes from within the body enables us to "see" what lies beneath the skin, just as the porpoise can identify objects in the water. To simplify as much as possible, A-mode is the graphic representation of two important pieces of sonographic information along a single line of sound. These two parameters are the time it takes for an echo to return to the transducer and the amplitude or strength of the returning sound beam (Fig. 4–1A). Because sound travels at a constant speed through soft tissue (1480 m/sec), one may tell how far an object lies from the transducer by how long it takes for an echo to return to the transducer. If the time it takes for an echo to return to the transducer is equated to the distance traveled within the body, amplitude spikes may be placed along the X-axis on a cathode ray tube (CRT) or a monitor that correspond to echoes returning to the transducer. Superficial structures return echoes quickly, and their corresponding dots are placed near the left of the screen. Similarly, sound takes much longer to travel to and return from structures located deep in the body, and these dots are placed at the right of the X-axis monitor. In this way, the depth of structures within the body can be determined by A-mode ultrasound.

The simple act of listening for one's own echo after shouting into a canyon is a similar process. Sound may travel undisturbed through the air and may strike the opposite side of a canyon, where an interface is encountered and much of the sound is reflected, returning to the shouter as an echo. In like fashion, as sound travels undisturbed through a full urinary bladder and strikes its posterior wall, a large amount of sound is reflected at this strong interface. Depending on the length of time elapsed, a dot is placed on the CRT along the X-axis at the corresponding depth. Repeating this process many times, if the transducer is moved in a transverse line across the skin, eventually yields the outline of the bladder (Fig. 4–1B).

Not all sound is reflected at the first interface, and

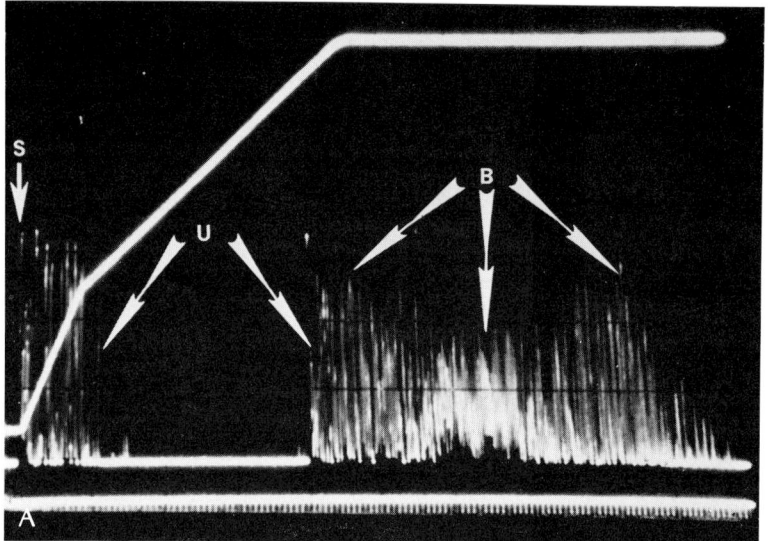
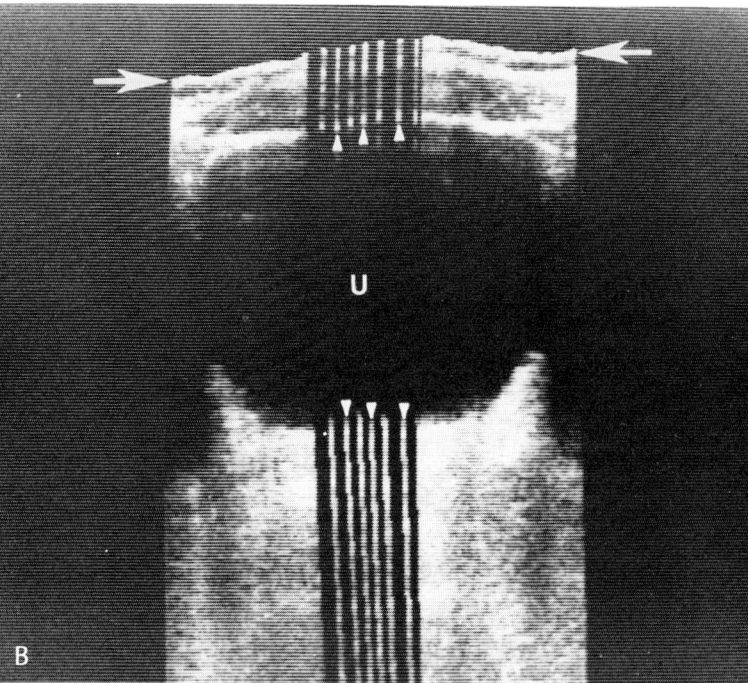
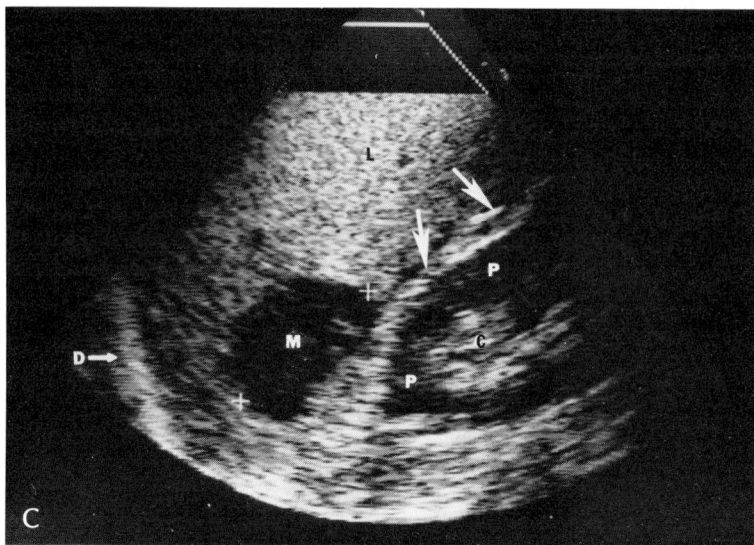

FIG. 4–1. *A,* A-mode ultrasound display; the X-axis represents the time elapsed since the transmission of the sound beam into the tissue and is proportional to the distance along the X-axis in centimeters. The Y-axis is proportional to the intensity of reflected sound returning to the transducer. This image is the graphic representation of a single path of sound from the patient's skin (S), passing through the filled urinary bladder without echoes (U) to the bowel behind the bladder, that produces scattered high-level reflections (B). *B,* Bistable ultrasound display; if the X-axis from *A* is turned on its side and if the amplitude spikes are reduced to dots, many such sound lines (arrowheads) will yield the outline of the urinary bladder (U) as the transducer is moved over the patient's skin (arrows). *C,* Gray-scale ultrasound; longitudinal section through the right upper quadrant: Note various shades of gray, each corresponding to a specific intensity of reflection by various structures. The whitest regions correspond to the most echogenic areas, such as the capsule of the kidney (arrows) or the diaphragm (D). Strong reflectors such as the liver (L) or collecting system echoes in the kidney (C) are grayer. Progressively less reflective tissues become blacker, such as the renal parenchyma (P) and, finally, the hypoechoic deposit of metastatic lymphoma (M) within the liver. Anechoic structures such as the bladder contain no echoes and are empty, or totally black, on the screen, as in *B.*

some continues deeper. If the patient is a female, the sound will then travel through the bladder and into the muscle of the uterus. Here, a second major interface will be encountered as the sound traverses the posterior wall of the uterus into the rectum. With only this mechanical adaptation of lining up many individual A-mode displays next to each other on a CRT, we have evolved to bistable ultrasound and are able to display simple organ outlines or cross-sectional anatomic features.

GRAY-SCALE IMAGING

Use of the second basic parameter of A-mode, which is reflection amplitude as seen on the Y-axis, as well as improvement of amplification approximately one million times, made gray-scale ultrasound possible in the mid-1970s.

It has undoubtedly long been obvious to porpoises that certain interfaces reflect sound better than others. In terms of physics, the amount of reflection is proportional to the acoustic mismatch of the substances on either side of an interface. This mismatch depends on two inherent properties of the substances, and when sound travels from one into the next, a reflection is produced. The greater the acoustic mismatch, the greater the reflection. This principle is simple when dealing with large, visible reflectors such as the posterior wall of the bladder or the capsule of the kidney; these strong interfaces are called specular reflectors.

As the technology of sound improved, it was realized that minute, invisible, and weak reflectors are present inside soft tissue and each type of tissue, such as liver, pancreas, or spleen, reflects a specific amplitude of sound. These weak, invisible reflectors are called nonspecular reflectors and are the heart of the modern gray-scale display. Each type of tissue reflects sound at a constant amplitude, for example, all normal liver tissue returns approximately the same proportion of sound to the transducer. Shades of gray are assigned to correspond to varying returning echo amplitudes, from no reflection, characterized by an anechoic image or no dots on the screen, to moderate reflection, with some shade of gray, to much reflection, manifested by hyperechoic image or bright white dots on the screen. The consequent cross-sectional image contains not only organ outlines, but internal parenchymal detail as well.

This major step forward, the ability to use nonspecular reflectors, has brought us gray-scale imaging and the ability to characterize both normal and abnormal tissue types acoustically. For example, a fatty liver reflects sound at a strength different from that of a normal liver; similarly, a hepatic metastasis reflects sound at an intensity different from that of surrounding normal liver tissue. The result is that the fatty liver or the metastatic lesion is assigned a different shade of gray from that of the normal hepatic parenchyma and therefore is visible (Fig. 4–1C).

REAL-TIME SCANNING

The most recent achievement in sonographic technology has been the introduction of real-time ultrasound. Real-time scanning depicts images as they occur. The two most common types of real-time units in use today are linear-array scanners and mechanical sector scanners. Linear-array devices consist of a multitude of miniature transducers arranged in a row, each producing its own line picture in sequence. These individual lines form a conglomerate picture on a CRT (Fig. 4–2A). Because each line constantly updates its information, any change in the picture, caused by moving the transducer (scan head) to a different part of the patient or by scanning moving objects (fetus, blood vessels), becomes immediately evident. This constant update of a large group of sound lines yields a real-time image.

Mechanical sector scanners have become popular in the past few years. These scanners consist of small transducers that change position rapidly within the scan head. This method also yields a constant update of information, and when the image is displayed rapidly on a CRT, the eye sees a smoothly moving picture. In addition to providing a rapid sweep through any given area, real-time scanners are maneuverable, and the scan plane can be changed instantly to fit the need of the operator. Consider the difficulty in obtaining the optimum scan plane to yield the accurate length of a moving 2-cm fetus with static scanning.

The real-time scanner has revolutionized modern sonography. For example, early reports showed that one could identify gallstones sonographically, but classic static scanning was tedious, and even using 5-mm sections through the gallbladder, small stones were easily missed.[2] By moving a real-time scanner over the length of the gallbladder, an almost infinite number of sections are available in minutes (Fig. 4–2B). The study is rapid, and small stones cannot hide between individual sections. Real-time ultrasound has made sonography the method of first choice in the evaluation of gallbladder disease. This example is only one of many in which real-time ultrasound has completely changed the diagnostic workup of certain organs; many other examples are given later in this chapter.

Although linear-array and sector scanners may often be used interchangeably, each has advantages in certain types of examinations. The linear-array scanner is most frequently used in obstetric sonography, in which a large field of view may be desirable. The sector scanner is well suited for the

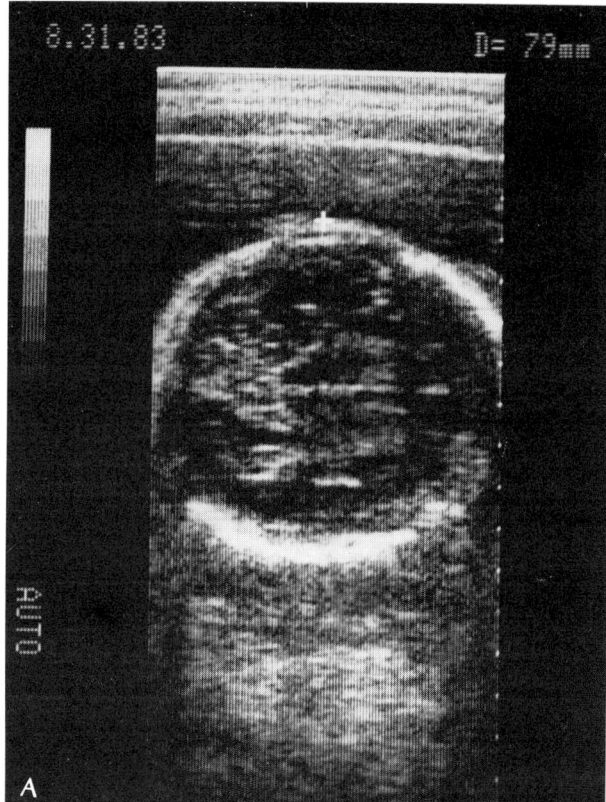

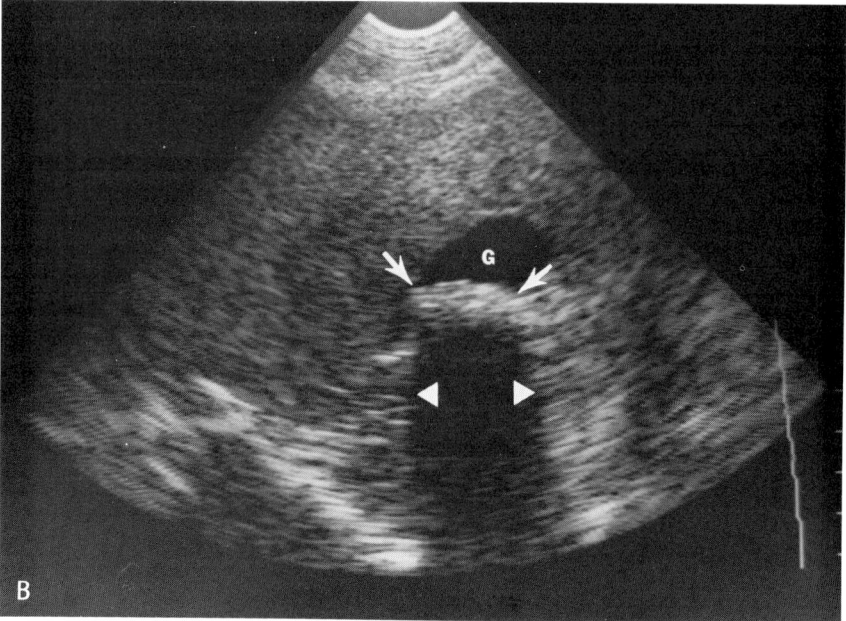

FIG. 4–2. *A,* Linear array real-time scan; normal fetal head, in the assessment of gestational age by biparietal diameter. Note the multiple fine lines that make up the picture. They are the result of many minute transducers in a row, each contributing a single line to the picture. The 79-mm measurement of the biparietal diameter corresponds to a 36-week gestational age. (Courtesy of Dr. Steven Warsof, Georgetown University Hospital.) *B,* Mechanical real-time sector scan; the "pie-shaped" image results as the individual transducers rotate in the scanning head. Note the anechoic gallbladder (G) and the echogenic gallstones (arrows) layering in a posterior position. Reflection of the sound by the stones leaves a scanning void or acoustic shadow (arrowheads).

upper abdomen, in which scanning through interspaces between overlying ribs requires a small scan head. The sector scanner's triangular field of view and limited surface contact is ideal.

The resolution of both linear-array and sector scanners is excellent and, in our opinion, often better than that of static scanners. Transducers with resolution of up to 10 MHz have recently become available.

The term "megahertz" means one million cycles per second. It is the measure of the frequency of a sound. As frequency increases, so does resolution, but increasing frequency leads to decreased penetration. Therefore, high-resolution scanners are currently only able to penetrate a few centimeters beneath the skin. These real-time small-parts scanners, as they are called, have completely changed our ability to image such superficial structures as the thyroid and parathyroid glands, the eyes, and the carotid arteries.

Finally, many real-time scanners are portable and are even inexpensive. The advantages of any inexpensive piece of equipment need not be further explained. Portability has made real-time ultrasound the examination of first choice in evaluation of the head of the premature neonate because it allows bedside ultrasonic examination in the intensive care unit. Another application is in the fluoroscopic suite, where portable ultrasound can be combined with radiography to give new dimensions to many invasive procedures.

M-MODE SONOGRAPHY

M-mode sonography has important applications in the evaluation of the heart. The information seen on an A-mode display is mechanically manipulated to produce the cross-sectional anatomic images with which we are so familiar, whereas a different type of manipulation of the A-mode display results in an M-mode (or motion mode) ultrasonic examination. If one compares the ultrasonic beam to an ice pick that can be pointed in any direction, then the resultant echo pattern along its path at any given instant is an A-mode display. Obviously, when the ultrasonic beam is aimed through the heart, it is aimed through structures that are constantly moving in changing patterns. Consequently, the resulting A-mode display is constantly changing. If one connects the A-mode display seen on the CRT to a strip-chart recorder, the changing echo pattern will then be displayed in a graphic format in which the Y-axis represents distance from the transducer at the skin surface and the X-axis represents time. This graphic display of the A-mode pattern changing with time is M-mode ultrasound.

Although the M-mode method was one of the earlier developments in ultrasound, it did not find its way to the ultrasonic scrap pile during the real-time revolution; instead, it has maintained its role in evaluating the heart by its fine temporal resolution, by which important information is obtained. M-mode ultrasound offers ease in making spatial and temporal measurements in the heart, in allowing determinations of wall thickness, valve opening distances and times, ejection fractions, chamber sizes, and cardiac output; however, some of this information can be obtained with a real-time evaluation of the heart using a phased-array or a mechanical sector scanner. In addition, real-time scanning allows one to observe complex anatomic relationships in easily understandable images. Because of the difficulty in interpreting M-mode echocardiograms by those unfamiliar with the technique, the evaluation of the heart in this chapter is discussed primarily as it applies to the more flexible and more easily understandable real-time image.

DOPPLER ULTRASOUND

Doppler blood flow detection is another important form of ultrasound and is used increasingly in the noninvasive cardiovascular laboratory. The Doppler effect is a phenomenon that occurs when sound is "piled up" by an approaching object. This compression of sound causes a change in its frequency. The opposite is true when an object has passed a source of sound. As it moves away, the sound is "pulled apart," also changing its frequency. This Doppler shift is best known to us as the sound of a train passing. We hear the result of sound compression and rarefaction as changing frequency. Inside the body, red blood cells act in a similar manner; they are moving objects altering the frequency of an approaching sound beam. This Doppler shift may be evaluated in two ways. First, experienced examiners can actually hear abnormal Doppler shifts when evaluating the blood flow in a vessel. Second, "spectral analysis" has become available. This term refers to the graphic representation of the sounds that are heard and are quantitatively displayed. As discussed in the section concerning carotid vascular disease and duplex scanning, areas of blood-flow turbulence and increased velocity may be accurately identified by the way in which they affect the Doppler shift. These areas of turbulence or increased velocity may then be used to identify the location and severity of vascular stenoses.

DIFFICULTIES IN ULTRASONIC IMAGING

Before describing the specific applications of modern ultrasound, we need to discuss those areas where one cannot scan using ultrasound. Bones and air are the enemies of reflective ultrasound, and ultrasonic scanning of fat patients is often difficult.

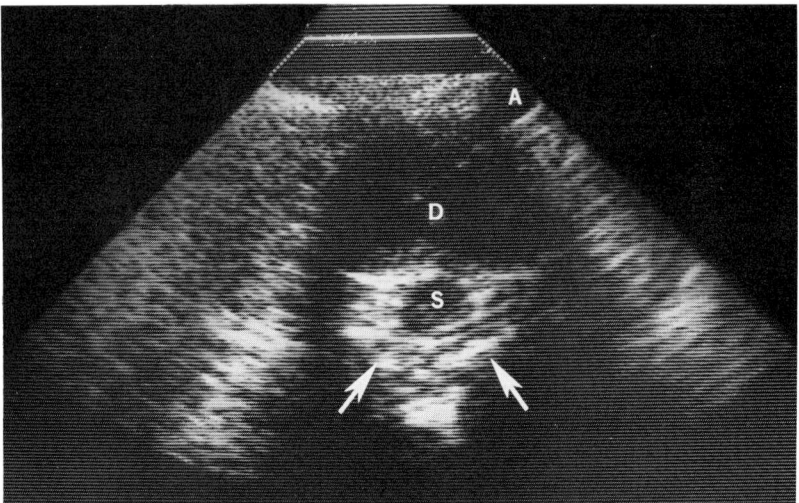

FIG. 4–3. Transverse section through the midabdomen of a thin patient almost places the scanner directly on top of the spine; one peers through the anechoic intervertebral disc (D) to see echogenic fat (arrows) around the spinal cord (S). Note the aorta, to the left of the spine (A).

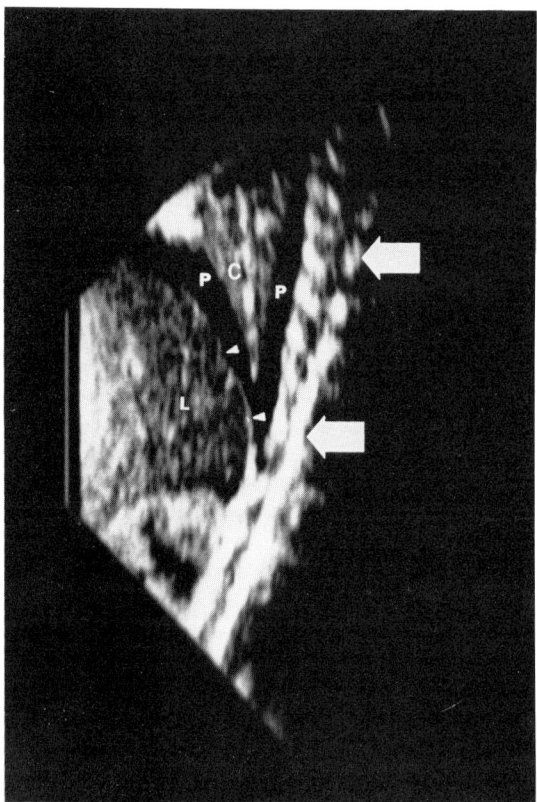

FIG. 4–4. Longitudinal section through the abdomen of a neonate; the liver (L) has an echogenicity similar to that of the consolidated lung (C). Pleural effusion (P) surrounds the lung, and the soft neonatal spine can be penetrated by the sound beam (arrows). Arrowheads diaphragm.

Although acoustic mismatch provides the interfaces that produce ultrasonic pictures, too great a mismatch causes complete reflection of sound at the interface. This phenomenon is well illustrated by the gallstones in Figure 4–2B. One cannot see beyond them. The acoustic properties that affect all interfaces are the density of a substance and the inherent speed at which sound travels through it. This product of density and sound velocity is termed acoustic impedance, which for bones, air, and any type of calculi is very different from that for soft tissues and causes a complete reflection of sound that makes it impossible to see beyond these entities. This makes the adult brain impossible to scan unless, for example, a bone flap has been removed or unless scanning takes place in the operating room during a craniotomy. In the head of an infant, nature has provided an acoustic window in the form of the fontanelle. A similar situation exists in the adult spinal canal. We may see only the point at which the disc spaces allow penetration of sound (Fig. 4–3). In the chest, pleural-based lesions are visible, but an abscess within the lung is inaccessible to the scanner because it is surrounded by air. The opposite situation may be found with pulmonary infiltrates. The normal lung sets up an inpenetrable barrier and reflects all sound, whereas a dense pulmonary infiltrate fills the alveoli with fluid and allows sound to pass inside. The consolidated lung has an ultrasonic appearance similar to that of the liver (Fig. 4–4), an interesting analogy to the pathologic term "hepatization."

Finally, the imaging of fat presents a problem. Although oil conducts sound as well as any other liquid medium, human fat scrambles the sound beam and degrades the ultrasonic image. One cannot scan around fat, and the organs of heavier patients are often better imaged by computed tomographic (CT) scanning. In radiography, fat is an excellent contrast medium, and high-quality CT scans are frequently obtained from obese patients who may be unsuited for ultrasonic examinations. Sonographic image quality may be degraded not only by superficial fat, but also by fat that may be present in large quantities within the abdomen and may not be expected by the overall appearance of the patient. Even routine gallbladder examinations become a problem. In one obese patient, a large gallstone was missed on a sonogram made prior to gastric partitioning. In such patients, the sonographer must make the clinician aware of the likelihood of a reliable examination.

SPECIFIC APPLICATIONS OF ULTRASONIC SCANNING

We should like to wander ultrasonically through the body, starting at the top, and to introduce our readers to the current applications of ultrasound.

Head: Neurosonography

The echoencephalogram is now only a memory from the diagnostic past. It was once used to locate a shift of the midline structures in the brain, such as is seen with intracranial tumors or subdural hematomas. With the advent of CT scanning, the previously well-hidden brain became easily accessible by a noninvasive technique. Echoencephalography was instantly outmoded, and CT scanning then dominated the techniques for evaluation of the brain. Ultrasound has since become the method of first choice in the evaluation of the neonatal and infant brain, however. Some investigators have also explored the use of ultrasound in specific situations in the adult brain, but in general, CT scanning remains the only technique by which to penetrate the adult skull effectively.

INTRACRANIAL APPLICATIONS. As far back as 1974, Kossoff and his Australian co-workers obtained high-quality images of the infant brain using an automated water-path scanner.[3] Neurosonography did not become established until 1980, however, when many American researchers began publishing high-resolution ultrasonic images of the young brain.[4-6] Although the water-path technique is still used, the stationary nature of the machine has limited its usefulness. What was really needed was an easily portable scanner that could be taken into a neonatal intensive care nursery. For this reason, the portable real-time sector scanner came into widespread use almost immediately. In addition to the device's portability, the patient's anterior fontanelle serves as an acoustic window almost perfectly suited to the sector scanner. One may look inside the skull and may obtain high-resolution images that often surpass those of CT scanning. In addition, the plane of section is limitless. With a turn of the transducer, one may change from coronal to sagittal views. In addition to portability, high resolution, and images in any scan plane desired, the sector scanner is constructed such that one may examine a moving patient, and sedation of the patient is unnecessary. Ultrasonic examination involves no ionizing radiation, and the scans may be repeated as frequently as needed. This feature has special importance in the premature infant, in whom weekly scanning is often required, to observe for rapid development of posthemorrhagic hydrocephalus. Ultrasound has found use in almost all areas of neuroimaging in infants, from evaluation of the premature infant with suspected intracranial hemorrhage or hydrocephalus to examination of the infant with possible neural malformations (Fig. 4–5). An intraoperative use of ultrasound has been in the localization of shunt catheters.[7] This examination is especially easy in infants with open fontanelles; one may scan through the fontanelle and not even enter the operative field.

By 2 years of age, the anterior fontanelle closes, sealing the brain in an envelope of bone. Under a number of unusual circumstances, however, the adult brain may be visible to the sonographer. In patients with bony defects in the skull, one may peer inside the head. More common is the use of ultrasound in the operating room. Craniotomy creates an acoustic window. One may therefore assist the surgeon in locating lesions that are not plainly visible on the surface of the brain. The utility of this technique has been well documented in locating deep-seated brain tumors.[8]

Neck: Scanning of Small Parts

Although high-resolution transducers have been in use for a number of years, the recent proliferation of high-resolution real-time scanners is changing the entire approach to the evaluation of many of the structures in the neck. As the frequency of a transducer increases and thereby wavelength decreases, the resolution of the resultant image improves. Unfortunately, the penetration of these higher-frequency transducers is limited to a few centimeters. Just a short time ago, a 5-MHz transducer was considered to have high resolution. With the newer machines, one may scan the abdomen of a thin patient with a transducer of such frequency. In today's terminology, high-frequency scanning generally means the use of 7.5- or 10-MHz transducers. These systems are currently of limited penetration, but the soft tissues of the neck are ideally located for such scanning. Other areas well situated for high-

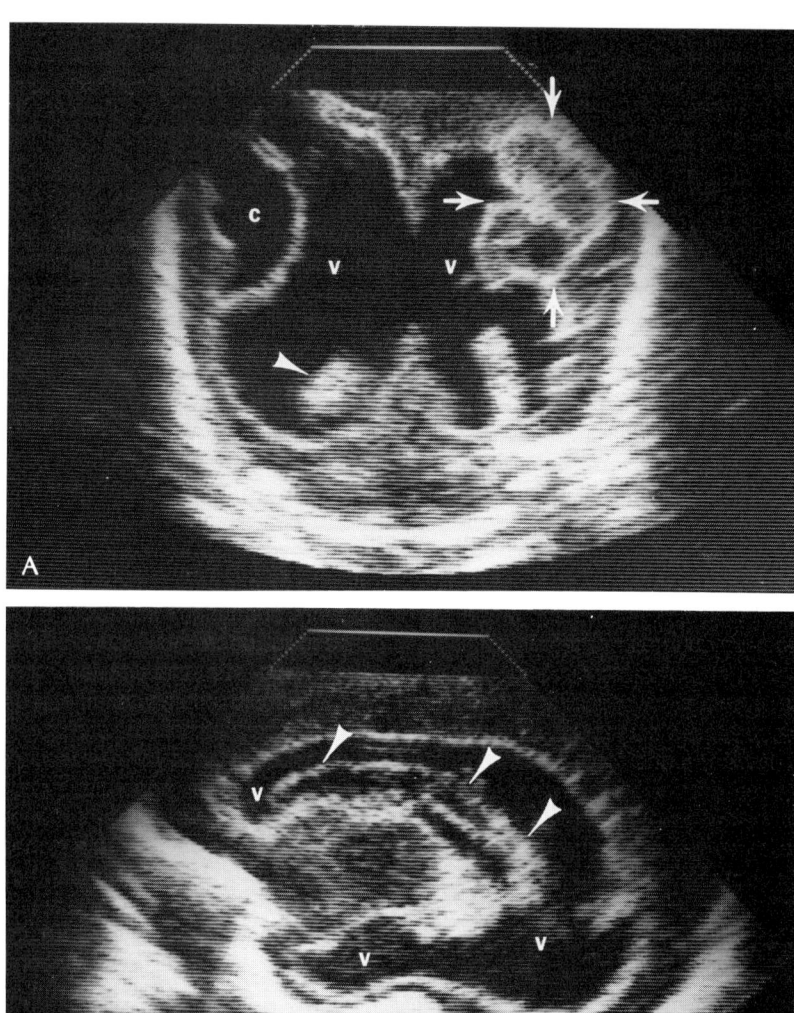

FIG. 4–5. Semiaxial (A) and parasagittal sections (B) of neonatal brain through the anterior fontanelle; enlargement of lateral ventricles (V) with a cast-like intraventricular hematoma (arrowheads) and a discrete area of intraparenchymal hematoma in the left frontoparietal area (arrows). C, Area of cystic periventricular leukomalacia.

resolution examination include the eye, breast, testicle, and many parts of the neonate.

THYROID GLAND. The thyroid has been evaluated sonographically for years, and the primary interest has always been the simple differentiation between a cystic and a solid mass. A large study by Simeone and colleagues, however, has shown that, with high-resolution scanning, true, simple, and therefore benign cysts do not exist.[9] The high-resolution scanner has shown that what were previously determined to be simple cysts by more routine scanning techniques actually were lesions with septa (Fig. 4–6A), debris, or mural nodules. By definition, such masses must be classified as solid and should therefore be removed. Has the high-resolution scanner rendered sonography obsolete in the diagnosis of thyroid lesions? The opposite is actually the case. This same study showed that high-resolution scanning is capable of identifying thyroid nodules too small to be felt or identified by radioactive isotope scan.[9] The importance of sonography lies not in differentiating between cystic and solid masses, but in classifying a thyroid nodule as either singular, therefore with a high (approximately 15%) chance of malignancy, or multiple, with a low (approximately 4%) probability of cancer.[10] These findings are controversial, however, and deserve more attention. On the basis of extensive personal experience, our results with thy-

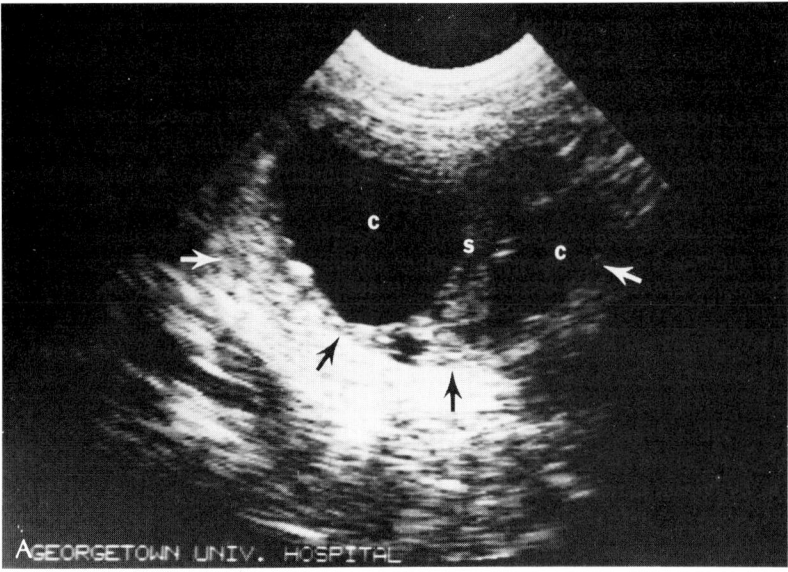

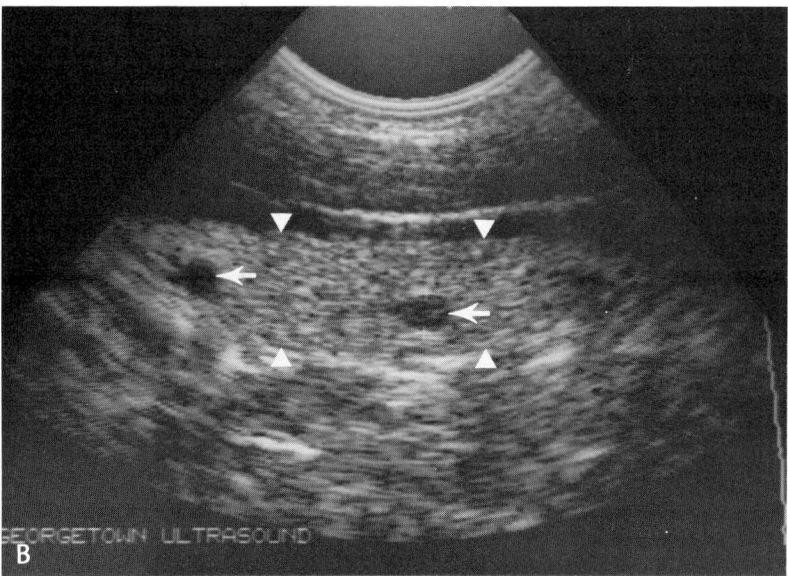

FIG. 4–6. *A,* Transverse 7.5-MHz scan through the right lower pole of the thyroid gland. A palpable nodule has 2 large cystic spaces (C), but the prominent septation (S) and the solid outer rind (arrows) indicate that this mass is sonographically "solid." Only simple cysts are benign by classic ultrasonic criteria. *B,* Longitudinal 7.5-MHz scan through the left lobe of the thyroid gland; no palpable abnormality; nuclear medicine scan of the left lobe had been normal. Sonogram shows two discrete hypoechoic nodules (arrows) within the thyroid (arrowheads).

roid sonography seem in keeping with those published by Simeone and co-workers.[9] True cysts are rare, and it is possible to identify minute thyroid nodules not seen by any other method (Fig. 4–6B). Many diagnoses are thereby changed from solitary to multiple nodules. At this point, we believe that one should still be cautious, but if the sonogram identifies multiple nodules, regardless of how small, the thyroid gland is truly multinodular. As proof of the accuracy of sonography in finding small nodules, many small thyroid nodules have been found incidentally at our institution when scanning patients for parathyroid adenomas. Such subclinical nodules have been proved to exist when patients undergo neck exploration.

PARATHYROID GLANDS. Moving directly posterior to the thyroid, we come to the parathyroid glands. These endocrine organs are closely bound to the calcium control of the entire body, and oversecretion of their principal product, parathormone, can lead to a host of medical problems. Abnormal calcium levels are usually identified by routine blood-chem-

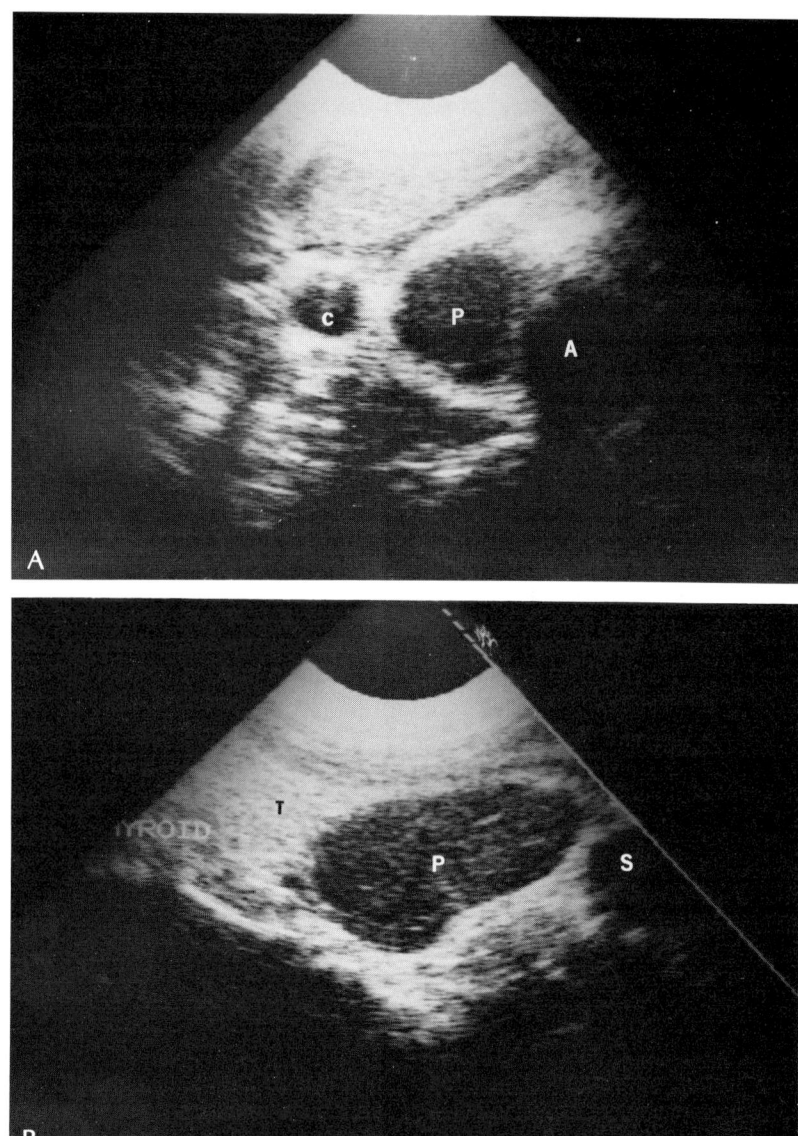

FIG. 4–7. Transverse (A) and longitudinal (B) 7.5-MHz scans in a young male with history of renal calculi and an elevated serum calcium level. A large parathyroid adenoma (P) is located inferior to lower pole of the thyroid gland (T). A, Air in the trachea; C, carotid artery; S, subclavian artery.

istry evaluations, and in most instances, a parathyroid adenoma is the underlying problem. Various methods of preoperative identification of parathyroid adenomas have been devised over the years, including scanning with radioactive selenomethionine, CT scanning, and angiographic localization. Radionuclide scanning is not effective, and angiography is obviously invasive and is time-consuming. With the help of high-resolution real-time scanning, investigators have reported a high degree of accuracy in localizing parathyroid adenomas or in identifying hyperplasia preoperatively. Reading and associates have reported a high success rate in identifying parathyroid enlargement and even better accuracy in locating adenomas not removed during prior neck exploration.[11] The preoperative localization of these adenomas is a tremendous aid and shortens the duration of the surgical procedure. The typical parathyroid adenoma is hypoechoic and is well defined. Such masses are usually located in the notch between the posterolateral edge of the thyroid and the common carotid artery in transverse scans and in the longitudinal planes about either the upper or lower pole of the thyroid glands (Fig. 4–7). We have found a surprising number located posterior to the carotid artery, often far inferior, almost at the branching of the carotid from the subclavian artery. Parathyroid scanning requires meticulous detail in scanning, but it can be gratifying because of its accuracy and its helpfulness to the surgeon. Even the largest parathyroid adenomas should be localized preoperatively because they are not usually palpable. The adenoma in Figure 4–7 measured 3 cm, but these soft masses are not usually felt, as a result of their extension along tissue planes.

CAROTID ARTERIES. The use of ultrasound in the evaluation of the carotid arteries is a vast subject. We shall mainly discuss our personal bias in this complicated field of noninvasive vascular diagnosis. Many methods, machines, and gadgets are available to the physician about to enter this field. Both indirect methods of evaluation of the carotid arteries, such as oculoplethysmography, and direct methods, which generally use some form of Doppler ultrasound, are in current use. The indirect methods are often said to be more physiologic, that is, reflecting the state of blood flow to the brain. Significant collateral circulation or bilateral disease may lead to false-negative results, however, because no actual images of the carotid arteries are obtained.[12]

Various types of Doppler scanners are available. Some actually make color printouts reflecting the state of blood flow in a given area of the artery. Some authors have reported success using duplex scanning, which is a combination of pulse-gated Doppler and simultaneous high-resolution real-time scanning,[13] whereas others have used real-time sonography alone.[14] In our experience, neither Doppler scanning nor real-time sonography alone is optimal; the two must be used together. We and our colleagues have become strong proponents of duplex scanning. The single greatest drawback to this method is the difficulty in learning the scanning technique. It may take a long time to develop confidence in one's diagnostic ability. We evaluated our first year's experience, as compared to our experience with digital subtraction angiography and conventional angiography, and found that our original accuracy was less than 65%. In the most recent group of our patients evaluated by duplex scanning, with a comparison of results with contrast studies, we are now 93% accurate.[15] This rate of accuracy has gradually improved in the course of an entire year. We have evaluated our many pitfalls in scanning, but perseverance with this technique does bring about accuracy. Other authors have published their results with this technique, and they report a similarly high degree of accuracy in identifying carotid stenoses.[13]

Duplex scanning itself is a combination of real-time scanning, which yields anatomic information about the vessel walls, such as calcific or soft plaque, and flow information in the form of Doppler shifts (Fig. 4–8A and B). The two most important Doppler changes in atherosclerotic disease are increased frequency shift, which is proportional to increased blood velocity, and spectral broadening,[13a] which is associated with flow turbulence (Fig. 4–8C to E). Duplex scanning remains to be further investigated. In experienced hands, duplex sonography is at least as accurate as digital subtraction angiography and is absolutely noninvasive. We have found digital angiography a great addition to the available diagnostic tools for evaluating carotid atherosclerotic disease, but we do not see it replacing all other noninvasive testing. In some instances, in fact, the sonogram has agreed more closely with the arteriogram than the digital study, and the Doppler scan often supplies much information about blood-flow dynamics. In general, duplex scanning seems to be a logical way to evaluate carotid atherosclerotic disease if it is performed by experienced examiners.

Thorax

Because ultrasound does not penetrate gas, the thorax is largely off limits to the sonographer, and cross-sectional thoracic imaging is best performed by the CT scanner. Although the contribution of ultrasound in the differentiation of solid and cystic pleural opacities and guidance in cases of difficult thoracentesis should not be overlooked, sonography plays a significant role in two specific areas of the thorax, namely, in breast examination and in echocardiography.

BREAST. As stated in the introduction, the breast was among the first areas of the body to be examined with ultrasound. Not until recently, however, was interest in sonographic evaluation of the breast renewed. Because the breast is not a fixed organ with relation to other constant structures, finding landmarks and scanning in general may be difficult. For this reason, dedicated breast scanners have been constructed, usually employing some form of water-path scanning where the breasts can be immersed freely and the nipple used as a landmark. These scanners are largely automated and are easy to operate. The patient lies on a padded table, and the breasts are immersed in body-temperature water. Most patients find the examination pleasant. A great advantage of ultrasonic examination of the breast is the lack of ionizing radiation. Women may be opposed to mammograms because of radiation. Nonetheless, mammography remains the method of choice in evaluation of the breast for carcinoma. The fatty breast offers excellent contrast with both microcalcifications, which are not seen at all sonographically, and with dense masses. Routine screening for breast carcinoma should be performed with mammography, not sonography.[16] In general,

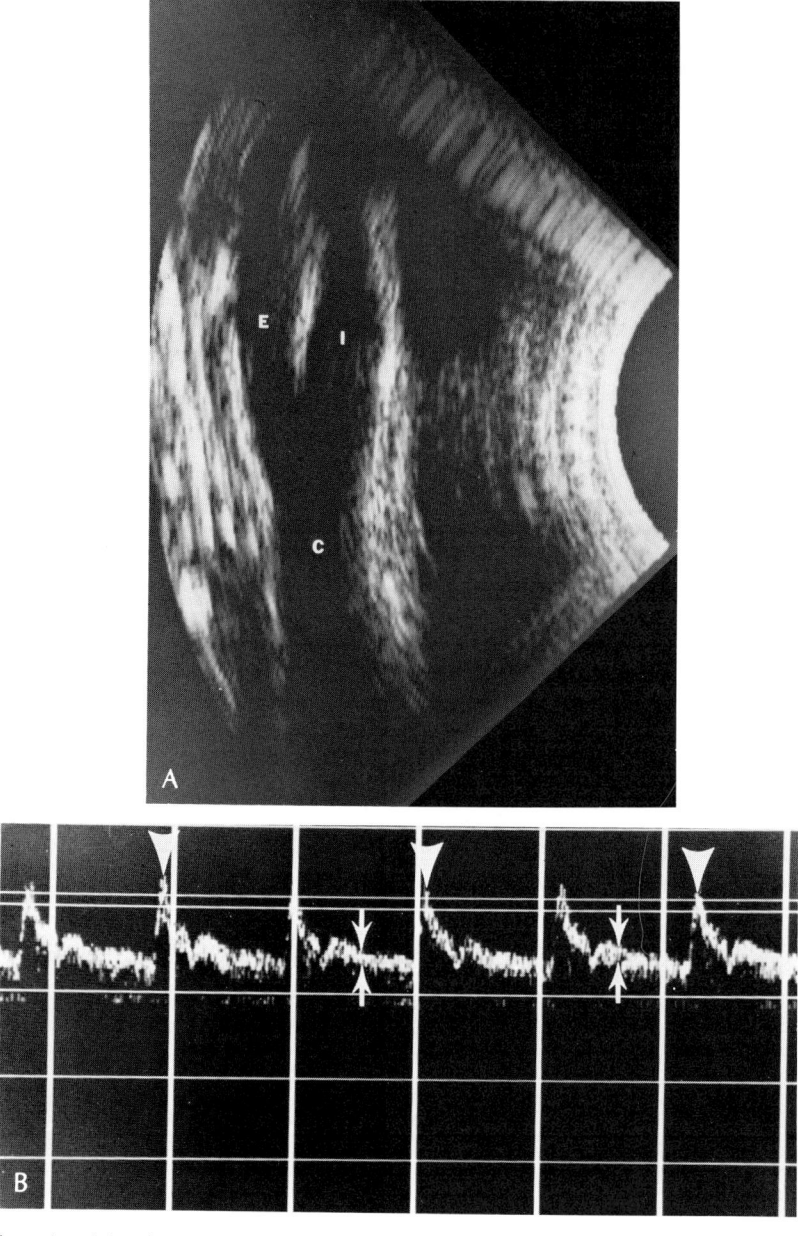

FIG. 4–8. *A,* Normal real-time image of the carotid bifurcation; smooth vessel walls are present in the common (C), internal (I), and external (E) carotid arteries. *B,* Simultaneous Doppler spectral analysis shows flow pattern at the internal carotid artery shown in A. Note the similarity of Doppler shifts as evidenced by a narrow sound spectrum (arrows). Similar Doppler shifts indicate that red blood cells travel at similar speeds (laminar flow). A low amplitude of Doppler shift (arrowheads) shows that red blood cells travel at normal or low velocity. *C,* Real-time image; the internal carotid artery (I) has a distinct area of plaque (arrowheads) at the bifurcation from the common carotid artery (C). The external carotid artery is not visible in this plane. *D,* Doppler evaluation; spectral analysis from internal carotid origin at the position of the Doppler sample in C shows marked broadening of the spectrum of sound (S), as opposed to the normal narrow spectrum in B. This pattern indicates flow turbulence. The extreme increase in frequency shift is shown by "aliasing," in which the signal goes off the scale at the top of the picture, and the rest is shown at the bottom of the image (arrows). This pattern indicates an abnormal increase in flow velocity. Real-time findings alone suggest stenosis, but Doppler findings show a high-grade lesion. *E,* Arteriogram; marked narrowing at the origin of the internal carotid artery (arrow).

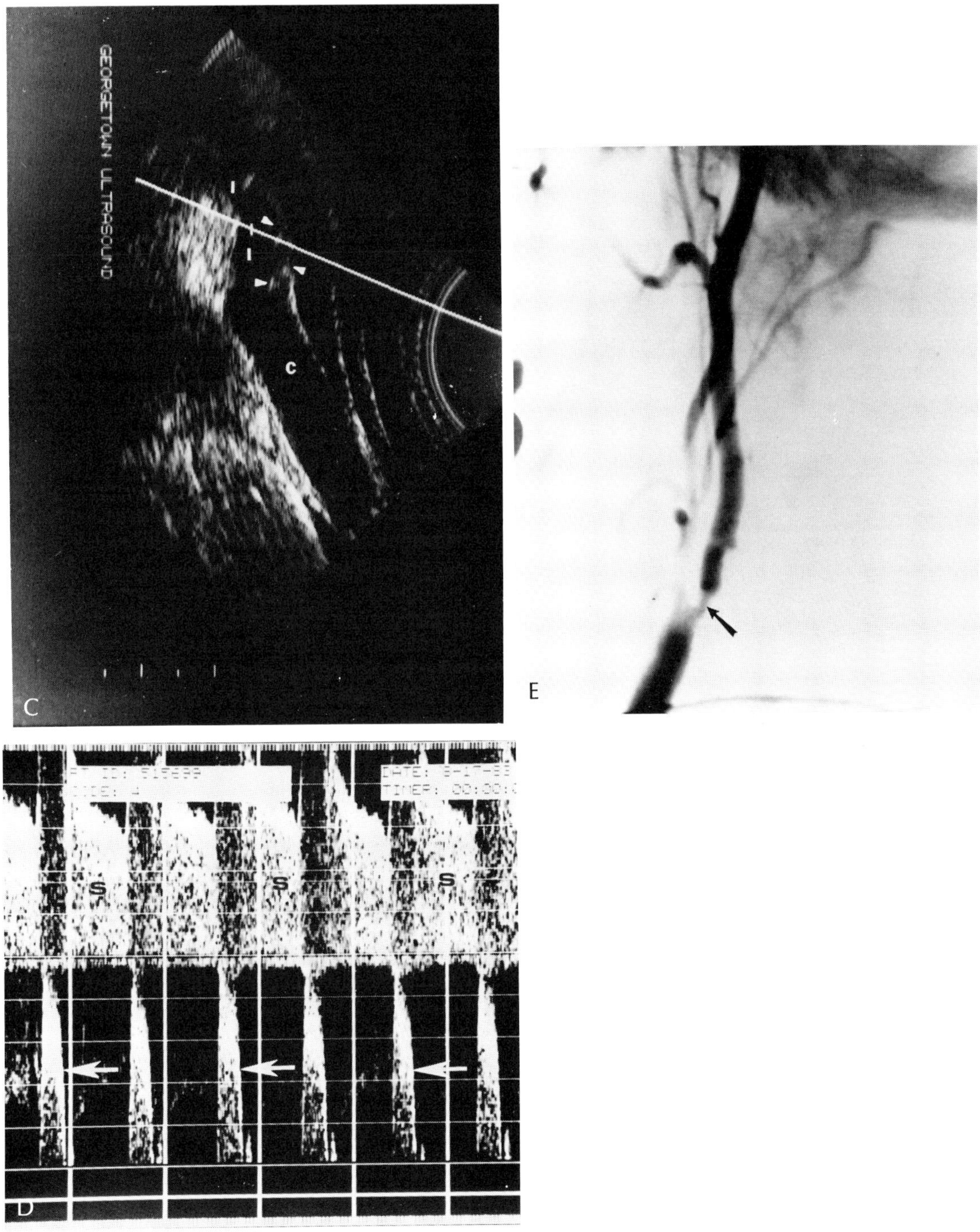

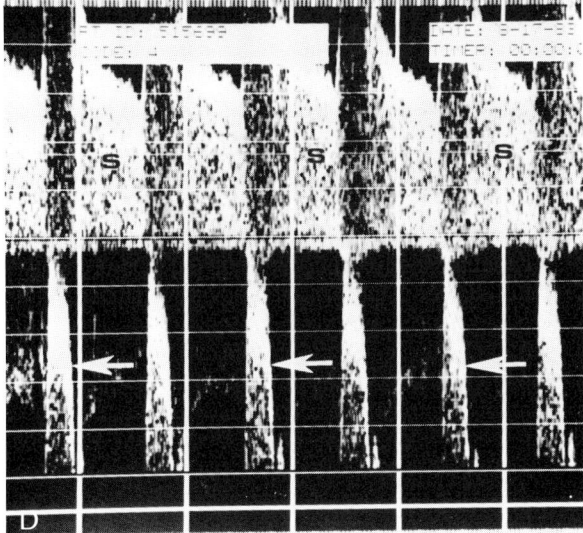

FIG. 4–8 *Continued.*

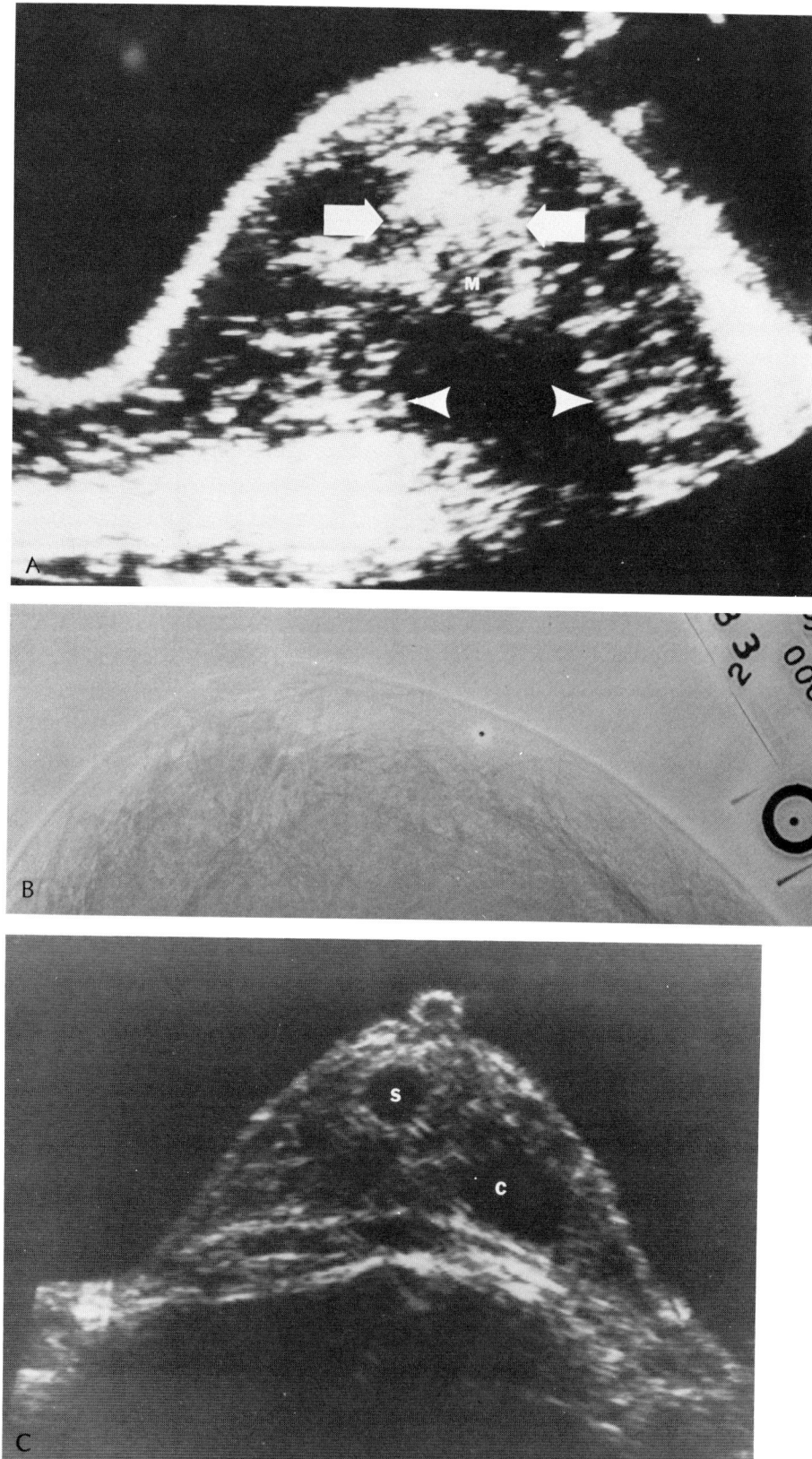

FIG. 4–9. Carcinoma of the breast; the sonogram *(A)* shows a dense area of acoustic shadowing (arrowheads) behind an echogenic area (arrows) containing a central hypoechoic mass (M), a common finding in carcinoma. The corresponding mammogram *(B)* shows no abnormality. *C,* Transverse waterpath sonogram of a 37-year-old patient with a palpable mass in the lateral central portion of the left breast. A 2.5-cm cyst is identified (C). Note the second cyst, found incidentally (S).

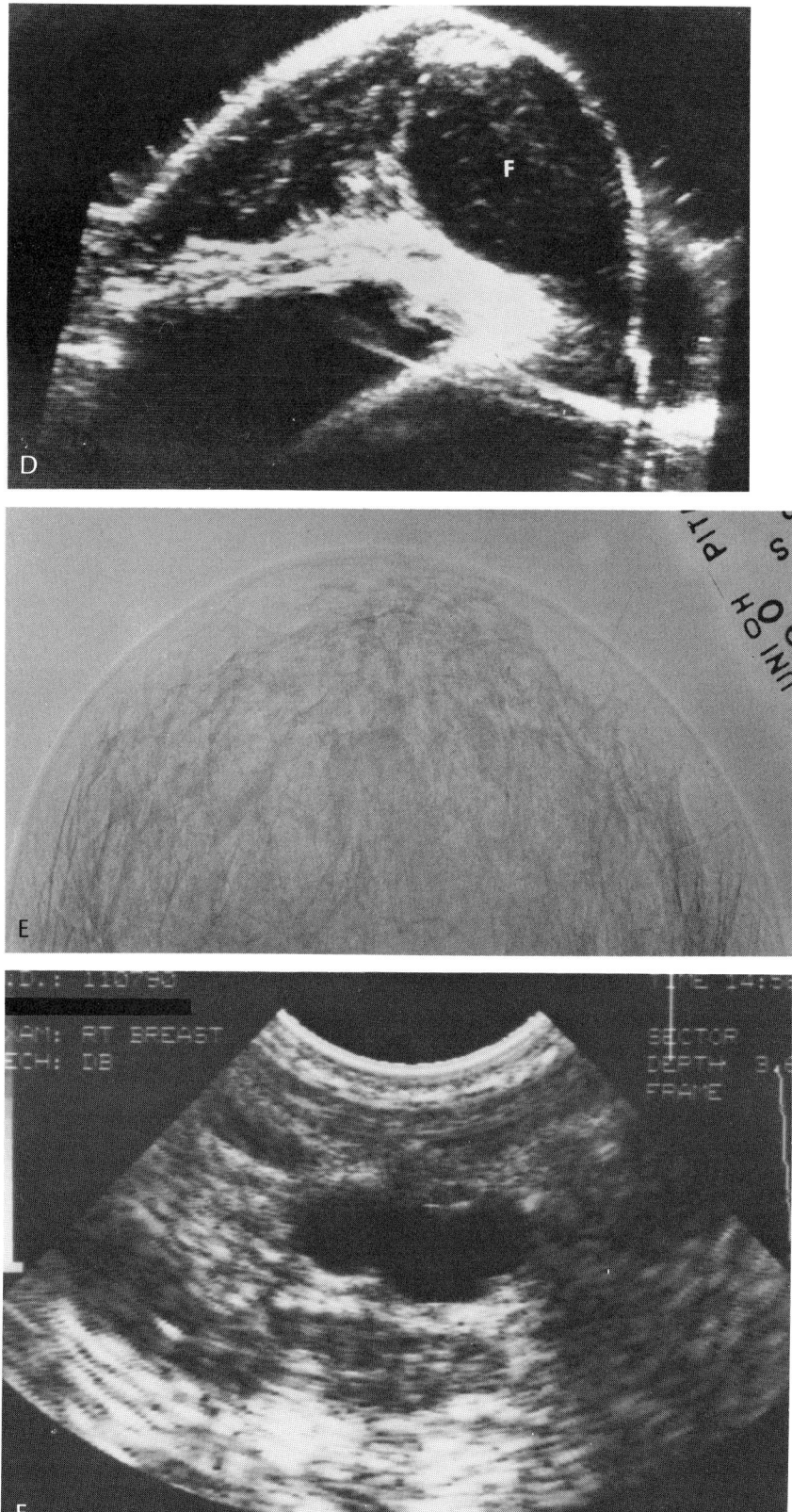

FIG. 4–9 Continued. *D,* Transverse waterpath sonogram of an 18-year-old patient with a palpable mass; the large, well-defined, solid mass with a homogeneous internal echo pattern is typical of a giant fibroadenoma (F). *E* and *F,* Nonpalpable breast cyst; screening mammogram *(E)* shows a central density, the posterior wall of which is not clearly defined. A sonogram *(F),* using a 7.5-MHz hand-held scanner, clearly shows this density to represent a lobulated cyst. The cyst was aspirated under real-time guidance.

mammography remains the primary diagnostic technique, and sonography plays a subordinate role.

In a number of areas, however, sonography can made a great contribution in breast diagnosis. In young, dense breasts, it may be difficult to identify masses with mammography (Fig. 4–9A and B), and sonography may be of particular value. Older patients with dense breasts may also be candidates for sonography. Another group of patients in whom sonography can be of benefit are those with palpable masses. The basic question to be answered for the surgeon about any breast mass is whether or not it is cystic. If cystic, such a mass can generally be considered benign and ignored, or aspirated if so desired. If it is solid, the mass must almost always undergo biopsy. Mammography can define the borders of a mass and may suggest a cyst on the basis of shape, but one cannot actually discern anything about the lesion's internal consistency, that is, whether it is cystic or solid. Sonography is ideally suited for this purpose and can easily differentiate between cystic and solid masses (Fig. 4–9C and D). Additionally, it often offers insight into the diagnosis of solid masses preoperatively. Although some solid breast masses have typical sonographic appearances, one cannot always classify a solid mass as definitely benign by ultrasound. Cole-Beuglet and associates have shown that the use of strict criteria for carcinoma increases the specificity of sonography, but it leads to an unacceptable number of carcinomas classified as benign. On this basis, most solid masses with a benign sonographic appearance should undergo biopsy.[17] Other groups of patients that should be considered for sonomammography are lactating and pregnant women and those with breast implants.

Although most research has been directed toward the use of the automated breast scanner, the real-time, hand-held scanner can also be of help in diagnosing breast disease. When no dedicated scanner is available, the internal characteristics of any palpable breast mass can easily be determined by scanning over it. In our experience, the majority of such breast masses are cysts, but the preoperative diagnosis of a number of solid masses has been aided by the use of real-time ultrasound in our laboratory as well. We have recently scanned nonpalpable breast masses that were identified on a xeromammogram, again to investigate their internal characteristics. When these masses were cystic, we have also successfully aspirated a number of such nonpalpable lesions under direct ultrasonic guidance (Fig. 9–4E and F).

HEART. Real-time scanning has dramatically changed imaging of the heart, where function and anatomic structure are so intimately associated. Although M-mode scanning still has its place with its graphic display of temporal and spatial resolution, most of this information and more can be easily obtained with real-time scanning, either on mechanical sector scanners or on phased-array equipment. An M-mode echocardiogram is comparable to looking at a scenic panorama through a drinking straw held close to the eye and panning in various directions, whereas a real-time echocardiogram is comparable to looking at the same panorama with a wide-angle lens on a movie camera. The information is essentially the same, but the presentation of the information is different. With its ability to sweep through the heart thoroughly and rapidly and to see chambers contracting and valves opening and closing while actually happening, real-time scanning has carved its niche as an invaluable tool in noninvasive cardiac evaluation. The information thus obtained may be unavailable by other means. The heart is ideally suited to ultrasound because it is positioned against the anterior chest wall, posterior to and slightly to the left of the sternum. Most patients have excellent "windows" to the heart, through the intercostal spaces or from inferior to the diaphragm in the subxiphoid region, looking through the left lobe of the liver. Occasionally, adipose tissue, overinflated lungs (air), a small left lobe of the liver with much abdominal gas, and a bony thorax with tight rib interspaces all interfere with a satisfactory image of the heart. Fortunately, these circumstances are rare in combination, and the cardiac examination usually provides the information requested.

Using the left parasternal and apical intercostal spaces and the subxiphoid region as windows, and by rotating the transducer from sagittal to transverse planes, one can evaluate the heart by looking at it from the many points where it is in contact with the chest wall. Sweeping views through the heart in several intersecting planes can be obtained, where all the walls of the heart can be covered. Conventionally, longitudinal and transverse views are taken while moving the transducer inferiorly along the left parasternal border to the apex. This technique provides views of the aortic root, the aortic and mitral valves, the left atrium posterior to the aorta, and the basal portion of the left ventricle, septum, and posterior wall, papillary muscles and chordae tendineae, as well as the right ventricular inflow and outflow tracts and the pulmonic and triscupid valves. The apical region is not always seen from this approach. The views from the apex show this region well and offer what is known as the four-chamber view, in which the lateral walls of the ventricles can be seen, as well as the septum, the aortic, mitral, and tricuspid valves, and the two atria with their interatrial septum. The apical views are basically at an intersecting right angle to the higher parasternal views. The subxiphoid view looks from across the left lobe of the liver through the right side of the heart to the left and is essentially at an intersecting right angle to the other views. Other views can be obtained through available windows such as the suprasternal area or the right parasternal area, if the examination must be tailored to an unusual and specific question.

The information available on real-time examination is plentiful and is beyond the scope of this chapter. The reader is referred to textbooks dedicated entirely to this one topic.[18,19] It should suffice to cover briefly some of the important and common entities that may be encountered.

Starting at the outside and working inwards, the pericardial space is easily evaluated for the presence or absence of an effusion. A small effusion appears only in systole, as the contracting heart with its covering layer of visceral pericardium pulls away from the parietal layer and reveals the fluid between; this space is then obliterated in diastole. In a large effusion, the heart bounces within the large, fluid-filled space. Because the pericardium is attached in the region of the atrioventricular groove, it is uncommon to see effusions posterior to the left atrium. It is also unusual to find an effusion anterior to the heart without any posterior component.

The walls of the heart are observed for their contractility. Akinetic areas, compatible with infarction, can be seen. Areas of hypokinesis are characterized according to whether they are focal, as in ischemic disease, or global, as in cardiomyopathy. Chamber size is assessed and is correlated with any associated wall-motion abnormalities, and the ejection fraction is calculated. Dyskinetic areas, as in ventricular aneurysms, in which the walls of the heart move paradoxically, are easily seen; the ventricles are evaluated for the presence of clots, which may be sources of emboli.

The thickness of the myocardium can be measured, and if hypertrophy is present, one should note whether it is concentric or asymmetric. Concentric left ventricular hypertrophy is seen in conditions such as aortic stenosis and hypertension and in infiltrative diseases such as amyloidosis. Amyloidosis adds a characteristic "sparkling" appearance to the thick muscle wall. Patients with concentric left ventricular hypertrophy often have high ejection fractions because the muscle of the heart enlarges at the expense of the chamber size, and the ventricular cavity can be almost completely obliterated in systole. Some patients with hypertrophic cardiomyopathy have asymmetric involvement of only the septum; if severe enough, it can cause left ventricular outflow tract obstruction and premature closure of the aortic valve. This condition, known as idiopathic hypertrophic subaortic stenosis (IHSS) reqires specific medical or even surgical management.

The valves of the heart are evaluated for abnormalities, and these findings are correlated with associated findings such as chamber size, wall thickness, and motion. The aortic valve can become thickened and sclerotic. In the presence of a severely sclerotic aortic valve and concentric left ventricular hypertrophy, a narrow opening suggests aortic stenosis, although hemodynamically significant stenosis should be confirmed by cardiac catheterization. In a bicuspid aortic valve, three normal leaflets and commissures are not identified, but instead, one sees an eccentrically closing valve with deformed leaflets and commissures. Mitral stenosis can be detected early, by evidence of valve thickening and abnormal motion, usually accompanied by left atrial enlargement, especially in advanced cases. Flail leaflets, torn chordae tendineae, and ruptured papillary muscles can be seen, although these lesions are uncommon. Although mitral valve prolapse continues to be a debatable issue, its characteristic appearance of a varying retreat into the left atrium beyond the plane of the mitral anulus in systole is easily seen. Tricuspid abnormalities are readily found, although the pulmonic valve may be difficult to see. The search for vegetations as sources of emboli in patients with endocarditis may be frustrating because small lesions can be missed. A negative search does not rule out vegetations, which must be 2 to 3 mm in size before they can be detected.

The presence of regurgitant valvular lesions can be inferred by enlarged chamber size, by hypercontractility, and by findings suggestive of elevated cardiac output, combined with associated valvular abnormalities. Recent advances in cardiac Doppler ultrasound allow blood flow to be assessed in systole and diastole on either side of any selected valve. This technique appears to have unusual sensitivity in the detection of regurgitant lesions.[20,21]

Cardiac tumors, although rare, are easily visible, whether they are primary or metastatic. Myxomas, which are usually found in the left atrium, can be seen as a well-defined, pedunculated mass attached to the wall of the atrium near the atrioventricular groove and mitral valve leaflets. In real-time scanning, the tumor moves back and forth from atrium to ventricle through the mitral valve in diastole and systole.

A final note relates to the use of ultrasonic contrast agents in the heart. While looking at the heart with a real-time scanner, any peripheral intravenous injection produces microbubbles that can be seen as fine, bright echoes suddenly filling the right-sided chambers as the bolus reaches the heart. With a

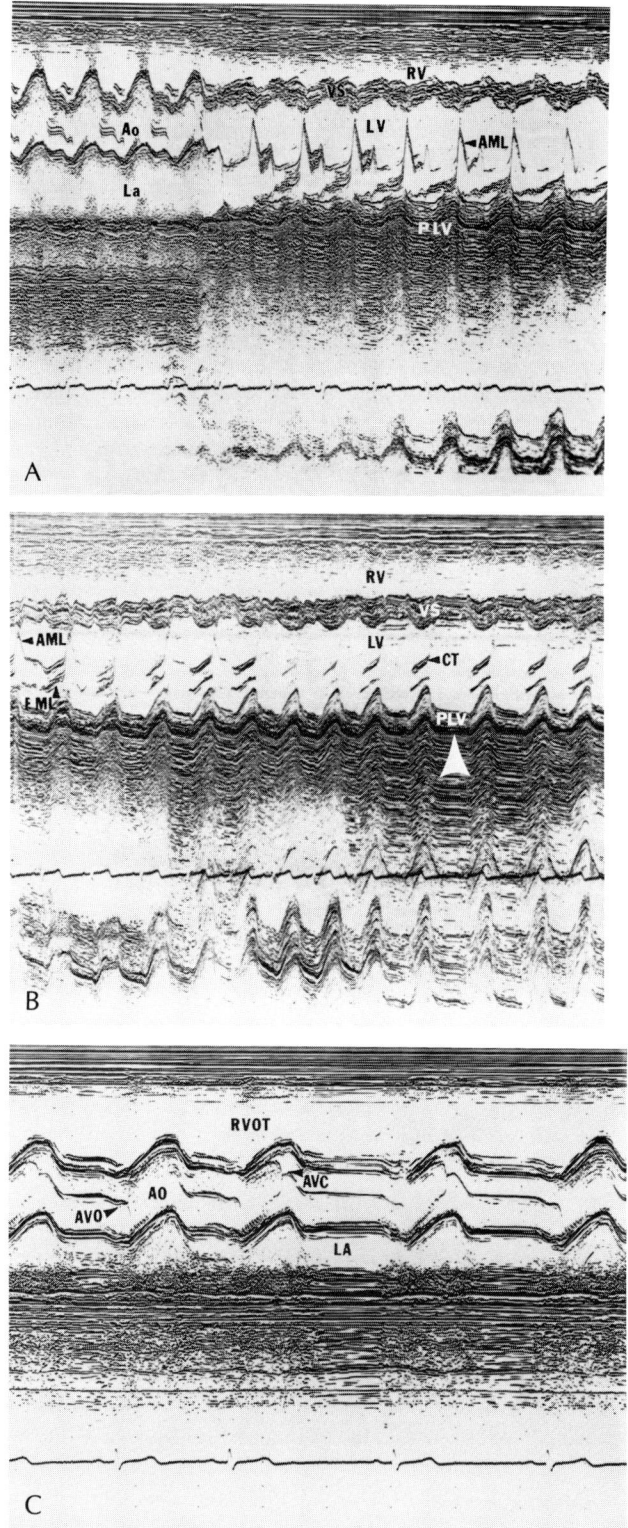

FIG. 4–10. *A,* M-mode sweep from the aortic root, at the left, through the mitral valve to the midportion of the left ventricle (LV), at the right. The X-axis is time, and the Y-axis represents the motion of the structures. AO, Aortic root with aortic valve; LA, left atrium; RV, right ventricle; VS, interventricular septum; AML, anterior mitral leaflet; PLV, posterior wall of left ventricle. *B,* M-mode sweep from the mitral valve through the left ventricle (LV) towards the apex. Note thickening of the wall during systole. AML, Anterior mitral leaflet; PML, posterior mitral leaflet; RV, right ventricle; CT, chordae tendineae; VS, interventricular septum; white arrowhead, pericardium; PLV, posterior left ventricle. *C,* M-mode view of the aortic valve. RVOT, Right ventricular outflow tract; AO, aorta between opened aortic valves; AVO, aortic valves opening; AVC, aortic valves closing; LA, left atrium.

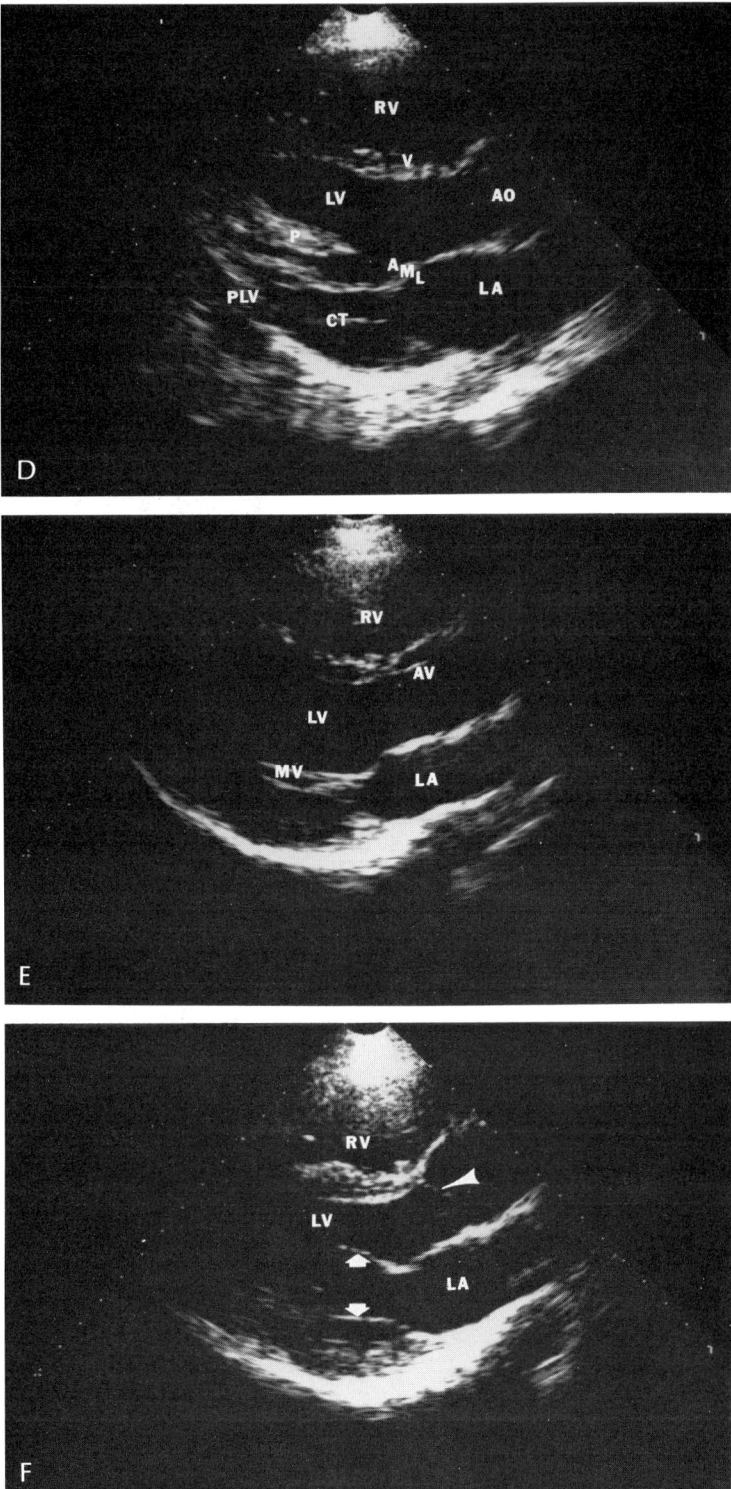

FIG. 4–10 Continued. *D,* Real-time B-mode scan of the parasternal long axis of the base of the heart in systole. RV, Right ventricle; V, interventricular septum; LV, left ventricle; AO, aorta; AML, anterior mitral leaflet; LA, left atrium; CT, chordae tendineae; PLV, posterior left ventricular wall; P, papillary muscle. *E,* Real-time B-mode scan of the long axis of the heart in systole. RV, Right ventricle; LV, left ventricle; AV, aortic valve leaflet open; MV, mitral valve leaflet closed; LA, left atrium. *F,* Real-time view of the long axis of the heart in systole. RV, Right ventricle; LV, left ventricle; arrowhead, aortic valve leaflets closed; arrows, mitral valve leaflets opened; LA, left atrium.

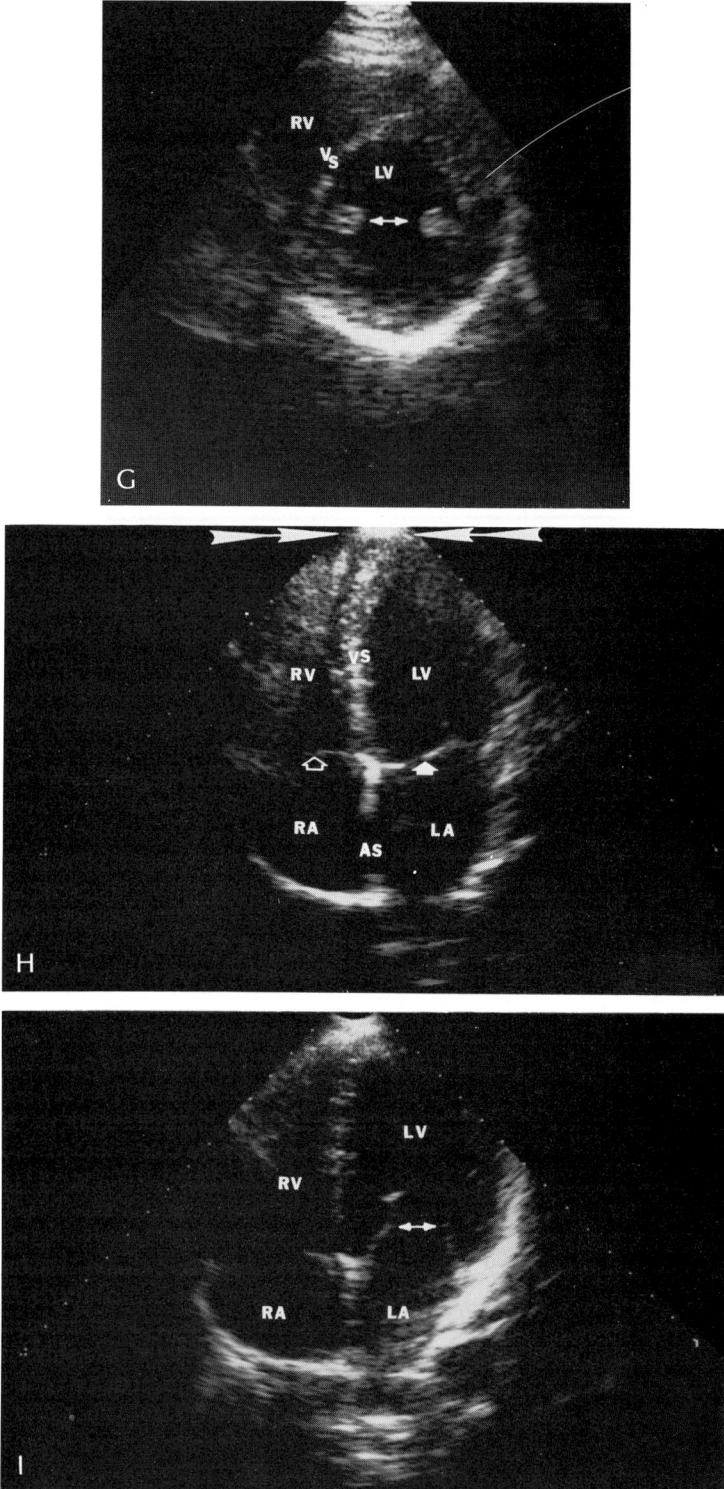

FIG. 4–10 Continued. *G,* Real-time view of the parasternal short axis of the left ventricle (LV) at the level of the papillary muscles (arrows). RV, Right ventricle; VS, interventricular septum. *H,* Real-time four-chamber view in systole. Large arrowheads, apex; VS, interventricular septum; RV, right ventricle; LV, left ventricle; open arrow, tricuspid valve; arrow, mitral valve closed; RA, right atrium; AS, interatrial septum; LA, left atrium. *I,* Real-time four-chamber apical view in diastole. RV, Right ventricle; LV, left ventricle; RA, right atrium; LA, left atrium; arrows, mitral valve opened.

real-time scanner, one sees the microbubbles and any abnormal flow patterns such as shunts.[22]

Because of the complexity and scope of echocardiography, we have limited this discussion to common acquired heart problems. The subject of congenital heart disease has been excluded, and only normal anatomic illustrations are presented, showing both M-mode and real-time scanning (Fig. 4–10).

Abdomen, Retroperitoneal Structures, and Testes

Many of the uses of ultrasound just discussed are still under investigation, if not openly controversial. Abdominal sonography is more proven ground, but even here, one encounters disputes over accuracy, technique, and other matters. For the remainder of this chapter, we shall try to give an up-to-date account of the applications and indications for sonography in the abdomen.

GALLBLADDER. In imaging the gallbladder, we have already discussed the way in which real-time sonography has made ultrasound a primary diagnostic technique.[23,24] Reasons include a high rate of accuracy in diagnosing gallstones, the absence of ionizing radiation, the lack of need to ingest medication, elimination of the "double-dose" examination, and the ease and rapidity of the examination itself. The surgeon must feel more secure when operating on a patient with a definite diagnosis of cholelithiasis than when the result of an oral cholecystogram is "nonvisualization of the gallbladder" and any number of things could have happened to the contrast agent. Did the patient take the pills? Were they absorbed?

The sonographic features of gallstones classically include the visualization of echogenic foci within the gallbladder, movement of these foci to the dependent part of the gallbladder when the patient changes position, and posterior acoustic shadowing (see Fig. 4–2B). "Shadowing" refers to the complete blockage of sound waves by the gallstone, similar to the effect of bones or air. The three findings of cholelithiasis are the same whether one uses real-time or static imaging, but they are usually more easily seen with real-time imaging. The ultrasonic diagnosis of cholelithiasis is straightforward in most cases, although other entities may cause intraluminal gallbladder echoes, including "sludge," which is a nonpathologic collection of inspissated bile probably associated with lack of emptying,[25] polyps and carcinoma,[26] mucosal desquamation,[27] hematoma,[28] and even metastasis.[29] Many of these entities can be differentiated, depending on whether or not they move within the gallbladder or exhibit posterior shadowing.

It is not clear which technique is best for diagnosing acute cholecystitis. Some authors argue that sonography is the imaging method of choice,[30] and specific sonographic signs are visible in the patient with acute cholecystitis, including a thickened or double wall, a tense or rounded appearance, and point tenderness over the gallbladder. Other authors advocate the use of radionuclide scanning, which has a high accuracy rate in acute cholecystitis.[31] Both examinations may have specific advantages, and the debate continues. Practically speaking, the ability to obtain a scan quickly, the competence of the sonographer or the physician, obtaining the radionuclide scan, and other similar reasons may affect one's choice of diagnostic methods. In some instances, both examinations are indicated.

In patients with chronic cholecystitis, however, gallstones are the hallmark of disease, and sonography has the decided edge. The contracted, chronically diseased gallbladder may be more difficult to evaluate sonographically because the calculi appear only as discrete foci of shadowing (Fig. 4–11). The accuracy of this once-difficult diagnosis has been improved by the use of real-time sonography.[32] Although the main thrust of the sonographic examination of the gallbladder has been the identification of intraluminal abnormalities, the technique plays a significant role in the evaluation of the gallbladder wall as well. We have already discussed wall thickening in acute cholecystitis. This sign alone is nonspecific, and a thickened gallbladder wall has also been associated with ascites, hypoproteinemia, and other abnormalities. The sonographic findings in other wall abnormalities such as gallbladder carcinoma and polyps are also well known. Some authors have found ultrasound, often in conjunction with oral cholecystography, to be of value in the diagnosis of cholesterolosis and adenomyomatosis.[33,34]

COMMON BILE DUCT. Evaluation of the common bile duct is another important application of ultrasound. Although the cause of jaundice can be determined on the basis of clinical presentation and laboratory data in the majority of patients, it may be a diagnostic problem. Additionally, in the patient with suspected obstructive jaundice, one should try to confirm the diagnosis prior to initiating more invasive procedures. Ultrasound is the first choice in these patients. The common bile duct can be identified in almost all patients, by real-time sonography, and if the duct is larger than 4 mm, obstruction should be suspected.[35,36] Occasionally, normal patients have common bile ducts larger than 4 mm, and one report suggests that up to 7 mm is the maximum width of a normal common bile duct.[37] This measurement may be greater in patients who have undergone cholecystectomy or who have gallstones or pancreatitis; the duct may measure up to 11 mm.[37] Although controversy exists as to the exact measure-

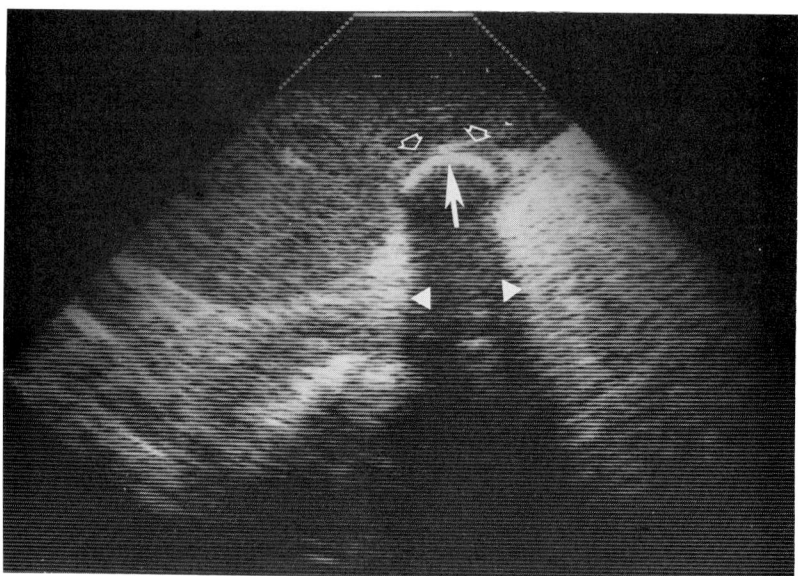

FIG. 4–11. Oblique real-time sector scan at the inferior edge of the liver showing a "double-arc" sign; dense gallstones block all sound and produce a shadow (arrowheads). So much sound is reflected that only the anterior surface of the gallstones are seen as a reflective arc (arrow). A second arc above it is the gallbladder wall (open arrows), which ensures that this echogenic area consists of gallstones and not air in the duodenum.

ment for the upper limit of normal, all authors have found sonography an accurate method of evaluating biliary obstruction, and most advocate it as the technique of first choice.[38]

Following identification of a dilated common bile duct, one must also look for dilated intrahepatic biliary radicals. The sonographic appearance of these enlarged ducts is distinct,[39] and the identification of enlarged intrahepatic biliary radicals should establish the diagnosis of obstruction (Fig. 4–12A). Ductal dilatation may be present only within the liver or one may see a disparate amount of dilatation when comparing ducts from the right and left lobes. Such obstruction high in the porta hepatis or at the junction of the main biliary ducts suggests Klatskin's tumor or metastases.

Occasionally, ductal dilatation is seen by ultrasound before elevation of serum bilirubin levels,[40] and if the sonographic findings are on the borderline, some authors have suggested giving a fatty meal and observing for an increase in the caliber of the common bile duct.[41] Another alternative is to wait a short time and to see what happens. The biliary tree may be dilated in patients who have undergone biliary bypass procedures. These patients often have air in the biliary tree, with attendant posterior shadowing, which may obscure the more posterior portions of the liver.[42]

Although ultrasound allows one to diagnose obstruction accurately, it is more difficult to determine the cause of such obstruction ultrasonically. The common bile duct passes posterior to the duodenum and may often be obscured by gas; one is thereby prevented from identifying the reason for the obstruction. Various authors have reported on this subject, and although the ability to identify pancreatic carcinoma or choledocholithiasis, for example, has been improved with real-time imaging, the accuracy rate of sonography continues to be disappointing in some series. In other reports, results have been excellent.[43,44] Our personal experience is that ultrasound is often helpful (Fig. 4–12B). Meticulous and often time-consuming real-time sonographic evaluation is of utmost importance in identifying the cause of the obstruction, but it is worthwhile because results are gratifying. Even with the most extensive sonographic evaluation, however, the cause of an obstruction cannot always be determined by ultrasound.

Additionally, an obstruction may arise from a stricture or a small ampullary tumor. In these patients, a transhepatic cholangiogram or an endoscopic retrograde cholangiopancreatogram is essential, to identify the cause of obstruction. Whether or not one has acceptable results with sonography in identifying the lesion in patients with biliary obstruction is a direct result of meticulous scanning technique.

Anomalies of the biliary tree are infrequent, but again, sonographic study may be diagnostic. Choledochal cyst, duplication cyst, and Caroli's disease have all been described in the sonographic literature.[45,46] The lack of a biliary system, biliary atresia,

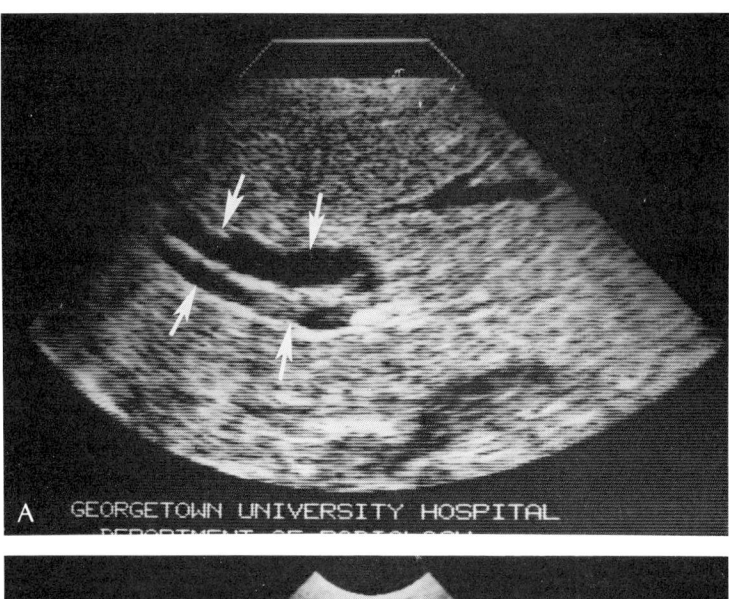
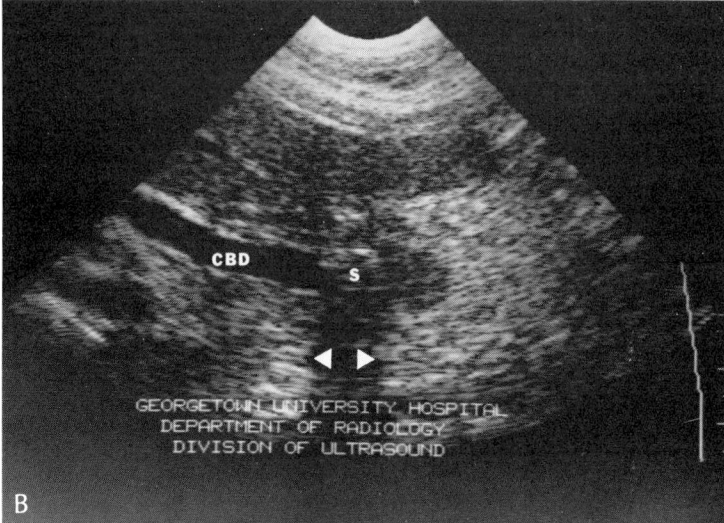

FIG. 4–12. *A,* "Shotgun" or double-channel sign; two parallel tubular structures in the liver beyond the area of the porta signify obstruction. Biliary radicals are normally not visible and, when dilated, lie next to the larger portal vein, giving the appearance of two parallel tubular structures (arrows). *B,* Oblique real-time scan through the right upper quadrant; dilated common bile duct (CBD) with stone (S) obstructing distal portion. Note the posterior shadowing (arrowheads).

on the other hand, is best detected with radionuclide scanning, although the presence or absence of a gallbladder can easily be determined sonographically.

LIVER. In the liver, various disease entities may be investigated with ultrasound. Focal lesions including metastases, abscesses, cysts, and hematomas are all well visualized sonographically (Fig. 4–13). Unlike radionuclide scanning, which can only show a photon-deficient area to indicate the presence of focal lesions, ultrasound yields information about the internal characteristics of a mass that can aid in differentiation. Additionally, the resolution of ultrasound is better than that of radionuclide scanning, and focal lesions under 1 cm in size within the liver are well visualized. Efficient follow-up of hepatic metastases for response to therapy is also possible with ultrasound and is much less expensive than with CT scanning. Cysts and abscesses may be punctured and drained under sonographic guidance. In patients with suspected hematoma, one may follow the original mass, and one may watch it change from hyperechoic to anechoic over time, thus proving it to be a hematoma without intervention.[47] One may adequately measure the size of the liver, but basic attempts at tissue characterization have been unrewarding, although active research continues in this field. In patients with fatty infiltra-

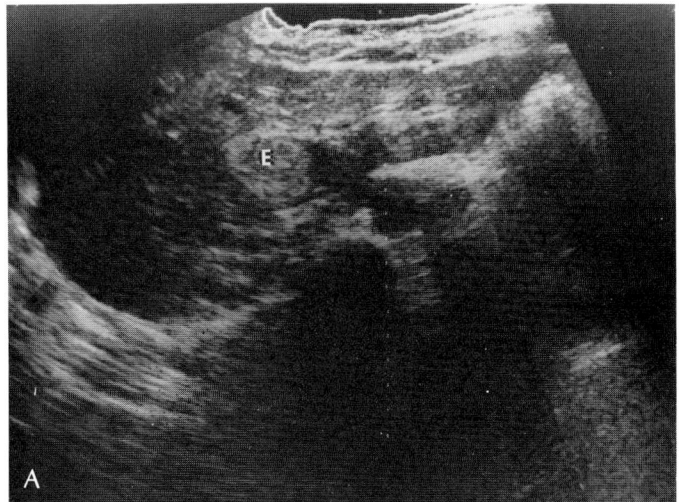

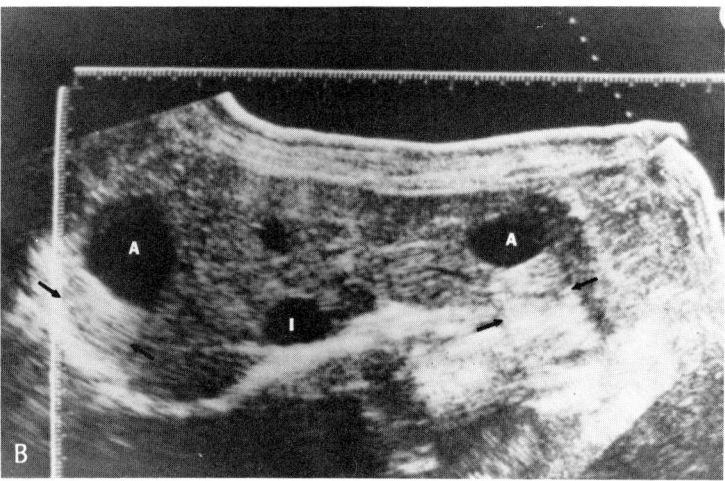

FIG. 4–13. *A,* Transverse static scan; single focal echogenic lesion in the liver (E). The patient is an asymptomatic young female examined for possible gallbladder disease. A computed tomographic scan with a bolus injection showed an increase in density typical of a hemangioma. *B,* Transverse static scan; 2 anechoic lesions in the liver (A) of a 54-year-old man with colon carcinoma and 2 matching defects on a radionuclide scan. Aspiration yielded clear fluid, and patient was clinically free of disease on follow-up. Note the increased "through transmission" behind lesions typical of cysts (arrows). I, Inferior vena cava.

tion, the liver may show increased echogenicity or a mottled echo pattern. This pattern may be confused with widespread metastatic infiltration, and CT scanning often provides the differentiation.

PANCREAS. Imaging of the pancreas is limited to CT scanning or ultrasound. Although CT scanning has been reported to be more effective than ultrasound in diagnosing pancreatic disease,[48] many factors may make sonography an attractive examination. Is the patient thin? Can one easily obtain a CT scan when needed? Is the sonographer at hand experienced enough to give dependable diagnoses? Another consideration is that CT scanning generally costs three to four times more than ultrasonic examination. The choice of examination may be difficult, and often one has no set answers.

Pancreatic disease, as seen by the sonographer, is straightforward. In acute pancreatitis, the gland is swollen and edematous. It may swell to huge proportions and may become phlegmonous (Fig. 4–14A). In patients with marked ileus, the examination may be impossible because of bowel gas and the inability to fill the stomach with fluid to act as an acoustic window. These patients are better evaluated by CT scanning. In chronic pancreatitis, the gland gradually shrinks and becomes hyperechoic, and the pancreatic duct may develop a beaded appearance. The major complication of pancreatitis, pseudocyst, is almost always adequately assessed using ultrasound. These anechoic collections may attain tremendous size rapidly and may dissect widely (Fig. 4–14B).

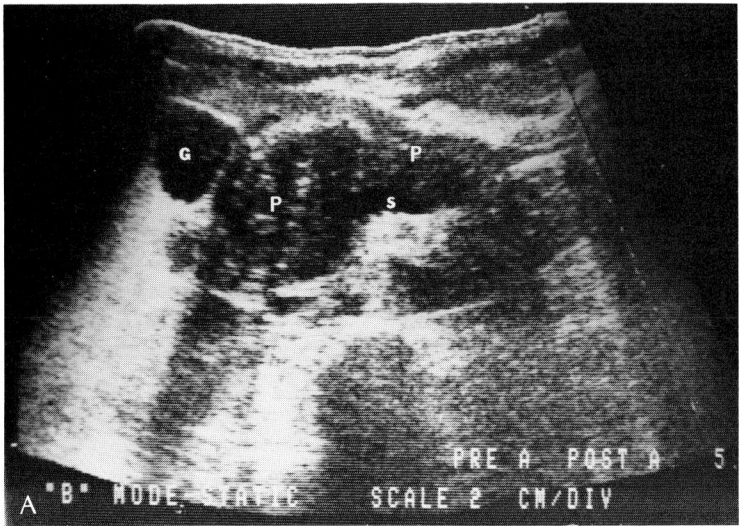

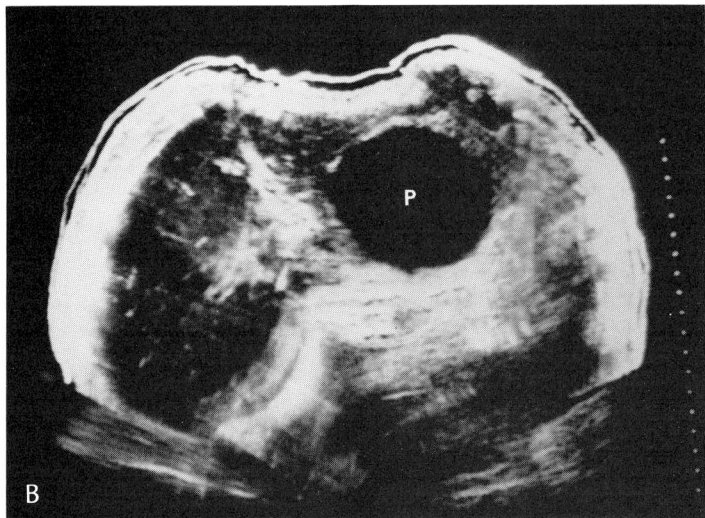

FIG. 4–14. *A,* Transverse static scan; huge, swollen, hypoechoic pancreas (P) in a patient with phlegmonous pancreatitis. G, Gallbladder; S, splenic vein. *B,* Transverse static sonogram; large anechoic pseudocyst (P) in the left upper abdomen.

Pancreatic carcinoma has specific sonographic features in addition to a focal enlargement of the gland by the tumor. Carcinoma is generally hypoechoic. This feature may be of great value when the tumor is small and does not enlarge the pancreas. With CT scanning, one cannot make this distinction because the technique depends only on contour, although CT scanning with a bolus of contrast material may enable one to identify small pancreatic carcinomas. One must carefully differentiate between carcinoma and focal pancreatitis. They may be identical on ultrasound and CT scanning, although the histories of these two diseases are usually different.

Other more unusual malignant tumors, including pancreatic cystadenocarcinoma, islet cell tumors, and lymphomas, are also readily identified with ultrasound. Shawker has described the accuracy of ultrasound as greater than that of angiography in identifying pancreatic islet cell tumors.[49] In the past, angiography was commonly used in the search for these sometimes elusive tumors because of their small size, but with improved resolution, one may now identify a high percentage of these lesions with ultrasonography.

SPLEEN. The spleen is often overlooked during ultrasonic examination. Information similar to that pertaining to the liver can be gleaned from ultrasonic examination of the spleen. Focal splenic lesions including metastases, cysts, paracystic infestations, and abscesses are all readily identified with sonography[50] (Fig. 4–15A). In general, we have found ultrasound to be a logical method of determining the origin of any left upper quadrant masses,

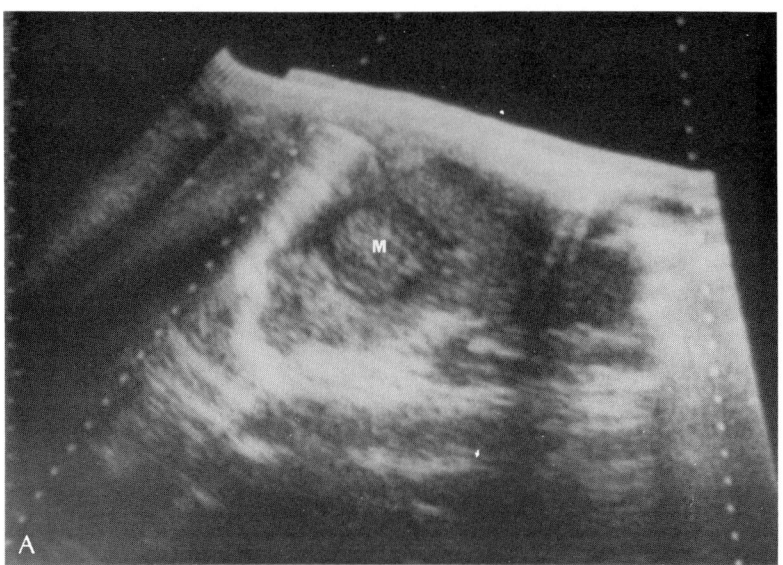

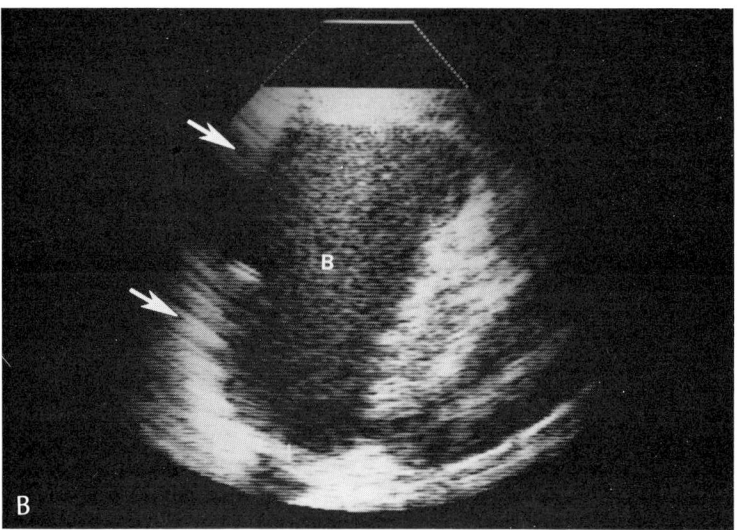

FIG. 4–15. *A,* Longitudinal scan through the left upper quadrant; large, solid metastatic focus of melanoma (M) in the spleen. *B,* Real-time sector scan through the left upper quadrant; homogeneous, bean-shaped collection (B) beneath the left hemidiaphragm (arrows) in a young male who had undergone splenectomy during staging laparotomy for lymphoma. Pus was obtained during percutaneous drainage.

especially in the pediatric patient, in whom the differentiation among splenomegaly, Wilms' tumor, and neuroblastoma can be so important. Again, real-time evaluation is the best ultrasonic technique for thorough examination of the spleen.

The left subphrenic space is a prime site for postsurgical collections, whether or not the patient has undergone splenectomy. Abdominal abscesses may have varied sonographic characteristics,[51] and in the left upper quadrant, they may actually have a sonographic appearance similar to that of the normal spleen, both in shape and in echo texture (Fig. 4–15B). The reason may have to do with the state of organization of the abscesses. Abscess is an acute surgical problem, and a diagnostic conclusion must be reached rapidly. The patient's medical history usually indicates whether the spleen is present. If one sees a spleen-like collection or a collection in addition to the spleen, subphrenic abscess should be considered. For diagnostic purposes or for drainage, a percutaneous puncture should be performed, guided either by real-time sonography or CT scanning.[52] This approach can eliminate second operations. More is said about the use of real-time ultrasound in guiding percutaneous procedures later in this chapter.

KIDNEYS. The kidneys and retroperitoneum were among the earliest areas investigated by ultrasound. Even in the sonographic dark ages of 10 years ago, the idea of evaluating renal cysts with ultrasound was accepted. Many other uses for sonography in the kidney have been developed since then, but the assessment of renal masses remains common. Sonography is the first choice in the differentiation between cystic and solid renal masses (Fig. 4–16A and B). The sonographic diagnosis of simple cysts may end the workup. Cysts with irregular walls, with septa, or with internal echoes should be punctured to prove their cystic content, and patients with solid masses should undergo arteriography or CT scanning. This simple scheme may vary with each particular lesion, radiologist, and urologist. Each patient must be treated on an individual basis, but the foregoing plan is usually effective. Cyst puncture is usually innocuous and may be performed as an outpatient procedure. It should always be done before proceeding to an arteriogram if one suspects the presence of a complicated cyst. Additionally, some physicians have found renal masses during CT scanning that do not have low enough CT numbers to be confidently classified as cysts, and they have performed arteriography without a prior ultrasonic examination. This procedure is a disservice to the patient because the majority of cysts are found ultrasonically and may be confirmed by puncture. The arteriogram is invasive and should be used last.

Aside from the evaluation of a typical renal mass, sonography can be of great value in examining other areas of the genitourinary system. The sonographer can, in minutes and without the aid of contrast material, determine whether renal failure is caused by medical renal disease or by obstruction, by identifying hydronephrosis (Fig. 4–16C). In patients with medical renal disease, the kidneys are often small, with or without an irregular outline, and may have increased echogenicity. The renal size and kidney outlines are readily identifiable sonographically in most patients. Various renal problems can be diagnosed, including renal abscess, pyonephrosis, perirenal hematoma, and calculi. In the follow-up of a filling defect in the renal collecting system, ultrasound plays a limited but important role. One may confidently differentiate a calculus, whether radiopaque or nonradiopaque, from other causes of the defect, by means of ultrasound (Fig. 4–16D and E). We have found static scanning inadequate in locating calculi; real-time imaging is a necessary indication. Many known calculi go unnoticed when one uses static scanning alone. We have used high-resolution ultrasound extensively in search of calculi in the pediatric kidney, and we have found the technique to be effective. In fact, a number of stones have been identified in children with hemocysteinuria that were not visible on a plain film or even on an intravenous pyelogram. Neonates are also well suited for ultrasonic examination of the kidneys. Neonatal kidneys are poorly visualized on an intravenous urogram. Ultrasound, frequently coupled with radionuclide scanning, often obviates the need for a urogram. A useful application of ultrasound is the evaluation of a neonate with a flank mass. One may immediately determine the internal characteristics of the mass by using ultrasound. The sonographic findings in the infantile polycystic kidney are diagnostic,[53] and the macroscopic cysts of multicystic dysplastic kidney are also specific and may be confirmed by following the ultrasonic examination with a radionuclide scan, to evaluate the blood flow[54] (Fig. 4–16F). Similarly, hydronephrosis is easily evaluated using a combination of ultrasound and radionuclide scanning. Screening for congenital renal malformations, including crossed-fused ectopia, renal agenesis, dysgenesis, and renal hypoplasia in the pediatric population is adequately performed using ultrasound and, if necessary, radionuclide scanning.

ADRENAL GLANDS. Sonographic evaluation of the adrenal glands is less helpful than that of the kidneys. Although some authors have reported favorable results with ultrasound,[55] our personal experience and that of other investigators indictate otherwise.[56] Certainly, one may identify large adrenal masses sonographically (Fig. 4–17), but the normal or slightly enlarged gland may be impossible to find. As usual, the patient's body habitus as well as the sonographer's experience must be taken into account. Although we advocate CT scanning as the most likely first choice for adrenal evaluation, ultrasound may play a role when a urogram shows a mass superior to the kidney, in children, and when following patients with known adrenal masses for response to therapy. We have successfully performed biopsies of adrenal masses under sonographic guidance, but overall, CT scanning seems the better imaging technique for evaluating the adrenal glands in most patients.

TESTES. High-resolution sonography is ideal for evaluating the testes. Images of high quality may be obtained, and some authors have shown that sonography may be of great value in detecting a variety of scrotal lesions, both cystic and solid[57,58] (Fig. 4–18). This feature may be of particular import in patients with overlying hydroceles or varicoceles in whom testicular masses are not palpable. Sonography should be the first choice for imaging the testes for almost any reason. The examination is painless and often yields valuable information.

RETROPERITONEUM. Various pathologic entities may affect the retroperitoneum, but the two most common are aortic atherosclerotic disease and associated aneurysms and retroperitoneal masses, either primary or metastatic. The abdominal aorta

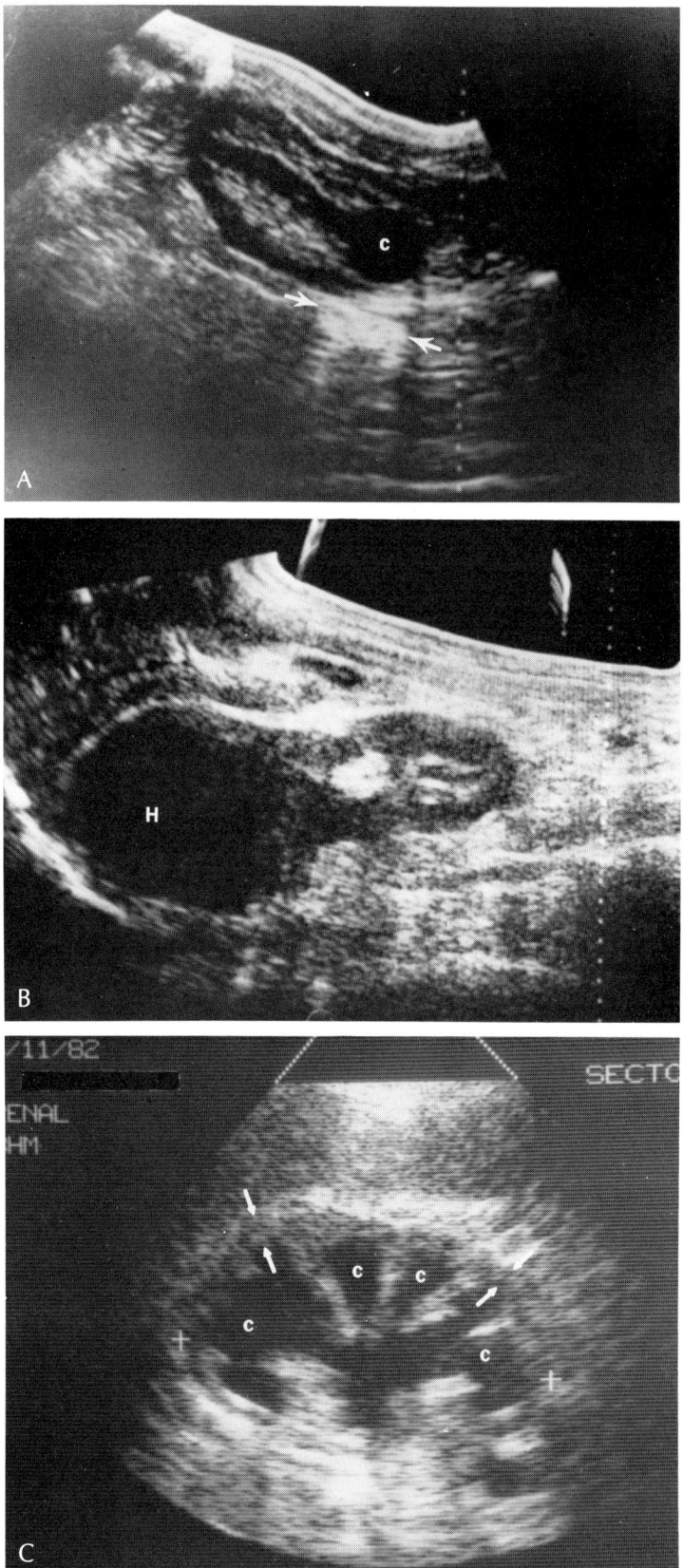

FIG. 4-16. *A*, Small, lower-pole kidney cyst (C), which is anechoic and has smooth walls and good "through transmission" (arrows). *B*, Larger, upper-pole hypernephroma (H), which clearly displays internal echoes and no increased transmission of sound. *C*, Real-time sector scan through the flank; marked dilatation of renal calices (C) and thinning of parenchyma (arrows) in chronic hydronephrosis.

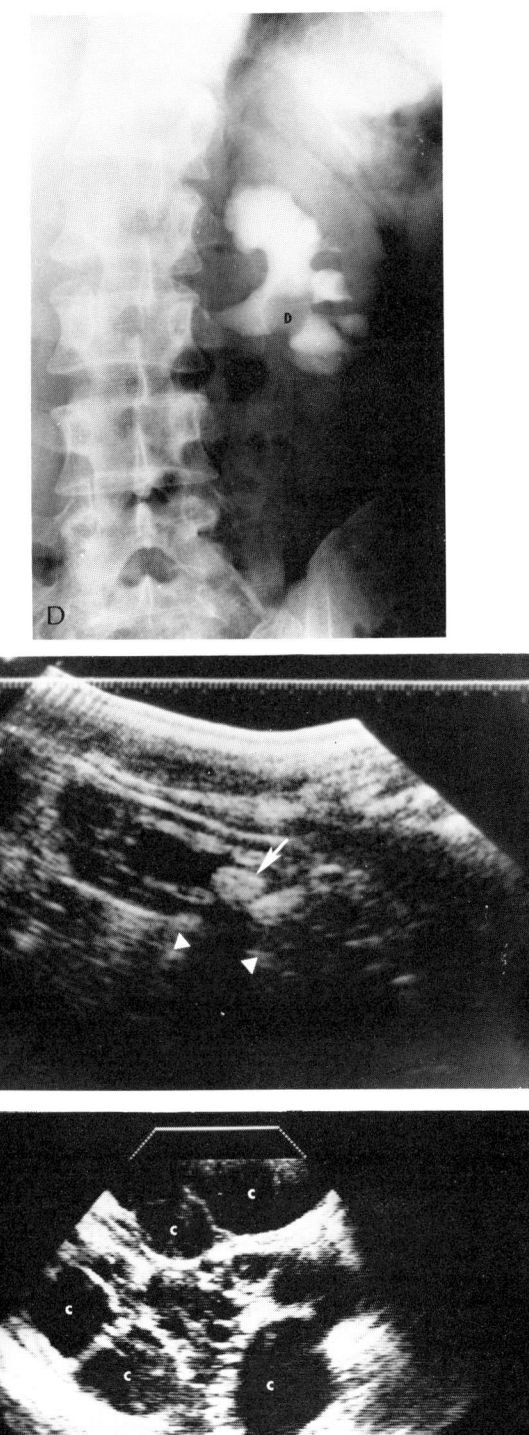

FIG. 4-16 Continued. *D,* Intravenous urogram showing a large filling defect (D) in the collecting system. *E,* Sonogram showing an echogenic focus (arrow) and posterior shadowing (arrowheads), confirming that the defect seen in *D* is a calculus. *F,* Neonate with a palpable flank mass; multiple cysts (C) of various sizes in a configuration typical of multicystic dysplastic kidney.

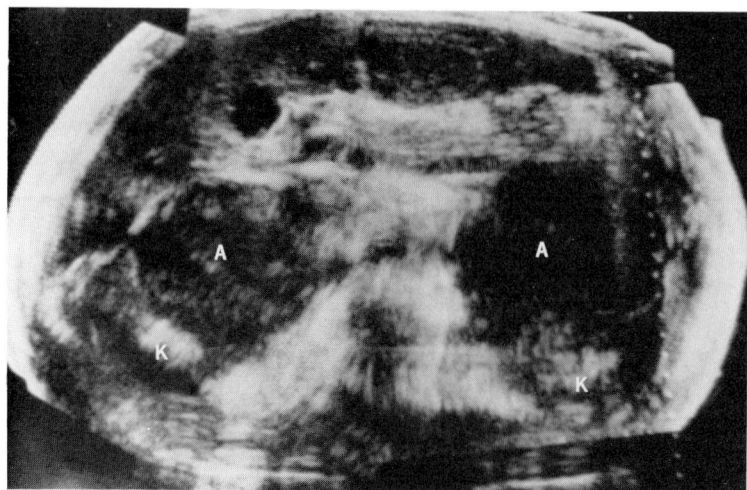

FIG. 4-17. Transverse static scan; large bilateral adrenal metastases (A) from primary lung carcinoma. K, Kidney.

can be evaluated to its bifurcation in almost every patient, even the most obese, although certain scanning tricks may be needed, such as pushing pannus aside with the hand-held transducer or even resorting to a bistable display to obtain vessel outlines. Aortic aneurysms are easily and accurately evaluated sonographically, and dimensions, internal thrombus, and size of the patent lumen are routinely determined (Fig. 4-19A and B). In slow leaks or tears of the aorta, CT scanning is preferred to sonography because of its superior ability to display density differences and thereby to show smaller amounts of blood that has dissected into the retroperitoneum.

CT and ultrasound may not allow one clearly to identify the origin of important vessels such as the renal arteries, and it may be difficult to determine whether these vessels are involved in an aneurysm. One should at least be able to approximate closely the level of the renal hila and their relationship to the superior extent of the aneurysm, using either CT or ultrasound. In many patients, the iliac vessels can be imaged for their entire course, although this procedure may be more challenging than imaging of the aorta. Femoral and iliac artery aneurysms and even occlusion may be evaluated using sonography,[59] and we are encouraged by preliminary findings using duplex scanning in the arteries of the pelvis and legs (Fig. 4-19C and D).

Adenopathy in the retroperitoneum is common. It may be primary, as in lymphoma, or metastatic, often from gynecologic or testicular neoplasms (Fig. 4-19E). Again, the basic principles apply; obese patients should undergo CT scanning, but thinner ones should benefit from ultrasound. The interaction of ultrasound, CT scanning, and lymphangiography in the evaluation of retroperitoneal adenopathy remains controversial, however. Ultrasound may be sufficient, and if the results are positive, the workup may end there. From this point, CT could be the next logical choice, with lymphangiography reserved for those patients with negative CT and ultrasonic findings. Evidence indicates that the CT scanning, and therefore probably ultrasound as well, should not replace the lymphangiogram entirely, however.[60]

Many retroperitoneal tumors are sarcomas, and the main diagnostic problem is in distinguishing them from other retroperitoneal processes. This process may be difficult, and sarcomas, other than liposarcomas, and, more notoriously, lymphomas may appear cystic ultrasonically. This appearance should not be a problem when the mass is large and cannot be mistaken for an aneurysm or a cyst. In smaller, more discrete masses, which by nature lie in direct proximity to the vessels, the sonographic differentiation among aneurysm, adenopathy, and sarcoma may be difficult. An aneurysm may be effectively ruled out if Doppler scanning is available. The differentiation between lymphoma and sarcoma is probably best left to the pathologist after percutaneous biopsy.

ULTRASONIC NEEDLE GUIDANCE. Percutaneous ultrasonically guided needle pucture techniques have gained wide acceptance during the past 10 or so years. The use of ultrasound as a method of guidance was successfully accomplished by Holm and his Danish co-workers as early as 1973.[61] This technique employed a specially built transducer with a slot or hole in the center that was aligned to the central beam of the ultrasonic device and served as a needle guide. Although this method has been successful in thousands of procedures, its major drawback is the inability to monitor the needle tip con-

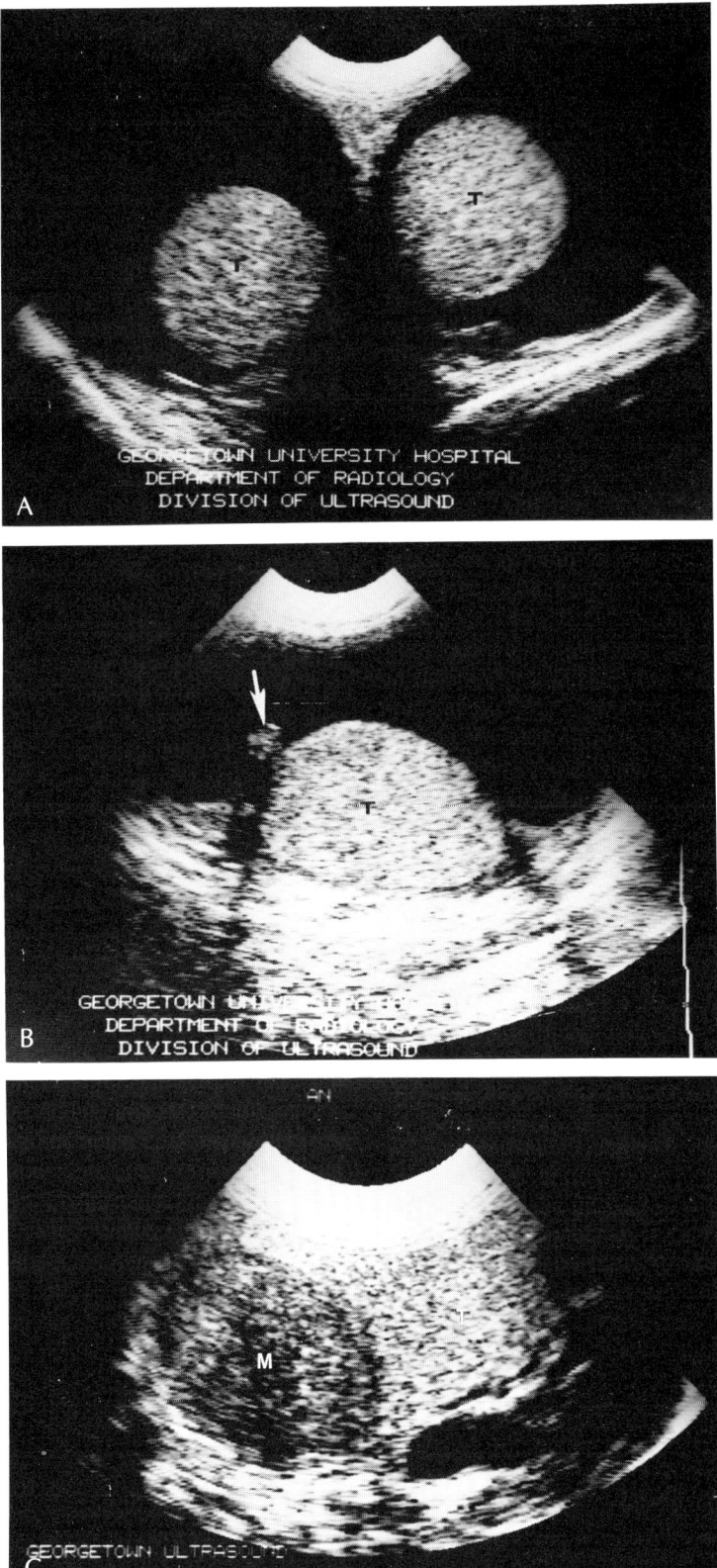

FIG. 4–18. Transverse (A) and longitudinal (B) sonograms in a young male who had undergone renal transplantation; fluid in the hydrocele separates the testes (T) from the scanner, to yield exceptional images. Arrow, Appendix testes. C, Longitudinal real-time scan through the left testis of a 23-year-old medical student; hypoechoic mass (M) typical of neoplasm, which was embryonal cell carcinoma. This mass was not palpable. T, Normal testis.

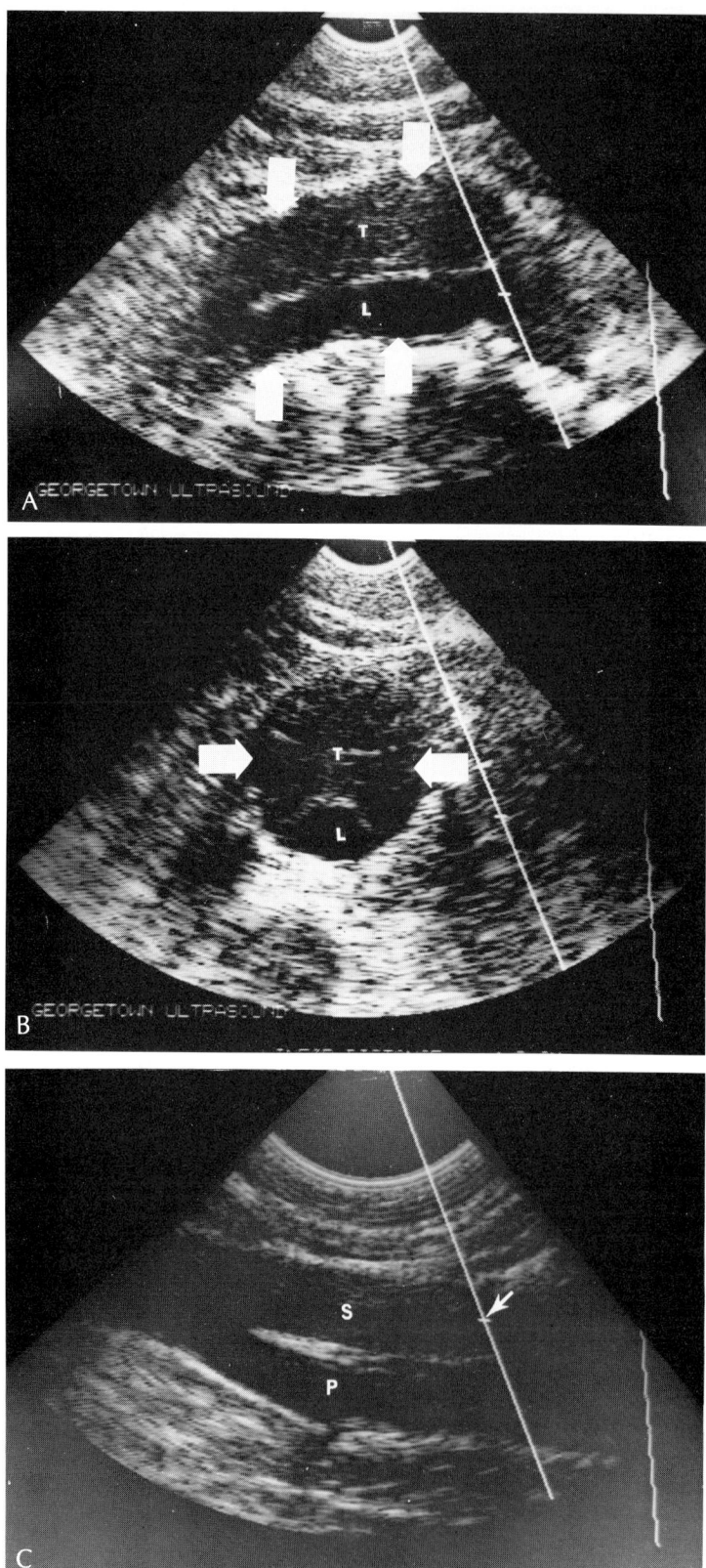

FIG. 4–19. Longitudinal *(A)* and transverse *(B)* real-time sections through an abdominal aortic aneurysm (arrows). Note the internal thrombus (T) and the anechoic lumen (L). *C* and *D*, Duplex scan through a normal left thigh. *C*, Real-time image showing the superficial (S) and deep (P) femoral arteries.

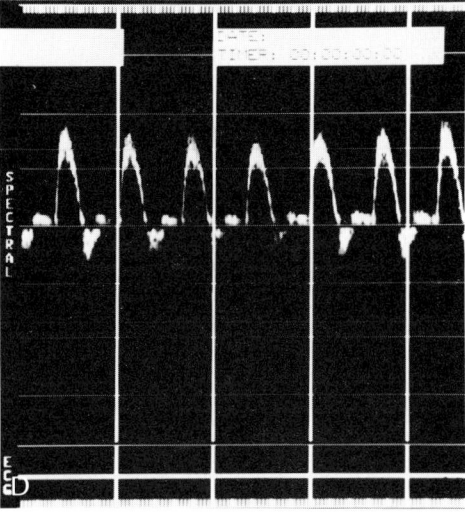

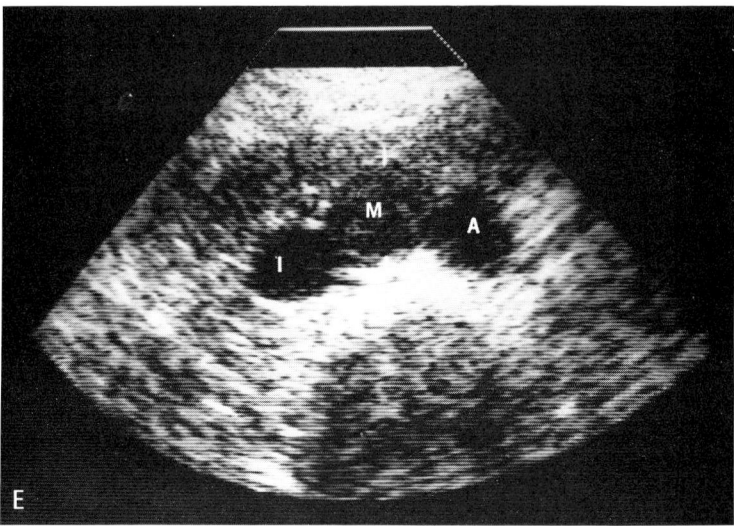

FIG. 4–19 Continued. *D,* Normal, sharp, triphasic Doppler wave form obtained from the superficial femoral artery at the region of the Doppler sample marker in *C* (arrow). *E,* Transverse real-time scan; anechoic aorta (A) to the left and inferior vena cava (I) to the right. Between is metastatic adenopathy (M) from testicular carcinoma.

stantly. Indeed, many authors advocate ultrasonic guidance for large masses only,[62] and CT is the needle-guidance technique of first choice in many institutions.

We evaluated a method of biopsy guidance coupling a neele guide to a commercially available real-time sector scanner (Fig. 4–20). Our results in percutaneous biopsy of a large group of patients with suspected abdominal neoplasms were good, with a 93.4% accuracy rate in successfully puncturing masses throughout the abdomen.[63] This system has definite advantages. It is rapid, portable, and inexpensive and multiple needle passes may be made in minutes. CT schedules are often already overburdened, and the addition of a 1- or 2-hour biopsy is prohibitively expensive. The real-time biopsy can be performed as rapidly as most abdominal scans, and the entire procedure can be moved outside the laboratory and into another room, if necessary. This feature is a particular advantage in procedures such as percutaneous nephrostomy or abscess drainage. The ultrasonic unit may be brought directly into the fluoroscopic suite, and the initial puncture may be performed under ultrasonic guidance. The injection of contrast material and the insertion of guide wires can then be monitored fluoroscopically without moving the patient. These biopsy guides are now commercially available for almost all newer real-time sector scanners. We believe that this method of guidance should be considered before any other, including CT, and with widespread availability of biopsy guides, its use will undoubtedly become commonplace.

In our own experience at a conservative institu-

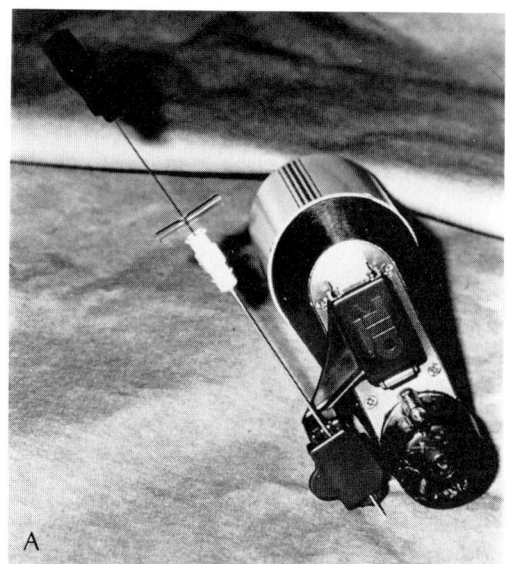
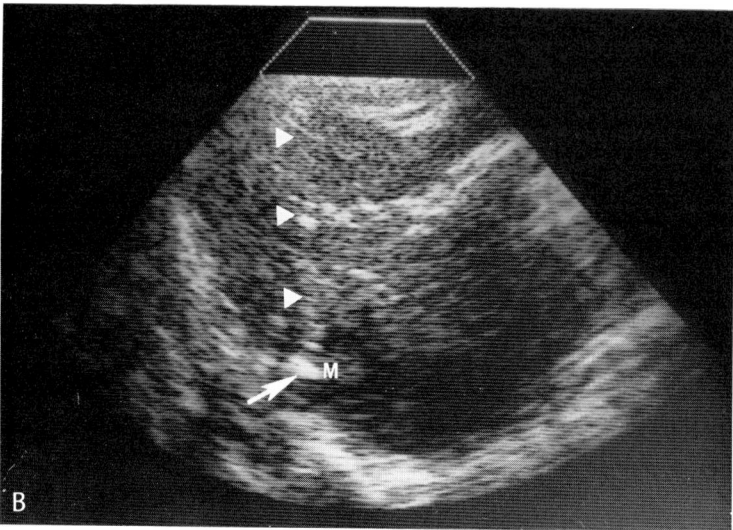

FIG. 4–20. A, Real-time biopsy guidance apparatus, with the guide and the biopsy needle in place. B, Real-time guidance of biopsy of liver metastasis (M); the brightly echogenic focus is the needle's tip (arrow). The entire needle is visible (arrowheads) on the monitor.

tion, percutaneous procedures were initially considered to be surgical heresy. Today, however, percutaneous biopsy of malignant masses is performed on an outpatient basis, and surgical consultants themselves often recommend percutaneous biopsy, for example, over laparoscopic biopsy. Even the most conservative surgeons acknowledge that percutaneous drainage of a postoperative abscess is far superior to a second trip to the operating room. Many patients attest to the immediate improvement in their condition following percutaneous evacuation of an abscess.

Pelvis

Ultrasound first came into widespread use in examination of the pelvis, and pelvic evaluation continues to be the most common use of the technique. Although the male pelvis is occasionally examined ultrasonically, such as for abscess, prostatic evaluation, or spread of neoplasm, most pelvic sonography is performed in women. In the pelvis, the problem of ionizing radiation is paramount, and ultrasound is an excellent means of avoiding such exposure. To date, no studies have indicated that ultrasound causes increased birth defects or is in any way teratogenic.[64] We do not advocate routine pregnancy scanning, however, because the cost is high and the diagnostic yield is low.

In the female pelvis, the organs of interest are ideally located for ultrasonic evaluation. The uterus and adnexal regions lie directly posterior to the uri-

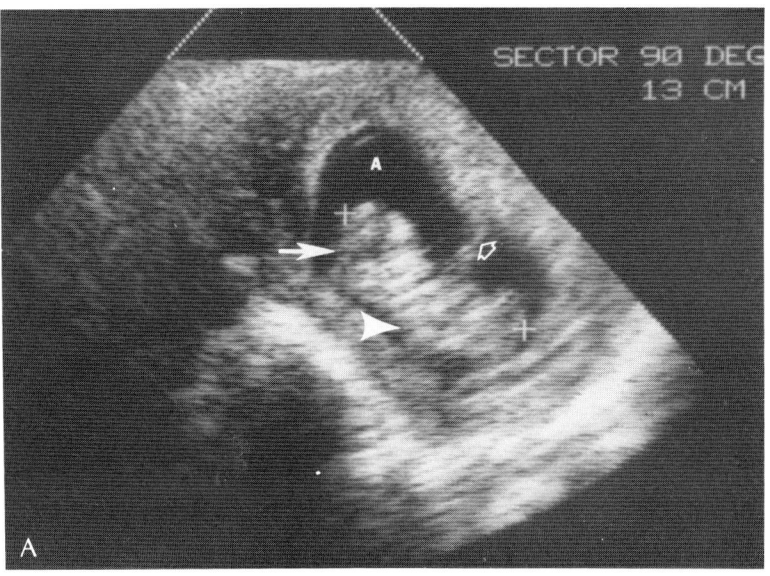

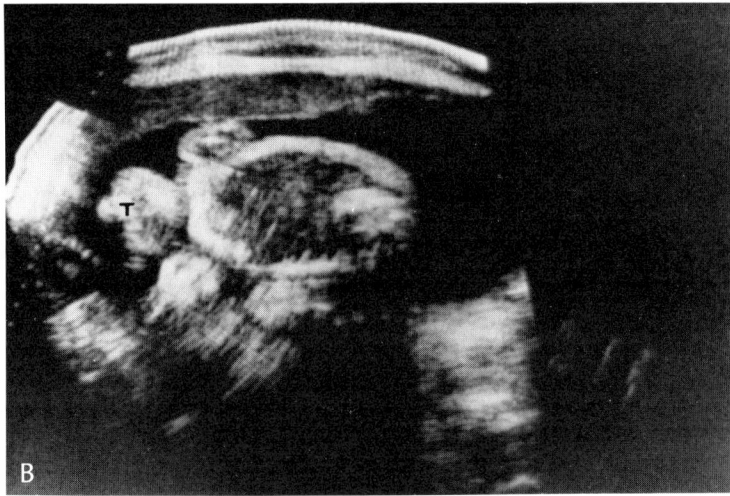

FIG. 4–21. A, Normal 12-week fetus; note the head (arrow), the body (arrowhead), and the umbilical cord (open arrow) suspended in anechoic amniotic fluid (A). B, Static sonogram; fetal body, but no evidence of normal head development in this 34-week gestation. The head is reduced to a mass of soft tissue (T) in this anencephalic fetus.

nary bladder. Therefore, having a full bladder is the only preparation essential for such an examination. The full urinary bladder not only acts as an acoustic window by transmitting sound undisturbed, but it also pushes the bowel out of the way and enables the sound beam to reach an area otherwise covered by the pubic symphysis and gas. So much has been written about the use of ultrasound in the evaluation of the female pelvis that any detailed account would be beyond the scope of this book. The reader is referred to excellent texts in both obstetrics and gynecology that deal thoroughly with these topics.[65,66]

A comparison of ultrasound with contrast radiography indicates that barium studies and intravenous urography have a different approach from the cross-sectional technique of sonography. Conventional contrast studies outline hollow organs such as the bowel or bladder and thereby imply the presence of a mass, for example, by extrinsic compression. Ultrasound, on the other hand, actually sees the mass. In some areas, barium studies and urography are superior to ultrasound. Certainly, the mucosal detail available from a properly done air-contrast barium enema is excellent. The ability of the urogram to identify a ureteral stricture remains unsurpassed, but in evaluating lesions and structures located beyond the mucosa, CT scanning and ultrasound are superior. The more difficult problem for many clinicians today is which of the cross-sectional imaging techniques, CT scanning or ultrasound, is best. One study has shown that either method is similar in accuracy and yield.[67]

Although either CT or ultrasound may be of value in the diagnosis of pelvic disorders, in the younger patient, ultrasonography has the great advantage of not using ionizing radiation. Additionally, the lower cost of an ultrasonic examination makes it a logical choice in evaluating almost any kind of pelvic disorder. One particular group of patients, however, are not candidates for pelvic ultrasonography. Patients who cannot fill their bladder, such as those with vesical fistulas or radiation-induced cystitis or those who have undergone cystectomy, should be evaluated routinely by CT scanning.

OBSTETRIC EXAMINATIONS. The area of obstetric ultrasound is a whole field in itself. Debate over which imaging technique to use is not an issue. The previous techniques, such as pelvimetry for fetal lie or multiple gestations or radionuclide placentography, are no longer performed. Modern ultrasound provides us with images that were considered fantasy just 5 years ago. We can see the fetal pole at 6 weeks and the fetal heart beat at 7 weeks, and we can identify most of the major internal organs of the fetus during the second trimester (Fig. 4–21). The fetus cannot hide much from the world any longer, and even the sex can be determined before birth, for better or worse. A whole new field of obstetric procedures has arisen, using ultrasound to guide a needle to a target. Earlier, amniocentesis was directed by ultrasonography to avoid puncturing the placenta or the fetus. Intrauterine transfusions and even correction of birth defects are now attempted under ultrasonic guidance.

ACKNOWLEDGMENTS

We wish to thank Gloria Wynn Lilly, Natesa Pandian, M.D., Richard Begin, Ria Barnett, and Sandra McInnes.

REFERENCES

1. Wild, J.J.: The use of ultrasonic pulses for the measurement of biologic tissue and the detection of tissue density changes. Surgery, 27:181, 1950.
2. Doust, B.D.: Ultrasonic B-mode examination of the gallbladder. Radiology, 110:643, 1974.
3. Kossoff, G., Garrett, W.J., and Radavanovitch, G.: Ultrasonic atlas of normal brain of infant. Ultrasound Med. Biol., 1:259, 1974.
4. Haber, K., et al.: Ultrasonic evaluation of intracranial pathology in infants: a new technique. Radiology, 134:173, 1980.
5. Babcock, D.S., Han, B.K., and LeQuesne, G.W.: B-mode gray-scale ultrasound of the head in the newborn and young infant. AJR, 134:457, 1980.
6. Grant, E.G., et al.: Real-time ultrasound of the neonatal and infant head. AJNR, 1:487, 1980.
7. Skolnik, A., and McLone, D.G.: Intraoperative real-time ultrasonic guidance of intracranial shunt tube placement in infants. Radiology, 144:573, 1982.
8. Gooding, G.A.W., et al.: Sonography of the adult brain through surgical defects. AJNR, 2:449, 1981.
9. Simeone, J.F., et al.: High-resolution real-time sonography of the thyroid. Radiology, 145:431, 1982.
10. Brown, C.L.: Pathology of the cold nodule. Clin. Endocrinol. Metab., 10:235, 1981.
11. Reading, C.C., Charboneau, J.W., and James, E.M.: High-resolution parathyroid sonography. AJR, 139:539, 1982.
12. Beach, K.W.: Non-invasive carotid diagnosis: entering the second decade. Bruit,4:132, 1980.
13. Blasberg, D.J.: Duplex sonography for carotid artery disease: an accurate technique. AJNR, 3:609, 1982.
13a.Sigel, B., et al.: A Doppler ultrasound method for distinguishing laminar from turbulent flow. J. Surg. Res., 10:221, 1970.
14. James, E.M., et al.: High-resolution dynamic imaging of the carotid bifurcation: a prospective evaluation. Radiology, 144:853, 1982.
15. Jacobs, E.M., et al.: Duplex carotid sonography—the Georgetown experience. Paper presented at the twenty-seventh Annual Meeting of the Radiologic Society of North America, New York, November 22, 1983.
16. Dodd, G.D.: The continuing challenge of mammography. Am. Coll. Radiol. Bull., 39:3, 1983.
17. Cole-Beuglet, C., et al.: Ultrasound mammography: a comparison with radiographic mammography. Radiology, 139:693, 1981.
18. Feigenbaum, H.: Echocardiography, 3rd Ed. Philadelphia, Lea & Febiger, 1981.
19. Weyman, A.E.: Cross-sectional Echocardiography. Philadelphia, Lea & Febiger, 1982.
20. Baker, D.W., Rubenstein, S.A., and Lorch, G.S.: Pulsed-Doppler echocardiography: principles and applications. Am. J. Med., 63:69, 1977.
21. Hatle, L.: Non-invasive assessment and differentiation of LV outflow obstruction with Doppler ultrasound. Circulation, 64:381, 1981.
22. Talanow, J., and Gardin, J.M.: Textbook of 2-Dimensional Echo-Cardiography. New York, Grune & Stratton, 1983.
23. Cooperberg, P.L., and Burhenne, H.J.: Real-time ultrasonography: diagnostic technique of choice in calculus gallbladder disease. N. Engl. J. Med., 302:1277, 1980.
24. Wolson, A.H., and Goldberg, B.B.: Gray-scale ultrasonic cholecystography: a primary screening procedure. JAMA, 240:2073, 1978.
25. Simeone, J.F., et al.: Significance of nonshadowing focal opacities at cholecystosonography. Radiology 137:181, 1980.
26. Ruiz, R., et al.: Ultrasonic diagnosis of primary carcinoma of the gallbladder: a review of 16 cases. JCU, 8:489, 1980.
27. Wales, L.R.: Desquamated gallbladder mucosa: unusual sign of cholecystitis. AJR, 139:810, 1982.
28. Grant, E.G., and Smirniotopoulos, J.G.: Intraluminal gallbladder hematoma, sonographic evidence of hemobilia. JCU. 11(9):507, 1983.
29. Bundy, A.L., and Ritchie, W.G.M.: Ultrasonic diagnosis of metastatic melanoma of the gallbladder presenting as acute cholecystitis. JCU, 10:285, 1982.
30. Laing, F.C., Federle, M.P., and Jeffrey, R.B.: Ultra-

31. Weissman, H.S., et al.: Spectrum of ⁹⁹ᵐTc-IDA cholecystoscintigraphy patterns in acute cholecystitis. Radiology, 138:167, 1981.
32. Raptopoulos, V., et al.: Dynamic cholecystosonography of the contracted gallbladder: the double arc shadow sign. AJR, 138(2):275, 1982.
33. Berk, R.N., van der Vegt, J.H., and Lichtenstein, J.E.: The hyperplastic cholecystoses: cholesterolosis and adenomyomatosis. Radiology, 146:593, 1983.
34. Raghavendra, B.N., et al.: Sonography of adenomyomatosis of the gallbladder: radiologic-pathologic correlation. Radiology, 146:747, 1983.
35. Niederau, C., et al.: Extrahepatic bile ducts in healthy subjects, in patients with cholelithiasis, and post-cholecystectomy patients: a prospective ultrasonic study. JCU, 11:23, 1983.
36. Cooperberg, R.L., et al.: Accuracy of common hepatic duct size in extrahepatic biliary obstruction. Radiology, 135:141, 1980.
37. Parulekar, S.G.: Ultrasound evaluation of common bile duct size. Radiology, 133:703, 1979.
38. Berk, R.N., et al.: Radiography of the bile ducts. Radiology, 145:1, 1982.
39. Weill, F., Eisencher, A., and Zeltner, F.: Ultrasonic study of the normal and dilated biliary tree: the "shotgun" sign. Radiology, 127:221, 1978.
40. Weinstein, B.J., and Weinstein, D.P.: Biliary tract dilatation in the nonjaundiced patient. AJR, 134:889, 1980.
41. Simeone, J.F., et al.: Sonography of the bile ducts after a fatty meal: an aid in the detection of obstruction. Radiology, 143:211, 1982.
42. Grant, E.G., et al.: Pneumobilia: a comparison of four imaging modalities. J. Comput. Assist. Tomogr., 4:630, 1981.
43. Koeningsberg, M., Wiener, S.N., and Walzer, A.: The accuracy of ultrasound in the differential diagnosis of obstructive jaundice: a comparison with cholangiography. Radiology, 133:157, 1979.
44. Haubek, A., et al.: Dynamic sonography in the evaluation of jaundice. AJR, 136:1071, 1981.
45. Richardson, J.D., et al.: Type II choledochal cyst: diagnosis using real-time sonography. J. Ultrasound Med., 3(1):37, 1984.
46. Mittelstaedt, C.A., et al.: Caroli's disease: sonographic findings. AJR, 134:585, 1980.
47. Wicks, J.D., Silver, T.M., and Bree, R.L.: Gray-scale features of hematomas: an ultrasonic spectrum. AJR, 131:977, 1978.
48. Hessel, S.J., et al.: A prospective evaluation of computed tomography and ultrasound of the pancreas. Radiology, 143:129, 1982.
49. Shawker, T.H., et al.: Ultrasonic investigation of pancreatic islet cell tumors. J. Ultrasound Med., 1:193, 1982.
50. Mittelstaedt, C.A.: Ultrasound of the spleen. Semin. Ultrasound, 2:233, 1981.
51. Subramanyam, B.R., et al.: Ultrasound analysis of solid-appearing abscesses. Radiology, 146:487, 1983.
52. Van Sonnenberg, E., et al.: Percutaneous drainage of abscesses and fluid collections: techniques, results and applications. Radiology, 142:1, 1982.
53. Boal, D.K., and Teele, R.L.: Sonography of infantile polycystic kidney disease. AJR, 135:575, 1980.
54. Stuck, K.J., Koff, S.A., and Silver, T.M.: Ultrasonic features of multicystic dysplastic kidney: expanded criteria. Radiology, 143:217, 1982.
55. Sample, W.F., and Sarti, D.A.: Computed tomography and gray-scale ultrasonography of the adrenal gland: a comparative study. Radiology, 128:377, 1978.
56. Abrahams, H.L., et al.: Computed tomography versus ultrasound of the adrenal gland: a prospective study. Radiology, 143:121, 1982.
57. Carroll, B.A., and Gross, D.M.: High-frequency scrotal sonography. AJR, 140:511, 1983.
58. Blei, L., et al.: Ultrasonic analysis of chronic intratesticular pathology. J. Ultrasound Med., 2:17, 1983.
59. Gooding, G.A.W.: Aneurysms of the abdominal aorta, iliac and femoral arteries. Semin. Ultrasound, 3:170, 1982.
60. Dunnick, N.R., and Javadpour, N.: Value of CT and lymphography: distinguishing retroperitoneal metastasis from non-seminomatous tumors. AJR, 136:1093, 1981.
61. Holm, H.H., Rasmussen, S.N., and Kristensen, J.K.: Ultrasonically guided percutaneous puncture technique. JCU, 1:27, 1973.
62. Ferucci, J.T., et al.: Diagnosis of abdominal malignancy by radiologic fine-needle aspiration biopsy. AJR, 134:323, 1981.
63. Grant, E.G., et al.: Fine-needle biopsy directed by real-time sonography: technique and accuracy. AJR, 141:29, 1983.
64. Baker, M., and Dalrymple, G.V.: Biological effects of ultrasound: a review. Radiology, 126:479, 1978.
65. Sanders, R.C., and James, A.E.: The Principles and Practice of Ultrasonography in Obstetrics and Gynecology. New York, Appleton-Century-Crofts, 1980.
66. Athey, P.A., and Hadlock, F.P.: Ultrasound in Obstetrics and Gynecology. St. Louis, C.V. Mosby, 1981.
67. Sanders, R.C., et al.: A prospective study of computed tomography and ultrasound in the detection and staging of pelvic masses. Radiology, 146:439, 1983.

5

Radionuclide Scanning

Bernard Shapiro

Radionuclide scanning is the production of images of normal and diseased tissues and organs by means of the gamma-ray emissions from radiopharmaceutical agents having specific distributions in the body. The gamma rays are detected at the body surface by a variety of instruments that convert the invisible rays into visible patterns representing the distribution of the radionuclide in the body. The patterns, or images, obtained can be interpreted to provide or to aid diagnoses, to follow the course of disease, and to monitor the management of various illnesses. In surgical diagnosis, radionuclide scanning can be valuable in helping one to determine whether a surgical procedure is indicated, when an operation is best performed, how the operation should be done, and what the surgical outcome actually is. Scanning is a sensitive technique, but its specificity may be low when interpreted alone. To be used most successfully, radionuclide scanning must be interpreted in conjunction with other techniques, such as bone radiographs with bone scans, chest radiographs with lung scans, and ultrasonic studies with thyroid scans. Interpretation is also enhanced by providing pertinent clinical information because the distribution of radiopharmaceutical agents can be altered by drugs and by various procedures besides physiologic and pathologic conditions. Discussion of the patient with the radionuclide scanning specialist prior to the study and review of the results with that specialist after the study are beneficial.

GENERAL PRINCIPLES

This section focuses on available radiopharmaceutical agents and on instruments in current use.

Agents

Radiopharmaceuticals are chemical agents that contain a radioactive isotope, or radionuclide. In scanning, they are used in trace amounts and do not have pharmacologic actions. The important characteristics of radiopharmaceutical agents are the nature of the emissions and the physical half-life of the incorporated radionuclide, the physical and chemical state and pharmacokinetics of the compound, and the sterility, pyrogenicity, isotonicity, pH, and purity of the agent as a pharmaceutical. For scanning, the optimal radionuclide emits a single gamma ray of 100 to 300 keV energy with no beta emission. The optimal radionuclide has an effective half-life equal to 0.693 of the time interval between the administration of the compound and the performance of the test. The optimal agent either forms a simple solution or a stable suspension in physiologic aqueous media and does not deteriorate rapidly on standing. This optimal agent concentrates instantly and for a sufficient time in normal or diseased tissue, clears quickly from background tissue, and is rapidly excreted from the body. ^{99m}Technetium (^{99m}Tc) sulfur colloid for liver scanning is an example of an excellent radiopharmaceutical agent. ^{99m}Tc has a 140-keV gamma ray only and a 6-hour half-life. The sulfur colloid can be stored at room temperature for hours; ^{99m}Tc sulfur colloid concentrates in the liver, spleen, and bone marrow in a few minutes after intravenous injection and is almost completely cleared from the blood in the same time. Although this agent is not rapidly excreted from the body, its short physical half-life keeps the radiation dose small.

Instruments

SCINTILLATION CAMERA. This instrument is the major imaging device used in radionuclide scanning. The detector head contains a large sodium iodide (NaI) crystal that may be 15 inches in diameter and half an inch thick. When a gamma ray strikes the crystal, a flash of light or scintillation occurs in the crystal and is localized by a battery of photomultiplier tubes arranged on the backside of the crystal. The scintillations in the NaI crystal are translated into pinpoints of light on an oscilloscope screen that can be accumulated photographically to provide an image on film. The scintillations can also be translated into digital signals for storage in the memory of a computer. This feature permits recall of the image, application of desired processing, and various forms of permanent storage. Important features of the scintillation camera besides the crystal and photomultiplier tubes are the collimator and the pulse-height analyzer. The collimator is a lead disc containing a network of holes, placed on the front side of the crystal, so only gamma rays from radionuclide directly in front of an area of the crystal can enter that area of the crystal. Gamma rays from other areas are absorbed by the lead septa between the holes in the collimator. The pulse-height analyzer checks the energy of each incoming gamma ray and rejects those of higher energy, which may be cosmic rays, and those of lower energy, which may be scattered gamma rays from distant parts of the body.

NEWER INSTRUMENTS. Several methods of tomographic imaging have recently come into use. One involves a collimator with a circular array of pinholes at various angles that projects multiple simultaneous images from different directions into the camera. The information is processed by a computer to give longitudinal tomography. The seven-pinhole system is used in cardiac tomography and provides image slices through the heart at various depths from the body wall.

Another tomographic system involves a rotating scintillation camera that moves 360° around the body and takes images continuously or in stepwise fashion. The computer processes the data to give transverse tomography known as SPECT (single-photo-emission computed tomography). Still another tomographic system involves a multiple crystal device with crystals and photomultiplier tubes in circular array around the body. It uses radionuclides that emit positrons and is known as the PETT (positron-emission transaxial tomography) scanner. The positrons result in annihilation radiation that consists of pairs of oppositely directed 0.51-MeV gamma rays striking opposing crystals in the scanner simultaneously. By registering and processing only such coincident emissions, background radiation is eliminated, and the source of the emanation is located. The computer provides transverse tomography in multiple slices. The advantage of PETT scanning is the ability to image with isotopes of carbon, nitrogen, and oxygen, which can be incorporated into natural compounds and their analogs to observe and to measure physiologic functions and their pathologic aberrations. A disadvantage is the need to have a cyclotron on site because of the short half-lives of the foregoing radionuclides. For the same reason, specialized synthetic chemistry must be available to incorporate the radionuclides into organic compounds. The expense of this procedure and its narrow range of routine applications have limited the number of PETT facilities currently in operation.

Procedures

Radionuclide scanning procedures usually involve an intravenous injection of the radiopharmaceutical agent and the collection of static images of areas of the body in multiple views at some fixed time or times after the injection. Some studies, such as gastrointestinal examinations, require oral ingestion of the radionuclide, and some, such as ventilation studies, require inhalation of the radionuclide as a gas. Dynamic studies usually involve an intravenous injection of a radiopharmaceutical agent and multiple images obtained at various time intervals. In some studies, pharmacologic agents may be used before, during, or after administration of the radiopharmaceutical, to achieve or to enhance the differential distribution of radioactivity necessary to obtain the desired information. Because radiopharmaceutical agents are administered in trace amounts, reactions are rare. Radiation from the diagnostic use of these agents is minimal, and no radiation effects have been reported. Some studies may deliver several rads to some tissues, but this dose is lower than that received during many standard radiologic procedures.

BRAIN

The purpose of brain scanning is to observe intracranial mass lesions and cerebrovascular disease. The visualization of mass lesions is based on a breakdown of the blood-brain barrier, which normally keeps most substances out of normal brain tissue. Tumors, infarcts, and abscesses develop new vasculature without a blood-brain barrier and therefore allow certain radiopharmaceutical agents to enter and to be imaged. The study of cerebrovascular disease is based on visualization of blood flow through cerebral vessels, as well as on the breakdown of the blood-brain barrier.

In the past, brain scanning was used to diagnose primary and metastatic brain tumors, subdural hematomas, arteriovenous malformations, abscesses, cysts, and ischemic and hemorrhagic infarcts. Because of the availability of transmission computed tomography (CT), the volume of radionuclide brain scanning in recent years has diminished. Radionuclide brain scanning is now used less for tumor, cyst, and abscess detection than for study of cerebrovascular disease. Magnetic resonance imaging (MRI) may make further inroads on brain scanning because this technique seems to be more sensitive and specific in the study of cerebrovascular disease than CT or radionuclide imaging. New radiopharmaceuticals, such as N-isopropyl ^{123}I p-iodoamphetamine, and single-photon-emission CT may reverse the trend because they provide valuable physiologic information not obtainable by other means.[1]

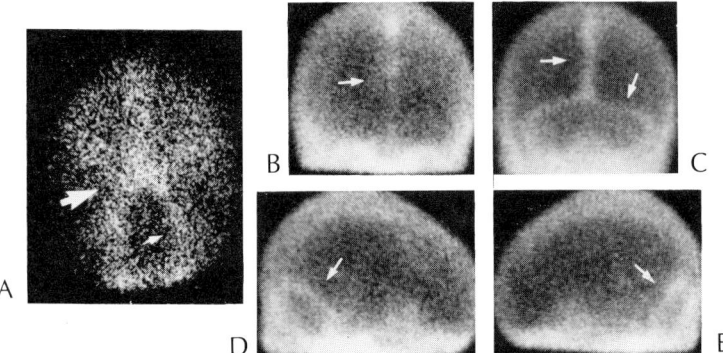

FIG. 5-1. Normal brain scan. *A,* One frame from the arterial phase of the flow study, an anterior view, with the large arrow pointing to the circle of Willis and the small arrow pointing to the left internal carotid artery; the anterior and middle cerebral arteries are radiating from the circle. Anterior *(B),* posterior *(C),* and lateral *(D* and *E)* views of the delayed, static study; the horizontal arrows *(B* and *C)* point to the sagittal sinus, and the diagonal arrows,*(C, D,* and *E)* point to the transverse sinuses.

Brain scanning with the PETT scanner and with positron-emitting analogs of metabolites provides much metabolic information of the brain, but it is unlikely that this technique will become available for routine use.[2]

Procedure and Interpretation

The brain scan is begun with an intravenous injection of ^{99m}Tc-glucoheptonate or ^{99m}Tc-DTPA (diethylenetriamine penta-acetic acid) and immediate collection of dynamic blood flow images at 2-sec intervals from the time of appearance of activity in the carotid arteries through the cerebral venous phase. The cerebral blood flow study is usually obtained in the anterior view. Static images are obtained in anterior, posterior, and both lateral projections 1 to 2 hours after injection.

The part of the study imaging cerebral blood flow usually yields one or two accurate arterial-phase images showing the carotid arteries, the circle of Willis, the anterior cerebral arteries, and the middle cerebral arteries (Fig. 5-1). Uniform diffuse activity in the cerebral hemispheres indicates normal flow in the small vessels. The beginning of the venous phase is indicated by the appearance of the sagittal sinus. The static images obtained at 1 to 2 hours show activity in the muscle of the face and neck, in the skull and scalp, and in the sagittal and transverse sinuses and the confluence of sinuses (torcular Herophili). The cerebral hemispheres in the static images show relative inactivity in the normal individual (Fig. 5-1).

Abnormal Manifestations

TUMORS. If hypervascular, primary or metastatic tumors may show an area of abnormally increased flow during the flow study and may show a "hot" area on the static study (Fig. 5-2). Not all tumors are visualized on flow or static images. Meningiomas show up the best, whereas low-grade gliomas may not show up at all. To be certain that an abnormality represents an intracranial lesion, it should be seen in two different views. Some indication of the nature of the lesion can be obtained from the shape, multiplicity, location, vascularity, and change in appearance with time, but a definite diagnosis is not always possible. Lesions with a "doughnut" appearance may represent a tumor with a necrotic center, but they may also indicate a cyst, an abscess, or a cerebrovascular accident.

CEREBROVASCULAR ACCIDENTS (CVA). Patients with this disorder often have a decreased flow pattern during the flow portion of the study and a wedge-shaped area of increased activity during the static portion of the study. The branches of the middle cerebral artery are most commonly affected (Fig.

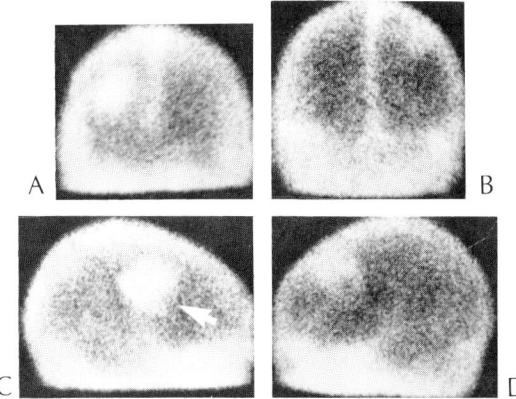

FIG. 5-2. Brain tumor. Anterior *(A),* posterior *(B),* and lateral *(C* and *D)* views of the delayed static study. Note the large, right parietal "hot" area *(C,* arrow), seen in all views, which is a meningioma.

5–3). The flow abnormality may be seen early after the stroke, but the area of increased activity on the static images is usually not detectable in the first few days. It is best seen at 2 weeks, and it usually has faded 2 months after the event. If the abnormality seen on the static images develops within a few days of the event, it may be due to intracerebral hemorrhage rather than to thrombosis. A subarachnoid hemorrhage does not usually produce an abnormality on a brain scan unless the patient has a large aneurysm that would be visualized on the flow study or an infarct or intracerebral hematoma that might be seen on the static images.

SUBDURAL HEMATOMAS. These lesions may be characterized by an absence of peripheral activity on the flow study producing a flattened or even concave shape to the head on the involved side on the anterior or posterior view (Fig. 5–4). On the static images, the same area shows increased activity. As with the CVA, subdural hematoma is often not seen for several weeks after the event. The lateral views are not as remarkable as the anterior or posterior views and often show only a diffuse increase in activity. Increased peripheral activity on static images can also be seen in extradural hematoma, scalp edema and hematoma, hyperostosis, Paget's disease, fibrous dysplasia, craniotomy, bruises, fractures, osteomyelitis, or metastasis to the skull.

ABSCESSES AND CYSTS. Patients with abscesses or cysts show an area of decreased activity on the flow study, but increased activity on the static images if a capsule has formed. Some cysts or abscesses have a clear central portion that has a "ring" or "doughnut" appearance.

OTHER DISORDERS. Meningitis may result in a diffuse increase in activity in the static images, or the scan may appear completely normal. Patients with arteriovenous malformations have an area of increased activity during the arterial phase of the flow study that fades during the venous phase. Such malformations may not appear at all in the static images.

Comparison with Computed Tomography

With the advent of CT, the use of radionuclide scanning of the brain has declined, although it is still helpful in many situations.[3] For primary brain tumors, CT is more sensitive because it can detect the low-grade cystic lesions that are often difficult to visualize with radionuclides. CT also has inherently better resolution, and even when radionuclide scans identify a tumor, one can see it more clearly on a CT scan. Small vascular meningiomas lying close to bone over the convexity or along the floor of the skull may be missed by CT but shown by radionuclides, however. Pituitary lesions and acoustic neuromas are better seen with CT scanning. The use of contrast infusion with CT is necessary in look-

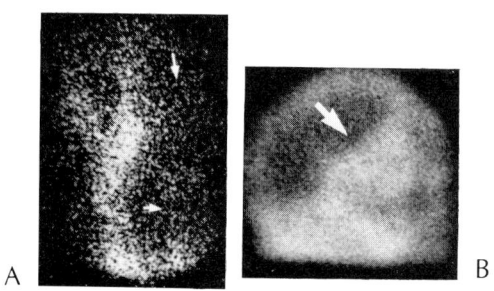

FIG. 5–3. Cerebrovascular accident. A, One frame from the arterial phase of the flow study; note the absence of flow through the left carotid and left middle cerebral arteries (arrows). B, Left lateral view from the delayed static study showing a large, fan-shaped infarct (arrow).

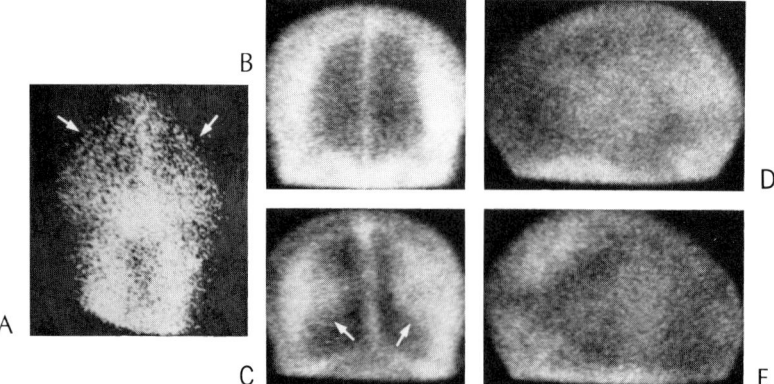

FIG. 5–4. Subdural hematomas. A, One frame from the arterial phase of the flow study; note the flattened lateral margins of the flow (arrows), caused by the presence of bilateral subdural hematomas. Anterior (B), posterior (C), and lateral (D and E) views of the delayed static study; the arrows in C point to the hematomas, which are seen best on anterior and posterior views.

ing for metastases, and with infusion, CT is more sensitive than radionuclide scanning in detecting brain metastases. Although both techniques have a high sensitivity, 85 to 95%, in the detection of intracranial mass lesions, CT is more sensitive than radionuclide scanning, and it provides much more information about the lesion.

One may identify intracerebral hemorrhage with greater sensitivity and more quickly with CT than with radionuclide scanning. On the other hand, radionuclide scanning may show an older hematoma better than CT after resorption of extravasated blood.[4] The radionuclide scan may also be more effective in demonstrating thrombotic infarcts, especially when the perfusion deficit covers a large area of the brain.

Subdural hematomas are better seen with radionuclides, although both radionuclide and CT scanning have significant false-negative rates. CT may show the lesion better early and late in the natural evolution of the subdural hematoma, whereas the radionuclide scan may be most sensitive in the interim, at about 2 weeks, when CT scanning may be least sensitive.[4]

Radionuclide imaging is more sensitive than CT in inflammation of the brain, except for abscess identification, in which they are equivalent.[4] If the inflammatory process is less intense, less discrete, and less well organized, such as in focal herpetic encephalitis, diffuse viral encephalitis, septic emboli, and bacterial meningitis, radionuclide scanning may show the lesion more clearly than CT.

Radionuclide scanning of the brain is a safe and effective procedure. One may thereby detect 90% of meningiomas, 80 to 90% of gliomas, 70 to 80% of metastases, and 58% of infarctions. Flow studies, or radionuclide angiographic studies, are important in the diagnosis of cerebrovascular disease and provide a sensitive method for the detection of decreased cerebral perfusion, for which CT is not effective. CT scanning is more expensive, but substitution of CT for radionuclide scanning in patients with neurologic signs or symptoms is beneficial despite the cost. Radionuclide brain scanning does offer advantages in some clinical circumstances and does not require the use of contrast material. Moreover, many institutions still do not have CT scanners.

Radionuclide Cisternography

Radionuclide cisternography is performed to observe cerebrospinal fluid (CSF) dynamics and is based on the same principle as other flow studies. The radionuclide introduced into the CSF moves with that fluid, and imaging at intervals can demonstrate the movement. Blockage of the fluid excludes the radionuclide from anticipated localization in certain normal sites, and leakage allows localization in abnormal sites.

Radionuclide cisternography is a major tool in diagnosing CSF leaks and in determining the patency of CSF shunts. Cisternography is also useful in evaluating low-pressure hydrocephalus for surgical shunting, although CT scanning is better suited to this purpose in some cases.[5]

Radionuclide cisternography usually involves a lumbar intrathecal injection of ^{111}indium-DTPA and images over the brain at 4, 24, 48, and possibly 72 hours. In 4 hours, the radioactivity is usually in the basal cisterns. By 24 hours, the radionuclide is usually over the convexities, and in 48 hours, it is partly reabsorbed (Fig. 5–5). If the injection is accidentally extra-arachnoid but subdural or even epidural, the radioactivity will be seen on imaging the spine, and little or none may reach the basal cisterns. For leakage studies, imaging of the suspected site and collection of fluid for counting (CSF rhinorrhea) may provide the diagnosis.

In normal-pressure hydrocephalus, the radionuclide appears in the ventricles (ventricular reflux) in 4 hours and remains there at 24, 48, and 72 hours without moving over the convexities (stasis) (Fig.

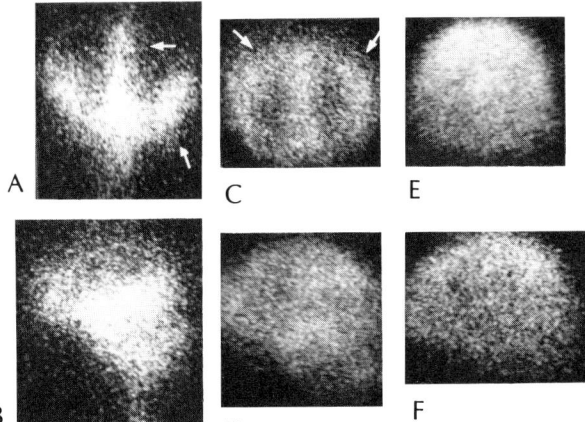

FIG. 5–5. Normal cisternogram. Anterior (A) and left lateral (B) views obtained 6 hours after intrathecal injection of ^{111}indium-DTPA into the lumbar spine; the horizontal arrow (A) points to the cisterna lamina terminalis, and the diagonal arrow (A) points to the left Sylvian cistern. Anterior (C), and left lateral (D) views obtained at 24 hours; the arrows (C) point to radioactivity in the subarachnoid space over the convexities; activity is also seen in the interhemispheric fissure. Anterior (E) and left lateral (F) views at 48 hours.

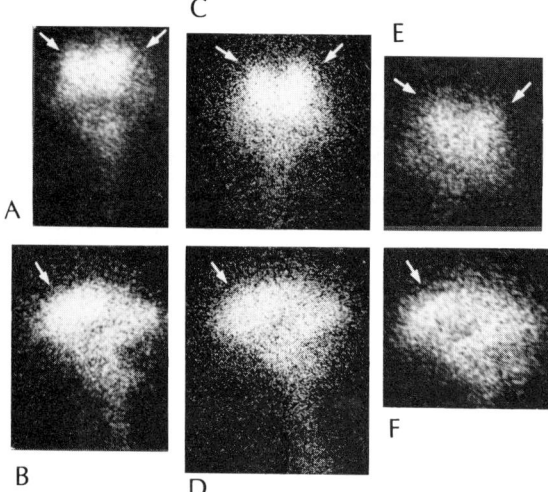

FIG. 5–6. Normal pressure hydrocephalus. Anterior (A) and left lateral (B) views obtained 6 hours after intrathecal injection of ¹¹¹indium-DTPA in the lumbar spine; the arrows point to the lateral ventricles. C and D, The same views at 24 hours. E and F, the same views obtained at 48 hours. Note that the radioactivity remains in the ventricles and does not appear over the convexities.

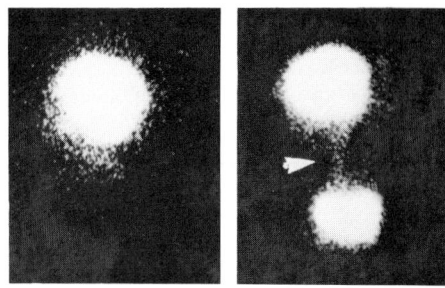

FIG. 5–7. Ventriculoperitoneal shuntogram. A, Image obtained immediately after intraventricular injection of ¹¹¹indium-DTPA. B, Image obtained an hour later, showing radioactivity in the shunt (arrow) and in the abdomen, indicating the patency of the shunt.

5–6). Whether or not the characteristic pattern is seen, however, surgical shunting may or may not be effective. Although the radionuclide may not move over the convexities, it may be absorbed from the ventricles. Measurement of this transventricular absorption may be of value. CT scanning appears to be more valuable in assessment of this disease because it can visualize dilated ventricles and also dilated subarachnoid sulci indicative of cerebral atrophy.[5] Such patients are not usually aided by shunting.

Most CSF leaks are post-traumatic. They may cause rhinorrhea, most often from leakage through the cribriform plate. Imaging in anterior and lateral projections 1, 2, 3, and 4 hours after injection is used to attempt to localize the leak. Appearance of radioactivity outside the normal subarachnoid space identifies the leak. The precise site of the leak may not be determinable, but the side of the leak and its approximate location can often be ascertained.[6]

Radionuclide cisternography may demonstrate other abnormalities such as subarachnoid blockage, arachnoid cysts, and porencephalic cysts. To demonstrate shunt patency, one injects the radionuclide into the ventricle and images the shunt (Fig. 5–7). Although it has limited applications, radionuclide cisternography may be valuable.

THYROID

Thyroid scanning is carried out to evaluate abnormalities in the size and shape of the thyroid gland and to evaluate masses, including nodules, in or near the thyroid gland. It is based on the principle that normal thyroid tissue concentrates certain radionuclides, whereas abnormal thyroid, thyroid carcinoma in the presence of normal thyroid, and nonthyroidal tissue does not.

The major use of thyroid scanning is to determine whether a thyroid nodule is likely to be malignant. Because nodule function, as characterized by concentration of radionuclide, is related to the possibility of malignancy, one must determine whether a nodule is functioning or nonfunctioning. Functioning nodules are rarely malignant. Solitary nonfunctioning nodules are malignant in 10 to 20% of the patients who have undergone operations in various series. Nonfunctioning nodules in multinodular thyroid glands are also rarely malignant. Thyroid scanning can identify a substernal mass, which causes tracheal deviation on a chest radiograph, or other masses palpated in the anterior neck. Scanning can distinguish diffuse hyperthyroidism of Graves' disease from Plummer's toxic nodular disease. If therapy with radioiodine (¹³¹I) is contemplated, scanning can help one to determine the dose. Thyroid scanning is used to aid in the diagnosis of acute thyroiditis. After total thyroidectomy for thyroid carcinoma, the technique is used to look for metastases.

Procedure and Interpretation

Thyroid scanning may be performed by oral administration of ¹²³iodine (¹²³I) or intravenous administration of ⁹⁹ᵐTc-pertechnetate. After ¹²³I administration, the scan is performed at 24 hours with a scintillation camera and pinhole collimator. At that time, a quantitative measurement of thyroid uptake can also be made as an indicator of thyroid function. If the scan is performed with ⁹⁹ᵐTc-pertechnetate, it can be carried out 15 minutes after injection. ⁹⁹ᵐTc scans provide better resolution with less radiation. Moreover, with ⁹⁹ᵐTc, the image is obtained so quickly that oblique views are feasible without much risk of the patient's moving. If an uptake measurement is desired, however, an iodine isotope must also be given, at a dose much smaller than for scanning, and the patient must return in 24 hours.

The thyroid scan is evaluated for size and position of the gland, shape of the gland, uniformity of distribution of activity, and function or nonfunction of nodules. Masses external to the thyroid are also evaluated for activity. Palpable nodules are localized in the gland by making a "marker image" with a radioactive marker held over the nodule. The normal gland has lobes about 3 to 4 cm long and 1.5 to 2 cm wide and shows uniform distribution of activity (Fig. 5–8). The isthmus is of varied size and position. A pyramidal lobe is sometimes seen connected to the upper pole of either lobe and extending medially and cephalad.

Abnormal Manifestations

NONFUNCTIONING NODULE. Such a nodule may represent a cyst, hemorrhage, or tumor. Ultrasound may help one to differentiate among these lesions (Fig. 5–9). Areas of degeneration and of acute thyroiditis may also appear as nonfunctioning portions of the thyroid gland. If scanning is carried out with ^{99m}Tc-pertechnetate, solitary nodules that seem to be functioning should be rescanned with ^{123}I. Several instances of thyroid carcinoma have been reported

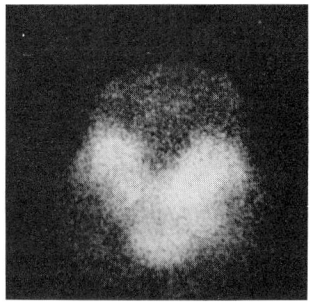

FIG. 5–10. Chronic thyroiditis. Anterior view showing an enlarged thyroid gland with irregular distribution of activity characteristic of this entity.

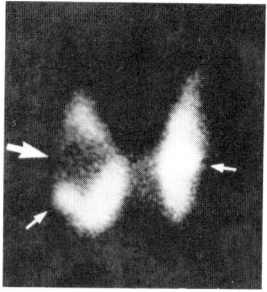

FIG. 5–11. Multinodular goiter. Anterior view showing an enlarged thyroid gland with a large, "cold," nonfunctioning nodule in the right lobe (large arrow) and "warm," functioning nodules in both lobes (small arrows).

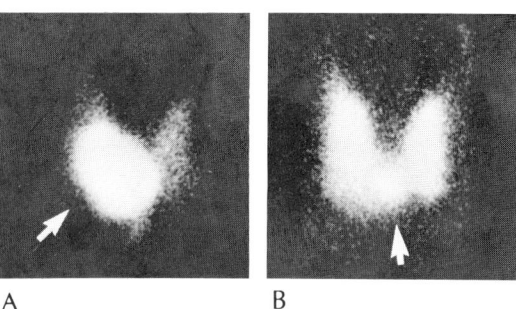

A   B

FIG. 5–12. Hot autonomous thyroid nodule. A, Anterior view showing a large, "hot" nodule (arrow) in the right lobe and isthmus; the suppressed normal gland is seen faintly at the edges of the nodule. B, The same patient, 3 months after a large therapeutic dose of ^{131}iodine; a small residual part of the nodule is seen in the isthmus (arrow), and the normal gland has resumed full activity.

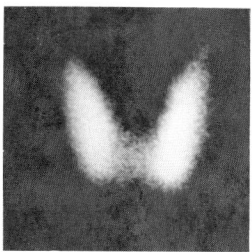

FIG. 5–8. Normal thyroid scan. Anterior view obtained 15 min after intravenous injection of ^{99m}technetium-pertechnetate. Both lobes and isthmus are visualized.

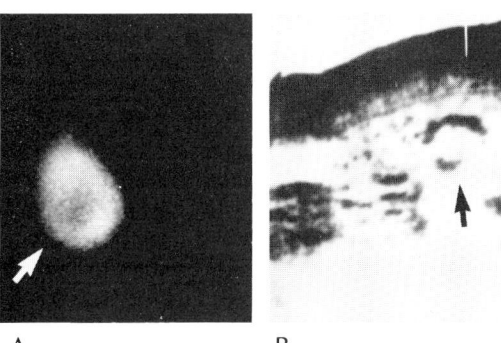

A   B

FIG. 5–9. Thyroid cyst. A, Radionuclide scan of right thyroid lobe only; the left lobe had been surgically removed. The "cold" area (arrow) is a cyst, as demonstrated on the ultrasonogram (B, arrow).

in which the lesion trapped ^{99m}Tc at 15 min but did not retain ^{123}I at 24 hours.

IODINE UPTAKE AND SERUM THYROXINE. The thyroid uptake of iodine and serum thyroid hormone levels may be helpful in interpreting the scan. A tender gland with low iodine uptake, nonfunctioning areas on the scan, and an elevated serum thyroxine (T-4) level is likely to represent acute thyroiditis. A large, irregular gland with normal or high uptake,

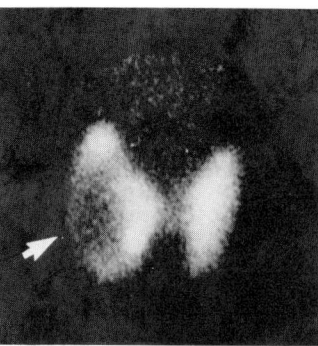

FIG. 5–13. Carcinoma of the thyroid. Anterior view showing a "cold" nodule (arrow) in the right thyroid lobe, which was a papillary adenocarcinoma of the thyroid.

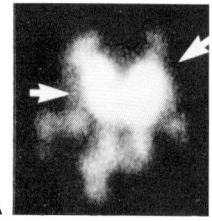 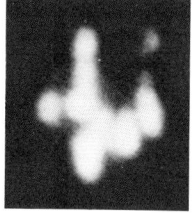

A B

FIG. 5–14. Metastatic thyroid carcinoma. A, Anterior view showing residual thyroid tissue (arrows) 6 weeks after surgical treatment for a follicular adenocarcinoma of the thyroid with lymph node metastases; visible at the periphery of the residual thyroid are metastatic lesions, which are unusual when significant thyroid tissue remains. B, The same view 3 months after ablation by ^{131}iodine of the residual normal thyroid tissue, showing uptake of the radioisotope by the metastases.

irregular distribution of radioactivity, and a low serum T-4 level is likely to represent chronic thyroiditis (Fig. 5–10). Multinodular glands are common and may have both functioning and nonfunctioning nodules (Fig. 5–11). Patients with Graves' disease usually have a large thyroid gland with uniform activity, high thyroid uptake, and a high T-4 level. Those with Plummer's disease also have a large gland with high uptake and a high T-4 level, but one will see one or more "hot" nodules and areas of suppressed uptake, giving the scan an irregular appearance (Fig. 5–12). In patients with thyroid carcinoma, the scan may appear normal, it may show a small, "cold" nodule, or it may show a nonfunctioning area of varying size (Fig. 5–13). Metastatic lesions rarely pick up radioactivity as long as a significant portion of functioning gland is present (Fig. 5–14).

METASTATIC LESIONS. In thyroid carcinoma, after operations other than total thyroidectomy, scanning shows only residual functioning tissue. After total thyroidectomy, metastatic lesions may pick up sufficient radioactivity to be visualized, whether in lymph nodes in the neck, in the lungs, or in bone. To increase the likelihood of such observation, patients who have undergone total thyroidectomy are given a large scanning dose of ^{131}I (5 to 10 mCi), and the whole body is scanned at 48 to 72 hours. If small bits of thyroid tissue remain in the thyroid bed or if metastatic lesions are seen, a therapeutic dose of ^{131}I (100 to 200 mCi) is usually given, and the patient is rescanned at 3 to 6 months. Prior to such scanning for metastases, the patient must discontinue thyroid replacement medication for 4 to 6 weeks to ensure maximum stimulation of the lesions to pick up radioactivity.

Screening of Persons at Risk for Cancer

Persons exposed to external X radiation of the neck in childhood have an increased incidence of thyroid carcinoma. Thyroid scanning of these individuals is recommended, to detect thyroid abnormalities that may require further investigation. The incidence of carcinoma in these patients has been reported to be 3 to 9%.[7] Because of the long latent period in thyroid carcinoma of 15 to 30 years, it is not known how long these patients should continue to be observed.

LUNG

Lung scanning, or V/Q (ventilation-perfusion) study of the lungs, is used to diagnose pulmonary emboli. Prior to lung operations, it may also be helpful. Relative quantitation of perfusion of each lung can be measured, to estimate the risk of pneumonectomy.[8]

The ventilation portion of the study is based on the distribution throughout the pulmonary alveoli of an inhaled radioactive gas and its clearance during subsequent breathing of air, or the distribution throughout the pulmonary alveoli of an inhaled radioactive aerosol. The perfusion portion of the study is based on the blockage of flow of radioactive albumin particles to the capillary bed by an embolus. The patent vessels of the lung permit flow of the labeled particles to their respective capillary beds, where they temporarily lodge and provide an image of the perfused portions of the lung.

Procedure for and Interpretation of Ventilation-Perfusion Study

The ventilation study using radioactive gas is performed by having the patient inhale a quantity of ^{133}xenon (^{133}Xe). Posterior images are obtained when the patient has taken a deep breath, after rebreathing the radioactive gas for 4 minutes to obtain equilibrium, and then at 45-sec intervals while breathing room air for 4 to 5 min to wash out the ^{133}Xe. The use of ^{99m}Tc-DTPA aerosol for ventilation scanning has become more common. The patient inhales the tiny radioactive monodisperse aerosol particles produced by a small atomizer, and images can then be obtained in multiple views. The ^{133}Xe ventilation scan has the advantage of providing information during the washout phase that is unavailable when using aerosols. The ^{99m}Tc-DTPA aerosol ventilation study has the advantage of providing multiple views not available when using ^{133}Xe.

The perfusion study is performed by intravenous injection of ^{99m}Tc-albumin macroaggregates or microspheres and by imaging in multiple views.

Interpretation of the V/Q study requires a chest radiograph obtained within a few hours of the study. Any abnormality seen on the chest radiograph may produce a perfusion defect. In the normal ventilation study, ^{133}Xe is uniformly distributed throughout both lungs on inspiration and at equilibrium and is uniformly cleared from both lungs during the washout phase (Fig. 5–15). Defects on the ventilation study indicate airway obstruction, which may be seen on any or all of the images. In obstructive lung disease, the ^{133}Xe fails to enter involved regions of the lung during the inspiratory phase, diffuses into those regions during equilibrium, and remains in those areas during the washout phase (Fig. 5–16). Compression, such as from pleural effusion, and consolidation such as from pneumonia or infarct, of portions of the lung or tumors or other masses restrict ^{133}Xe through all the ventilation images. Pulmonary emboli do not produce ventilation defects.

In the normal perfusion scan, radioactivity is uniform throughout both lung fields (see Fig. 5–15). Defects on the perfusion study may or may not match ventilation defects and chest radiography abnormalities. If the perfusion scan is entirely normal or if it shows small peripheral defects or only abnormalities that match ventilation defects, the patient probably (90 to 95%) does not have pulmonary emboli. If the perfusion scan shows defects that conform to anatomic lobes or segments of the lung, and if these are not matched by ventilation defects or chest radiograph abnormalities, the patient probably (80 to 90%) has pulmonary emboli (Fig. 5–17). Between these interpretations is a range of diagnostic uncertainty that may require pulmonary angiography. In some instances, the clinical and laboratory information, in conjunction with a V/Q study providing an intermediate probability of a pulmonary embolus, may help one to make the decision. In other situations, the ventilation study demonstrates so much chronic disease that the diagnostic probability of pulmonary embolism cannot be determined, and pulmonary angiography is necessary.

Repeat perfusion scans can be helpful in verifying the impression of pulmonary emboli. Disappearance of the defects suggests pulmonary embolism (Fig. 5–17E, F). Significant resolution can occur in 48 to 72 hours and is almost always apparent in 7 to 10 days. Rapid change can be a problem, however. If the first V/Q study is not obtained for 2 to 3 days after the onset of pulmonary embolism, the diagnosis may be missed because the pattern may no longer be characteristic. The presence of a chest radiograph abnormality does not necessarily render the perfusion scan useless. When perfusion defects are much larger than chest film abnormalities indicative of infiltrates, atelectasis, or effusion, an absence of matching ventilation defects has frequently been associated with angiographically confirmed pulmonary emboli. On the other hand, when perfusion defects are much smaller than the radiographic abnormalities, the incidence of pulmonary emboli is low.

The V/Q study, or at least the ventilation portion, requires co-operation from the patient that is not always possible. The study has limited usefulness

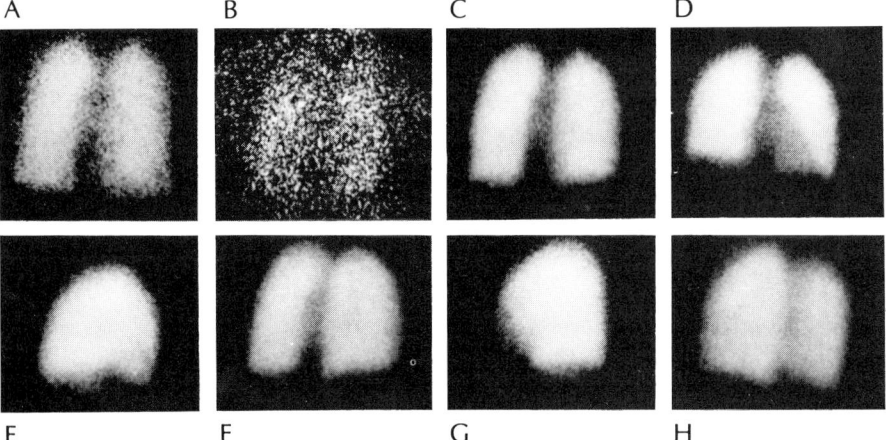

FIG. 5–15. Normal V/Q lung scan. Posterior inspiratory *(A)* and posterior late washout *(B)* images of the ventilation study and posterior *(C)* and anterior *(D)* views of the perfusion study; note the uniform distribution of ^{133}xenon on inspiration and the uniform clearance on washout. Right lateral *(E)*, right posterior oblique *(F)*, left lateral *(G)*, and left posterior oblique *(H)* views of the perfusion study; note the uniform distribution of activity and smooth edges of the images.

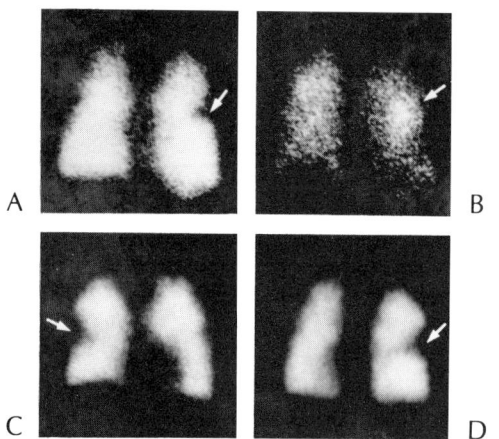

FIG. 5–16. Obstructive pulmonary disease. Posterior inspiratory (A) and late washout (B) views of the ventilation study; note the defect in the right lung (arrows), where ^{133}xenon diffusion is obstructed. This defect fills in on equilibrium (not shown) and remains at the site during the washout phase. Anterior (C) and posterior (D) views of the perfusion study, showing the matching abnormality (arrows).

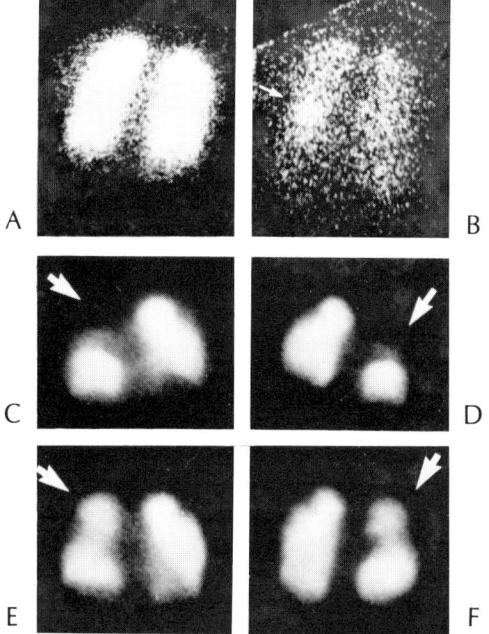

FIG. 5–17. Multiple pulmonary emboli. Posterior inspiratory (A) and late washout (B) views of the ventilation study; the small area of ^{133}xenon hangup (arrow) represents air trapping in the left lung, but the remainder of the ventilation is normal. C and D, The perfusion scan carried out at the same time (C, anterior view; D, posterior view); arrows point to the large perfusion defect representing most of the right lung. E and F, Partial resolution of the embolization a week later.

without the ventilation portion, however. The V/Q study is not difficult to perform, it provides much valuable information, and it often obviates the need for an invasive pulmonary angiogram.

Gallium Scanning

One other type of lung scanning that has proved to be of value uses ^{67}gallium (^{67}Ga).[10] This study relies on ^{67}Ga uptake by areas of infection, inflammation, and neoplasm (Fig. 5–18). Gallium scanning can distinguish active tuberculosis, with a 97% sensitivity rate. Patients with inactive tuberculosis do not have gallium uptake. From 61 to 97% of patients with active sarcoidosis show gallium uptake in pulmonary parenchyma or hilum, but many patients with inactive sarcoidosis also show gallium accumulation; however, a normal scan suggests the absence of disease. The gallium scan can differentiate between pneumonia, which takes up the isotope, and pulmonary infarcts, which do not, except infarcts from septic emboli. Many conditions cause diffuse pulmonary uptake of ^{67}Ga, including Pneumocystis carinii infection, bleomycin therapy, cyclophosphamide therapy, vascular talc granulomatosis in drug addicts, radiation therapy to the lungs, interstitial lung disease, and pneumoconiosis. Gallium scanning for tumor detection has not lived up to its original promise. Although ^{67}Ga scans are positive in 85% of patients with primary lung cancers, the use of the scan to detect mediastinal or hilar involvement for staging purposes is not reliable. In one series, sensitivity was only 55%. Gallium has been used successfully to detect sites of tumor in-

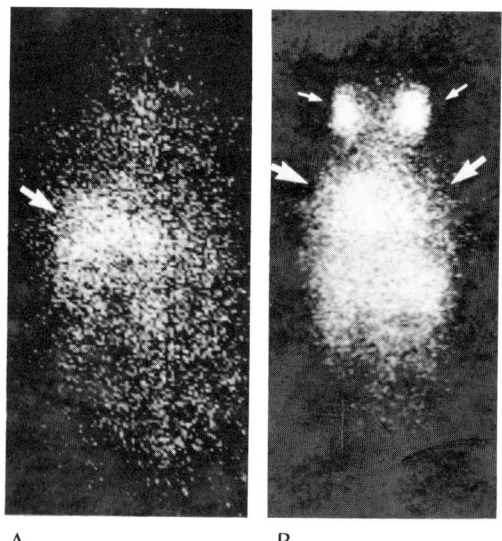

FIG. 5–18. Gallium scan for sarcoidosis. A, Normal whole-body gallium scan at 24 hours; the arrow points to normal uptake by the liver. B, Abnormal uptake in the lungs (large arrows) and in the parotid glands (small arrows) in a patient with sarcoidosis.

volvement in patients with lymphoma, particularly Hodgkin's disease and histiocytic lymphoma; sensitivity for thoracic and mediastinal involvement was 78 to 100%, with a specificity of 84 to 94%.

LIVER

Liver scanning, carried out to detect and to monitor hepatic disease, is based on the uptake of radioactive colloid by functioning reticuloendothelial cells distributed throughout normal liver tissue. Tumors, cysts, abscesses, infiltrating fat, and fibrous tissue do not contain these cells and appear as "cold" areas in the liver. Alterations in the blood flow through the liver may reduce the function of the reticuloendothelial cells or may impair delivery of the radioactive colloid by the circulation, with consequent, irregular patterns on imaging. Reduced uptake of radioactive colloid in the liver may result in increased uptake in the spleen and bone marrow.

The major use of liver scanning is in the detection of metastatic disease. The sensitivity for this purpose is 85 to 95%, with a specificity of 75 to 85%.[11] Scanning is done for staging purposes and for evaluation of hepatomegaly. In the patient with known cancer, the scan, if negative, may be a control for follow-up studies and, if positive, may be useful for monitoring therapy. The liver scan is also used to detect lacerations or hematoma following trauma, abscesses with evidence of sepsis, hepatoma in the cirrhotic patient, and benign tumors. The liver scan is helpful in the investigation of hepatomegaly. It may either verify or contradict the clinical finding. Often, the position or shape of the liver leads to a misinterpretation of size on physical examination. Although hepatomegaly may be due to focal lesions, it is usually caused by diffuse hepatic disease. The liver scan is sensitive, but it is also nonspecific in identifying diffuse hepatic disease. Cirrhosis is the most common cause of hepatomegaly, but often it cannot be distinguished from passive congestion, hepatitis, lymphoma, or fatty infiltration. The accompanying clinical and laboratory findings help one to establish the proper diagnosis. The liver scan may enable the physician to determine the stage and severity of the disease process.

Procedure

The liver scan is performed by intravenous injection of 99mTc-sulfur colloid and by imaging 15 to 20 min later. Multiple views are obtained, some of which include the spleen and vertebral bone marrow. A marker film shows the position of the costal margin and a centimeter scale to more accurately estimate the dimensions of the liver and spleen.

Interpretation

The scan interpretation includes evaluation of the size, shape, and position of the liver and spleen,

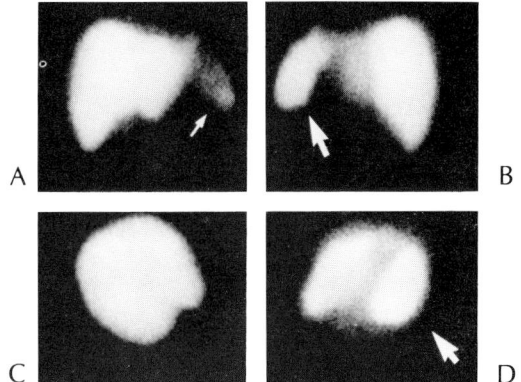

FIG. 5–19. Normal liver-spleen scan. Anterior (A), posterior (B), right lateral (C), and left lateral (D) views of the liver and spleen. The arrows point to the spleen, which appears more active than the liver in D because of its proximity to the scintillation camera.

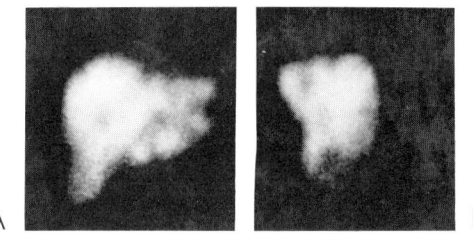

FIG. 5–20. Metastatic liver disease. Anterior (A) and right lateral (B) views of the liver in a patient with carcinoma of the breast. The "cold" areas represent multiple metastatic lesions.

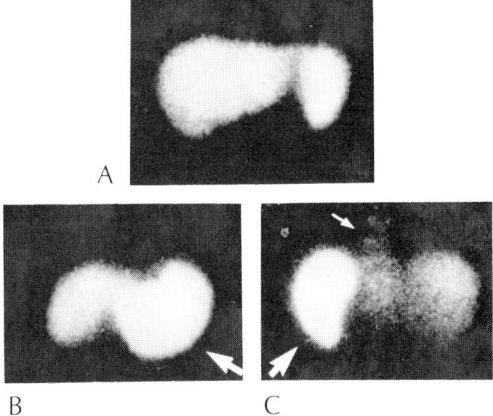

FIG. 5–21. Cirrhosis of the liver. A, Anterior view showing a liver with reduced activity and an enlarged spleen with increased activity. The same features are illustrated in the left lateral (B) and posterior (C) views. The large arrows (B and C) point to the spleen; the small arrow (C) points to radioactivity in the vertebral bone marrow. Reduced liver uptake results in increased uptake in the spleen and bone marrow.

estimation of the uniformity of distribution of the radioactivity, and a search for focal lesions (Fig. 5–19). Also noted is the relative distribution of radioactivity among liver, spleen, and bone marrow. Focal lesions may be single or multiple, round, linear or irregular, and sharply or poorly defined. Dilated biliary ducts, prominent porta hepatis, gallbladder fossa, breasts, ribs, kidneys, and ascites may all produce defects that need to be distinguished from pathologic space-occupying lesions. Metastases from some primary tumors may be characteristic (Fig. 5–20). Metastases from colorectal and renal cell carcinoma are usually well-defined focal lesions, whereas metastases from lung and breast carcinoma are often small and widespread, appearing as an irregular distribution of radioactivity in the liver. Cysts and abscesses cannot be distinguished from tumors on the basis of the liver scan alone. Diffuse disease has few differentiating characteristics. Cirrhosis usually is characterized by an enlarged liver and spleen; the spleen may have greater uptake of radioactivity than the liver, and the uptake of colloid in the vertebral bone marrow may be significant (Fig. 5–21). In patients with progressive disease, the liver may become smaller and may take up less radioactivity. The distribution in the liver may be either mottled or irregular in appearance.

Comparison with Other Techniques

Other imaging techniques may be helpful in the diagnosis of liver disease. Ultrasound can distinguish the nature of a focal lesion and enables one to identify it as a cyst, an abscess, or a tumor.[12] CT scanning can do the same and is comparable to radionuclide scanning in the detection of focal lesions. One can detect smaller lesions that are more centrally located with CT scanning, but one cannot see lesions of isodensity with the liver. When used together, CT and radionuclide scanning miss few lesions.[13]

BILIARY TRACT

The purpose of biliary tract scanning is to determine the patency of various portions of the biliary system. It is based on the uptake and excretion of a radiopharmaceutical agent by the polygonal cells of the liver. The radionuclide then moves through hepatic ducts to the common hepatic duct, through the cystic duct, to the gallbladder, and through the common duct to the duodenum. Sequential imaging thereby enables one to visualize the integrity of the system, and obstruction is manifested by failure of the radioactivity to appear distally.

The major use of biliary tract scanning is in the diagnosis of acute cholecystitis, as indicated by obstruction of the cystic duct. The overall accuracy of diagnosis in a large series was 97.6%.[14] The false-positive rate was 0.6%, and the false-negative rate was 4.8%. The study has also been used to diagnose acute common bile duct obstruction, patency of and leakage from biliary-enteric anastomoses, and functional ampullary stenosis. Radionuclide scanning is not helpful in the diagnosis of chronic cholecystitis and does not indicate the cause of obstructive jaundice.

Procedure

The study is performed by intravenous injection of ^{99m}Tc-di-isopropyl iminodiacetate (DISIDA) or other IDA analog and imaging at 5, 15, 30, 60 and 240 min in the anterior and, occasionally, in the right lateral and left anterior oblique views. It is important that the patient fast for at least 2 and preferably 4 hours prior to the test. Images can be obtained in the jaundiced patient, even with serum bilirubin levels of 20 to 30 mg/100 ml.

Interpretation

The scan interpretation is based on visualization of the gallbladder (Fig. 5–22). If the gallbladder is seen within 60 min, the cystic duct will be patent, and the patient will not have acute cholecystitis. An occasional patient with acute acalculous cholecystitis has a normal DISIDA scan. If the gallbladder is not visualized in 60 min but appears by 240 min, the patient probably has chronic cholecystitis, although 18% of patients with this pattern have acute disease. If the gallbladder is not visualized in 240 min, despite common duct and duodenal visualization, the patient will have cystic duct obstruction and acute cholecystitis (98%) (Fig. 5–23). If hepatic

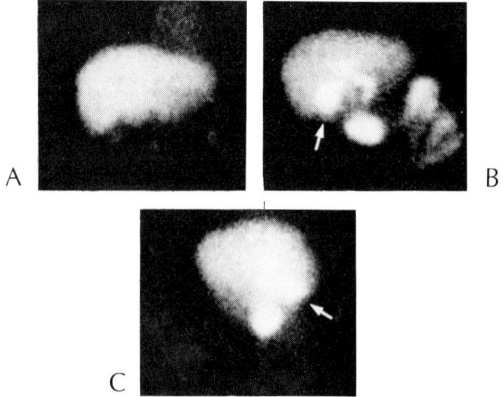

FIG. 5–22. Normal biliary scan. Anterior views at 5 min (A) and at 60 min (B) and a right lateral view at 60 min (C) after intravenous injection of DISIDA. The 5-min image shows the liver only because the parenchymal cells concentrate the contrast agent. The 60-min images (B and C) show the gallbladder (arrows), the common duct to the right of the gallbladder, and radioactivity in the duodenum, inferior to the common duct.

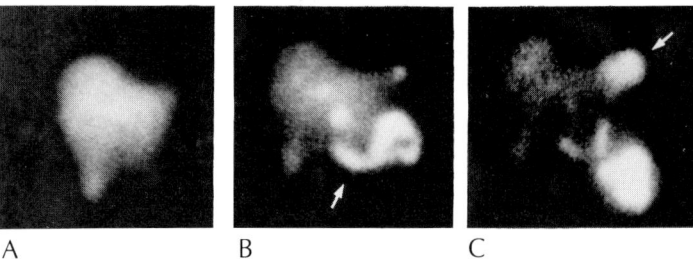

FIG. 5–23. Acute cholecystitis. Anterior views of the biliary system at 5 min *(A)*, 60 min *(B)*, and 4 hours *(C)* after intravenous injection of DISIDA. Radioactivity is seen in hepatic and common ducts and in the intestinal tract (*B*, arrow). Activity is also seen in the stomach (*C*, arrow) because of retrograde movement from the duodenum. That the gallbladder is not visualized indicates obstruction of the cystic duct.

uptake is adequate but no ducts, gallbladder, or duodenum are seen, common duct obstruction will be suggested, and one will not be able to evaluate cystic duct patency. When the ducts and gallbladder are visualized but no radioactivity is noted in the duodenum, functional common bile duct obstruction will usually be present. The administration of intravenous cholecystokinin may overcome this problem, depending on the severity of the ampullitis.

Comparison with Other Techniques

Other imaging methods may be helpful in evaluating chronic cholecystitis, but none have the sensitivity and specificity of DISIDA scanning in patients with acute cholecystitis.[15] The DISIDA scan may also be useful in the assessment of defects in the liver scan, which may represent gallbladder fossa, prominent porta hepatis, or dilated bile ducts.

KIDNEYS

Kidney scanning is performed to assess renal morphologic features and function, obstructive uropathy, and renovascular disease. Scanning is based on the concentration and excretion, by renal filtration and tubular mechanisms, of radiopharmaceutical agents that move through the collecting system, renal pelves, ureters, and bladder at convenient rates for imaging. Blood-flow images use agents that can be imaged during the first pass through the kidneys. Function and excretion images use agents that are rapidly concentrated and excreted. Obstruction is identified by the failure of radioactivity to pass from the superior to the inferior portions of the tract. Morphologic information is provided by agents that concentrate in the kidneys and remain long enough to allow background clearance for optimal imaging.

The major use of kidney scanning is for evaluation of obstruction. Although radionuclide scans have less resolution and provide less anatomic information than corresponding radiographic studies of the kidney, they are a safe and convenient way to assess obstructive uropathy. Scans not only show the location and degree of obstruction, but also they indicate the effect of the obstruction on renal function. Kidney scanning is used to evaluate suspected renal masses and gross effects on renal blood flow. In recent years, renal scans have been used extensively to assess kidney transplants, to identify acute tubular necrosis, rejection, and anatomic integrity.[16]

Procedure and Interpretation

Information on renal blood flow or on renal morphologic features is provided by the intravenous injection of ^{99m}Tc-glucoheptonate or ^{99m}Tc-dimercaptosuccinate. Immediately after injection, rapid sequential images of the renal area are obtained for blood-flow information. Delayed static images at 2 or more hours show renal morphologic features. When information on renal function or obstruction is required, the scan is performed by intravenous injection of ^{131}I-iodohippurate or ^{99m}Tc-DTPA. Images are made at 3-min intervals for 24 min in the supine position and then once again when the patient has been in the upright position for 5 min. Kidney-transplant patients receive ^{99m}Tc-pertechnetate for blood-flow information and ^{131}I-iodohippurate for tests of function and excretion. Images are obtained immediately for blood flow and at 4-min intervals up to 20 min for function and excretion determinations.

Renal blood flow on the scan is compared to the appearance of the abdominal aorta (Fig. 5–24). Poor aortic flow caused by an injection that does not produce an adequate bolus, by cardiac failure, or by aortic aneurysm must be recognized, to prevent misinterpretation of the scan. In patients with renal transplants, the flow study is recorded on computer, and curves of activity from areas of interest in the aorta and the transplant are generated. A high aortic peak, followed in 3 to 5 sec by an even higher renal peak, is normal. Delayed images show morphologic kidney features (Fig. 5–24). These images can be compared with the flow study, to determine whether renal masses are vascular, such as in renal column hypertrophy or tumors, or avascular, such as in cysts or abscesses or avascular tumors. The size, shape, and position of the kidneys, and the

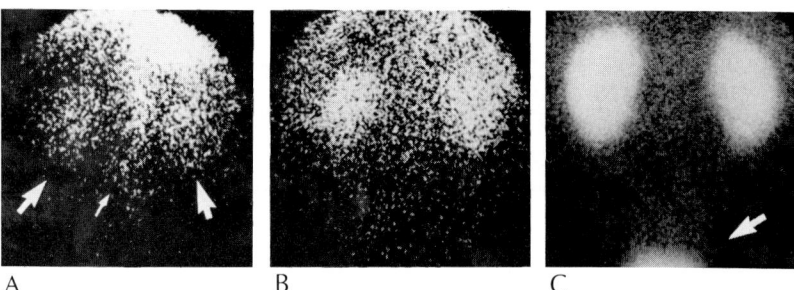

FIG. 5-24. Normal renal flow and scan. Posterior views obtained seconds (A), minutes (B), and hours (C) after intravenous injection of 99mtechnetium-glucoheptonate. A, The large arrows point to the kidneys, and the small arrow points to the abdominal aorta. The arrow in C points to the bladder.

presence of a horseshoe kidney, may be determined in the delayed images with 99mTc-glucoheptonate or dimercaptosuccinic acid.

A normal hippuran study shows a peak concentration of radioactivity in the first or second 3-min image and then gradual clearance bilaterally with little or no activity remaining in the 21- to 24-min image (Fig. 5-25). If a small amount of activity remains in the renal pelvis at 24 min, it may be due to drainage inhibition by the patient's position, and it should clear after 5 min in the upright position. Retention of radioactivity in either renal pelvis at 24 min that does not clear when the patient is upright indicates obstruction (Fig. 5-26). Sometimes, obstruction is shown by a visualized dilated ureter, and the site of a stone may be indicated. Longstanding obstruction may result in parenchymal renal damage and progressive decline in renal concentration of radionuclide; however, this finding is not completely predictive of a return of function following decompression.[17]

Patients with chronic renal disease show a pattern of poor concentration by both kidneys, no peak concentration, and no evidence of excretion. Concentration of the radionuclide is so slow that the excretion is not visualized. Quantitation of radioactivity over the kidneys produces a low, flat curve. Hepatorenal syndrome, renal cortical necrosis, and renal arterial occlusion show an extreme reduction of renal blood flow and poor-to-absent hippuran uptake.

Use in Kidney Transplantation

In the patient with a kidney transplant, activity does not usually peak early, but a kidney-to-background-radioactivity ratio is calculated on the computer for the 1- to 4-min image as a measure of function (Fig. 5-27). Ratios of 5:1 and above are satisfactory. Excretion by the transplanted kidney is measured by the bladder-to-background-radioactivity ratio in the 16- to 20 min image. Ratios of 10:1 or better are satisfactory. Acute tubular necrosis has a characteristic pattern of high concentration of the radionuclide, but absence of any excretion. This pattern may be difficult to distinguish from obstruction in some cases, but ultrasound may assist in differentiating between these conditions. Rejection of the transplant is usually characterized by poor blood flow to the transplant and poor radionuclide concentration and excretion. Consecutive studies may produce an identifiable pattern.

Gallium Scanning

Kidney scanning with 67Ga is another procedure that has proved to be of value. This study is performed by the intravenous injection of 67Ga and by imaging over the kidneys at 24 and 48 hours. Inflammatory disease of the kidneys results in uptake of gallium (Fig. 5-28). Acute interstitial nephritis

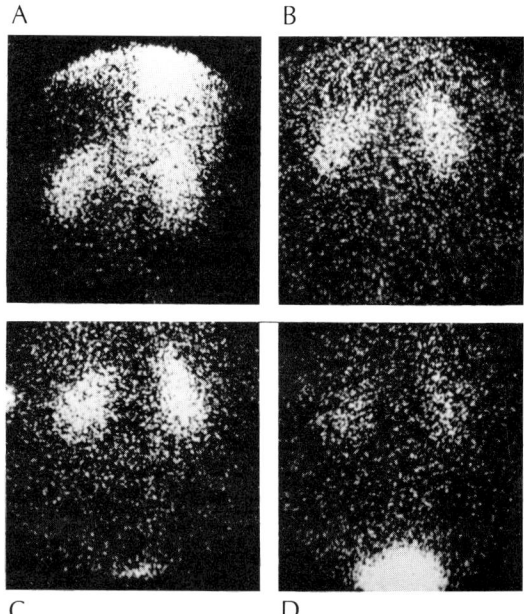

FIG. 5-25. Normal hippuran renogram. A, A frame from the flow study. Posterior views obtained 0 to 3 min (B), 3 to 6 min (C), and 21 to 24 min (D) after intravenous injection of 131iodine-iodohippurate. Normally, activity peaks at about 3 to 6 min and is almost completely cleared at 21 to 24 min. The bladder is seen at the bottom of both C and D.

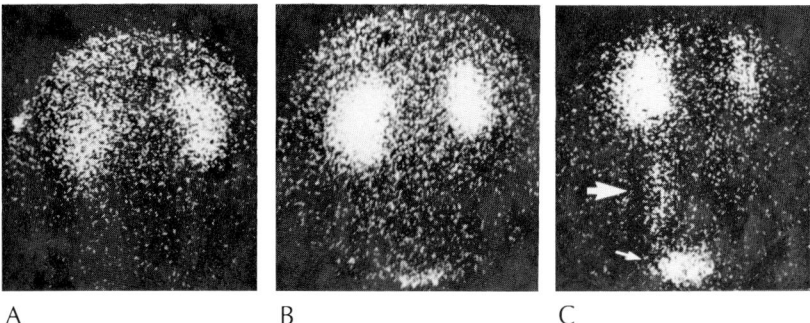

FIG. 5–26. Ureteral obstruction. Posterior views 0 to 3 min *(A)*, 3 to 6 min *(B)*, and 21 to 24 min *(C)* after intravenous injection of ^{131}iodine-iodohippurate. Concentration in both kidneys is normal in *A* and *B* images, but retention of radioactivity is seen in the left renal pelvis and the left ureter in *C* (large arrow); the small arrow in *C* points to the bladder.

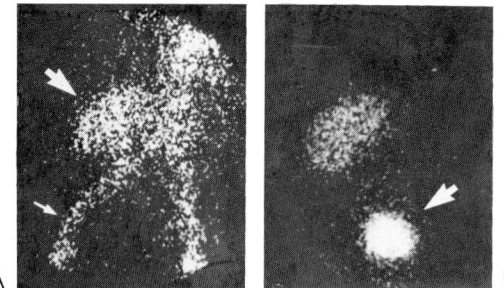

FIG. 5–27. Transplant scan. *A,* Anterior view obtained seconds after intravenous injection of ^{99m}technetium-pertechnetate showing flow in the abdominal aorta and iliac vessels. The small arrow points to right iliac artery, and the large arrow points to the perfused transplanted kidney. *B,* A similar view 20 min after intravenous injection of ^{131}iodine-iodohippurate showing kidney transplant uptake and excretion; the arrow points to radioactivity in the bladder.

causes a diffuse, intense renal uptake of gallium that can be used to differentiate this condition from acute tubular necrosis.[18] Gallium scanning may also be useful in the detection of acute pyelonephritis; however, it is difficult to distinguish acute pyelonephritis from perinephric abscess. The use of ^{99m}Tc-glucoheptonate delayed images to show typical cortical abnormalities, such as a striated or "flare" pattern of defects in the cortex radiating from the pelvicalyceal structures toward the periphery, may provide the additional specificity needed to diagnose acute pyelonephritis.[19]

BONES

Bone scanning can enable one to detect and to monitor bone and joint disease. The technique is based on adsorption of radionuclide on bone crystal surfaces or bone collagen sites, particularly where active osteoblastic activity is in progress. Such adsorption also depends on blood flow to an area and possibly on calcium concentration in soft tissue deposition. The bones normally pick up a certain amount

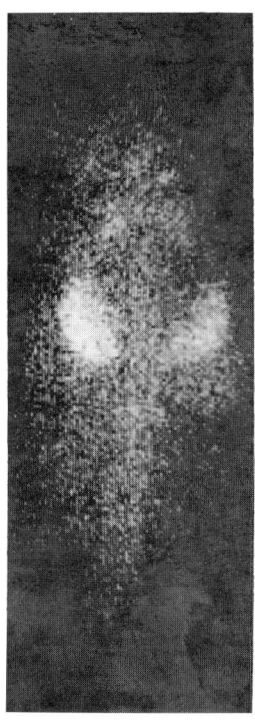

FIG. 5–28. Glomerulonephritis. This whole-body posterior image was obtained 24 hours after intravenous injection of ^{67}gallium-citrate. The scan shows increased uptake in the kidneys because of the presence of inflammatory cells.

of the radionuclide, but abnormal areas of increased bone turnover have a much higher concentration.

Bone scanning is used primarily for the detection of metastatic disease. It is more valuable in cancer metastases with a preference for bone, such as from tumors of the breast (50 to 85%), prostate (50 to 70%), Hodgkin's disease (50 to 70%), lung (30 to 50%), and kidney (30 to 50%).[20] The yield of positive results in the early stages of these cancers may be low, but the bone scan is valuable as a baseline study. Bone scanning is also used to identify primary bone tumors, benign bone lesions, osteomyelitis, Paget's disease of bone, fractures, and joint disease that tends to involve bone.[21] Although bone scanning is sensitive, it is nonspecific and requires inspection of bone and joint radiographs for increased specificity. In searching for metastatic disease, one should perform a bone scan first, to determine which bone radiographs are needed.

Procedure and Interpretation

Bone scanning is performed by the intravenous injection of ^{99m}Tc-methylenediphosphonate (MDP) and by whole body imaging at 2 hours. For magnification and greater detail, images of local areas may be obtained using a scintillation camera and a high-sensitivity or a pinhole collimator. If determinations of blood flow and vascularity of the area are also needed, such as in patients with osteomyelitis or periarticular calcification, a "triple-phase" study should be done. This examination includes imaging of the first pass of blood flow through the area, of the blood pool 1 to 2 min after appearance of the flow, and of the bone-joint uptake at 2 hours.

Bone scan interpretation involves comparison of areas of abnormal uptake on the scan with recent radiographs of the same area. The normal bone scan shows increased uptake of radioactivity in the facial area, sternum, tips of the scapulae, spine, and sacroiliac joints (Fig. 5–29). Scans of children's bones also show increased uptake in active epiphyseal bone-growth centers such as knees, ankles, elbows, and wrists. Most abnormalities result in increased uptake, but some lesions, such as multiple myeloma, irradiated bone, neuroblastoma metastases, and bone infarcts, may produce areas of decreased activity on bone scanning. Although the bone scan has limited specificity, the number, character, and location of the abnormalities may help one to identify the cause. Multiple, irregular lesions of intense activity scattered throughout the skeleton have a high probability of being metastases (Fig. 5–30). Metastases are most often found in the vertebrae (39%), ribs and sternum (28%), and pelvis (12%).

Abnormal Manifestations

METASTATIC LESIONS. Routine bone scanning for staging and follow-up is recommended for patients with some cancers.[20] Although in stage I or II breast cancer, only 2% of patients are likely to have metastases, 28% of those with stage III disease have bone metastases at the time of initial treatment. A preoperative scan is recommended. If normal, the scan serves as a baseline study, bone scans should be repeated every 6 months. In patients with stage I or II prostatic cancer, only 7% have bone metastases, but 18% of those with stage III disease have

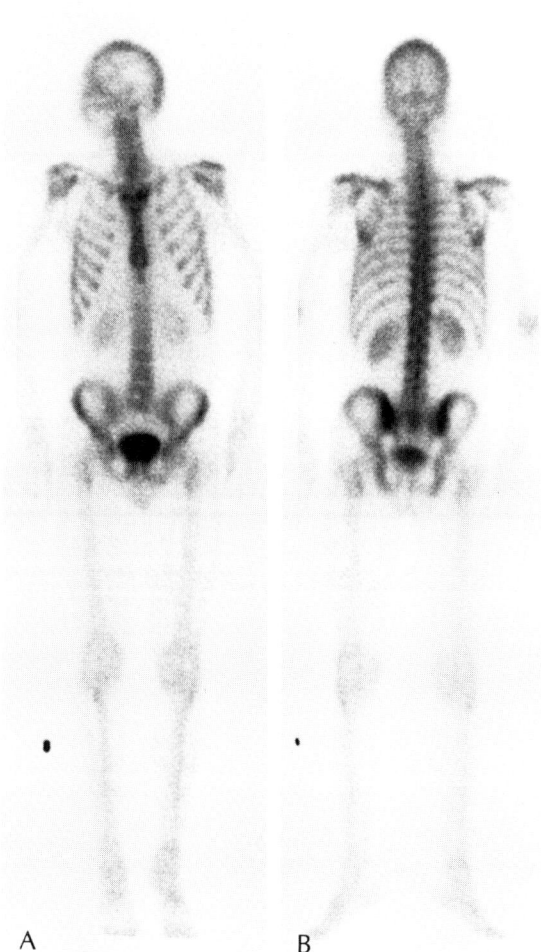

FIG. 5–29. Normal bone scan. Anterior *(A)* and posterior *(B)* whole-body views obtained 2 hours after intravenous injection of ^{99m}technetium-methylenedisphonate. Besides the bony structures, the kidneys and bladder are visualized because of the renal excretion of the agent.

such lesions. Preoperative scanning is recommended because it affects the choice of therapy. Follow-up scans are an objective measure of remission of the disease. In patients with osteogenic sarcoma, the bone scan is a guide to excision and an indicator of distant metastases. Fifty percent of these patients develop lung metastases in the first year, which can be visualized on the bone scan. Furthermore, 15% develop bone metastases in the absence of or prior to lung metastases. In patients with lung cancer, renal cancer, Ewing's sarcoma, and neuroblastoma, bone scanning for staging is considered important. In those with gastrointestinal tract, gynecologic, and bladder cancers, however, bone scanning is only recommended when one suspects the presence of bone metastases because the

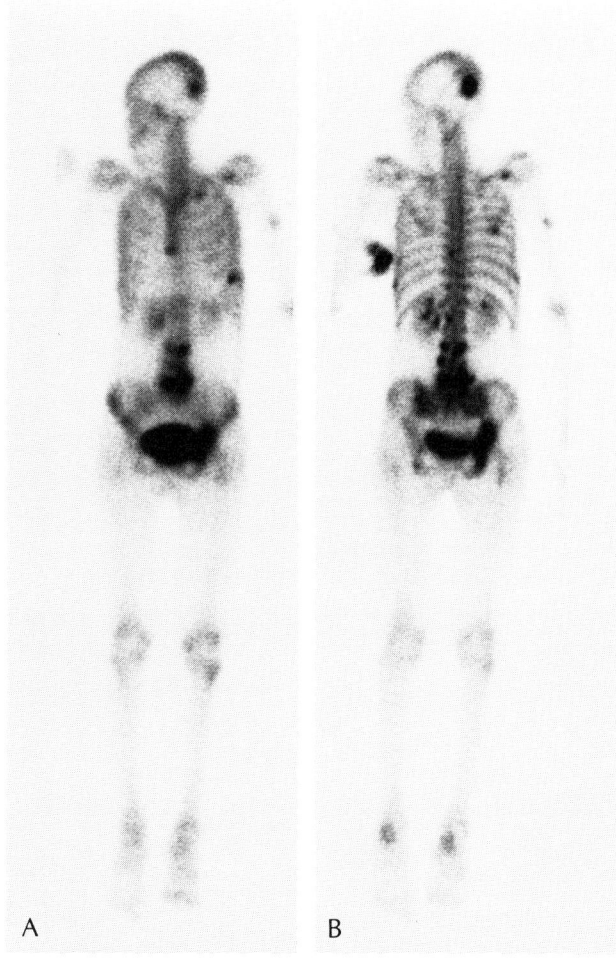

FIG. 5-30. Metastatic bone disease. Anterior (A) and posterior (B) whole-body views showing "hot spots" in the skull, left humerus, left shoulder, ribs, thoracic and lumbar spine, pelvis, and left proximal femur, all representing metastases from breast carcinoma.

patient is in pain or has an elevated alkaline phosphatase level.

BENIGN BONE NEOPLASMS. Lesions such as osteoid osteomas, nonossifying fibromas, and osteochondromas all concentrate bone radionuclides to some degree, whereas bone cysts show little or no uptake.[22] Low-grade bone uptake rules out sarcoma. Patients with fibrous dysplasia, hyperostosis, and Paget's disease may show intense radionuclide uptake (Fig. 5-31). Bone scanning in patients with suspected fractures can be useful because fractures may appear on scans prior to appearing on radiographs (Fig. 5-32). The age of the fracture cannot be estimated from the scan; such sites may remain "hot" years after healing.[22] Patients with osteomyelitis usually have intense uptake of bone nuclides in the region and also show increased vascularity and greater uptake of ^{67}Ga at the site of the disease (Fig. 5-33). Combined techniques are sometimes necessary to distinguish among cellulitis, bone marrow infarcts, and osteomyelitis.

JOINT DISEASES. In joint disease, bone scanning again is limited by its nonspecificity, but the localization of activity within the joint, usually requiring pinhole imaging, or the distribution of radioactivity among all the joints may provide important information for diagnosis and management (Fig. 5-34). In early stages of avascular necrosis, one may note an absence of radioactivity at the site of disease. During the reactive stage, activity in the area is increased (Fig. 5-35). Evaluation of joint prostheses is another application of joint scanning.

HEART

Heart scanning is carried out to evaluate ventricular wall perfusion and ventricular wall motion. The study is based on the active transport of a radionuclide into viable cells of the myocardium and on the changing configuration of the ventricular blood pool containing a radionuclide during the beating of the heart. If the circulation to an area is compromised, or if the myocardial cells are not able to engage in active transport, then the radionuclide will not be transported into the cells. If the muscle of the ventricular wall does not contract normally, then the configuration of the labeled blood pool will not

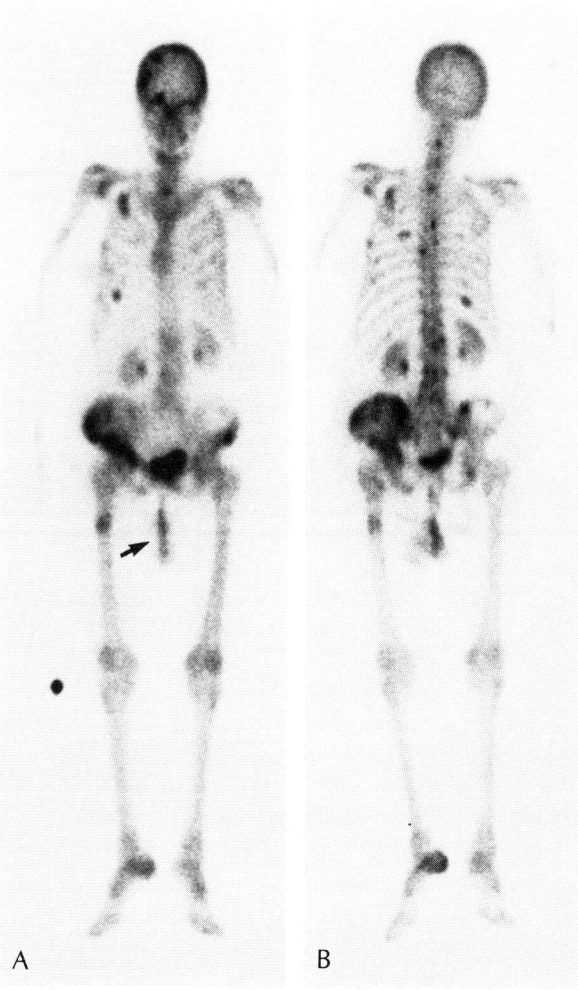

FIG. 5–31. Paget's disease of bone. Anterior (A) and posterior (B) whole-body views showing intense uptake of radioactivity in the right hemipelvis and the right calcaneus secondary to Paget's disease. The patient also has metastatic bone disease in the ribs, spine, skull, right shoulder, pelvis, and right femur from prostatic carcinoma. The arrow in A points to radioactivity in the catheter.

change normally with each beat. The quantitative changes of the blood pool between systole and diastole, measured as the ejection fraction, provide additional information. Another type of heart scanning, "hot-spot" scanning, directly shows myocardial infarcts and is based on the localization of a radionuclide in infarcted tissue.

Heart scanning is used primarily to identify coronary artery disease. To achieve this end, it is usually necessary to observe ventricular wall perfusion both "under stress" and "at rest." Areas that do not concentrate the radionuclide during exercise, but do concentrate it well at rest, represent areas of ischemia and indicate disease in the vessels supplying that portion of the myocardium. Areas that do not concentrate the radionuclide even at rest usually represent an infarct, except in instances of coronary artery spasm, cardiomyopathy, or left bundle branch block.

Ventricular wall motion studies aid in the detection of myocardial infarction and in the determination of its extent. These tests are also used to detect aneurysms, to confirm cardiomyopathies, to evaluate pharmacologic agents, to investigate persistent congestive failure, and to assess valvular disease. This study also yields important information during exercise, as compared to resting conditions.

To diagnose acute myocardial infarction, all three tests may be used. The "hot-spot" scan may actually show the infarct, but it must be done 24 hours to 7 days after the infarction. The perfusion scan may show the defect representing the infarct, but it does not indicate its age. Wall motion studies may show the effect of the infarct on the local wall motion, and on the ejection fraction, but they cannot indicate age, either.

Procedure

Heart scanning is more complex than most radionuclide studies because of the need to use a computer. It may also require an exercise-stress facility for use in conjunction with the imaging process. For the hot-spot scan, an intravenous injection of ^{99m}Tc-pyrophosphate is given, and imaging is carried out

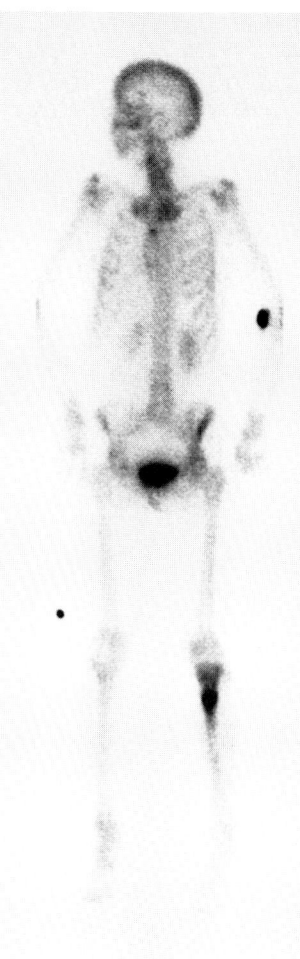

FIG. 5–32. Fracture of the tibia. Anterior view of the whole body showing a "hot spot" at the site of a stress fracture of the left tibia not visualized on initial x-ray films.

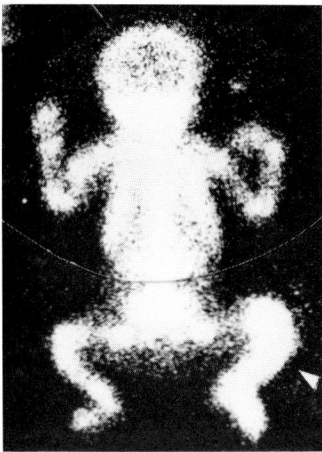

FIG. 5–33. Osteomyelitis. Anterior whole-body view of an infant 2 hours after intravenous injection of ^{99m}technetium-methylenediphosphonate showing a "hot" tibia (arrow) due to osteomyelitis.

in several views 4 to 5 hours later. For the perfusion scan, the patient is given an intraveneous injection of ^{201}thallium (^{201}Tl)-chloride, either at rest or during maximum exercise a minute before stopping. Imaging should begin within 5 to 10 min and at least two views, anterior and left anterior oblique, should be obtained. Tomographic or planar images are used for interpretation (Fig. 5–36). For wall motion studies, ^{99m}Tc-labeled albumin or red blood cells are injected, and either rapid sequential images are obtained during first pass of the radionuclide through each chamber or, once the radionuclide has come to equilibrium in the total-body blood pool, images are obtained during 16 equal time segments (gates) between R waves on the electrocardiograph for a certain number of beats. In equilibrium gated studies, the respective segments for all the beats are collected and are summed by the computer to produce a composite beat that is replayed repetitively, simulating the beating heart. The gated study can be displayed by a composite image using color or shades of a color to indicate areas of different movement (Fig. 5–36). The gated study may be done during stress as well as at rest. First-pass studies can also be performed during stress and then at rest using ^{99m}Tc-DTPA to allow the kidneys to reduce the background radioactivity between studies. During first-pass studies, the bolus may be in each cardiac chamber for only 4 to 8 beats. With the proper equipment, ejection fraction and wall motion can be obtained for each ventricle. It is also possible to obtain a gated first-pass study by summing respective gated segments of the beats while the bolus is in each ventricle.

Interpretation

Interpretation of heart scanning involves reviewing static images, moving images, and quantitative information. The hot-spot scan is considered positive if definite focal actvity is seen in the region of the heart (Fig. 5–37). Slight diffuse activity in the heart may represent a subendocardial infarct, but it is sometimes seen in patients with unstable angina, cardiomyopathy, ventricular aneurysm, certain arrhythmias, left bundle branch block, and acute left heart failure, as well as after cardioversion. Normal uptake of ^{99m}Tc-pyrophosphate in the sternum and ribs may make interpretation more difficult.

The ^{201}Tl scan is considered positive if one sees a significant defect in the "doughnut"-shaped left anterior oblique or "horseshoe"-shaped anterior projection (Fig. 5–38). In the resting ^{201}Tl study, this pattern usually indicates infarction. The presence of a wall motion abnormality at the site of the thallium defect may confirm the suspicion of infarct (Fig.

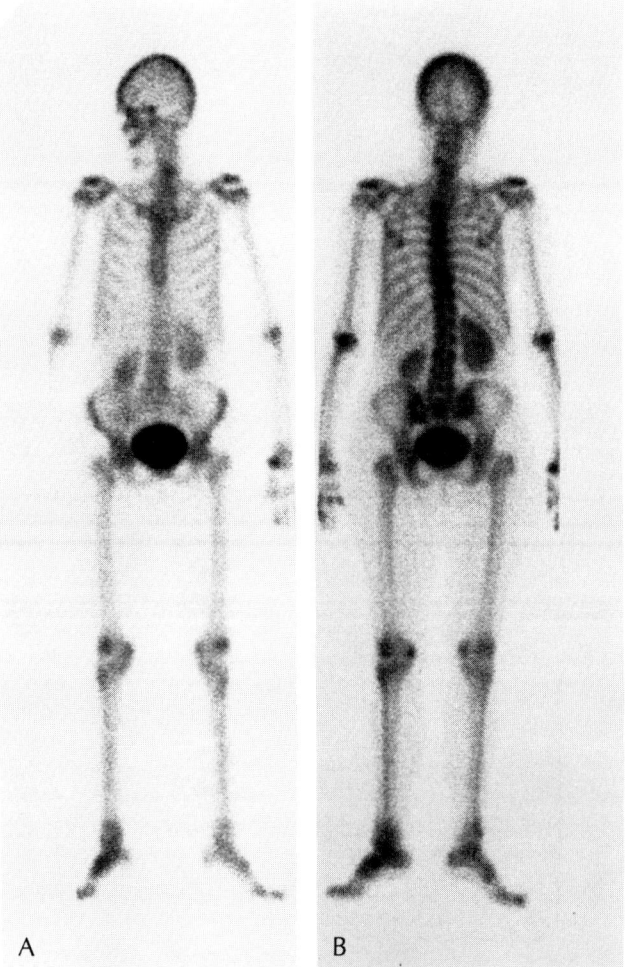

FIG. 5-34. Polyarthritis. Anterior (A) and posterior (B) whole-body views showing increased activity in the shoulders, elbows, temporomandibular joint, wrists, phalangeal joints, knees, and ankles because of rheumatoid arthritis.

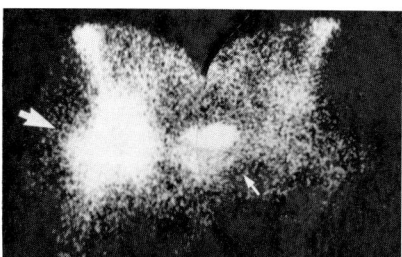

FIG. 5-35. Aseptic necrosis of the hip. Anterior view of the pelvis showing increased uptake in the right hip (large arrow) representing the reactive phase of aseptic necrosis. The small arrow points to the bladder.

5-38). Defects without wall motion changes may represent subendocardial infarcts or old infarcts of small size. Thallium scans carried out within a few days of infarct may have close to 100% sensitivity because the infarcted area, in addition to the surrounding ischemic tissue, produces a visible defect. Later, the ischemia improves, and the defect become smaller. The resting thallium study is also useful in the diagnosis of right ventricular hypertrophy, asymmetric septal hypertrophy, as in idiopathic hypertrophic subaortic stenosis, and cardiomyopathy, and in the pre- and postoperative evaluation of coronary bypass patients.

In the stress study, a thallium defect can indicate ischemia or infarction (Fig. 5-39). For the stress to be meaningful, it must be sufficient to produce a heart rate that is at least 80% of the predicted maximum.[23] The thallium stress study is more sensitive than the exercise electrocardiogram (ECG) in the detection of single-vessel disease (^{201}Tl, 71%, versus ECG, 46%), but its sensitivity equals that of the ECG in multiple-vessel disease (^{201}Tl, 77%, versus ECG, 80%). The two tests together enable one to detect 83 to 89% of coronary artery disease, more than either technique alone.[24] Although many physicians use planar images successfully, the tomographic systems offer some advantages. They facilitate interpretation and increase sensitivity, but they also reduce specificity.[25] The time course of clearance of

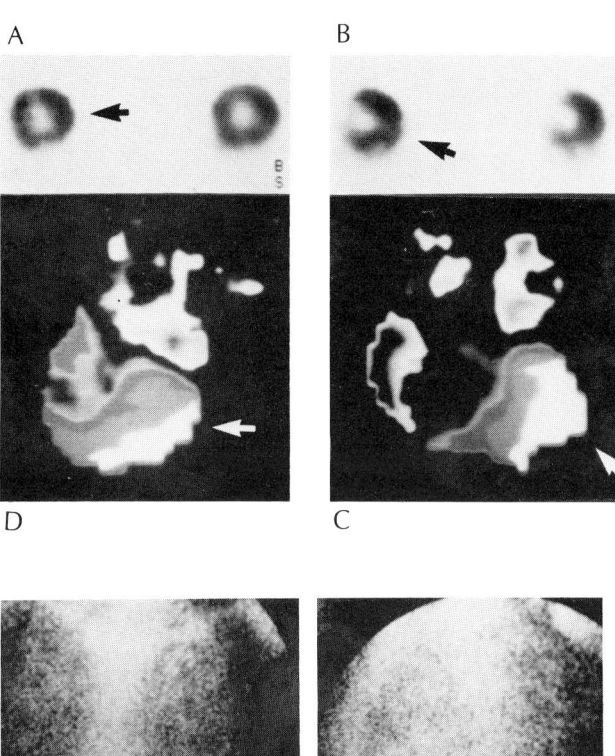

FIG. 5-36. Normal thallium and gated heart scans. *A*, Seven-pinhole tomographic cuts of a left anterior oblique view of the left ventricle after intravenous injection of ^{201}thallium. The arrow points to the posterior wall; the inferior wall is at the bottom, and the septum is the left part of the "doughnut." *B*, Similar cuts of an anterior view. The arrow points to the apex; above the apex is the anterior wall, and below it is the inferior wall. *C* and *D*, Composites of an equilibrium gated study after the patient's red cells were labeled with ^{99m}technetium. *C*, Anterior view, with the arrow pointing at the apex; the white area indicates good wall motion of the anterior wall and the apex. *D*, Left anterior oblique view, with the arrow pointing at the posterior wall; the white area indicates good wall motion of the posterior and inferior walls.

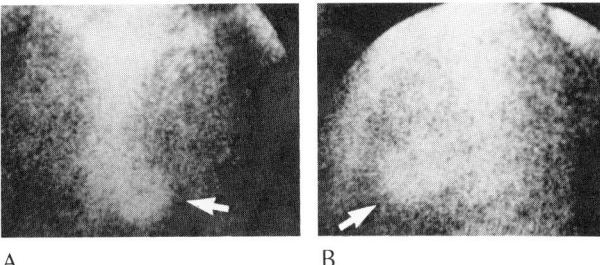

FIG. 5-37. Acute myocardial infarct. Anterior *(A)* and left anterior oblique *(B)* views of the chest 6 hours after intravenous injection of ^{99m}technetium-pyrophosphate. The arrows point to the abnormal uptake of radioactivity in the inferior left ventricular wall that indicates an infarct.

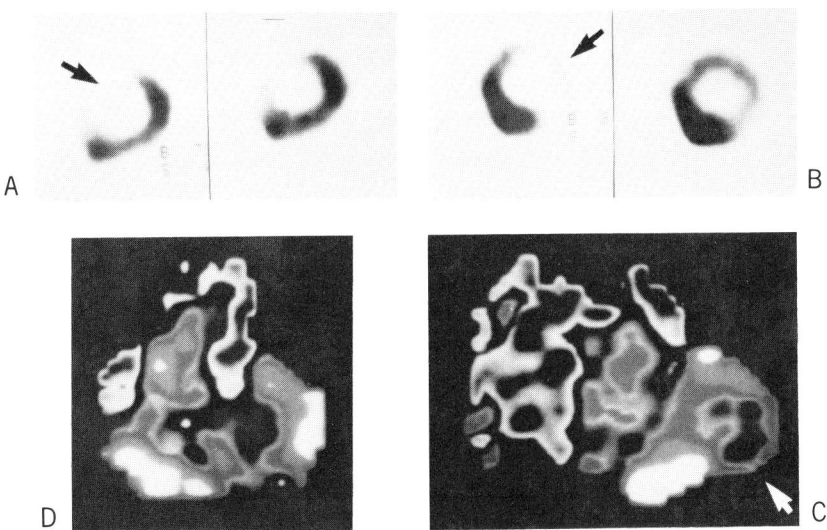

FIG. 5-38. Anterior wall and septal infarct. *A*, Left anterior obligue tomographic cuts of a ^{201}thallium scan showing a large defect involving the septum (arrow). *B*, Anterior tomographic cuts showing a large anterior wall defect (arrow). The second of the two cuts in *B* is 1 cm deeper and begins to show perfused wall. The composite gated anterior view *(C)* shows anterior wall hypokinesia (absence of white area at apex (arrow) and above). *D*, The gated left anterior oblique view also shows some inferior wall hypokinesia (white area does not extend inferiorly).

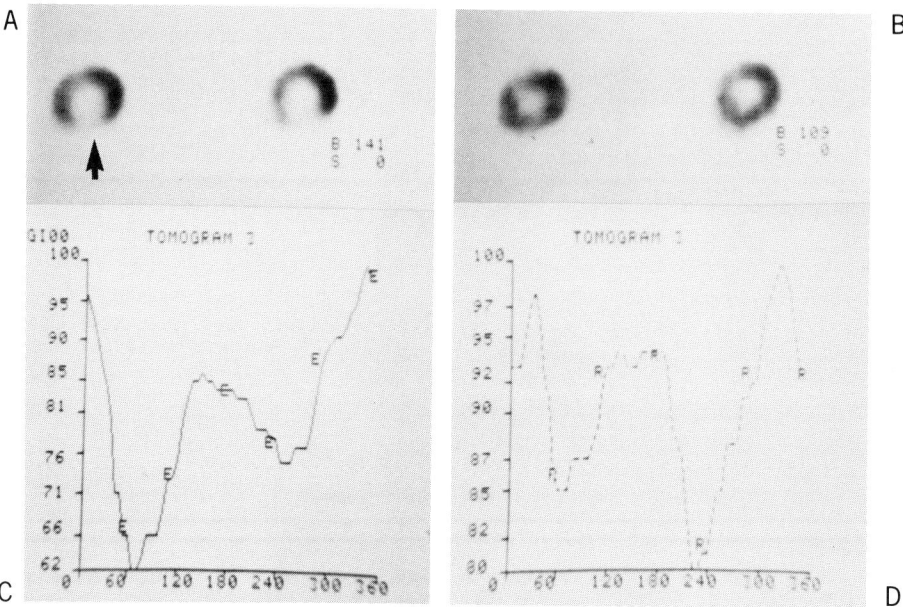

FIG. 5-39. Inferior wall ischemia. *A,* Left anterior oblique tomographic cuts of a ^{201}thallium scan immediately after stress (treadmill) and showing an inferior wall defect (arrow). *B,* The same cuts of a ^{201}thallium scan performed at rest. The reversibility of the inferior wall defect indicates ischemia. *C,* Graphic representation of *A; D,* graphic representation of *B.*

^{201}Tl may also provide useful information concerning coronary artery disease.[26]

One may interpret wall motion studies by observing the video display of the repeating composite heart beat or the composite images (see Figs. 5-36 and 5-38). Normal, hypokinetic, akinetic, and dyskinetic regions of the left ventricular wall can be seen. Aneurysms and pseudoaneurysms can be observed. In the left anterior oblique view, the right ventricle and its wall motion are visible, and in the anterior view, the right atrium and pulmonary outflow tract may be seen. Numerous computer programs have been developed to present wall motion in a single static image using a color scale to indicate differences in degree and direction of motion. For interpretation, one must become familiar with the color pattern and its significance. Computers can automatically find the ventricular edge and can calculate the ejection fraction; they can also calculate regional ejection fractions for various segments of the ventricle and can display these by color scale. Ejection fractions over 50% are considered normal, and those under 40% are considered abnormal; 40 to 50% is the borderline zone. Ejection fractions may be used for early diagnoses of cardiac pump failure, for prognosis in patients with acute myocardial infarction, for decision-making concerning cardiac operations, for estimating cardiotoxicity from chemotherapeutic agents, for evaluating the effects of cardiac medication, and for assessing cardiomyopathy. Patients with cardiomyopathy usually have normal or patchy ^{201}Tl studies, except patients with ischemic cardiomyopathies, and poor, diffusely abnormal wall motion with low ejection fractions (20 to 30%).

Cardiac studies are expensive because of the high cost of ^{201}Tl and of computer hardware and software. They also require a high degree of expertise on the part of the technician and more of the physician's time. Nevertheless, radionuclide cardiac studies provide a wealth of information and are noninvasive.

SPLEEN

One performs spleen scanning to confirm the size and integrity of the spleen and to obtain evidence of splenic disease. The study is based on the uptake of radioactive colloid by the reticuloendothelial cells located there or by the trapping of damaged red blood cells tagged with a radionuclide. Radiocolloid

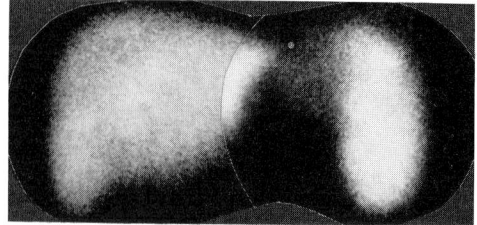

FIG. 5-40. Splenomegaly. Anterior view of a liver-spleen scan showing a normal liver and an enlarged spleen.

images the liver and bone marrow as well as the spleen, but for most purposes, this feature does not interfere with splenic visualization. The use of labeled heat-damaged red blood cells places more of the radionuclide in the spleen, but the technique may be unpredictable. Overdamaged cells may appear in the liver, and underdamaged cells may remain in the circulation, raising the background radioactivity.

Spleen scans are usually done to evaluate splenomegaly (Fig. 5–40). In adults, splenic size should be 10.0 ± 1.5 cm. Splenomegaly may have many causes, some of which can be seen on a scan, such as tumor, cyst, abscess, diffuse infiltration, and infarcts. In some conditions, one may see only enlargement without a characteristic pattern. Spleen scanning is also performed to rule out splenic tears, rupture, or hemorrhage following trauma. Spleen scanning with labeled cells is usually done to visualize accessory spleens following splenectomy if the patient continues to show manifestations of hypersplenism. With labeled cells, less chance exists that the liver will be able to obscure an accessory spleen.

Procedure

Spleen scans are performed by intravenous injection of ^{99m}Tc-sulfur colloid and by imaging in multiple views at 15 to 20 min. For spleen scanning with red blood cells, a sample of the patient's blood (20 ml) is drawn, and the red blood cells are labeled with ^{99m}Tc. The blood is then heated at 50° C for 30 min and is reinjected. Scanning is carried out in multiple views 1 to 2 hours later.

Interpretation

Interpretation of the spleen scan involves observation of size, shape, and position of the spleen. A marker film with a centimeter scale is obtained for accurate measurement. Wedge-shaped defects along the margin may represent infarcts (Fig. 5–41). Blurring of the margin may represent a subcapsular hemorrhage. Irregular linear defects may be tears or "bleeds" when found after known trauma. Except in patients with lymphoma, it is rare to see metastases to the spleen before they appear in the liver; however, malignant melanoma and chorioepithelioma are known to involve splenic tissue. Failure to visualize the spleen in the absence of splenectomy or congenital asplenia occurs occasionally. Such functional asplenia is seen in patients with sickle cell disease, mixed hemoglobinopathies in crisis, Thorotrast intoxication, celiac-sprue disease, and some immunologic disorders.[27]

Other Studies

Other radionuclide spleen studies include measurements of splenic sequestration of red blood cells using tagged, undamaged red cells and measurements of splenic hematopoiesis using ^{59}iron.

BONE MARROW

Bone marrow scanning is used to determine the location and distribution of bone marrow and to detect bone marrow infarcts.[28] It is based on the uptake of radiocolloid by reticuloendothelial cells in the bone marrow or uptake of ^{111}indium (^{111}In)-chloride by erythropoietic cells. The problem with using radiocolloid is the overwhelming uptake of the agent by liver and spleen that obscures a large area of bone marrow in the lower ribs, lower thoracic spine, and lumbar spine. Although the liver takes up some indium, the degree of uptake is not sufficient to obscure bone marrow.

Bone marrow scans are usually done when radiation and chemotherapy have destroyed much bone marrow and when an assessment of the residual functioning bone marrow is needed before further therapy is undertaken. It can be useful in finding a fertile site for bone marrow biopsy. In patients with sickle cell anemia, bone marrow scanning can show an infarcted area that may explain sites of pain.[29]

Procedure

The scans are performed by intravenous injection of ^{99m}Tc-sulfur colloid and whole-body imaging 15 to 20 min later or by injection of ^{111}In-chloride and whole-body imaging in 48 hours.

Interpretation

Interpretation of the bone marrow scan involves localization of bone marrow. In the normal adult, bone marrow is seen in the trunk, but not in limbs or skull. Extension into these areas follows destruc-

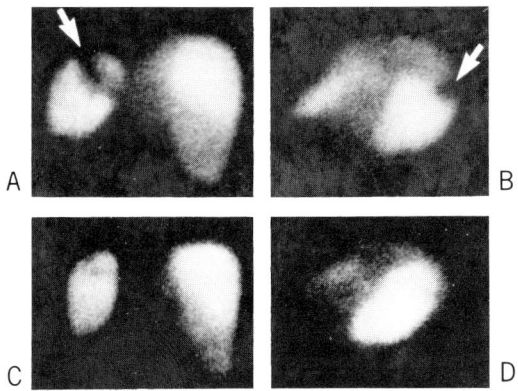

FIG. 5–41. Splenic infarct. Posterior (A) and left lateral (B) views of a liver-spleen scan showing a large defect (arrows) in the upper portion of the spleen. C and D, The same views a month later, showing almost complete healing.

tion of the central bone marrow. Defects in the limbs may mean tumor, infarct, or infection. ^{67}Ga scanning can help one to make the distinction because the radionuclide concentrates in infections and not in infarcts.

ABSCESS LOCALIZATION

Scanning of abscesses is based on uptake of a radionuclide by inflammatory cells in vivo or accumulation at an abscess site of whole blood cells labeled in vitro with a radionuclide.

Procedure and Interpretation

Scanning is usually performed by intravenous injection of ^{67}Ga-citrate and whole-body scanning at 24 and, possibly, 48 hours (Figs. 5–42 and 5–43). Diagnosis of abdominal and pelvic abscesses is frequently sought, and these areas are the most difficult to interpret. During the first 24 hours after injection of the radionuclide, the kidneys are the major excretory organ, and the bladder may obscure an abscess. After 24 hours, the large intestines represent the excretory site, and pooled ^{67}Ga in the bowel may be misinterpreted as an abscess. One may need to administer laxatives and enemas to ensure that the activity visualized in the abdomen does not represent a lesion in the colon.

Abscess scanning with labeled leukocytes is not yet routine, but it is reported to be effective.[30] The procedure requires separation of white blood cells and labeling with ^{111}In in vitro, followed by reinjection and scanning between 4 and 24 hours. This technique has the advantage of low abdominal background radioactivity.

In several studies of ^{67}Ga scanning of abdominal abscesses, the sensitivity of the technique was 91%, and its specificity 93%.[31] Ultrasound and CT should be used initially if the patient has acute, localizing signs and symptoms. One should then use ^{67}Ga scanning if results of the other techniques are negative. ^{67}Ga scanning should be used first if the patient has nonlocalizing signs and symptoms. False-negative results can occur in leukopenic patients.

In the diagnosis of abscesses, ^{111}In leukocyte scintigraphy is as sensitive as ^{67}Ga, but with greater specificity. Scanning with ^{111}In is recommended for localizing, acute infections of under 2 weeks' duration, but ^{67}Ga scanning is reported to be better for patients with chronic infections of more than 3 weeks' duration. ^{111}In leukocyte scanning appears promising in the evaluation of osteomyelitis and inflammatory bowel diseases.[30]

STOMACH AND INTESTINES

Gastrointestinal scans are carried out to observe gastroesophageal reflux, to measure gastric emptying, to localize intestinal bleeding, and to detect Meckel's diverticulum. The gastroesophageal reflux study is based on the visualization of movement of a radionuclide from the stomach into the esophagus under imposed external epigastric pressure. The gastric emptying study is based on the measurement of the quantity of a radionuclide in liquid or solid form moving from the stomach into the duodenum during a certain time interval. The intestinal bleeding study is based on the extravasation of a circulating radionuclide into the bowel lumen.

Procedure and Interpretation

GASTROESOPHAGEAL REFLUX STUDY. The gastroesophageal reflux study is performed by oral administration of acidified orange juice containing ^{99m}Tc-sulfur colloid. As soon as the radioactive material has left the esophagus, the patient is put into a supine position with a pressure cuff about the abdomen and the balloon centered over the epigastrium. Images of the stomach and lower esophagus are obtained as pressure is applied in 20-mm Hg increments. If regurgitation into the esophagus occurs before the 100-mm Hg mark has been reached, then the study is positive and indicates gastroesophageal reflux (Fig. 5–44). The study can

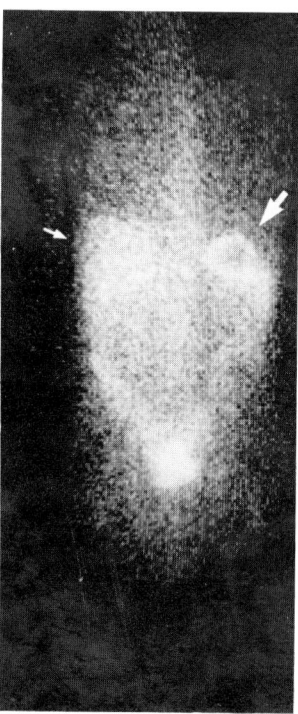

FIG. 5–42. Subphrenic abscess. Anterior view of the whole body 24 hours after intravenous injection of ^{67}gallium-citrate showing a doughnut-shaped area of activity (an abscess) in the left upper quadrant of the abdomen (large arrow). The small arrow points to normal activity in the liver. A concentration of activity is also present in the bladder.

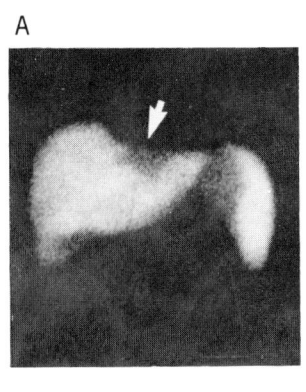
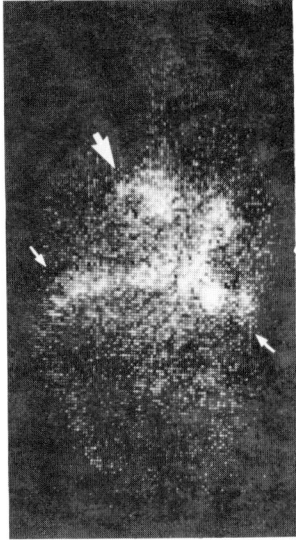

FIG. 5–43. Hepatic abscess. *A,* A liver-spleen scan showing a defect in the superior surface of the liver (arrow). *B,* A ^{67}gallium scan of the abdomen at 48 hours showing concentration of the radioisotope in the area of the liver defect (large arrow), representing an abscess; the small arrows point to normal ^{67}gallium activity in the colon.

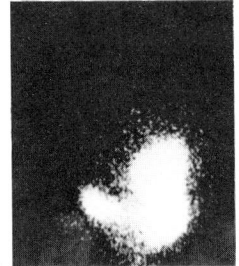
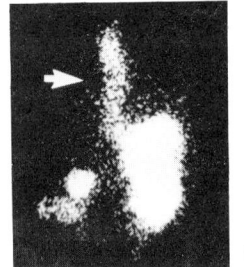

FIG. 5–44. Gastroesophageal reflux. *A,* Anterior view showing radioactivity in the stomach immediately after oral administration of ^{99m}technetium-sulfur colloid in acidified orange juice. *B,* The same view after application of pressure (40 mm Hg) over the epigastrium; the arrow points to radioactivity refluxing into the esophagus.

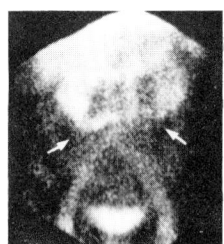

FIG. 5–45. Gastrointestinal bleeding. *A,* Anterior view of the abdomen immediately after labeling the patient's red blood cells with ^{99m}technetium. Activity is seen in the aorta and iliac vessels, as well as in heart and liver above. *B,* The same view 4 hours later, showing radioactivity (blood) in the transverse colon (arrows); radioactivity at the bottom of *B* is ^{99m}technetium in the bladder.

be quantitated if a computer is available. The technique is useful in the initial diagnosis of reflux esophagitis, as well as in the quantitative evaluation of response to therapy.[32]

GASTRIC EMPTYING STUDY. This test is performed by oral administration of either ^{111}In-DTPA in water, for measuring liquid gastric emptying, or ^{99m}Tc-sulfur colloid prepared in a scrambled egg, for measuring solid gastric emptying. Images are obtained at 5 min and at 30 and 90 min, and computer processing is used to calculate the percentage of original activity left in the stomach. Normally, 50% of the liquid activity leaves the stomach in 30 min, and 50% of the solid activity leaves the stomach in 90 min. Delayed gastric emptying has many causes, whereas rapid gastric emptying has few. The test does not indicate the cause of the disorder, but it is useful in confirming the diagnosis and in monitoring management.[33]

INTESTINAL BLEEDING STUDY. This examination is performed by intravenous injection of ^{99m}Tc-sulfur colloid or ^{99m}Tc-labeled red blood cells.[34,35] Immediately after the injection, images are obtained every 1 to 2 min over the pelvis and mid-abdomen for 10 to 15 min. If no bleeding is seen, more superiorly oriented images, including the lower liver and spleen, should be obtained, followed by a left anterior oblique image. The study is continued for another 10 to 15 min, to permit bleeding hidden by the liver or spleen to move along the bowel into sight. If the patient moves his bowels during the study, the stool should also be imaged; rectal or rectosigmoid junction bleeding may appear in the stools. The test is only positive if the activity detected moves from its site of origin. This test is excellent for localization of intestinal bleeding. If ^{99m}Tc-sulfur colloid is used, one has only a short time during which to observe the bleeding because the colloid is cleared by the liver in a matter of minutes. If tagged red blood cells are used, one can image at various times up to 24 hours, but visualization of radioactivity in the intestines does not indicate the point of origin (Fig. 5–45).

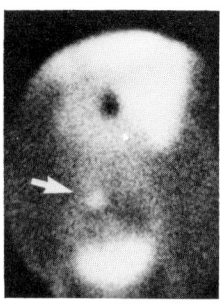 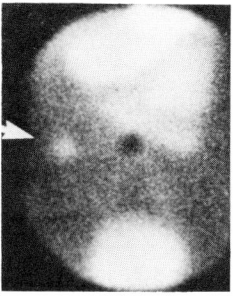

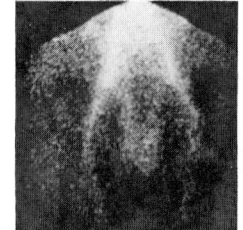 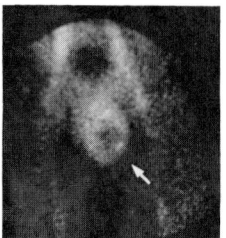

FIG. 5-46. Meckel's diverticulum. *A,* Anterior view of the abdomen 15 min after intravenous injection of 99mtechnetium-pertechnetate. The "hot spot" (arrow) is 99mtechnetium in the Meckel's diverticulum; the black spot is a lead marker on the umbilicus. Radioactivity visible above is in the stomach and below is in the bladder. *B,* The same patient 3 days later; one notes movements of the diverticulum.

FIG. 5-47. Missed testicular torsion. *A,* Anterior view of a normal scrotum and iliac vessels immediately following intravenous injection of 99mtechnetium-pertechnetate. *B,* The same view of a patient with testicular torsion; the clear area in the scrotum (arrow) is caused by the absence of blood flow to the left testicle; the increased peripheral activity represents tunica dartos hyperemia, which takes a day or more to develop.

MECKEL'S DIVERTICULUM STUDY. This test is based on the concentration of a radionuclide in the ectopic gastric mucosa of Meckel's diverticulum. Such gastric mucosa occurs in 50 to 60% of diverticula. The study is performed by intravenous injection of 99mTc-pertechnetate and imaging at 2-min intervals for 12 min and then at 15, 30, and 60 min. An abnormal study shows accumulation of radioactivity, usually as a small, round area distinct from the stomach, in the right lower quadrant. Radioactivity appears simultaneously with the stomach, that increases in intensity in the stomach and persists through the study (Fig. 5-46). A diagnostic accuracy rate of 90 to 98% has been reported.[36] False-positive results have several causes. Inflammatory conditions such as regional enteritis and ulcerative colitis, intussusception, and intestinal obstruction may localize pertechnetate. These lesions are usually larger than Meckel's diverticulum and often assume the shape of the bowel.

SCROTUM

Scrotal scanning is used to evaluate conditions involving the testis and its appendages and is based on blood flow to and vascularity of these tissues. Blood flow and vascularity are visualized by means of radionuclide in the circulation that diffuses slowly into the tissues. The major use of the scrotal scan is to differentiate testicular torsion from epididymitis. The rate of sensitivity for detecting torsion is 93%, with similar specificity.[37] Other information can be obtained from the scrotal scan in patients with scrotal trauma, hydrocele, and testicular tumors, but radionuclide scanning of patients with these conditions is rare.

Procedure

The scrotal scan is performed by intravenous injection of 99mTc-pertechnetate, with immediate rapid-

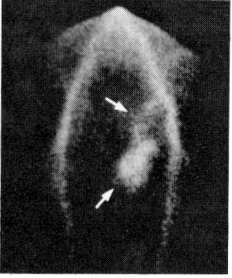

FIG. 5-48. Epididymitis. Anterior view of the scrotum and iliac vessels after intravenous injection of 99mtechnetium-pertechnetate showing increased flow in the left testicular and deferential vessels (upper arrow) and the epididymis (lower arrow) due to inflammation.

sequence imaging of the area for blood flow and then static imaging for blood-pool information.

Interpretation

Interpretation of the scan requires observation of the testicular-deferential vessels and the appearance of activity in the epididymal and testicular regions. Patients with testicular torsion may have an obvious interruption of blood flow through the vessels between the iliac artery and the testicle. The testicle shows no radioactivity, although uptake of the radionuclide in the tunica dartos may give a "halo" of activity around the "cold" testicle (Fig. 5-47). In epididymitis, the testicular-deferential vessels are usually prominent, and one sees intense radioactive uptake superiorly and laterally to the testicle at the location of the epididymis (Fig. 5-48). The study is simple and can be done quickly as an emergency procedure.

SALIVARY GLANDS

Scanning of the salivary glands is carried out to obtain functional information concerning the parotid

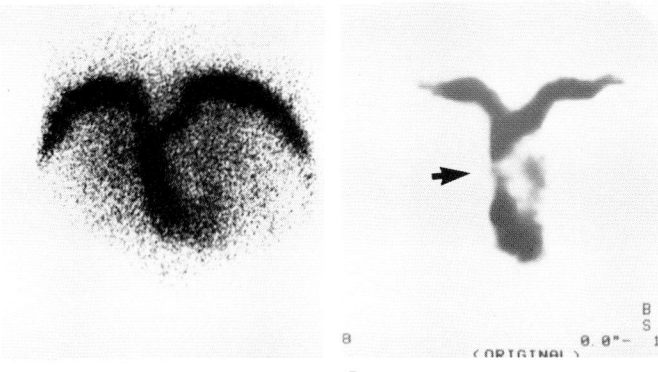

FIG. 5–49. Superior vena cava obstruction. *A,* Anterior view showing normal flow through subclavian and innominate vessels and vena cava following bilateral injection of 99mtechnetium-pertechnetate into antecubital veins. *B,* A similar study in a patient with narrowing (arrow) of the superior vena cava.

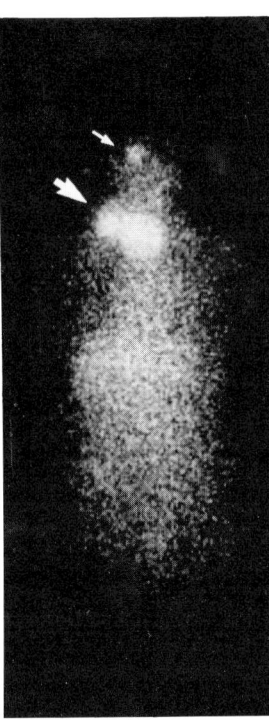

FIG. 5–50. Lymphoma. Anterior whole-body view 24 hours following intravenous injection of 67gallium-citrate. Note the concentration of the radioisotope in the right supraclavicular lymph nodes (large arrow) and in the mediastinal lymph nodes; such a pattern represents lymphoma. Note the involvement of the right maxillary sinus (small arrow).

Procedure and Interpretation

The salivary gland scan is performed by intravenous injection of 99mTc-pertechnetate, with imaging at 2-min intervals for 10 min and then at 20, 30, and 60 min. The normal scan shows a high concentration of radionuclide in the salivary glands, with bilateral symmetry in the first few images, and the appearance of radioactivity in the mouth by 10 or 20 min. In patients with mild-to-moderate disease, one sees decreased, late concentration of radioactivity, or almost no activity, in the glands, but radioactivity is visible in the mouth by 60 min. In those with severe disease, no radioactivity is seen in the glands or in the oral cavity. The scan does not add much to the clinical evaluation of tumors of the salivary glands. Major salivary duct obstruction can be visualized, but this technique is of limited value for this indication.

VASCULAR SYSTEM

Vascular scanning is done to evaluate vascular obstruction, aneurysms, and patency of vascular shunts and is based on dynamic flow of blood containing a radionuclide. Visualization of vascular flow depends on imaging of the bolus of radionuclide on its first pass though the vessels in question. The study requires an adequate bolus injection and sufficient cardiac output. Vascular scanning is usually used to observe blood flow through the carotid and cerebral vessels (see the section of the chapter on brain scanning), flow to the kidneys (see the section on kidney scanning), absence of flow in superior vena cava obstruction, abnormal flow in aortic aneurysms, and evidence of flow in femoropopliteal or brachioiliac shunts.

Procedure and Interpretation

Vascular scans are performed by intravenous injection of 99mTc-pertechnetate or another 99mTc radiopharmaceutical agent and by rapid sequential imaging over the area of interest. Computerized motion views are especially useful. For superior vena cava obstruction, simultaneous injections are

and submandibular glands and is based on the trapping and excretion of a radionuclide in the circulation. Some anatomic information is also obtained, but this indication has not proved valuable. Salivary gland scanning is most often used to evaluate collagen vascular disorders that may be detected before clinical manifestations occur.[38] Such salivary glands may show increased trapping of the radionuclide in the initial phase of disease, but may later show decreased trapping and failure to discharge the trapped radionuclide into the oral cavity.

usually given in both arms (Fig. 5–49). The images are inspected for narrowing or complete obstruction of vessels. The images do not have the resolution of x-ray angiography, but the study is simple, noninvasive, and without associated morbidity. Vascular scanning is not helpful in the visualization of aortic aneurysms. Turbulent flow through aneurysms breaks up the bolus, and the aneurysm may not be visualized. If a clot is present in the aneurysm, the image may appear normal as blood flows through the available channel. Resolution is not clear enough to enable one to see small irregularities even in large vessels. Sometimes, clear-cut widening of the aorta is observed, but the sensitivity of the study is low. For visualization of shunts and evaluation of peripheral vascular injuries, vascular scanning is helpful.[39] Because it is noninvasive and can be repeated frequently, it can be used for monitoring purposes.

SOFT TISSUE NEOPLASMS

Identification of soft tissue tumors has always been a cherished goal in radionuclide scanning. Various mechanisms have been explored, but none have had unqualified success. The most useful agents have been ^{67}Ga and ^{99m}Tc-diphosphonate compounds.[40,41] Almost any tumor may take up gallium, but the technique is limited by its variable sensitivity. The highest sensitivity has been in pulmonary carcinoma (80 to 95%) and in hepatoma (86 to 95%). Sensitivity in Hodgkin's disease is 87% overall, but it is only 50% for lesions inferior to the diaphragm (Fig. 5–50).

Although a bone-scanning agent, ^{99m}Tc-diphosphonate is taken up by a number of benign and malignant tumors, infarcted tissue, soft tissue calcifications, abscesses, and surgical wounds. The mechanism of concentration of ^{99m}Tc-diphosphonate in these lesions is unknown, but it may have to do with calcium localization.

Another scanning agent for soft tissue tumors is bleomycin labeled with various radionuclides; it has not been widely used. Most recently, work in this field has concentrated on labeled antibodies specific for certain tumor markers or tumor-associated antigens. Some investigators have had preliminary success in the concentration of these labeled antibodies in tumors, both primary and metastatic.[42]

ACKNOWLEDGMENT

I wish to thank B. Graubard for her assistance in the preparation of this chapter.

REFERENCES

1. Holman, B.L., et al.: Brain imaging with radiolabeled amines. Nucl. Med. Ann., 1983, p. 131.
2. Alavi, A., et al.: Functional imaging of the brain with positron emission tomography. Nucl. Med. Ann., 1982, p. 319.
3. Alderson, P.O., Gado, M.H., and Siegel, B.A.: Computerized cranial tomography and radionuclide imaging in the detection of intracranial mass lesions. Semin. Nucl. Med., 7:161, 1977.
4. Fordham, E.W.: The complementary role of computerized axial transmission tomography and radionuclide imaging of the brain. Semin. Nucl. Med., 7:137, 1977.
5. Harbert, J.C., McCullough, D.C., and Schellinger, D.: Computed cranial tomography and radionuclide cisternography in hydrocephalus. Semin. Nucl. Med., 7:197, 1977.
6. Salar, G., Certeri, A., and Zampieri, P.: The diagnosis of CSF fistulas with rhinorrhea by isotope cisternography. Neuroradiology, 15:185, 1978.
7. Wilkins, R.T., and Sandifer, S.H.: Follow-up on the problem of increased incidence of thyroid carcinoma from the effects of childhood irradiation. J. Fam. Pract., 8:265, 1979.
8. Boysen, P.G., et al.: Prospective evaluation for pneumonectomy using the 99m-technetium quantitative perfusion lung scan. Chest, 72:422, 1977.
9. Biello, D.R., et al.: Interpretation of the indeterminate lung scan. Radiology, 133:189, 1979.
10. Bekerman, C., et al.: Gallium-67 citrate imaging studies of the lung. Semin. Nucl. Med., 10:286, 1980.
11. Drum, D.E.: Current status of radiocolloid hepatic scintiphotography for space occupying disease. Semin. Nucl. Med., 12:64, 1982.
12. Taylor, K.J.W., Sullivan, D., and Rosenfield, A.T.: Grey-scale ultrasound and isotope scanning: complementary techniques for imaging the liver. AJR, 128:277, 1977.
13. Friedman, M.L., et al.: Computerized tomography and radionuclide scanning in hepatic disease: a retrospective study. Clin. Nucl. Med., 3:318, 1978.
14. Weissmann, H.S., et al.: Spectrum of cholescintigraphic patterns in acute cholecystitis. Radiology, 138:167, 1981.
15. Weissmann, H.S., et al.: Cholescintigraphy, ultrasonography and computerized tomography in the evaluation of biliary tract disorders. Semin. Nucl. Med., 9:22, 1979.
16. Kirchner, P.T., and Rosenthall, L.: Renal transplant evaluation. Semin. Nucl. Med., 12:370, 1982.
17. Sherman, R.A., and Blaufox, M.D.: Obstructive uropathy in patients with nonvisualization on renal scan. Nephron, 25:82, 1980.
18. Linton, A.L., et al.: Acute interstitial nephritis due to drugs. Ann. Intern. Med., 93:735, 1980.
19. Hurwitz, S.R., et al.: Gallium-67 imaging to localize urinary tract infections. Br. J. Radiol., 49:156, 1976.
20. McNeil, B.J.: Rationale for the use of bone scans in selected metastases and primary bone tumors. Semin. Nucl. Med., 8:336, 1978.
21. Rosenthall, L., and Lisbona, R.: Role of radionuclide imaging in benign bone and joint diseases of orthopedic interest. Nucl. Med. Ann., 1980, p. 267.
22. Matin, P.: Bone scanning of trauma and benign conditions. Nucl. Med. Ann., 1982, p. 81.
23. McLaughlin, P.R., et al.: Reproducibility of thallium-201 myocardial imaging. Circulation, 55:497, 1977.
24. Ritchie, J.L., et al.: Myocardial imaging with thallium-201 at rest and during exercise. Comparison with coronary arteriography and resting and stress electrocardiography. Circulation, 56:66, 1977.
25. Rize, H.R., et al.: Thallium-201 myocardial scintigra-

phy: a critical comparison of seven-pinhole tomography and conventional planar imaging. J. Nucl. Med., 22:493, 1981.
26. Berman, D.S., et al.: Rate of redistribution in thallium-201 exercise myocardial scintigraphy: inverse relationship to degree of coronary stenosis. Circulation, 58 (Suppl. 2):63, 1978.
27. Spencer, R.P., et al.: Causes and temporal sequence of onset of functional asplenia in adults. Clin. Nucl. Med., 3:17, 1978.
28. Gilbert, E.H., et al.: [111]Indium bone marrow scintigraphy as an aid in selecting marrow biopsy sites for the evaluation of marrow elements in patients with lymphoma. Cancer, 38:1560, 1976.
29. Alavi, A., et al.: Bone marrow scan evaluation of arthropathy in sickle cell disorders. Arch. Intern. Med., 136:436, 1976.
30. Froelich, J.W., and Swanson, D.: Imaging of inflammatory processes with labeled cells. Semin. Nucl. Med., 14:128, 1984.
31. Biello, D.R., Levitt, R.G., and Melson, G.L.: The roles of gallium-67 scintigraphy, ultrasonography and computed tomography in the detection of abdominal abscesses. Semin. Nucl. Med., 9:58, 1979.
32. Malmud, L.S., and Fisher, R.S.: Quantitation of gastroesophageal reflux before and after therapy using the gastroesophageal scintiscan. South. Med. J., 71 (Suppl. 1):10, 1978.
33. Malmud, L.S., et al.: Scintigraphic evaluation of gastric emptying. Semin. Nucl. Med., 12:116, 1982.
34. Alavi, A.: Detection of gastrointestinal bleeding with ^{99m}Tc-sulfur colloid. Semin. Nucl. Med., 12:126, 1982.
35. Marking, J.A.: Evaluation of ^{99m}Tc-labeled red blood cell scintigraphy for detection and localization of gastrointestinal bleeding sites. Gastroenterology, 83:394, 1982.
36. Sfakianakis, G.N., and Conway, J.J.: Detection of ectopic gastric mucosa in Meckel's diverticulum and in other aberrations by scintigraphy. 1. Pathophysiology and 10-year clinical experience. J. Nucl. Med., 22:647, 1981.
37. Tanaka, T., Mishkin, F.S., and Datta, N.S.: Radionuclide imaging of the scrotal contents. Nucl. Med. Ann., 1981, p. 195.
38. Daniels, T.E., et al.: An evaluation of salivary scintigraphy in Sjögren's syndrome. Arthritis Rheum., 22:809, 1979.
39. Rudavsky, A.Z., and Moss, C.M.: Radionuclide angiography for the evaluation of peripheral vascular injuries. Nucl. Med. Ann., 1981, p. 315.
40. Halpern, S., and Hagan, P.: Gallium-67-citrate imaging in neoplastic and inflammatory disease. Nucl. Med. Ann., 1980, p. 219.
41. Chew, F.S., Hudson, T.M., and Enneking, W.R.: Radionuclide imaging of soft tissue neoplasms. Semin. Nucl. Med., 11:266, 1981.
42. Larson, S.M., and Carrasquillo, J.A.: Nuclear Oncology: current perspectives. Nucl. Med. Ann., 1983, p. 167.

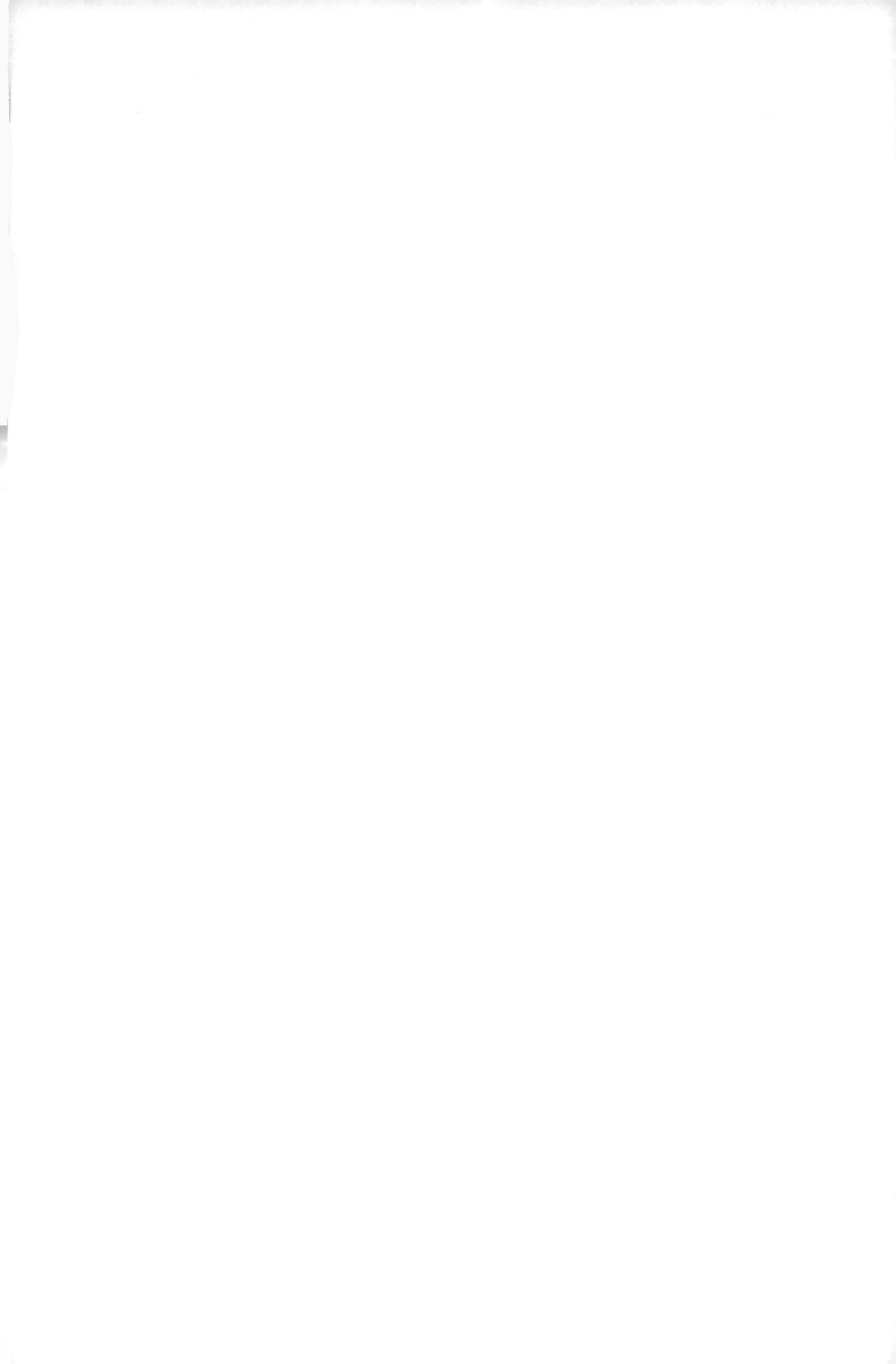

6

Computed Tomography

Carl L. Schultz ■ John R. Haaga

During the past 10 years, progress in the development and refinement of radiologic imaging systems has been remarkable. Computed tomography (CT) has had the greater clinical significance of these imaging techniques. In this chapter, we discuss the basic principles of CT and its applications to surgical diagnosis.

BASIC PRINCIPLES

The basic principle of computed tomography is the ability to reconstruct the internal structure of the body by multiple measurements of radiation transmission.[1,2] The measurements are obtained by scanning a thin cross section of the body with a narrow x-ray beam and by measuring the transmitted radiation with sensitive radiation detectors. The amount of radiation reaching the detectors depends on the density of the structures scanned. A high-density material, such as bone, absorbs more x-ray photons than a low-density material, such as air. This absorption of x-rays is called attenuation. The computer divides the area scanned into tiny blocks of tissue called voxels and then calculates an attenuation number, or CT number, for each voxel. CT numbers range from −1,000 Hounsfield units (HU) (air) to +1,000 (dense bone), with water at 0. The CT numbers are displayed as small squares called pixels on the video monitor; different CT numbers are represented by varying shades of gray. The composite picture of these pixels is the CT image. Permanent images are obtained by making a photographic recording of the image on the video monitor.

Table 6–1 shows the CT numbers of various structures in the body. The CT number of any structure can be obtained from the computer, but this determination is not usually necessary. Visual inspection usually suffices to ascertain whether a structure is fat, water, soft tissue, or calcific density.

CT scanning has several advantages over conventional radiography. Its cross-sectional images allow internal structures to be visualized without superimposition, and one is also able to detect much smaller differences in density. Because conventional

Table 6–1. Computed Tomography Numbers in Hounsfield Units (HU) on Nonenhanced Scans

Air	−1,000	
Fat	−60 −	−100
Water	0	
Cerebrospinal fluid	0 −	+20
Cysts	0 −	+20
Brain		
White matter	+20 −	+34
Gray matter	+34 −	+60
Pancreas	+30 −	+50
Kidney	+30 −	+50
Spleen	+30 −	+60
Liver	+40 −	+70
Acute hemorrhage	+45 −	+100
Calcification	+65 −	+1,000
Bone	+200 −	+1,000

radiographs cannot show a density difference under 10%, they are limited to 4 basic densities: air, fat, water, and bone. All soft tissue structures appear to have the density of water on conventional radiographs. CT can determine density differences of .5% or less, and so it can better distinguish among, for example, fluid, soft tissue, and fat. These small density differences are best appreciated by manipulation of the image on the video monitor.

Each CT examination should be monitored by the radiologist. Specific clinical information is needed from the referring physician, to tailor the examination to the individual patient. Based on the clinical information provided, the radiologist must decide the section thickness, the number of sections to be obtained over the area of study, and the use of intravenous, oral, or rectal contrast agents. Special indications may also require intrathecal contrast agents or bolus injections of intravenous contrast agents with sequential scans.

Despite the multiple sections required for each CT examination, the radiation dose to the patient is often comparable to that of other, less-informative radiologic procedures. For example, the radiation dose to the patient from a CT scan of the head is

127

about the same as from a standard series of radiographs of the skull.[1] Whereas the entire head is irradiated during each exposure for a skull film, only a thin section of the head is directly exposed to radiation during each CT scan. Scatter radiation from contiguous slices also contributes to the total dose of radiation received by each area during a CT examination.

Each CT examination takes 15 to 60 min to complete, depending on the number of sections needed and the speed of the scanner. The patient must lie still because motion can seriously degrade the image. Sedation is required for uncooperative patients and for young children.

CT scanning is usually more expensive than other imaging techniques, such as ultrasound and radionuclide scanning, because of the higher cost of CT equipment. In 1981, the average total cost of a CT scan of the head, with and without the use of contrast agents, was $324.[3] The cost of a body scan was $362. Despite the higher cost, CT is often the imaging method of choice. Indications for CT are compared to those for other radiologic procedures throughout this chapter, in relation to specific clinical problems.

Before describing the scanning of specific areas of the body, it may be helpful to discuss an approach to viewing CT scans. One should always view the scans in a systematic order, beginning with the most inferior section and continuing superiorly. The identity of a structure on a single CT slice may not be apparent until one examines the sections superior and inferior to it. All the structures on the slice should be examined, not just the organ of interest or the obvious abnormalities. Most abnormalities are detected on CT by an alteration of the normal attenuation (density) of a structure or by a change in size or contour. One should use symmetry to detect these abnormalities whenever possible. Finally, the scans should be reviewed with the radiologist. The interaction between the surgeon and the radiologist may improve their understanding of the case and may facilitate the diagnosis.

SCANNING OF THE HEAD

CT scanning of the head is the method of choice for evaluation of almost all intracranial abnormalities. Since its introduction in 1973, this technique has rendered pneumoencephalography and radionuclide brain scanning obsolete. Angiography is now reserved for the evaluation of primary vascular abnormalities and the preoperative evaluation of tumors. CT has become the method of choice because of its ability to show fine anatomic detail. A knowledge of normal anatomic structures is therefore basic to understanding CT examinations of the head.

Anatomic Structures

Each CT examination of the head requires 12 to 17 sections; Figure 6–1 shows 6 of these sections. The ventricular system and the cerebrospinal fluid (CSF) cisterns appear as low-density areas with a CT number slightly greater than that of water. The most inferior sections are beneath the level of the ventricles. At this level, the medulla oblongata is seen posteriorly. Anterior to the medulla are the clivus, sphenoid bone, and orbits (Fig. 6–1A). On slightly higher sections (Fig. 6–1B), the fourth ventricle is visualized. The fourth ventricle separates the brain stem from the cerebellum. At this level, the suprasellar cistern and the temporal and frontal lobes are also seen.

The third ventricle appears on higher sections as a slit-like midline structure (Fig. 6–1C). Lateral to the third ventricle is the thalamus; posterior to the third ventricle are the pineal gland, the midbrain, and the quadrigeminal plate cistern. The frontal horns of the lateral ventricles are also seen on this section. Tucked within the concavity of the frontal horn is the caudate nucleus. Lateral to the caudate nucleus and thalamus are the internal capsule and the lentiform nucleus. Anterior to the frontal horns is the genu of the corpus callosum. The gray and white matter of the frontal, temporal, and occipital lobes are also seen on this section.

On a higher section (Fig. 6–1D), the body of each lateral ventricle is seen. Figure 6–1E shows a section superior to the level of the ventricles. On this section, the centrum semiovale and the frontal, parietal, and occipital lobes are seen.[4]

Each examination is usually done first without contrast agents and is then repeated after the intravenous administration of an iodine-containing contrast agent. The contrast medium causes an increase in the density of the gray matter that is greater than that of the white matter, and so it accentuates the gray-white junction. It also allows visualization of the major arteries and the venous sinuses (Fig. 6–1F). The falx cerebri, tentorium cerebelli, and choroid plexus also show marked contrast enhancement.

Intracranial calcifications are frequently seen in normal patients in the pineal gland, falx cerebri, choroid plexus, and habenula. These calcifications should not be confused with other causes of increased attenuation, such as hematoma.

Pathologic Findings

TRAUMA. CT scanning should be the initial radiologic examination in all patients suspected of intracranial abnormalities following head trauma. With CT, one can rapidly demonstrate intracranial abnormalities that are life-threatening but treatable. Al-

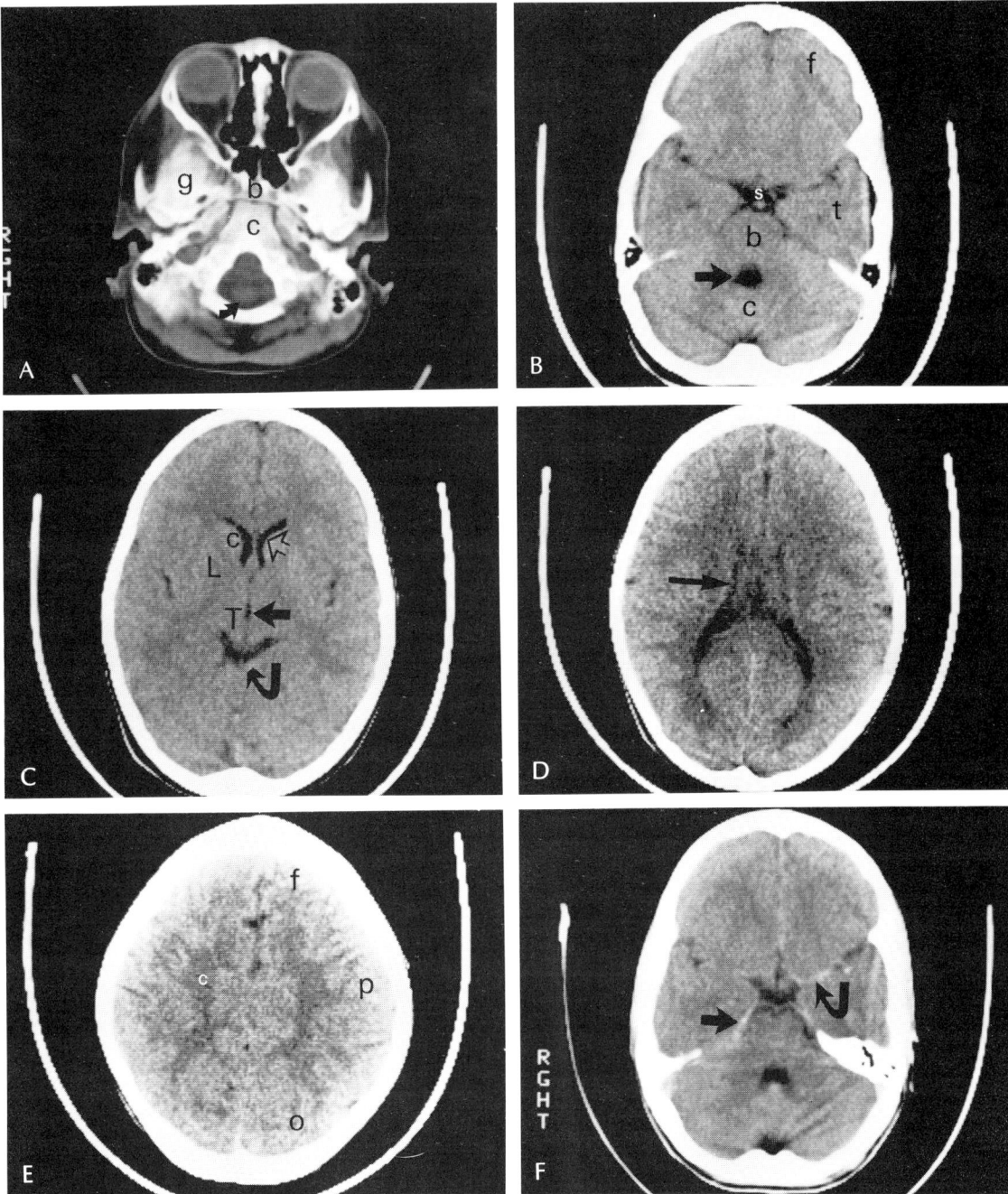

FIG. 6–1. Normal head scan. *A* to *E* show progressively higher sections without contrast; *F* is a contrast-enhanced scan at the same level as *B*. *A,* Medulla oblongata (arrow), clivus (c), and body (b) and greater wing (g) of the sphenoid bone. *B,* Fourth ventricle (arrow), brain stem (b), cerebellum (c), suprasellar cistern (s), and temporal (t) and frontal (f) lobes. *C,* Third ventricle (arrow), frontal horn of the lateral ventricle (open arrow), quadrigeminal plate cistern (curved arrow), caudate nucleus (c), thalamus (T), and lentiform nucleus (L). *D,* Body of the lateral ventricle (arrow). *E,* Centrum semiovale (c) and frontal (f), parietal (p), and occipital lobes (o). *F,* The linear enhancing structures are the arteries in the circle of Willis; posterior cerebral artery (arrow) and middle cerebral artery (curved arrow) are visible.

though CT does not always show linear, nondepressed skull fractures, these injuries are usually of no clinical significance in the absence of intracranial abnormalities. Plain films may be completely normal despite significant intracranial injury and cause needless delay in the initial management of a severely injured patient.

Subdural Hematomas. Most subdural hematomas occur supratentorially over the convexity and are the result of tears of the bridging cortical veins or lacerations of the dura and the dural venous sinuses. Subdural hematomas have a semilunar configuration with a convex lateral border, which conforms to the calvaria, and a concave medial border. The hemetoma is usually diffuse, covering most of the hemisphere. Acute subdural hematomas are hyperdense, when compared to the adjacent brain (Fig. 6–2). The hyperdensity of the hematoma is related to hemoglobin concentration.[5] Acute isodense or hypodense subdural hematomas are rare, but they can occur in patients with severe anemia or when the lesion comprises a mixture of hemorrhage and CSF. The density within a subdural hematoma may be layered, with the denser portion of the hematoma in the dependent region.

Subdural hematomas decrease in density with time and gradually become hypodense, relative to the adjacent brain. Between 1 and 3 weeks after the initial injury, the hematoma passes through an isodense phase. During this phase, a subdural hematoma may be less obvious on a CT scan, but virtually all such lesions can still be detected by CT if one pays careful attention to diagnostic features other than abnormal density.[6] Isodense subdural hematomas displace the parenchyma away from the calvaria. The sulci do not extend all the way to the calvaria if a subdural hematoma is present (Fig. 6–3A), and the white matter may be displaced medially or may be "buckled."[7]

Chronic subdural hematomas appear as hypodense collections (Fig. 6–3B). They usually retain a semilunar configuration, but some chronic subdural hematomas may acquire a biconvex configuration. Repeated episodes of bleeding may cause a chronic subdural hematoma to appear hyperdense or to have areas of different density. These changes may complicate the determination of the age of the hematoma, but this factor is not of clinical significance. The patient's clinical status, along with the CT determination of the size of the hematoma and the mass effect, should determine whether surgical treatment is necessary.

Epidural Hematomas. These lesions result from tears of the meningeal arteries. Almost all epidural hematomas are associated with skull fractures. Epidural hematomas appear on CT scans as biconvex lesions of blood density (Fig. 6–4). Because they expand rapidly, they are almost always evaluated in the acute phase when the hematoma is hyperdense. Epidural hematomas usually remain more localized than subdural hematomas because dural attachments and sutures limit their spread. Mass effect is usually present.

Injuries of the Brain Parenchyma. Trauma to the brain parenchyma may result in cerebral edema, contusion, or hematoma.[8] Post-traumatic edema may be either focal or diffuse. Focal areas of edema show decreased density and mass effect (see Fig. 6–2). Diffuse cerebral edema causes a generalized decrease in density of the brain parenchyma and compression or obliteration of the ventricles, sulci, and cisterns.

Cerebral contusions have a "salt-and-pepper" appearance, from small punctate hemorrhages interspersed with normal or edematous brain tissue. Contrast-enhanced scans in patients with cerebral contusion may show marked contrast enhancement

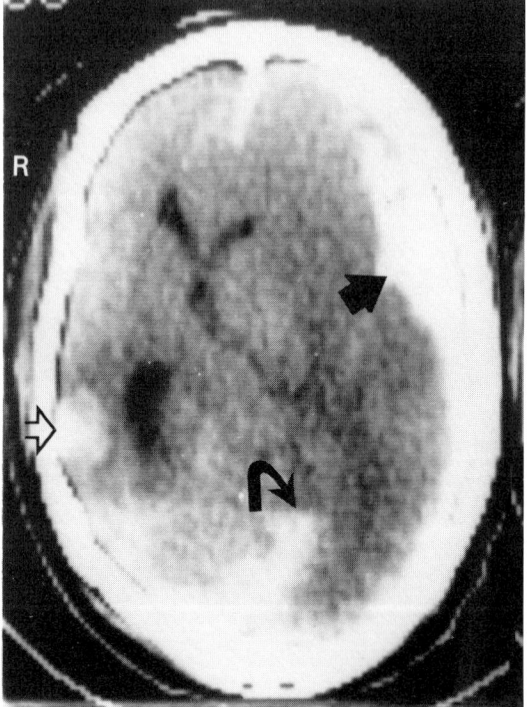

FIG. 6–2. Acute subdural hematoma, intracerebral hematoma, and subarachnoid hemorrhage. Acute hemorrhage appears hyperdense; a hyperdense subdural hematoma (arrow) is present on the left. A generalized decrease in the density of the brain parenchyma is seen on the left because of edema. This edema has shifted the ventricles to the right (R). The subarachnoid hemorrhage posteriorly (curved arrow) appears as increased density in the superior cerebellar cistern. An intracerebral hematoma is also seen on the right (open arrow).

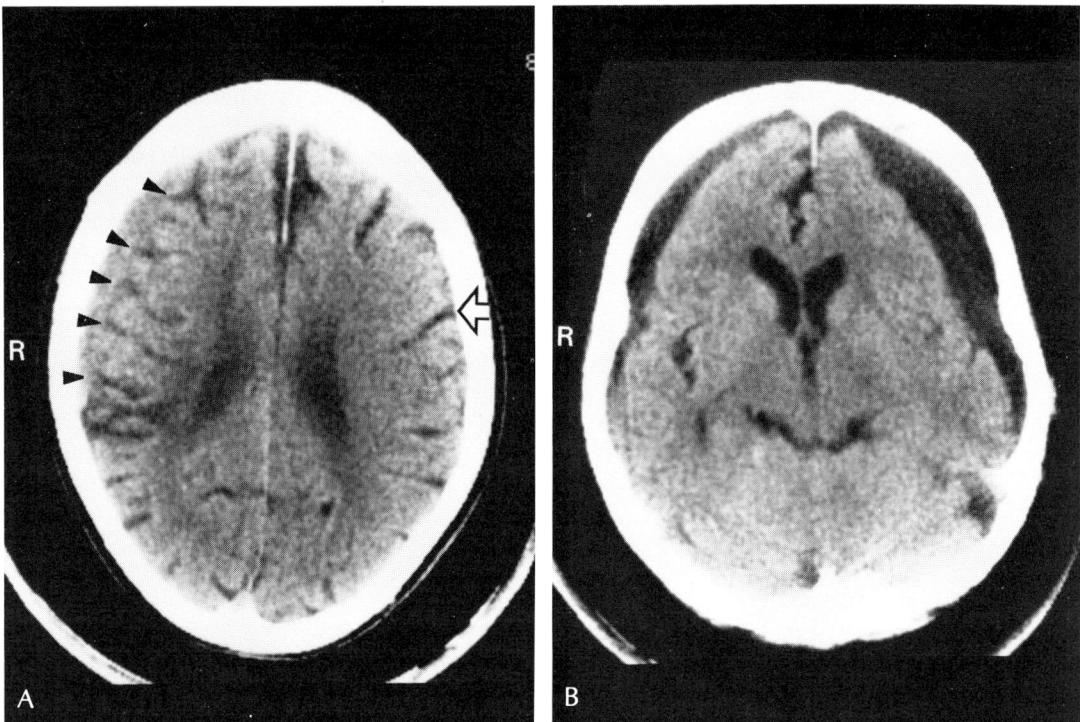

FIG. 6–3. *A,* Isodense subdural hematoma. On the left the sulci extend to the calvaria (open arrow); on the right (R), the sulci stop at the site of the subdural hematoma (arrowheads). The hematoma has the same density as the brain parenchyma. *B,* Bilateral hypodense subdural hematomas. Low-density fluid collections, which have the typical semilunar configuration of subdural hematomas, are present on both sides. R, Right.

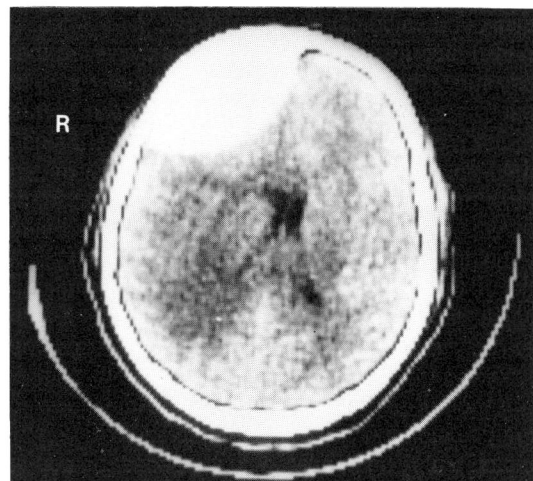

FIG. 6–4. Epidural hematoma. The hyperdense hematoma has the characteristic biconvex shape of an epidural hematoma. The right lateral ventricle appears compressed and pushed to the left. R, Right.

in the area of the contusion, caused by disruption of the blood-brain barrier.

Cerebral hematomas are hyperdense and are well circumscribed on CT scans (see Fig. 6–2). They produce mass effect and are often surrounded by a region of low density due to edema. Cerebral hematomas decrease in density with time, as do all hematomas. This change should not be interpreted as resolution because a large isodense or hypodense hematoma may still be present. Determination of resolution should be based on changes in mass effect, not CT density.

BRAIN TUMORS. CT scanning is accurate in the detection and localization of brain tumors. Intracranial tumors are detected on CT scans by mass effect, altered parenchymal density, and abnormal contrast enhancement. The mass effect of the tumor may produce midline shift, compression or obliteration of the sulci, cisterns, and ventricles, and displacement of parenchymal structures. Altered parenchymal density due to brain tumors often appears as areas of decreased density on nonenhanced scans. Small calcifications, many of which are not seen on skull films, may appear as areas of increased density. Most brain tumors show some contrast enhancement because of pooling of the contrast agent in the extravascular compartment secondary to blood-brain barrier disruption. The enhancement may be uniform or inhomogeneous, or it may appear as enhancement of a capsular ring around a low-density core. The tumor may be surrounded by edema.

Frequently, the specific type of tumor may be suggested by its CT appearance and location, in conjunction with appropriate clinical data such as the patient's age and symptoms. Low-grade astrocytomas appear as poorly marginated areas of decreased attenuation with prominent mass effect. Contrast enhancement is frequently absent with low-grade astrocytomas, and when it does occur, it is mild in degree and irregular in distribution. Glioblastomas show marked contrast enhancement and prominent peritumoral edema. The contrast enhancement of glioblastomas frequently appears as an enhanced rim of viable tumor surrounding a hypodense, necrotic center (Fig. 6–5A). This necrotic center may show contrast enhancement on delayed scans.

Meningiomas usually occur in the parasagittal region, the cortical convexities, and along the sphenoid wings. They appear on nonenhanced scans as well-circumscribed masses of slightly increased density (Fig. 6–5B). The increased density is due to psammomatous calcification. Meningiomas frequently provoke thickening and sclerosis of the adjacent calvaria. After injection of the contrast agent, one sees intense, homogeneous enhancement of the meningioma.[9]

Intracranial metastases usually appear on CT scans as multiple, round, enhancing lesions (Fig.

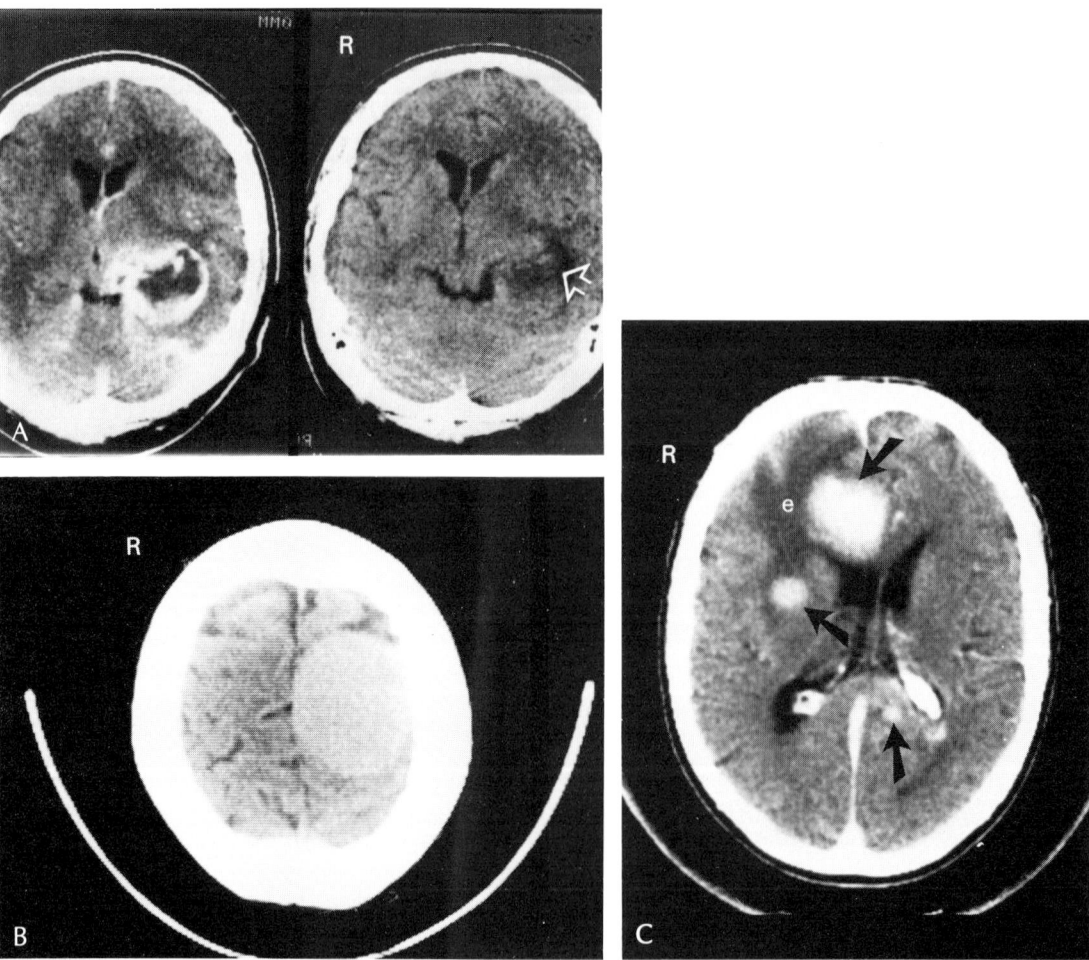

FIG. 6–5. *A,* Glioblastoma. The unenhanced scan on the right shows a low-density lesion in the left temporal lobe (open arrow). The enhanced scan at the same level shows an enhancing ring surrounding a low-density core. *B,* Meningioma. The unenhanced scan shows a well-circumscribed lesion that is denser than the brain parenchyma. The enhanced scan (not shown) showed intense, homogeneous enhancement. *C,* Metastases. An enhanced scan shows three enhancing metastatic lesions (arrows). The area of low density adjacent to the metastases on the right is due to edema (e). The increased density in the lateral ventricles is due to calcification in the choroid plexus. R, Right.

6–5C). Metastases occur most commonly at the junction of the gray and white matter. Edema of the adjacent white matter may be disproportionately severe in relation to the size of the metastasis. As metastatic lesions grow, they may develop necrotic, nonenhancing centers.

INTRACRANIAL VASCULAR DISEASE. Subarachnoid hemorrhage is most commonly due to rupture of a berry aneurysm. Arteriovenous malformations, trauma, and hypertensive hemorrhage are other causes.

Subarachnoid Hemorrhage. CT scanning should be the initial diagnostic test in all patients suspected of subarachnoid hemorrhage. The CT scan can show the presence and extent of a subarachnoid hemorrhage and associated abnormalities, such as hydrocephalus, parenchymal hemorrhage, and infarction.

The CT scan in patients with subarachnoid hemorrhage shows increased density within the cisterns, fissures, and ventricles on nonenhanced scans (see Fig. 6–2); enhanced scans are not needed. In one study, the CT scan showed the presence of subarachnoid hemorrhage in 75 to 85% of the patients scanned within the first 4 days.[10] Because a small subarachnoid hemorrhage can be missed on a CT scan, a spinal tap is necessary to exclude the diagnosis of subarachnoid hemorrhage if the CT scan is normal. The location of the blood within the subarachnoid space is helpful in determining the site of the ruptured aneurysm. In patients with multiple aneurysms, this information may help to determine which aneurysm has bled. Angiography is needed for the actual visualization of the aneurysm because most ruptured aneurysms are too small to detect on CT scans.

Vascular Malformations. Patients with vascular malformations may present with subarachnoid or intraparenchymal hemorrhage. In addition to showing the intracranial hemorrhage, CT scans often demonstrate the malformation as an enhancing region with ill-defined margins. Sometimes, one sees serpiginous structures that represent enlarged arteries or veins (Fig. 6–6). A vein of Galen aneurysm is due to a malformation that increases blood flow through the vein of Galen; the dilated vein is seen on enhanced scans as a round, midline structure of uniform enhancement located posterior to the third ventricle.

Cerebral Infarction. Early CT evaluation of suspected cerebral infarction is important in establishing the correct diagnosis and in excluding hemorrhage, neoplasm, and other abnormalities. Newer-model scanners have shown 80% of infarcts within the first 24 hours, and in some patients the infarct may be seen after only 3 hours.[11,12] Early infarcts appear as ill-defined areas of decreased attenua-

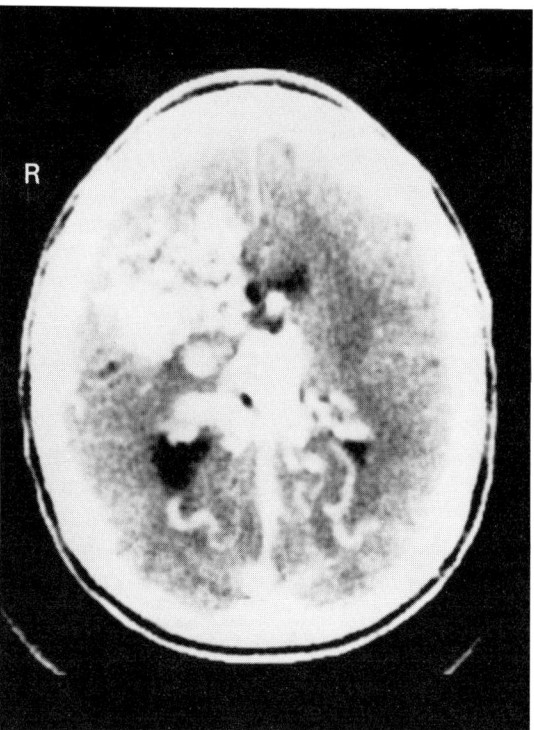

FIG. 6–6. Arteriovenous malformation. The enhanced scan shows a huge arteriovenous malformation involving both the right and the left hemispheres. R, Right.

tion. In some cases, subtle mass effect, such as effacement of sulci or slight compression of cisterns, may be the only finding in the first 24 hours. In 2 to 5 days, the area of decreased density becomes more homogeneous and better defined. At this time, the maximal mass effect due to edema is noted. The mass effect quickly subsides and is usually resolved by the end of the first week. Several months later, the attenuation in the region of the infarct may return to normal, and ipsilateral ventricular dilatation and enlargement of adjacent sulci may be seen. It may then be difficult to distinguish an old infarct from localized atrophy. Contrast enhancement in the region of the infarct does not occur until 4 to 5 days after infarction and it may persist for 3 to 4 weeks. The enhancement occurs in the gray matter and is due to disruption of the blood-brain barrier.

CT has been reported to show 75 to 98% of all infarcts. The ability of CT to demonstrate the infarct is related to the age and size of the infarct and the resolution of the scanner. A small infarct in the internal capsule or brain stem that may be undetectable on a CT scan may still produce catastrophic symptoms.[13]

CEREBRAL ABSCESS. Such a lesion may result from direct extension through the paranasal sinuses or mastoid processes, from hematogenous spread, or from penetrating wounds or surgical procedures. CT scans show an area of low density surrounded by an enhancing ring. This appearance is not specific for abscess because ring-enhancing lesions can also represent primary and metastatic tumors, infarct, resolving hematoma, and giant aneurysm.[14]

HYDROCEPHALUS AND ATROPHY. Increased ventricular size is readily apparent on CT scans. In addition to showing the degree of ventricular dilatation, CT also shows the site of obstruction in intraventricular (noncommunicating) hydrocephalus. The site of obstruction is identified as the point of transition from dilated to nondilated CSF spaces. The cause is usually a tumor or other mass lesion easily seen on a CT scan.

Extraventricular obstructive (communicating) hydrocephalus most commonly is due to posthemorrhagic or postinfectious fibrosis in the cisterns or in the arachnoid granulations of the parasagittal region. In about 25% of patients with extraventricular obstruction, the fourth ventricle is not dilated, and this feature may complicate localization of the site of obstruction.[15]

After shunting, the decrease in ventricular size is easily monitored by CT. The decrease in size may be asymmetric, with the shunt-containing ventricle smaller than the other lateral ventricle. Complications of shunting procedures and shunt malfunction can be quickly and reliably detected on CT scans. For follow-up of shunt therapy, one usually needs only a nonenhanced CT scan.

Enlargement of the CSF-containing spaces can have many causes other than obstruction of the CSF pathways; almost all degenerative diseases of the brain eventually enlarge the ventricles and sulci (Fig. 6–7). Because findings of atrophy also occur in normal individuals as they age,[16] the usefulness of these findings in the evaluation of dementia depends in part on the age of the patient. Some reports have attempted to define CT findings of Alzheimer's disease, which is the most common cause of dementia in elderly patients. These reports have stressed a correlation between ventricular size, especially the width of the third ventricle, and dementia, and loss of discrimination of the gray-white junction.[17,18] Although such findings are of interest, dementia cannot be reliably predicted by a CT scan at this time. In the assessment of patients with dementia, CT is used primarily to exclude treatable causes, such as neoplasm, obstructive hydrocephalus, and chronic subdural hematoma.

Atrophic changes are also produced by alcohol abuse, ingestion of various drugs and toxins, especially corticosteroids, and malnutrition. The "atrophy" may be reversed by removal of the offending substance or restoration of normal nutrition.

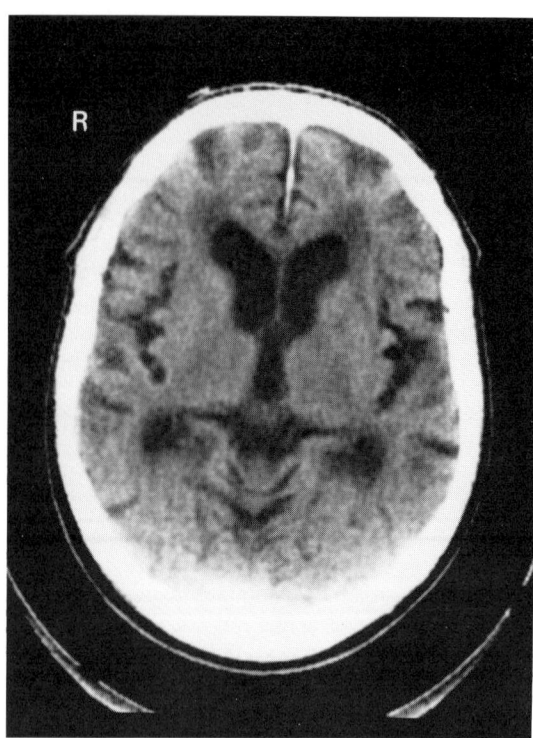

FIG. 6–7. Atrophy. The ventricles and sulci are enlarged. Compare this scan to Figure 6–1C, which is at the same level. R, Right.

SCANNING OF THE CHEST

Standard posteroanterior and lateral chest roentgenograms remain the initial radiographic examination of choice in patients with suspected chest disease because they are readily available and inexpensive. CT scans of the chest provide additional information about abnormalities detected on chest radiographs.[19] CT scans can also enable one to detect abnormalities not seen on standard radiographs or tomograms; therefore, CT is useful when one suspects the presence of a chest lesion, such as in myasthenia gravis. Additional indications for chest CT scanning include preoperative staging of lung and esophageal carcinoma and evaluation of patients with tumors that have a high incidence of chest metastases.

Anatomic Structures

Cross-sectional CT images provide an excellent view of the normal mediastinal structures superimposed on standard chest roentgenograms. In almost all adult patients, enough fat is present in the mediastinum to allow distinction of the margins of the normal structures and vasculature. The major vascular structures can be recognized on nonenhanced scans, but differentiation of the vascular structures is better if an intravenous infusion of urographic con-

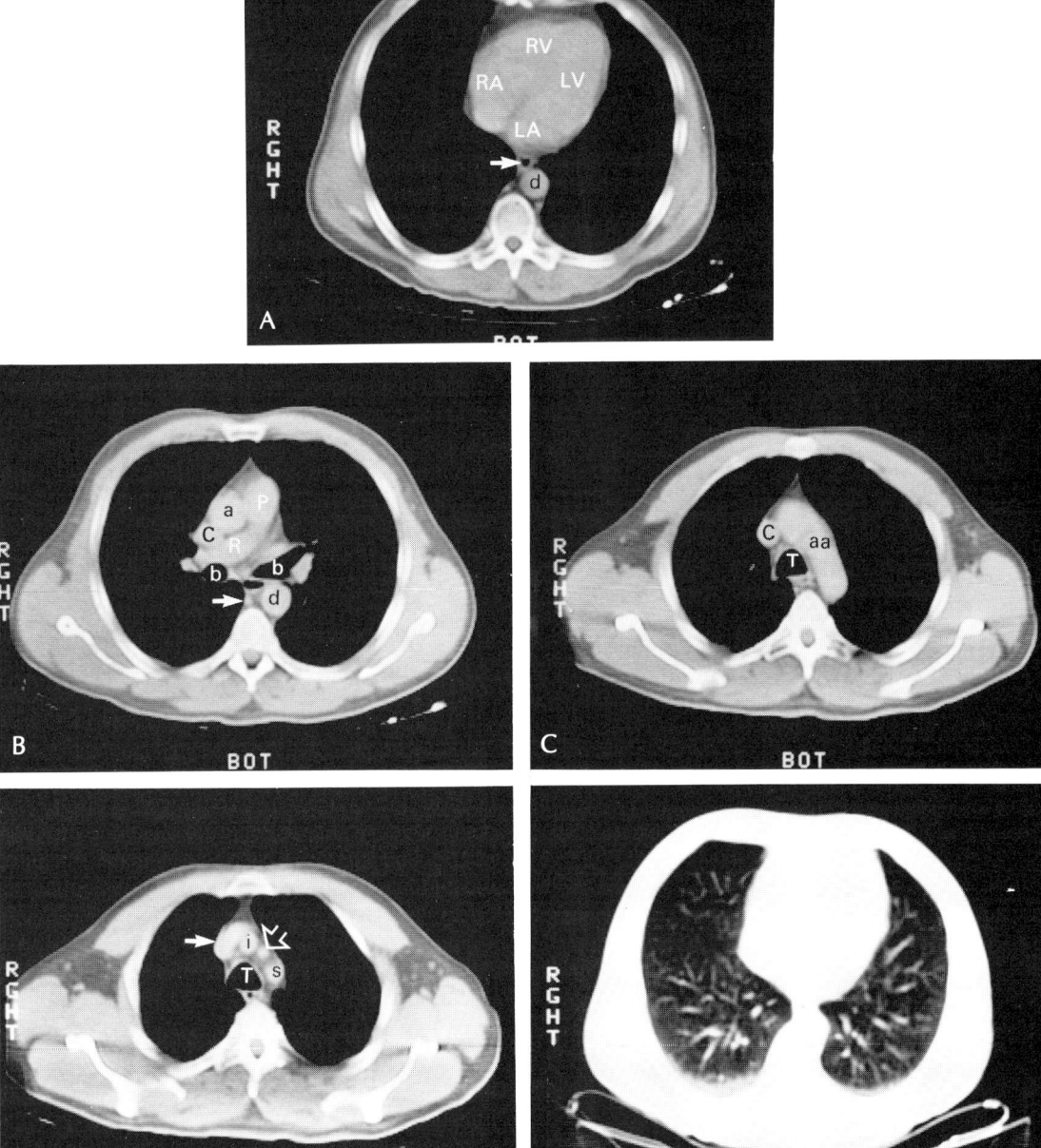

FIG. 6–8. Normal chest. *A* to *D* show progressively higher sections of a chest scan; *E* shows the same scan as *A*, with adjustments of the video monitor to demonstrate the lung parenchyma. *A,* At the level of the heart. Right atrium (RA), right ventricle (RV), left atrium (LA), left ventricle (LV), descending aorta (d), and esophagus (arrow). *B,* At the level of the hila. Main pulmonary artery (P), right pulmonary artery (R), superior vena cava (C), ascending aorta (a), descending aorta (d), and main stem bronchi (b). The soft tissue density lateral to the left bronchus is the left interlobar pulmonary artery. The esophagus is the air-filled structure medial to the descending aorta. Posterior to the esophagus is the azygous vein (arrow). *C,* At the level of the aortic arch (aa). Superior vena cava (C), trachea (T). *D,* Superior to the aortic arch. The arrow points to where the left and right brachiocephalic veins meet to form the superior vena cava. The other three vascular structures are the innominate artery (i), left common carotid artery (open arrow), and the left subclavian artery (s). The esophagus is seen posterior to the trachea (T). *E,* The lung shows increased vascularity in the dependent region, which is posterior.

trast material is given. Occasionally, a bolus injection of contrast material with rapid sequential scanning is needed for better evaluation of a specific area. Figure 6–8 shows normal mediastinal anatomic features.

In evaluating the lung parenchyma on a chest CT scan, the settings on the video monitor are different from those used for the mediastinum. Pulmonary vessels, bronchi, and interlobar septa are seen (Fig. 6–8E). As in standard chest radiographs, one sees preferential blood flow to the dependent portion of the lungs when the patient is supine.

Chest CT scans are obtained during suspended respiration in the inspiratory phase. Approximately the same depth of inspiration should be taken for each scan, to minimize missing a small lesion because of a varied depth of inspiration.

Mediastinum

Diagnoses can be made using CT by providing precise localization of mediastinal abnormalities and information about tissue density, which cannot be obtained by standard chest radiographs or conventional tomography.[20] In some cases, the CT appearance and attenuation value are so characteristic that a specific diagnosis can be made, and the patient can be spared invasive procedures.

LIPOMATOSIS VERSUS CYSTIC LESIONS. The characteristic attenuation value of fat (−80 HU) allows epicardial fat pads and mediastinal lipomatosis to be distinguished from cystic or solid masses. Epicardial fat pads are seen as localized collections of fatty tissue in the cardiophrenic angles. Mediastinal lipomatosis causes widening of the mediastinum due to generalized fat deposition and is the result of obesity, Cushing's syndrome, or exogenous corticosteroids. Benign cystic lesions, which are well-defined masses with thin walls, have an attenuation value of +5 to +25 HU, or just greater than that of water. Bronchogenic cysts are most commonly located in the subcarinal area (Fig. 6–9). Pericardial cysts are found in the pericardiophrenic angles and are more common on the right side than on the left.

VASCULAR ANOMALIES AND ANEURYSMS. Anomalies and aneurysms of the thoracic aorta can also be confidently diagnosed on CT scans by their characteristic enhancement after the administration of a contrast agent.[21] The role of CT in the diagnosis of aortic dissection is controversial, however. With CT, one can see aortic dissections as reliably as with angiography.[22,23] Both the true and false lumens and even the intimal flap can be seen on CT scans. On nonenhanced scans, the false lumen can be either hyperdense or hypodense relative to the true lumen, depending on the age of the clot in the false lumen. Pleural and pericardial leakage from the aorta can also be identified (Fig. 6–10). With a bolus injection of contrast material, one sees differential enhancement of the true and false lumens because of delayed or decreased flow through the false lumen. "Aortic wall thickening" and compression of the true lumen can also be seen. The site of intimal tear and the re-entry site are not visible on CT scans, but these same features are often missed on angiograms. The major disadvantage of CT scanning of dissecting aortic aneurysms is the inability to detect aortic valvular dysfunction and involvement of the major arterial branches. We therefore recommend angiography as the initial study in patients with suspected dissecting aortic aneurysm.

SOLID MASSES. The origin and extent of solid mediastinal masses can be evaluated by CT, but a specific histologic diagnosis is not possible.[24] Solid mediastinal masses may appear as a homogeneous mass of soft tissue density or as an inhomogeneous mass with some areas of low density. Invasion of mediastinal fat or extension into the pleura, pericardium, or lung suggests a malignant process. Thymoma, lymphoma, substernal thyroid, and teratoma are the most common anterior mediastinal masses. Thymomas can be seen on CT scans in patients with myasthenia gravis more often than on chest radiographs or conventional tomograms (Fig. 6–11). Teratomas may sometimes be distinguished from other mediastinal masses by the presence of fat, peripheral calcifications, and a "tooth" or bony element in the mass. Ectopic parathyroid adenomas may also be found in the anterior mediastinum or in the paratracheal region of the middle mediastinum. Solid tumors in the posterior mediastinum are usually neurogenic.

LYMPH NODES AND TUMOR STAGING. Mediastinal lymph nodes are easily visualized on CT scans. Nor-

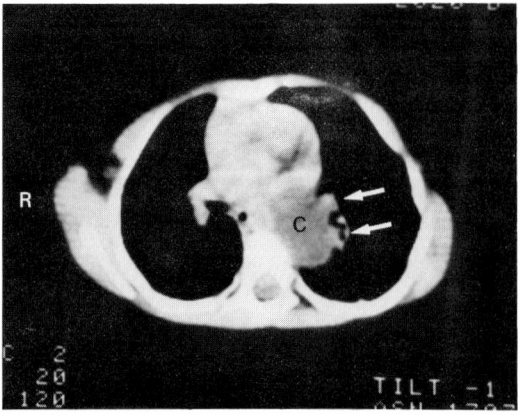

FIG. 6–9. Bronchogenic cyst. The scan demonstrates a well-defined, low-density fluid collection posterior to the heart in the subcarinal area. Lateral to the bronchogenic cyst (C), pulmonary vessels are seen (arrows). R, Right.

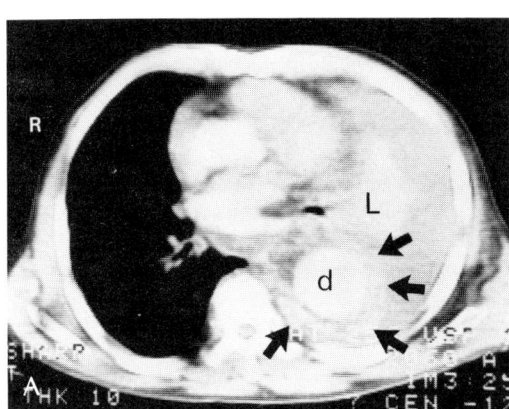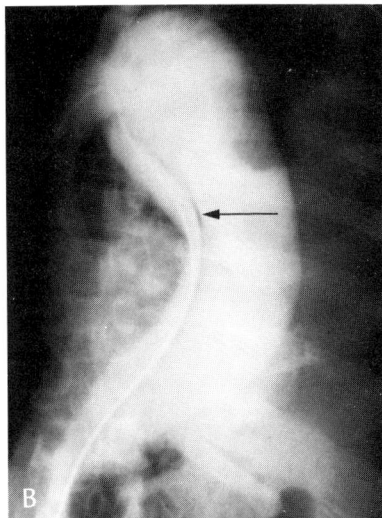

FIG. 6–10. Dissecting aortic aneurysm. A, The enhanced scan shows that the true lumen of the descending aorta (d) is greater in density than the false lumen (arrows) because of decreased flow through the false lumen. Leakage from the dissection has collapsed the lung (L) and has caused fluid to collect throughout the left pleural space. R, Right. B, The angiogram shows the dilated aorta and the lucent line that represents the intimal flap (arrow).

mal lymph nodes, which measure less than 1 cm, are seen in about 20% of all patients. Enlarged lymph nodes in the range of 1 to 2 cm may be due to neoplasm or inflammatory disease. If lymph nodes are larger than 2 cm, the cause is almost always neoplastic.[20] The ability of CT to show enlarged nodes is of great value in staging lymphoma and bronchogenic carcinoma. Preoperative staging of bronchogenic carcinoma by CT enables one to determine resectability accurately in most patients.[25] With CT, one may see invasion of the tumor into the mediastinum or chest wall (Fig. 6–12), mediastinal and hilar lymph node enlargement, and metastatic lung nodules. Direct mediastinal invasion is diagnosed when one sees tumor interdigitation with the mediastinal fat or tumor surrounding the great vessels on a CT scan. Visualization of enlarged mediastinal lymph nodes can guide the surgeon in the choice of lymph nodes for biopsy prior to thoracotomy. Because of the many causes of enlarged lymph nodes, no patient should be assumed to have metastatic lymph nodes without histologic proof. CT is limited in the staging of bronchogenic carcinoma because one cannot thereby detect metastases in lymph nodes of normal size. Moreover, if the tumor abuts the mediastinum or pleura without the foregoing evidence of direct invasion, such invasion may or may not be present.

Hilum

Abnormalities of the hilum can be evaluated either with CT scans or with 55° oblique tomograms. Results with tomograms have been more successful than with CT scans in the detection of hilar lymph nodes in some series, whereas others have reported equal accuracy.[19,26] Hilar prominence thought to be due to an enlarged pulmonary artery can best be evaluated by CT scanning, in which contrast enhancement can verify the vascular nature of the abnormality.

Lung

CT is more sensitive than plain radiography and conventional tomography in detecting pulmonary nodules. This feature makes CT valuable in the evaluation of patients with malignant tumors that have a high incidence of chest metastases, such as primary bone tumors, soft tissue sarcomas, and melanoma. CT is also useful in the further assessment of a nodule that is detected on chest radiographs. Evidence of calcification within the nodule by conventional tomography or by CT indicates a benign process. Siegelman and associates have used CT numbers to distinguish benign from malignant nodules in the absence of macroscopic calcifications,[27] but we have not found this method to be helpful. Until CT numbers become more accurate and more easily reproducible,[28] and until more extensive clinical experience has been reported, we believe that the distinction between benign and malignant should be left to the pathologist, unless macroscopic calcifications are evident.

In the evaluation of parenchymal lung lesions, CT is more helpful than conventional tomography. CT scanning allows one to define the nature of a mass, whether solid, cystic, or vascular, and to detect small cavitary lesions. With CT, one can also detect a

IMAGING

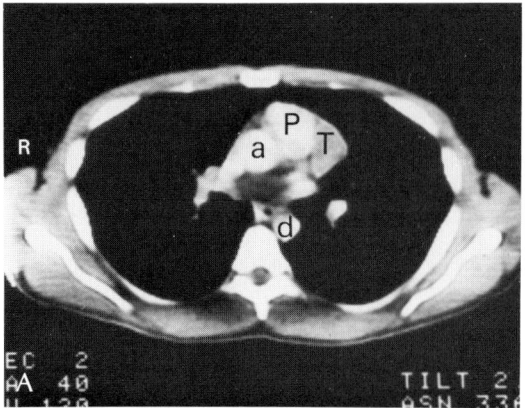

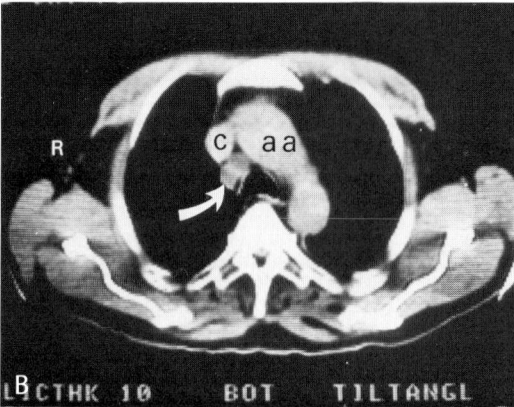

FIG. 6–11. *A*, Thymoma. The scan shows a soft tissue density (T) lateral to the main pulmonary artery (P) in a patient with myasthenia gravis. The chest films were negative. Ascending aorta (a), descending aorta (d). *B*, Enlarged lymph node. A scan at the level of the aortic arch (aa) shows an enlarged azygous lymph node (arrow) caused by metastatic lung carcinoma; the superior vena cava (c) is also visible. R, Right.

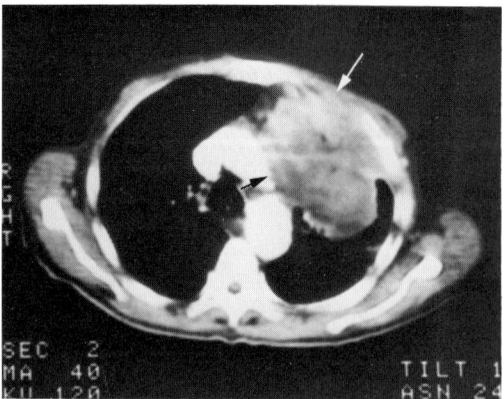

FIG. 6–12. Bronchogenic carcinoma. The scan shows invasion of both the mediastinum (black arrow) and the chest wall (white arrow).

mass that is obscured by fluid in an "opaque" hemithorax.[29]

Pleura and Chest Wall

The cross-sectional images of CT provide the best visualization of the pleura and chest wall, to aid in the distinction between parenchymal and pleural disease and to allow detection of pleural abnormalities that would otherwise be missed.[30] Extension of a tumor or infectious process into the pleura or chest wall can also be assessed by CT (Fig. 6–12).

SCANNING OF THE ABDOMEN AND PELVIS

With CT, one can visualize virtually every organ in the abdomen and pelvis. As in CT scanning of the chest, the patient should suspend respiration for each scan. Intravenous and gastrointestinal contrast agents are usually used. A steady infusion of contrast material appears to be the best method of intravenous contrast enhancement.[31] A dilute suspension of barium is ingested prior to scanning to better delineate the gastrointestinal system. Rectal contrast is often employed if a pelvic mass is suspected.

Liver

The normal nonenhanced liver has a uniform appearance, except for low-density defects, which represent the venous system. When intravenous contrast enhancement is used, the venous structures are no longer visualized, and the liver appears totally uniform (Fig. 6–13*A*). The separation of the left lobe of the liver into the medial and lateral portions is demarcated by the fat-density falciform ligament. The right and left lobes are not clearly separated on a CT scan, but this separation can be closely approximated by an imaginary line from the gallbladder to the inferior vena cava. The caudate lobe is located between the vena cava and the porta hepatis; the portal vein is consistently visualized in the porta hepatis. The hepatic artery and the undilated biliary system are only occasionally seen.

BENIGN LESIONS. A variety of benign lesions are encountered in the liver as incidental findings. The most common of these is the simple cyst. Most hepatic cysts occur as isolated defects, but some are due to polycystic kidney disease. Cysts are well circumscribed and are low in attenuation, with a CT number near 0. They have thin walls and show no contrast enhancement. The CT appearance of most hepatic cysts is characteristic enough that no further evaluation is necessary, unless the patient's medical history suggests the presence of a cystic neoplasm or an abscess.[32]

Hemangioma, a common benign tumor of the liver, appears as a low-density lesion on nonen-

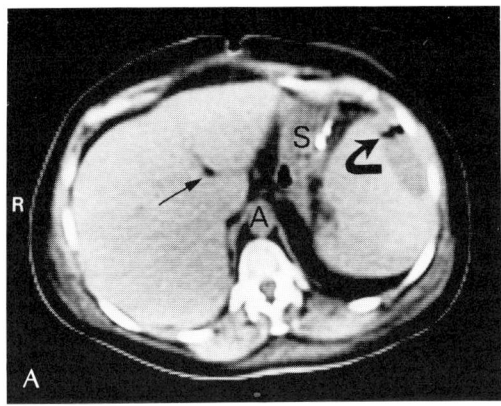

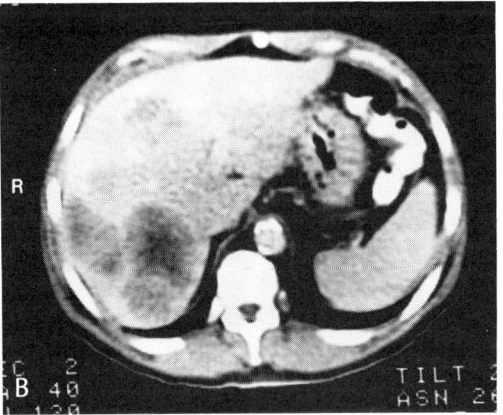

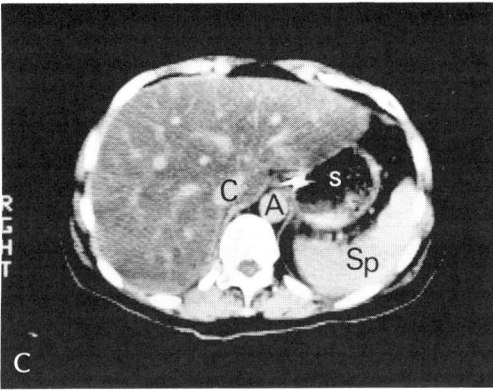

FIG. 6–13. *A,* Normal liver; left subdiaphragmatic abscess. The liver has a homogeneous appearance, except for the falciform ligament, which has the density of fat (arrow). The intrahepatic portion of the inferior vena cava and the portal venous system are isodense with the liver parenchyma on enhanced scans. On the left side is a subdiaphragmatic abscess (curved arrow), which appears as a fluid collection containing gas. The stomach (S) and the aorta (A) are also visible. *B,* Liver metastases. Multiple low-density metastatic lesions are seen. R, Right. *C,* Fatty infiltration of the liver. The liver is much less dense than the spleen (Sp) and the intrahepatic vascular structures on this enhanced scan. The aorta (A), the intrahepatic vena cava (C), and the stomach (s) are also seen.

hanced scans. A hemangioma undergoes a characteristic pattern of enhancement with a bolus injection of contrast material. Immediately after the bolus injection, the rim of the lesion becomes dense. During the next few minutes, the zone of enhancement extends centrally. In 10 to 15 min, the entire lesion becomes isodense.[33] We believe that this characteristic appearance is less common than some authors state; if the identity of such a lesion is in doubt, an angiogram should be performed.

Hepatic adenomas and focal nodular hyperplasia typically resemble each other on a CT scan. Both are seen as a homogeneous mass that may be slightly lower in density than the normal liver parenchyma. These lesions often are isodense and can only be detected by a change in contour of the liver. They cannot usually be differentiated from other solid tumors by CT, but some reports have noted the presence of a central scar that does not enhance as a characteristic feature of focal nodular hyperplasia.

MALIGNANT LESIONS. With CT, one can detect primary and metastatic disease of the liver. Hepatomas (hepatocellular carcinoma) may be focal or diffuse and are frequently found in association with other parenchymal liver disease, such as cirrhosis. Hepatomas typically appear as an area of low density, although some are isodense. The diffuse form of this tumor may be especially difficult to detect on a CT scan.[34] CT and radionuclide scanning have been compared in regard to hepatoma. For detection of hepatoma, radionuclide scanning is more accurate than CT. CT is better suited for determining the presence of mutiple lesions and for evaluating operability, based on lobar anatomy, however. For these reasons, the two examinations are complementary.

Metastases are typically multiple, low-density lesions (Fig. 6–13*B*). Because most metastatic lesions have a similar CT appearance, the primary tumor cannot be determined from the appearance of the metastases. Calcific metastases are usually of colorectal origin, but they may also result from ovarian or islet cell tumors or teratomas. The detection rate of hepatic metastases with CT is well over 90%. CT, ultrasound, or radioisotope scans can all be used to screen reliably for metastases. Some recent reports have indicated that CT has a higher sensitivity than the other methods.[35,36] CT and ultrasound have additional advantages over radionuclide scanning. One may thereby be able to distinguish benign lesions, such as a simple cyst or an intrahepatic gallbladder, from metastases, and one may thereby detect extrahepatic disease.

FATTY INFILTRATION. This disorder, the most common diffuse disease of the liver, results from a variety of causes including alcohol abuse, diabetes, obesity, corticosteroid therapy, endocrine disease, and parenteral hyperalimentation. Diffuse fatty infiltration causes a generalized decrease in the density of the liver that is recognized on CT scans when the density of the liver is less than that of other solid organs, such as the spleen, and when the enhanced vascular structures are denser than the liver parenchyma (Fig. 6–13C). Focal areas of fatty infiltration cause a localized area of decreased attenuation, which may be difficult to differentiate from other focal lesions, such as metastatic disease.[37]

CIRRHOSIS. This disease is best detected by radionuclide scan. CT scans may appear completely normal in patients with early cirrhosis, or scans may show signs of fatty infiltration.[38] In the late stages of cirrhosis, CT scans show lobulation of the hepatic contour due to regenerating nodules, hypertrophy of the caudate lobe, and atrophy of the right lobe of the liver. Secondary effects of cirrhosis, such as ascites, splenomegaly, and varices, can also be detected on a CT scan.

Biliary System

The gallbladder appears on a CT scan as an oval, low-density structure on the undersurface of the right lobe of the liver. The intrahepatic biliary radicles are not visualized, and the normal, unobstructed common duct is only occasionally visualized. When the common bile duct is seen, it should not exceed 6 to 8 mm.[39] Dilatation of the intrahepatic biliary system appears as low-density branching structures converging on the porta hepatis. The dilated intrahepatic radicles can be distinguished from blood vessels because the density of bile is much less than that of blood (Fig. 6–14).

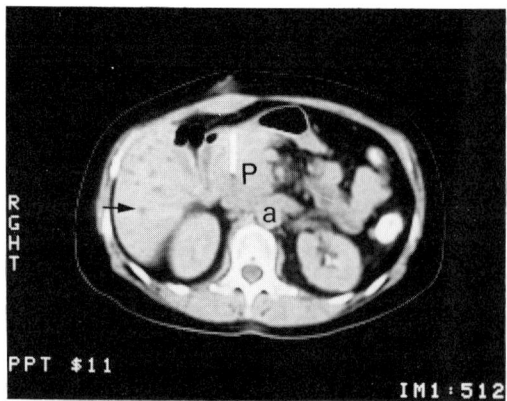

FIG. 6–14. Dilated intrahepatic ducts secondary to pancreatic carcinoma. The scan shows a biopsy needle within the head of the pancreas (P), which is massively enlarged. The needle has passed through the gastric antrum. The dilated intrahepatic ducts (arrow) are lower in density than the blood vessels, such as the aorta (a).

CT is not recommended for evaluation of routine gallbladder disease, such as cholelithiasis. Calculi can be detected on CT scans, but ultrasound is the method of choice for the detection of cholelithiasis because its accuracy approaches 99%. In the evaluation of patients with jaundice, either CT or ultrasound can enable one to determine whether the biliary system is obstructed. CT is more accurate in determining the site of obstruction (88 versus 60%) and the cause of obstruction (70 versus 38%), however.[40] The site of obstruction is identified as the point of transition from a dilated to a nondilated biliary system. The cause of obstruction may be identified as a stone in the common bile duct or a mass in the porta hepatis or pancreas. When no mass or stone is present, the appearance of the extrahepatic ducts may distinguish benign from malignant processes. Pancreatitis and benign strictures usually cause gradual tapering of the common bile duct over serial CT sections. Neoplasms usually produce abrupt termination and allow a presumptive diagnosis of cholangiocarcinoma or small pancreatic carcinoma in the absence of a detectable mass.[41,42]

Pancreas

CT or ultrasound can provide rapid, accurate, and noninvasive imaging of the pancreas, but ultrasonic examinations are frequently technically unsatisfactory because of the patient's obesity or overlying bowel gas. Even when suboptimal examinations are excluded, CT is more accurate than ultrasound in the detection of pancreatic lesions, in the assessment of their extent, and in the determination of their cause.[43] CT is therefore the method of choice for evaluating the pancreas.

The pancreas is located in the anterior pararenal space, immediately anterior to the superior mesenteric artery (Fig. 6–15A). The head of the pancreas is located anterior to the vena cava and medial to the descending portion of the duodenum. The uncinate process of the pancreas, congenitally the ventral pancreas, is the most inferior portion of the head of the pancreas and it is situated just posterior to the superior mesenteric artery and vein. The body and tail of the pancreas are situated posterior to the stomach and anterior to the splenic vein. The normal pancreatic duct is not usually visualized on a CT scan. The texture of the normal pancreas is typically uniform, but the margins may be irregularly interspersed with fat. Although measurements have been determined for the normal pancreas, we have found the simplest method of determining pancreatic enlargement is to use the vertebral body as a "yardstick." The anteroposterior diameter of the head of the pancreas should not exceed the transverse diameter of the vertebral body, and the anteroposterior diameter of the body and tail should not exceed two-thirds of that same transverse diameter.[44]

MALIGNANT LESIONS. Adenocarcinoma of the pancreas enlarges the gland and changes its contour (see Fig. 6–14). Although the enlargement is usually focal, it may be generalized.[45] When the tumor involves the head of the pancreas, changes may be noted distal to the carcinoma, such as a dilated pancreatic duct or atrophy of the tail of the pancreas. The density of most adenocarcinomas is usually the same as that of the normal gland, but cystadenocarcinomas and mucinous adenocarcinomas are of low density and may contain calcifications.

In addition to detection of the neoplasm, CT is also important in the staging of pancreatic carcinoma. One may thereby ascertain invasion of the surrounding tissues and metastases to regional lymph nodes and the liver. Although CT detection of pancreatic carcinoma has not improved survival rates, staging of the neoplasm by CT can at least guide appropriate treatment for each patient.

PANCREATITIS. The diagnosis of pancreatitis is usually established by laboratory and clinical data. CT is indicated when complications are suspected. In most patients with pancreatitis, the gland becomes diffusely increased in size, and the margins become poorly defined because of edema, fluid, and inflammation[46] (Fig. 6–15B). In some cases, focal enlargement is present, and the CT appearance mimics that of carcinoma. Thickening of the left anterior perirenal fascia occurs in patients with pancreatitis; this reliable sign distinguishes pancreatitis from neoplasm.[44]

The development of a pseudocyst is the most common complication of pancreatitis. Pseudocysts appear as low-density fluid collections with walls of variable thickness. These lesions are usually found within or adjacent to the pancreas (Fig. 6–15C), but they are occasionally seen in the perinephric region, subdiaphragmatic space, mediastinum, or lower abdomen.[47] A pseudocyst may become superinfected. If the infecting organisms are gas-producing, tiny gas bubbles may be noted on a CT scan. These gas bubbles are not usually discernible on plain films or ultrasonic scans.

In patients with chronic pancreatitis, the gland may be normal in size, enlarged, or atrophic. Calcifications may be noted in the parenchyma or the ductal system. If the calculi obstruct the pancreatic duct, dilatation will result in visualization of the duct on a CT scan.

Gastrointestinal System

Barium studies and endoscopic examinations are used to detect primary tumors of the gastrointestinal

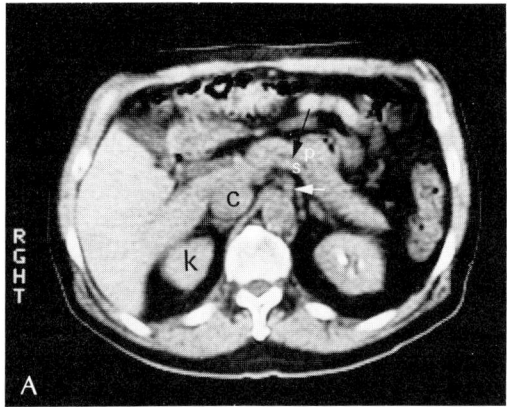
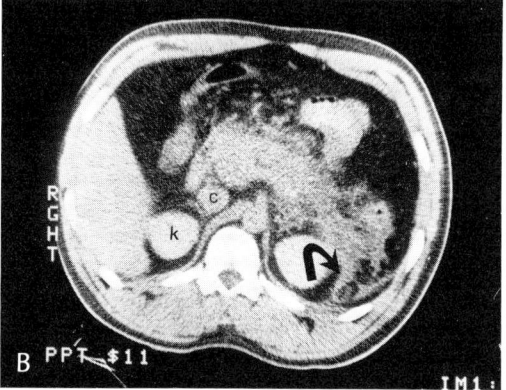
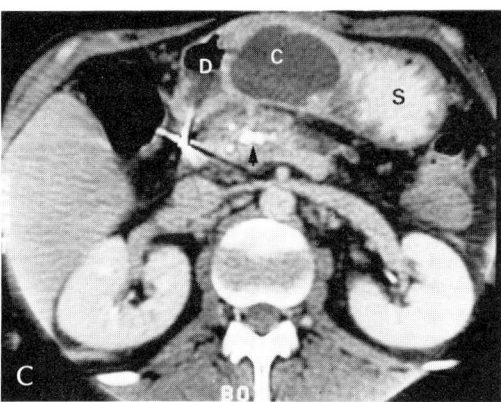

FIG. 6–15. *A*, Normal pancreas. The white arrow points to the superior mesenteric artery, which is an important landmark in identifying the pancreas. The black arrow points to the fat that separates the splenic vein (s) from the pancreas (p). This fat density should not be confused with a dilated pancreatic duct. The inferior vena cava (c) and the kidney (k) are also visible. *B*, Pancreatitis. The pancreas is diffusely enlarged, and the margins are poorly defined. Thickening of the left anterior perirenal fascia (curved arrow) is visible. Also seen are the inferior vena cava (c) and the kidney (k). *C*, Pancreatic pseudocyst. A pseudocyst is present in the lesser sac (C). The arrow is pointing to calcifications within the pancreas. The stomach (S) and the duodenum (D) are also visible.

tract. These examinations are limited in that they can only show the intraluminal extent of the disease. CT scanning enables one to stage gastrointestinal tumors accurately because it shows extraluminal extension of tumors, regional adenopathy, and distant metastases. CT staging of cancer of the esophagus, stomach, and colon is closely correlated with surgical findings.[48-51] By facilitating accurate preoperative assessments of the size and extent of malignant gastrointestinal tumors, CT can aid the surgeon or radiation therapist in planning appropriate treatment.[52]

Kidneys

The kidneys characteristically appear as "U"-shaped structures on CT scans. Renal sinus fat is usually abundant enough to outline portions of the pelvocaliceal system without intravenous contrast material. When a urographic contrast agent is administered, the excreted agent highlights the pelvocaliceal system. If dynamic scanning is done after a bolus injection of contrast material, the cortex, medulla, and papillae can be distinguished. The hilum of each kidney faces anteromedially, and the renal arteries and veins can usually be discerned. The veins lie anterior to the arteries. The left renal vein is much longer than the right, and it passes anterior to the aorta before entering the vena cava. The normal fascial borders of the perirenal space and retroperitoneum are also seen on CT scans. The anterior perirenal fascia forms the anterior border of the perirenal space and the posterior boundary of the anterior pararenal space; the posterior perirenal fascia forms the posterior boundary of the perirenal space and the anterior border of the posterior pararenal space.

Although excretory urography and ultrasound are the primary methods of evaluating renal disease, the kidneys are visualized on all abdominal examinations and should be carefully evaluated. The primary indications for CT scanning of the kidneys are evaluation of solid tumors and staging of renal neoplasms.

RENAL CYSTS. These lesions are often noted as incidental findings on abdominal CT scans (Fig. 6-16A). Simple cysts can be diagnosed confidently when they have the following criteria: (1) uniform, near-water attenuation value; (2) a thin, imperceptible wall; (3) sharp separation from normal renal parenchyma; and (4) lack of contrast enhancement.[53] Strict adherence to these criteria should enable one to avoid mistaking an abscess or a necrotic tumor for a simple cyst.

MALIGNANT LESIONS. Renal cell carcinoma appears on CT scans as a mass with a discrete alteration in the normal contour of the kidney (Fig. 6-16B). The attenuation of the mass, much higher

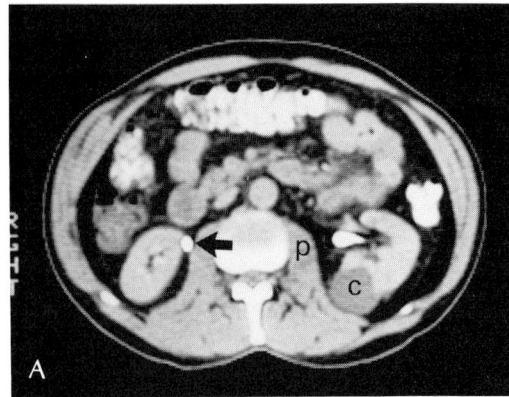

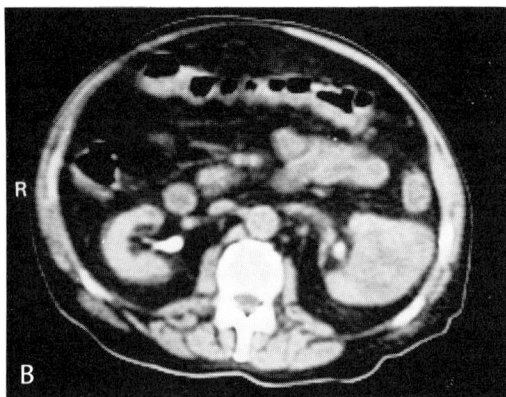

FIG. 6–16. *A,* Renal cyst. The scan shows a typical renal cyst (c), which has a uniform, low-density appearance and an imperceptible wall. The psoas muscle (p) and the right ureter (arrow) are also seen. *B,* Renal cell carcinoma. The mass in the left kidney distorts the lateral contour. The density of the mass is not homogeneous and is less than that of the normal renal parenchyma. R, Right.

than that of a cyst, is closer to that of normal renal parenchyma. The attenuation is often inhomogeneous because of areas of necrosis or hemorrhage. Renal cell carcinomas also show contrast enhancement and poor delineation from the surrounding renal parenchyma.

Preoperative staging of renal cell carcinoma can be guided by CT scanning, which often eliminates the need for angiography.[54,55] CT is more accurate than angiography in showing tumor bulk and extracapsular spread because it provides visualization of the tumor and fascial planes independent of vascularity. With appropriate use of contrast material, results of CT are comparable to those of angiography in the evaluation of main renal vein and vena cava involvement. Venography is sometimes needed in equivocal cases,[55] but routine angiography is no longer necessary in most patients with renal cell carcinoma.

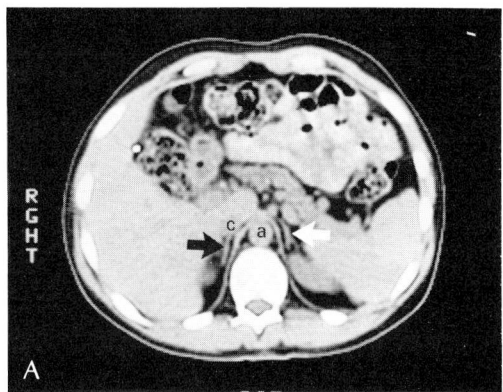

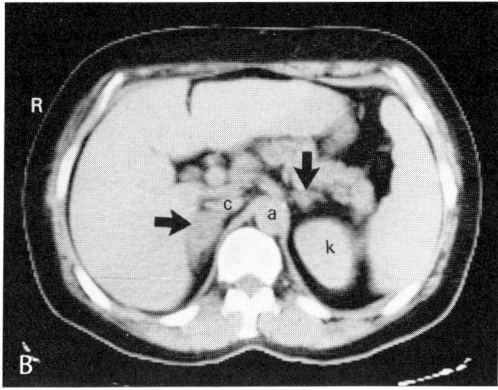

FIG. 6–17. *A*, Normal adrenal glands. The right adrenal gland (black arrow) is linear in shape and is posterior to the inferior vena cava (c). The left adrenal gland looks like an inverted "Y" (white arrow). The aorta (a) is also seen. *B*, Bilateral adrenal metastases. Both adrenal glands are enlarged (arrows), and they have lost their normal configuration. The right adrenal gland is larger than the left. Also visible are the inferior vena cava (c), the aorta (a), and the kidney (k). R, Right.

Adrenal Glands

The adrenal glands are located within the perirenal space, anterior and superior to the kidneys. The right adrenal gland is usually linear in shape, whereas the left adrenal gland looks like an inverted "Y" (Fig. 6–17*A*). The margins of the normal adrenal glands are straight or concave. In patients with hyperplasia, the glands may appear prominent, but they retain their normal configuration. When a mass is present within the adrenal gland (Fig. 6–17*B*), the margins of the gland are externally convex and give a spherical or oval appearance.[56]

TUMORS. The ability to visualize normal and abnormal adrenal glands on a CT scan has made CT the imaging technique of choice for localizing suspected adrenal tumors.[57] It has eliminated the need for arteriography and venography in almost all cases. In patients with hypercortisolism, CT is virtually 100% accurate in detecting an adrenal adenoma.[58] Visualization of normal or hyperplastic glands in these patients establishes the diagnosis of adrenocorticotropic hormone-dependent Cushing's syndrome, and no further adrenal studies are needed. In patients with hyperaldosteronism (Conn's syndrome) the adenomas are frequently undetected by CT scanning because of their small size, and so a negative CT examination must be followed by bilateral venous sampling and venography. Intra-adrenal pheochromocytomas are usually large at the time of clinical presentation and are readily detected by CT scanning. The CT examination for pheochromocytoma should extend into the pelvis; pheochromocytomas have been identified in the renal hilum, the organ of Zuckerkandl, and the urinary bladder. A recurrent pheochromocytoma may be difficult to identify on a CT scan because of artifacts produced by surgical clips and distorted tissue planes due to the previous dissection.

METASTATIC LESIONS. The adrenal gland is a common site for metastatic disease, especially metastatic lung carcinoma. CT scanning of the adrenal glands enables one to detect adrenal metastases reliably and should be performed as part of the preoperative evaluation in patients with lung carcinoma.[56]

OTHER MASSES. An adrenal mass is sometimes noted as an incidental finding on a CT scan.[59] This fact is not surprising because autopsy series have documented grossly visible adenomas in 2 to 9% of all patients. If clinical and biochemical findings indicate normal adrenal function and if no primary malignant tumor exists, a small adrenal mass, under 6 cm, will almost certainly be a nonfunctioning adenoma. Two approaches have been proposed for the evaluation of a small, nonfunctioning mass: percutaneous biopsy or a follow-up CT examination in 2 to 3 months. Either approach is reasonable.

Retroperitoneal Lymph Nodes

Para-aortic lymph nodes surround the aorta and inferior vena cava and are continuous with the iliac lymph nodes. In the normal adult, the aorta and vena cava have sharp contours on a CT scan because of the presence of fat along the posterior and lateral surfaces. Normal para-aorta lymph nodes are routinely visualized as small, oval structures contained within this retroperitoneal fat. Enlargement of the para-aortic lymph nodes obliterates the "fat angle" around the aorta and vena cava and obscures the vessel margins. Although loss of the vessel margins on a CT scan is usually due to enlarged lymph nodes, it can also occur in patients with primary retroperitoneal tumors, hematoma, or retroperitoneal fibrosis. In healthy patients with little retroperitoneal fat, the borders of the aorta and vena cava may be difficult to visualize. An enlarged lymph node may also be simulated by an adjacent bowel loop that does not contain oral contrast material.

Para-aortic lymph nodes smaller than 1 cm are considered normal, whereas those larger than 2 cm are always abnormal. Lymph nodes in the range of 1 to 2 cm are regarded as suspicious (Fig. 6–18A). Although enlarged para-aortic lymph nodes may appear as discrete, solitary masses, they often comprise a bulky conglomerate mass that forms a mantle across the prevertebral space (Fig. 6–18B).

COMPARISON OF CT WITH LYMPHANGIOGRAPHY. Prior to the development of CT, bipedal lymphangiography was required to visualize retroperitoneal lymph nodes. Lymphangiography is a tedious procedure for both the patient and the radiologist, and it is difficiult to interpret. Lymphangiography can only opacify certain groups of lymph nodes, and abnormal nodes within these groups may not fill with contrast material. CT has the advantage of showing all lymph nodes in the abdomen, and it is quick and reproducible. Because non-Hodgkin's lymphomas and testicular carcinoma usually produce large, bulky lymph nodes that are easily seen on a CT scan, lymphangiography is seldom required in patients with these diseases.[60] One cannot, however, detect with CT architectural changes in unenlarged lymph nodes, which are visible with lymphangiography. Lymphangiography is recommended for evaluation of Hodgkin's lymphoma if the CT scan shows an increased number of normal sized lymph nodes or minimally enlarged nodes; involvement by Hodgkin's disease frequently occurs without a marked increase in the size of lymph nodes.[61]

Pelvis

The pelvis can be evaluated by CT because the pelvic organs are sufficiently outlined by extraperitoneal fat. In addition to the bladder and reproductive organs, the pelvis also contains small bowel, colon, and rectum, as well as blood vessels, lymphatic vessels, and nerves. Figure 6–19 shows normal male and female pelvic anatomic structures.

The initial evaluation of suspected abnormalities involving the uterus, ovaries, or adnexa should be done with ultrasound rather than with CT. Ultrasound provides better delineation of the normal female pelvic anatomic features, and it is more accurate than CT in the detection of cystic structures or free fluid. Ultrasound has the additional advantage of not subjecting the patient to ionizing radiation, especially important in women of child-bearing age.

MALIGNANT LESIONS. The main role of CT in both male and female pelvic tumors is in evaluating the extent of a known malignant process. CT is more accurate than ultrasound in determining local extension of tumor. Extension of a bladder tumor into the perivesical fat is first manifested as a hazy, ill-defined increase in the density of the perivesical fat adjacent to the bladder wall;[62] as the tumor progresses, a soft tissue mass is often identified. Extension of prostate carcinoma into the seminal vesicles obliterates the intervening fat plane.[63] In patients with cervical carcinoma, CT is valuable in assessing parametrial and sidewall tumor extension.[64] CT is also superior to ultrasound in showing metastases to the pelvic lymph nodes, although false-negative results do occur because of tumor

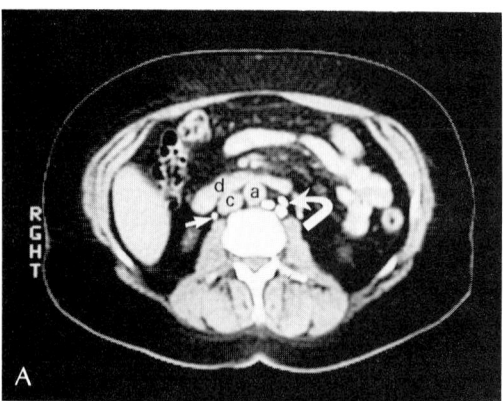

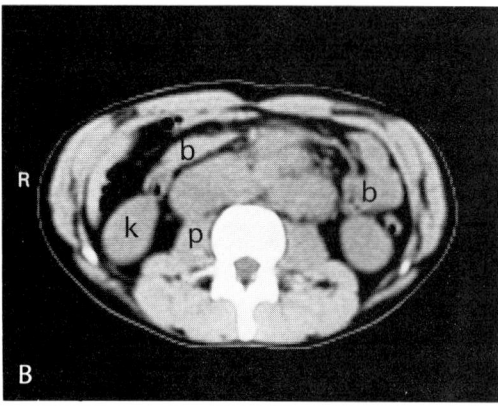

FIG. 6–18. A, Retroperitoneal lymph nodes. The patient previously had a lymphangiogram, which made the lymph nodes dense. The lymph node (arrow) posterior to the vena cava (c) is normal in size. The lymph nodes lateral to the aorta (curved arrow) are enlarged and are increased in number and must therefore be regarded as suspicious in this patient with Hodgkin's disease. The aorta (a) and the duodenum (d) are also seen. B, Massive paraaortic adenopathy. The enlarged lymph nodes form a bulky, conglomerate mass that creates a mantle across the prevertebral space and obliterates the vascular angles. Other visible structures are the kidneys (k), the psoas muscle (p), and the small bowel (b).

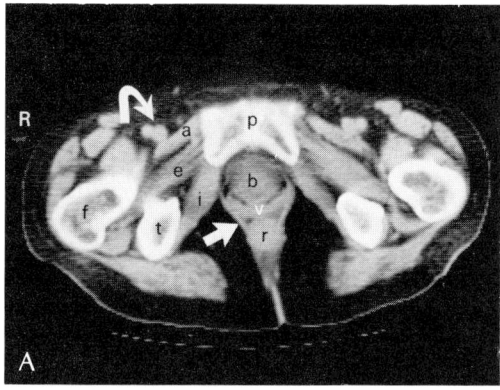

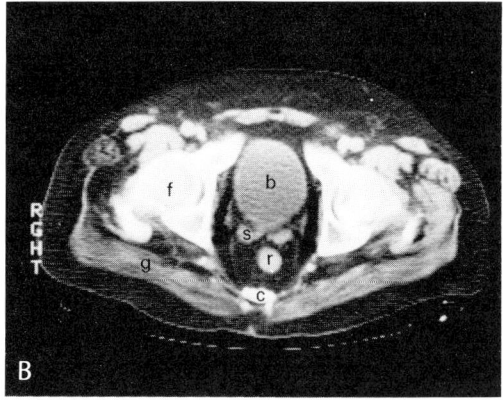

FIG. 6–19. *A*, Normal female pelvis. Posterior to the pubic symphysis (p) are the bladder (b), vagina (v), and rectum (r). The arrow points to the levator ani muscle, whereas the curved arrow indicates the femoral artery and femoral vein. Other visible structures are the obturator internus (i) and obturator externus (e) muscles, the adductor muscles (a), the ischial tuberosity (t), and the femur (f). *B*, Normal male pelvis, viewed at a higher level than in *A*. The femur (f) is seen within the acetabulum. The seminal vesicles (s) are seen between the bladder (b) and the rectum (r). The coccyx (c) and the gluteus maximus muscle (g) are posterior.

involvement in lymph nodes that are only minimally enlarged.[65]

Evaluation of recurrent tumor following therapy is best achieved with CT. Pelvic recurrence of carcinoma of the rectosigmoid colon, bladder, or cervix is usually identified as a localized soft tissue mass deep within the pelvis or along the pelvic sidewall. The mass usually has irregular margins and may contain low-density areas. Biopsy is sometimes required to distinguish recurrence from postoperative scar tissue or radiation-induced fibrosis.

Abdominal and Pelvic Abscesses

With CT, one may accurately detect and localize an abscess in the parenchymal organs, retroperitoneum, or peritoneal spaces. An abscess may be either ill defined or well circumscribed. Depending on the amount of debris, blood, and proteinaceous material present, an abscess may be of the same attenuation as water or higher than water. Usually, the wall of the abscess shows enhancement after the intravenous injection of contrast material. An abscess may contain gas, if gas-forming organisms are present or if a fistulous tract exists (see Fig. 6–13*A*). The gas may produce an air-fluid level or may be scattered throughout as small bubbles. The presence of gas is identified in 30% of all abscesses. In the absence of gas, many lesions can have a CT appearance similar to that of abscess, including urinoma, lymphocele, hematoma, pancreatic pseudocyst, loculated ascites, and even a necrotic neoplasm. The clinical setting usually leads one to a correct radiologic diagnosis of abscess, but if any question arises, percutaneous aspiration provides a rapid, safe, and accurate method for establishing the diagnosis.

An abscess within the peritoneal cavity may be confined to one compartment by inflammatory adhesions, or it may spread to other compartments by well-known and predictable pathways.[66] It is essential to evaluate all the compartments on CT scans, to plan appropriate therapy.

The accuracy of CT in showing abdominal and pelvic abscesses is about 95%.[67,68] CT is slightly more accurate than ultrasonic and radioisotope studies, but it has additional advantages as well. CT can be performed within minutes, rather than the hours or days required for radionuclide studies. Unlike with ultrasound, a satisfactory CT examination can be obtained in all patients despite wounds, dressings, ostomy sites, and large amounts of bowel gas.[69]

Abdominal and Pelvic Trauma

A number of radiologic techniques can be used in the evaluation of abdominal trauma, including plain films, excretory urograms, radionuclide scans, ultrasound, and angiography. None of these methods have the anatomic precision or multiorgan imaging characteristics of CT. This ability to examine the entire abdomen is important because multiple injuries are frequently present, and the site and extent of injury is sometimes difficult to determine by physical and laboratory examinations. CT provides a rapid and accurate appraisal of the entire abdomen and usually eliminates the need for angiography and other radiologic procedures.[70,71]

CT examinations for abdominal trauma must be done with intravenous contrast enhancement. Abdominal hematomas vary in attenuation with age, but most are lower in density than the parenchymal organs of the abdomen. Contrast enhancement facilitates the diagnosis by providing a greater difference in density between the normal parenchyma and the hematoma.[71,72] Contrast enhancement also allows evaluation of renal function and detection of extravasated urine.

In all solid organs, including liver, spleen, and kidneys, certain features are shared. A subcapsular hematoma appears as a peripheral mass that flattens the parenchyma of the organ. The density of hematomas varies with the age of the lesion. An intraparenchymal hematoma (laceration) appears as an irregular high- or low-density area within the organ. Splenic lacerations involve the lateral contour of the spleen and are associated with free intraperitoneal hemorrhage, which is easily identified as fluid within the peritoneal spaces.[73] Renal lacerations may be either complete or incomplete; the laceration is considered complete when it extends into the renal collecting system and produces extravasation of urine. Extravasated urine is much easier to detect on CT scans than on excretory urograms.[74]

Retroperitoneal hemorrhage may appear as a well-defined mass or as diffuse soft tissue thickening. The diffuse appearance is more common because of bleeding throughout the tissues. Hemorrhage may be confined to one retroperitoneal compartment, or it may extend into other compartments and the psoas muscle.[67]

SCANNING OF THE SPINE AND THE MUSCULOSKELETAL SYSTEM

Spine

CT scanning of the spine shows not only the osseous structures, but also the paraspinal and intraspinal soft tissues. The best differentiation of the intraspinal soft tissues is achieved in the lumbar region. The abundance of epidural fat in this region allows visualization of the subarachnoid space, nerve root sleeves, and ligamentum flavum, without intrathecal contrast agents (Fig. 6–20A and B). Sometimes, the cauda equina and conus medullaris can also be demonstrated. In the thoracic and cervical spine, the intraspinal soft tissues are not as clearly delineated as in the lumbar region, because of the difference in the size and configuration of the spinal canal and the relative paucity of epidural fat in these regions. An exception is at C1 and C2 where the spinal canal is large, and the spinal cord can be visualized within the surrounding subarachnoid fluid. Visibility of intraspinal structures can be improved with water-soluble myelographic contrast material, such as metrizamide. The metrizamide diffuses evenly throughout the subarachnoid space and outlines the spinal cord, nerve roots, and cauda equina. This procedure provides better delineation of the spinal cord and subarachnoid space from the surrounding epidural tissue (Fig. 6–20C). Metrizamide is needed in the cervical and thoracic regions, but

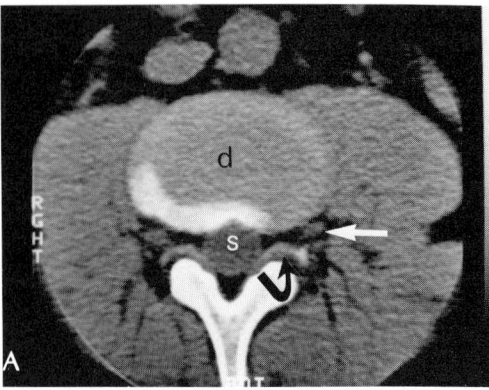

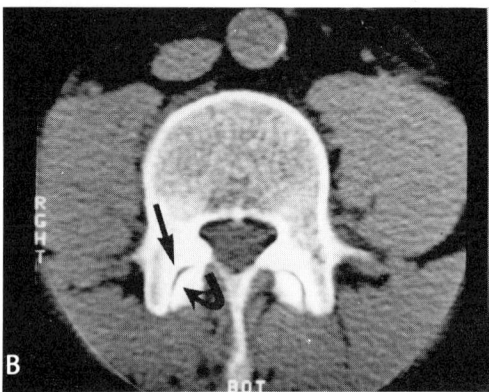

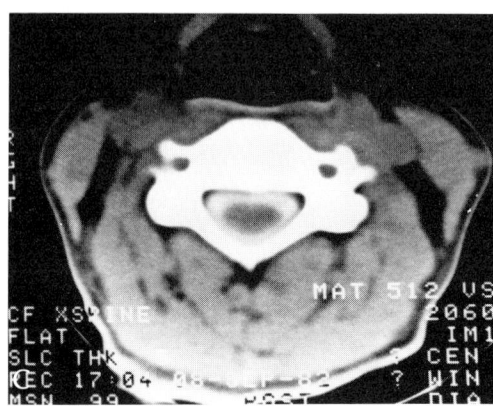

FIG. 6–20. Normal spine. A, Unenhanced scan at the level of L3 to L4. Disc (d), subarachnoid space (s), ligamentum flavum (curved arrow), nerve roots (arrow) are seen. B, Unenhanced scan at the level of L3. The inferior articulating facet of L2 (curved arrow) and the superior articulating facet of L3 (arrow) are visible. C, A metrizamide-enhanced scan of the cervical spine shows the spinal cord within the subarachnoid space.

it is often not required in the lumbar region. The exact size of the spinal cord can be determined, and thickening of the spinal cord by an intramedullary tumor or syringomyelia can be detected.

HERNIATED LUMBAR DISCS. Both unenhanced

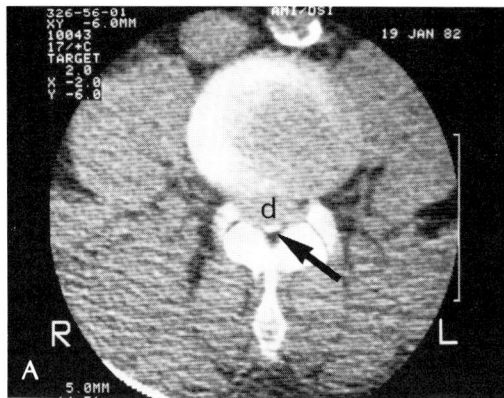

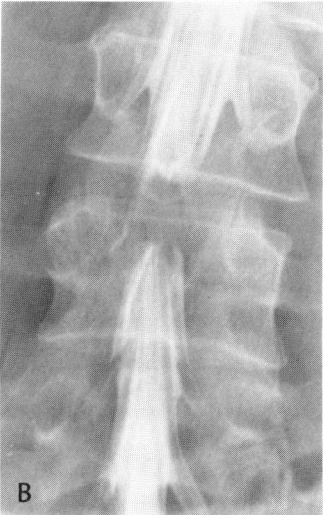

FIG. 6–21. Herniated lumbar disc. *A,* The metrizamide-enhanced scan shows a large herniated disc (d), which almost completely obliterates the subararachnoid space (arrow). The subararachnoid space is dense because of the intrathecal contrast. *B,* The myelogram shows the herniated disc as a defect in the metrizamide column.

and metrizamide-enhanced CT scans can diagnose herniated lumbar discs (Fig. 6–21). Criteria for diagnosis include: (1) focal protrusion of the disc margin; (2) compression of the dural sac; (3) displacement of epidural fat; and (4) displacement or obliteration of the nerve root sleeve. Some authors have reported results with unenhanced CT scans that are comparable to or even better than myelographic studies.[75,76] Others believe that contrast enhancement of the subarachnoid space is necessary for more accurate diagnosis.[77,78] Some discrepancies in results may be due to differences in resolution of various CT scanners or technical factors in obtaining the image. Most workers agree that CT is more accurate than myelography in the detection of lateral herniations and in the evaluation of the L5 to S1 disc, where a large epidural space may obscure disc compression on the subarachnoid space.[79]

Most physicians request an unenhanced CT scan as the initial radiologic test in patients in whom a herniated disc is suspected. Because routine lumbar CT scans usually include L3 to S1, higher levels must be specifically requested if clinically indicated. If a metrizamide study is needed prior to a surgical procedure, we usually perform myelography first and then, if necessary, follow the myelogram with a CT scan while the intrathecal contrast agent is still in place. The CT scan is done at L5 to S1 and at any level at which a questionable myelographic finding is present or a strong clinical suspicion of an abnormality exists despite a negative myelogram.

LUMBAR SPINAL STENOSIS. CT is the most accurate method for confirmation and localization of lumbar spinal stenosis.[80] Lumbar spinal stenosis may be congenital, degenerative, or a combination of the two. In the degenerative disorder, CT scans show narrowing of the lumbar spinal canal by hypertrophic degenerative changes of the laminae and articular processes and thickening of the ligamentum flavum. In patients with severe stenosis, the normally triangular spinal canal resembles a cloverleaf. Facet arthropathy is often a major contributor to lumbar spinal stenosis, but it may cause pain without significant narrowing of the spinal canal. CT findings of facet arthropathy are focal loss of articular cartilage, hypertrophy of the articular processes, osteophyte formation, and subchondral erosion.[81]

TRAUMA. In patients who have sustained trauma to the spine, CT scanning can enable one to assess the integrity of the spinal canal. Fractures of the posterior elements, often missed on plain films, can be detected on CT scans, as well as fractures of the vertebral body. Bone fragments or foreign bodies are easily visible within the spinal canal on CT scans. This information may be critical in determining the need for immediate surgical intervention. Compared to conventional tomography, CT can decrease the time, hazard, and discomfort of evaluating patients with acute spinal injury.[82]

OBSTRUCTING LESIONS. In patients with a myelographic block, the metrizamide-enhanced CT scan is valuable in determining the full extent of the disease. Even when a "complete" block is seen on a myelogram, enough metrizamide is usually visible beyond the obstruction on a CT scan to fully delineate the obstructing lesion. This information is of obvious importance in planning surgical therapy or radiation therapy for metastatic disease of the spine.

Musculoskeletal System

CT examination of the musculoskeletal system enables one to evaluate the soft tissue structures, which are not well visualized by any other radiographic method, as well as bone. Individual muscles, fascial planes, and the neurovascular bundle can be seen. Differentiation of these structures requires adequate fat. In thin patients and young children, CT examination of the musculoskeletal system may be compromised. When evaluating the musculoskeletal system on a CT scan, one should compare findings on both sides. Small asymmetric changes may be the only abnormalities detectable in significant soft tissue lesions.

SOFT TISSUE TUMORS. Such lesions are detected on CT scans by differences in tissue density and distortion of the normal tissues by the mass. With CT, one may determine the extent of the tumor and its relation to bone, muscles, and neurovascular bundle. The intra- or extracompartmental tumor localization provided by CT scanning often obviates the need for preoperative angiography.

It is difficult to distinguish between benign and malignant soft tissue tumors, but some diagnostic features are useful. Malignant tumors invade the adjacent tissues and blur and obliterate the soft tissue planes. Benign lesions are usually more homogeneous in density and have sharp boundaries, but some malignant lesions have these characteristics. Although the CT appearance of most soft tissue tumors is nonspecific, the appearance of fatty tumors and hemangiomas is characteristic enough to suggest the diagnosis.[83] Lipomas have sharply circumscribed borders and a density equal to that of normal fat. Liposarcomas have areas of higher density intermixed with fat density and often show evidence of invasion. Hemangiomas show calcification and enhancement with intravenous contrast material. Even though the CT appearance of lesions may be characteristic, final confirmation should be obtained by biopsy of fatty tumors and angiography for hemangiomas.

ABNORMALITIES OF BONE. Although plain films and radionuclide bone scans remain the primary method of detecting osseous abnormalities, several indications exist for CT in the skeletal system. CT scans can show metastatic lesions when plain films are normal and bone scans are nonspecific.[84] In patients with primary bone tumors, CT may show soft tissue and medullary extension that is not evident on plain radiographs or tomograms. CT is also useful in the evaluation of trauma in anatomically complex areas such as the spine, acetabulum, orbits, and facial bones.[82,85–87] CT can show the fracture site, extent of displaced bone fragments, and intra-articular fragments. Soft tissue injuries in the adjacent region are also visible.

INTERVENTIONAL PROCEDURES

In addition to diagnosis, CT is excellent for percutaneous guidance of interventional procedures. Such procedures include retrieval of material for cytologic, histologic, or bacteriologic study and therapeutic drainage of abscesses or other fluid collections. CT has several advantages over ultrasound in interventional techniques. Unlike ultrasound, CT provides direct visualization of the needle, and the CT image is unaffected by bowel gas or bone. This feature allows precise localization of the needle in relation to normal and abnormal structures. Ultrasound also requires acoustic coupling of the transducer to the skin that is sometimes not possible in patients with healing wounds or sinus tracts. For these reasons, we perform most interventional procedures under CT guidance. In the lung, however, fluoroscopic guidance is usually sufficient for biopsy of parenchymal lesions.

Biopsy

Prior to biopsy, we obtain rapid sequential scans after the bolus injection of contrast material. These scans provide information about the vascularity of the lesion and prevent inadvertent biopsy of unsuspected aneurysms or ectopic vascular structures. When a lesion is vascular or when cytologic study is all that is required, we perform the biopsy with a 22-gauge "skinny" needle. This needle has a high safety factor, and it can be passed through bowel or solid parenchymal organs with only a minimal chance of bacterial contamination or bleeding. For cystic lesions, we do not traverse bowel because of possible contamination. Because of its complication rate of about 2%, biopsy with the 22-gauge needle is commonly used in the pancreas (see Fig. 6–14), para-aortic tumors, and vascular lesions of the liver and kidney.[88]

The cytologic specimen obtained with this needle is sufficient for the diagnosis of metastatic disease or recurrence of tumor in a patient with a known malignant disease. In patients with a suspicious lesion in whom no diagnosis has been established, we prefer to obtain a histologic specimen by using a large, cutting needle such as a Menghini or a "Tru-Cut" needle. The larger core specimen provided by these needles allows a definitive diagnosis, rather than a simple cytologic confirmation of malignancy.[89] These large, cutting needles can only be used when the lesion is avascular and when the biopsy can be performed without penetration of bowel or other organs. By adhering to these strict criteria, our complication rate has been comparable to that with the 22-gauge needle because CT techniques eliminate inadvertent puncture of vascular lesions and normal adjacent structures.

CT visualization of the needle tip within the lesion confirms that the sample has been obtained from the desired area. Biopsy of a tumor mass, however, may fail to show tumor cells if the mass is composed of an admixture of neoplastic and inflammatory tissue, necrotic debris, and hemorrhage. We usually obtain at least two biopsy specimens from different areas of the mass, to reduce "sampling error." Negative cytologic and histologic reports must be evaluated in light of this possible source of error.

Percutaneous Drainage

Accurate localization with CT can provide the information necessary for percutaneous aspiration and drainage of an abdominal or pelvic abscess. Localization of the abscess within the peritoneal spaces is precise, and all parts and extensions of the abscess are visualized. Under CT guidance, puncture of bowel and other organs can be avoided; penetration of bowel may result in superinfection of a previously sterile fluid collection or may cause contamination of the specimen for culture. Specimens obtained by careful aseptic technique provide conclusive proof that a suspected fluid collection is an abscess and provide material for Gram staining and culture and antibiotic sensitivity studies.

Before recommending percutaneous drainage of an abscess, we consider the clinical status of the patient, the character and anatomic location of the abscess, and the nature of the purulent material.[67] In patients who are poor operative candidates, percutaneous drainage should be attempted in almost all cases. In patients who are good surgical candidates, we recommend percutaneous drainage if the abscess is unilocular and is confined to one or two anatomic spaces. Moreover, percutaneous drainage of an abscess should only be attempted if the abscess can be approached without penetration of an uninvolved organ. At the time of the initial placement of the catheter, the radiologist should make certain that the fluid is not too viscous for percutaneous drainage. In addition, a causative surgical condition should not be present. When any of these criteria are not met, we believe that surgical drainage is the method of choice for patients who are good surgical candidates. The criteria outlined are conservative and are not adhered to by all radiologists; some believe that percutaneous drainage should be attempted in virtually all patients. We believe that our approach for operative candidates is proper, considering the high surgical success rates.

Two methods can be used for percutaneous drainage: a modified Seldinger technique and a trocar technique.[67,90] A modified Seldinger technique is used in patients with abscesses that are small and centrally located. With this technique, a needle is inserted into the abscess. An angiographic guidewire is passed through the needle. The needle is then removed, and an 8-French angiographic catheter is inserted over the guidewire. A trocar is used when the abscess is large, superficial, and easily accessible. The trocar consists of a sharp central cannula covered by a plastic sheath. A 12- to 16-French trocar is used. When the abscess has been punctured with the trocar, the central cannula is removed, and the plastic sheath is left in place for drainage. Similar techniques have also been successful in drainage of pancreatic pseudocysts,[91] but the appropriateness of pseudocyst drainage is not yet known.

Regardless of whether percutaneous or surgical drainage of the abscess is performed, follow-up CT examinations are needed for any patients who fail to show clinical improvement after 48 hours. Such follow-up examinations may show fluid collections or loculations despite initial, adequate drainage.

REFERENCES

1. Christensen, E.E., Curry, T.S., and Dowdey, J.E.: An Introduction to the Physics of Diagnostic Radiology. Philadelphia, Lea & Febiger, 1978, p. 329.
2. Miraldi, F.: Physics. In Computed Tomography of the Whole Body. Edited by J.R. Haaga. St. Louis, C.V. Mosby, 1983.
3. Evans, R.G., and Jost, R.G.: CT utilizations and charges in 1981. Radiology, 145:427, 1982.
4. Kieffer, S.A., and Heitzman, E.R.: An Atlas of Cross-sectional Anatomy. Hagerstown, MD, Harper and Row, 1979.
5. Norman, D., et al.: Quantitative aspects of computed tomography of the blood and CSF. Radiology, 123:335, 1977.
6. Zimmerman, R.D., and Danziger, A.: Extracerebral trauma. Radiol. Clin. North Am., 20:105, 1982.
7. George, A.E., Russel, E.J., and Kricheff, I.I.: White matter buckling: CT sign of extraaxial intracranial mass. AJR, 135:1031, 1980.
8. Dublin, A.B., French, B.N., and Rennick, J.: Computed tomography in head trauma. Radiology, 122:365, 1977.
9. Kieffer, S.A., and Seunglo, H.L.: Neoplastic tumors of the brain. In Computed Tomography of the Whole Body. Edited by J.R. Haaga. St. Louis, C.V. Mosby, 1983.
10. Davis, K.R., et al.: A neuroradiologic approach to a patient with a diagnosis of subarachnoid hemorrhage. Radiol. Clin. North Am., 20:87, 1982.
11. Inone, Y., et al.: Sequential computed tomography scans in acute cerebral infarction. Radiology, 135:655, 1980.
12. Wall, S.D., et al.: High frequency CT findings within 24 hours after cerebral infarction. AJR, 138:307, 1982.
13. Modic, M.T., and Weinstein, M.A.: Cerebrovascular disease of the brain. In Computed Tomography of the Whole Body. Edited by J.R. Haaga. St. Louis, C.V. Mosby, 1983.
14. Bonstelle, C.T.: Infectious processes of the brain. In Computed Tomography of the Whole Body. Edited by J.R. Haaga, St. Louis, C.V. Mosby, 1983.

15. Naidich, T.P., Schott, L.H., and Baron, R.L.: Computed tomography in evaluation of hydrocephalus. Radiol. Clin. North Am., 20:143, 1982.
16. Hughes, C.P., and Gado, M.: Computed tomography and aging of the brain. Radiology, 139:391, 1981.
17. deLeon, M.J., et al.: Correlations between CT changes and behavioral deficits in senile dementia. Lancet, 2:859, 1979.
18. George, A.E., et al.: Parenchymal CT correlates of senile dementia (Alzheimer disease): loss of gray-white matter discriminability. AJNR, 2:205, 1981.
19. Sones, P.J., et al.: Effectiveness of CT in evaluating intrathoracic masses. AJR, 139:469, 1982.
20. Solomon, E., and Haaga, J.R.: Mediastinum. In Computed Tomography of the Whole Body. Edited by J.R. Haaga. St. Louis, C.V. Mosby, 1983.
21. McLoughlin, M.J., et al.: Computed tomography in congenital anomalies of the aortic arch and great vessels. Radiology, 138:399, 1981.
22. Heiberg, E., et al.: CT findings in thoracic aortic dissection. AJR, 136:13, 1981.
23. Moncada, R., et al.: Diagnosis of dissecting aortic aneurysm by computed tomography. Lancet, 1:238, 1981.
24. Heitzman, E.R.: Computed tomography of the thorax. AJR, 136:2, 1981.
25. Baron, R.L., et al.: Computed tomography in the preoperative evaluation of bronchogenic carcinoma. Radiology, 145:727, 1982.
26. Mintzer, R.A., et al.: Computed vs. conventional tomography in evaluation of primary and secondary pulmonary neoplasms. Radiology, 132:653, 1979.
27. Siegelman, S.S., et al.: CT of the solitary pulmonary nodule. AJR, 135:1, 1980.
28. Levi, C., et al.: The unreliability of CT numbers as absolute values. AJR, 139:443, 1982.
29. Cohen, A.M., and Haaga, J.R.: Parenchyma of the lungs. In Computed Tomography of the Whole Body. Edited by J.R. Haaga. St. Louis, C.V. Mosby, 1983.
30. Pugatch, R.D., et al.: Differentiation of pleural and pulmonary lesions using computed tomography. J. Comput. Assist. Tomogr., 2:601, 1978.
31. Burgener, F.A., and Hamlin, D.J.: Contrast enhancement in abdominal CT: bolus vs. infusion. AJR, 137:351, 1981.
32. Barnes, P.A., Thomas, J.L., and Bernardino, M.E.: Pitfalls in the diagnosis of hepatic cysts by computed tomography. Radiology, 141:129, 1981.
33. Johnson, C.M., et al.: Computed tomography and angiography of cavernous hemangiomas of the liver. Radiology, 138:115, 1981.
34. Stephens, D.H.: Liver. In Computed Tomography of the Whole Body. Edited by J.R. Haaga. St. Louis, C.V. Mosby, 1983.
35. Snow, J.H., Goldstein, H.M., and Wallace, S.: Comparison of scintigraphy, sonography, and computed tomography in the evaluation of hepatic neoplasm. AJR, 132:915, 1979.
36. Knopf, D.R., et al.: Liver lesions: comparative accuracy of scintigraphy and computed tomography. AJR, 138:623, 1982.
37. Halvorsen, R.A., et al.: CT appearance of focal fatty infiltration of the liver. AJR, 139:277, 1982.
38. Haaga, J.R., and Reich, N.E.: Computerized Tomography of Abdominal Abnormalities. St. Lous, C.V. Mosby, 1978.
39. Haaga, J.R., Alfidi, R.J., and Ament, A.: Biliary system. In Computed Tomography of the Whole Body. Edited by J.R. Haaga. St. Louis, C.V. Mosby, 1983.
40. Baron, R.L., et al.: A prospective comparison of the evaluation of biliary obstruction using computed tomography and ultrasonography. Radiology, 145:91, 1982.
41. Pedrosa, C.S., et al.: Computed tomography in obstructive jaundice. Part I. The level of obstruction. Radiology, 139:627, 1981.
42. Pedrosa, C.S., et al.: Computed tomography in obstructive jaundice. Part II. The cause of obstruction. Radiology, 139:635, 1981.
43. Hessel, S.J., et al.: A prospective evaluation of computed tomography and ultrasound of the pancreas. Radiology, 143:129, 1982.
44. Haaga, J.R.: Pancreas. In Computed Tomography of the Whole Body. Edited by J.R. Haaga. St. Louis, C.V. Mosby, 1983.
45. Wittenberg, J., et al.: Non-focal enlargement in pancreatic carcinoma. Radiology, 144:131, 1982.
46. Mendez, G., Isikoff, M.B., and Hill, M.C.: CT of acute pancreatitis: interim assessment. AJR, 135:463, 1980.
47. Siegelman, S.S., et al.: CT of fluid collections associated with pancreatitis. AJR, 134:1121, 1980.
48. Moss, A.A., et al.: Esophageal carcinoma: pretherapy staging by computed tomography. AJR, 136:1051, 1981.
49. Balfe, D.M., et al.: Computed tomography of gastric neoplasms. Radiology, 140(2):431, 1981.
50. Mayes, G.B., and Zornoza, J.: Computed tomography of colon carcinoma. AJR, 135:43, 1980.
51. Thoeni, R.F., et al.: Detection and staging of primary rectal and rectosigmoid cancer by computed tomography. Radiology, 141:135, 1981.
52. Moss, A.A., et al.: A uniform, CT-based staging system for malignant neoplasms of the alimentary tube. AJR, 136:1251, 1981.
53. Mauro, M.A., et al.: Computed tomography in the diagnosis and management of the renal mass. JAMA, 248:2894, 1982.
54. Weyman, P.J., et al.: Comparison of computed tomography and angiography in the evaluation of renal cell carcinoma. Radiology, 137:417, 1980.
55. Mauro, M.A., et al.: Renal cell carcinoma: angiography in the CT era. AJR, 139:1135, 1982.
56. Sandler, M.A., et al.: Computed tomographic evaluation of the adrenal glands in the preoperative assessment of bronchogenic carcinoma. Radiology, 145:733, 1982.
57. Abrams, H.L., et al.: Computed tomography vs. ultrasound of the adrenal glands: a prospective study. Radiology, 143:121, 1982.
58. Dunnick, N.R., et al.: Localization of functional adrenal tumors by computed tomography and venous sampling. Radiology, 142:429, 1982.
59. Glazer, H.S., et al.: Nonfunctioning adrenal masses: incidental discovery on computed tomography. AJR, 139:81, 1982.
60. Thomas, J.L., Bernardino, M.E., and Bracken, R.B.: Staging of testicular carcinoma: comparison of CT and lymphangiography. AJR, 137:991, 1981.
61. Castellino, R.A., Marglins, S., and Blank, N.: Hodgkin's disease, the non-Hodgkin's lymphomas, and the leukemias in the retroperitoneum. Semin. Roentgenol., 15:288, 1980.
62. Bryan, P.J.: Pelvis. In Computed Tomography of the Whole Body. Edited by J.R. Haaga. St. Louis, C.V. Mosby, 1983.
63. Morgan, C.L., et al.: Computed tomography in the evaluation, staging, and therapy of carcinoma of the bladder and prostate. Radiology, 140:751, 1981.

64. Walsh, J.W., and Goplerud, D.R.: Prospective comparison between clinical and CT staging in primary cervical carcinoma. AJR, 137:997, 1981.
65. Walsh, J.A., et al.: Computed tomographic detection of pelvic and inguinal lymph-node metastases from primary and recurrent pelvic malignant disease. Radiology, 137:157, 1980.
66. Meyers, M.A.: Dynamic Radiology of the Abdomen: Normal and Pathologic Anatomy. New York, Springer, 1982.
67. Haaga, J.R., and Weinstein, A.J.: CT-guided percutaneous aspiration and drainage of abscesses. AJR, 135:1187, 1980.
68. Knochel, J.Q., et al.: Diagnosis of abdominal abscesses with computed tomography, ultrasound, and ^{111}In leukocyte scans. Radiology, 137:425, 1980.
69. Haaga, J.R.: Peritoneum, including abscesses and other disorders. In Computed Tomography of the Whole Body. Edited by J.R. Haaga. St. Louis, C.V. Mosby, 1983.
70. Federle, M.P., et al.: Evaluation of abdominal trauma by computed tomography. Radiology, 138:637, 1981.
71. Sandler, C.M., and Toombs, B.D.: Computed tomography of blunt renal injuries. Radiology, 141:461, 1981.
72. Alexander, E.S., and Clark, R.A.: Computed tomography in the diagnosis of abdominal hemorrhage. JAMA, 248:1104, 1982.
73. Jeffrey, R.B., et al.: Computed tomography of splenic trauma. Radiology, 141:729, 1981.
74. Federle, M.P., et al.: The role of computed tomography in renal trauma. Radiology, 141:455, 1981.
75. Haughton, V.M., et al.: A prospective comparison of computed tomography and myelography in the diagnosis of herniated lumbar discs. Radiology, 142:103, 1982.
76. Raskin, S.P., and Keating, J.W.: Recognition of lumbar disc disease: comparison of myelography and computed tomography. AJR, 139:349, 1982.
77. Amand, A.K., and Lee, B.C.: Plain and metrizamide CT of lumbar disc disease: comparison with myelography. AJNR, 3:567, 1982.
78. Dublin, A.B., McGrahan, J.P., and Reid, M.H.: The value of computed tomographic metrizamide myelography in the neuroradiologic evaluation of the spine. Radiology, 146:79, 1983.
79. Williams, A.L., et al.: CT recognition of lateral lumbar disc herniation. AJR, 139:345, 1982.
80. Cacayorin, E.D., and Kieffer, S.A.: Applications and limitations of computed tomography of the spine. Radiol. Clin. North Am., 20:185, 1982.
81. Carrera, G.F., et al.: Computed tomography in sciatica. Radiology, 137:433, 1980.
82. Handel, S.F., and Lee, Y.Y.: Computed tomography of spinal fractures. In Computed Tomography of the Whole Body. Edited by J.R. Haaga. St. Louis, C.V. Mosby, 1983.
83. Eglung, N., et al.: CT of soft tissue tumors. AJR, 137:725, 1981.
84. Harbin, W.P.: Metastatic disease and the nonspecific bone scan: value of spinal computed tomography. 145:105, 1982.
85. Harley, J.D., et al.: CT of acetabular fractures: comparison with conventional radiography. AJR, 138(3):413, 1982.
86. Hammerschlag, S.B., et al.: Blow-out fractures of the orbit: a comparison of computed tomography and conventional radiography with anatomic correlation. Radiology, 143:487, 1982.
87. Zilkha, A.: Computed tomography in facial trauma. Radiology, 144:545, 1982.
88. Isler, R.J., et al.: Tissue core biopsy of abdominal tumors using a 22 gauge cutting needle. AJR, 136:725, 1981.
89. Haaga, J.R., et al.: Clinical comparison of small- and large-caliber cutting needles for biopsy. Radiology, 146:665, 1983.
90. van Sonnenberg, E., et al.: Percutaneous drainage of abscesses and fluid collections: technique, results, and applications. Radiology, 142:1, 1982.
91. Karlson, K.B., et al.: Percutaneous drainage of pancreatic pseudocysts and abscesses. Radiology, 142:619, 1982.

7

Angiography

Andrew C. Wilbur ■ Dimitrios G. Spigos

Angiography is the radiographic study of the arteries and veins following introduction of contrast material into the lumen. For the diagnosis of many diseases, angiography is considered to be the most definitive procedure available. All angiographic procedures carry certain inherent risks, however, and some special circumstances may further increase the risk to the patient.

RISK FACTORS AND COMPLICATIONS

In a large survey, the rate of significant complications of angiography was 1.86%, and the mortality rate was 0.03%.[1] Consultation between the referring physician and the angiographer should include assessment of the risks and benefits of the procedure and consideration of noninvasive diagnostic methods. One must avoid angiographic procedures when the risk to the patient is excessive and when the results will not alter the treatment plan.[2] Informed consent is a prerequisite for any angiographic procedure.

Many of the risks of angiography are related to the potential pathophysiologic effects of iodinated contrast media. In general, the risks increase with higher concentrations of contrast medium, longer duration of exposure, and greater total dosage. Potential hematologic effects of intravascular contrast agents include red blood cell hemolysis and sludging in patients with sickle cell anemia and increased thromboembolic complications in patients with homocystinuria.[3] Potential cardiopulmonary effects include a greater susceptibility to cardiac arrhythmia and to vasovagal bradycardia with hypotension. Patients with pheochromocytoma are at significant risk of contrast-induced hypertensive crisis. Potential neurotoxic effects of contrast media include seizures, paresis, and cortical blindness. Renal toxicity from contrast agents is related to the total dose, the degree of pre-existing renal failure, and the state of hydration of the patient.[3,4] Patients with pre-existing renal failure, diabetes, proteinuria, and low-renal-flow states are at an increased risk, particularly if they are dehydrated. Patients scheduled for angiographic testing, or any other indication for intravascular iodinated contrast agents, must be well hydrated before and after the procedure.[3,4]

All procedures using intravascular contrast media carry a definite risk of adverse "hypersensitivity" reactions, and severe, life-threatening reactions may occur at any time.[5] Minor, self-limited reactions to contrast media include nausea, vomiting, itching, and transient urticaria. More significant responses that require treatment include vasovagal reaction with hypotension, and mild bronchospasm. Severe, life-threatening reactions include cardiac arrest, severe hypotension, pulmonary edema, convulsions, laryngeal edema, and severe bronchospasm. In general, severe contrast reactions are idiosyncratic and are not dose-related. Milder reactions are about twice as frequent in atopic as in nonatopic individuals. Although no conclusive proof exists that premedication is useful in preventing contrast reactions, patients with a history of severe contrast reaction are often premedicated with corticosteroids or antihistamines if the use of contrast material is unavoidable.[6]

Angiographic complications from catheter effects include hemorrhage, thrombosis, thromboembolism, vascular wall damage, and pseudoaneurysm or arteriovenous fistula formation. Puncture-site bleeding with hematoma formation is the most common complication and occurs more frequently in patients with hypertension or coagulopathy. In general, catheter-related complications are more likely with long and complex procedures, with large catheters, and with an axillary, as opposed to femoral, approach.[1]

After an arteriographic examination, bedrest with restricted motion at the arteriotomy site is prescribed, to prevent the complications of hematoma or thrombosis. Pressure dressings are usually unnecessary and may actually do more harm than good by concealing slow bleeding until a significant hematoma has formed.[7] One should monitor the distal pulses in the limb frequently after arteriography, to detect arterial occlusion due to hematoma compression or thrombosis as early as possible.

Table 7-1. Patients at Increased Risk from Angiography

Predisposing Factors	Major Angiographic Risks
Advanced age	All complications, including fatal reactions
Acute systemic illness	
Ischemic cardiovascular disease	Cardiovascular complications
Ischemic cerebrovascular disease	Central nervous system complications; vasovagal reaction
Atopy	Idiosyncratic contrast reactions, including fatal reactions
Previous major contrast reaction	
Asthma	Bronchospasm
Diabetes	Nephrotoxicity; acute renal failure
Multiple myeloma	
Proteinuria	
Pre-existing renal disease	
Dehydration	
Bleeding diathesis or anticoagulation	Hemorrhage
Blood dyscrasia	Thromboembolism
Homocystinuria	Thromboembolism
Hypertension	Hemorrhage; arteriovenous fistula
Severe vascular disease	All catheter-related complications
Cystic medial necrosis	Vascular damage by catheter
Valvular heart disease	Bacterial endocarditis

Those categories of patients at predictably increased risk from angiographic procedures are summarized in Table 7-1.

ANGIOGRAPHIC TECHNIQUE

The basic technique of vascular radiology is percutaneous catheterization, as described by Seldinger.[8] Percutaneous catheterization requires the following steps: (1) insertion of a needle into the vessel; (2) passage of a flexible guidewire through the needle into the vessel; (3) withdrawal of the needle, leaving the guidewire in the vessel; (4) passage of a catheter over the guidewire into the vessel; (5) withdrawal of the guidewire, leaving the catheter in the vessel. For arteriography, the femoral artery in the groin is the most useful access site; the axillary artery is chosen when the femoral artery cannot be used. The femoral vein in the groin and the basilic vein in the antecubital fossa are the most useful catheter access sites for central venography and for central venous injections for digital subtraction angiographic procedures.

After initial insertion of the catheter, one positions its tip in the appropriate vessel or portion of a vessel to be studied by careful advancement of the catheter and by manipulation under fluoroscopic guidance. Specially shaped catheters facilitate catheterization of specific vessels. "Superselective catheterization" usually refers to catheterization of second- or third-order arterial branches and is used to study small abnormalities or to perform therapeutic vascular procedures.

Biplane filming, using two sets of x-ray tubes and film changers, allows one to make two views in planes at right angles to each other during the same injection. This technique maximizes the information obtained per dose of contrast material and provides two views at right angles for better interpretation of abnormalities.

An important principle of angiography is to obtain and record multiple sequential exposures before, during, and after maximum contrast concentration. Special pressure injectors are used for most angiographic injections. The iodine content of contrast agent and the rate of injection depend on the size and the flow rate of the vessel. For most arteriograms and many venograms, one uses rapid serial films with automatic film changers. Special x-ray tubes, capable of repetitive, high-power exposures, as well as fine focus, are also needed for most arteriographic studies. Magnification and subtraction techniques may be used to enhance visualization of vascular structures. Diagnostic pharmacoangiography involves selective injection of a vasoconstrictor, such as epinephrine, or a vasodilator, such as tolazoline, to enhance filling of certain vessels. For example, if renal arterial inflow is decreased by a selective renal-artery injection of epinephrine immediately prior to renal venography, enhanced retrograde filling of the renal veins will be possible.

Technologic advances in x-ray generators and tubes, fluoroscopy, automatic film changers, pressure injectors, and shapeable catheters promoted the rapid development of angiography in the 1960s and 1970s. More recently, innovations and modifications in catheter design have accompanied the rapid growth of therapeutic angiographic techniques.[9] Balloon catheters, based on the work of Grüntzig and used for dilation of arterial stenoses, have increased the applicability of percutaneous transluminal angioplasty. Balloon catheters, coaxial catheter systems, and detachable balloons have increased the safety and selectivity of transcatheter embolization and occlusion procedures. Arteriography using temporary balloon occlusion can enhance visualization of vessels with low flow. Small-diameter catheters now permit some conventional and digital subtraction arteriograms to be performed on an outpatient basis in some centers.

DIGITAL SUBTRACTION ANGIOGRAPHY

In digital subtraction angiography (DSA), the images are converted into an array of numbers in a computer. This array of numbers is obtained by digitizing a television picture, to "subtract" the images without contrast medium in the vessels from the images that contain contrast medium in the vessels. Thus, new images are produced in which the density of the contrast agent in the vessels is more easily seen because nonvascular background densities have been removed.

Procedure

As currently performed, DSA involves the making of a preinjection mask frame. The mask is then stored in the computer's digital memory. When contrast material is injected, images are produced at a rate of up to 30/sec, and the mask is subtracted from each. This technique eliminates bones and soft tissues and highlights the contrast agent in the blood vessel. The resulting subtracted images are available for immediate viewing.

For the subtraction method to be successful, the patient must remain motionless during data acquisition. If the patient does not move, then the density of contrast agent in multiple postinjection images can be added together and then subtracted from the preinjection mask; the result is a higher-density (contrast) resolution for the amount of contrast material used than in conventional angiography. Although the contrast resolution of DSA is higher than that of conventional angiography, the spatial resolution is lower: the vessels are not as sharply outlined, and small vessels cannot be resolved.

DSA may be performed using either intravenous or intra-arterial injection of contrast media. Judicious selection of the route of injection used is important. Intravenous DSA may be performed by peripheral or central venous injection. Injection through a catheter in the vena cava or right atrium results in a more compact bolus, with less dilution of the contrast agent during passage through the cardiopulmonary circulation. Dilution of the contrast bolus when the injection is made in an antecubital vein may be acceptable for pulmonary DSA or for screening studies of the aortic arch. Central venous or intra-arterial injection is needed for most DSA examinations, however. Low cardiac output may cause such dilution that diagnostic visualization of arteries is impossible with intravenous injection.

Comparison with Conventional Angiography

The major advantage of DSA is that it is less invasive than conventional angiography and therefore has fewer risks and a lower cost. That intravenous DSA studies are routinely performed on outpatients saves the cost of hospitalization. The low-volume contrast injections used in intra-arterial DSA allow the use of smaller French catheters and thereby lessen the risk of complications from the arterial puncture site and permit intra-arterial studies to be performed on an outpatient basis in some centers. Intra-arterial DSA may produce satisfactory studies of arteries such as the carotid and coronary arteries without selective catheterization; the risk of thromboembolic complications is thus decreased. The small volume of contrast agent required for intra-arterial DSA lowers the risk of renal, cardiac, or neurologic contrast toxicity, an especially important consideration in compromised patients. Intravenous DSA requires large doses of contrast material, however.

The small image intensifiers used in DSA create a limited field of view for each injection, and biplane imaging is possible only with the most sophisticated equipment. A greater number of injections are therefore needed to study a given anatomic area than with conventional angiography. For example, three or four injections are required for a study of both carotid bifurcations with DSA, as compared with two selective injections in conventional biplane filming. The major disadvantage of DSA is the low spatial resolution, which is caused by noise in the electronic imaging system and by motion artifacts and which limits evaluation of small vessels and fine details. Most DSA studies are nonselective; vessel overlap may obscure pathologic features. DSA studies are also more dependent on the patient than comparable conventional angiograms. Patients who are uncooperative, who cannot hold their breath, or who have low cardiac output may be impossible to study with DSA.

HEAD AND NECK STUDIES

Extracranial Arteriography

PROCEDURE. Carotid angiography is now most commonly performed by a transfemoral route using preshaped catheters. Some older or hypertensive patients with tortuous arteries may be difficult or impossible to study this way. Direct percutaneous puncture of the common carotid arteries, or direct puncture of the left carotid artery combined with retrograde injection of the right brachial artery, also may be used. Vertebral angiography is almost exclusively performed by transfemoral catheterization. Arch aortography is included in the evaluation of most patients with suspected extracranial occlusive disease because of the possibility of symptomatic lesions at the origins of the common carotid and vertebral arteries. The aortic arch is usually studied using transfemoral catheterization. If occlusive disease in the aorta or iliac arteries prevents the femoral approach, the aorta and common carotid arteries may be catheterized through the right axillary artery. Complete cerebral angiography with arch aortography requires a moderate dose of contrast medium of approximately 100 ml or 20.2 g iodine.

INDICATIONS. Angiography is the most reliable method for demonstrating the anatomic status of the brachiocephalic and cerebral arterial tree. The usual indication for arteriography in cerebrovascular disease is to determine whether the patient has an operable lesion of the carotid, vertebral, brachiocephalic, or subclavian arteries. Angiography is also necessary in the detection of intracranial stenotic lesions that might be amenable to an external carotid-internal carotid bypass operation.[10] To detect carotid occlusion prior to considering a surgical procedure, one should use less invasive methods, with lower morbidity and mortality rates than arteriography. Noninvasive testing is helpful in the diagnosis of hemodynamically significant stenoses in the neck, especially at the carotid bifurcation.[11] DSA enables one to detect stenoses in the brachiocephalic vessels and carotid bifurcations.[12] We have found a combination of DSA and duplex ultrasound to be particularly useful in screening evaluation of the carotid bifurcation.

A complete evaluation of the arteries of the neck and head is usually needed if surgical correction of a stenosis is contemplated. Arteriographically, this evaluation usually includes arch aortography and bilateral selective injections of the common carotid arteries (Fig. 7–1). The arch aortogram permits an assessment of the origins of the brachiocephalic vessels that is particularly important in patients with suspected vertebrobasilar disease because of the high incidence of stenosis of the origin of the vertebral artery. A study of the aortic arch also provides useful information about collateral circulation patterns and can show stenoses at the brachiocephalic vessel origins that could compromise surgical results. Biplane filming during the carotid arteriogram provides lateral and frontal views of the carotid bi-

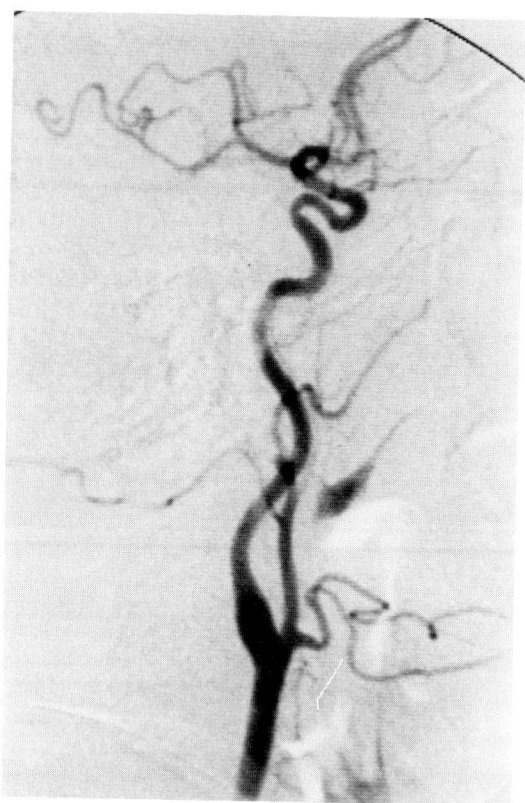

FIG. 7–1. Normal intra-arterial carotid digital subtraction angiography. Selective left carotid injection with excellent visualization of the major branches of the internal and external carotid arteries.

furcation and intracerebral vessels. With DSA, visualization of the carotid bifurcation is achieved by multiple injections in both oblique projections, following the angiographic principle that at least two views at right angles to each other are necessary for accurate detection and assessment of stenoses.

ABNORMAL FINDINGS. These findings include stenosis, plaques, subclavian steal phenomenon, and tumors.

Stenosis. Arteriosclerotic narrowing is generally most severe at sites of vessel branching or curving. The most common site of extracranial narrowing is at the carotid bifurcation and the origin of the internal carotid artery[13] (Fig. 7–2). Significant stenoses in other portions of the common or internal carotid arteries are much less common. The second most frequent site of extracranial stenosis is at the origin of the vertebral artery; this lesion is amenable to surgical treatment. Unlike the carotid artery, the vertebral artery often shows arteriosclerotic narrowing at any point along its course. After stenosis at its origin, stenosis of the vertebral artery is most common where it curves and enters the foramen magnum.

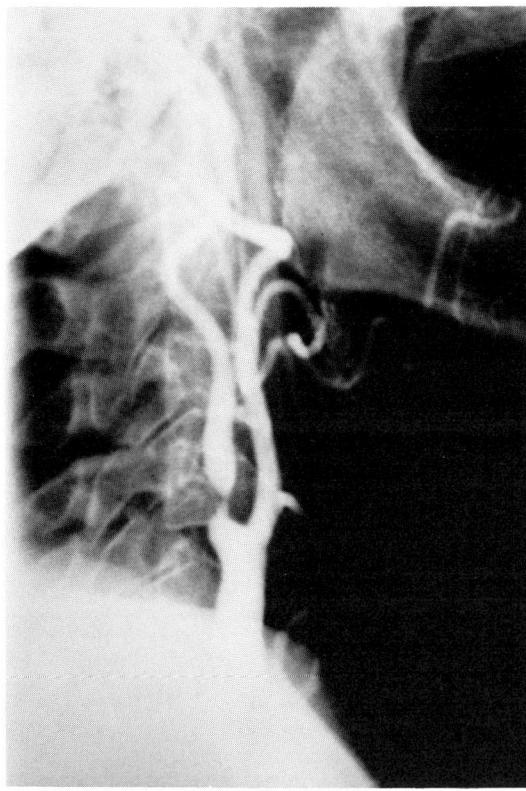

FIG. 7–2. High-grade carotid stenosis. One sees marked narrowing of the proximal internal carotid artery with slight poststenotic dilation.

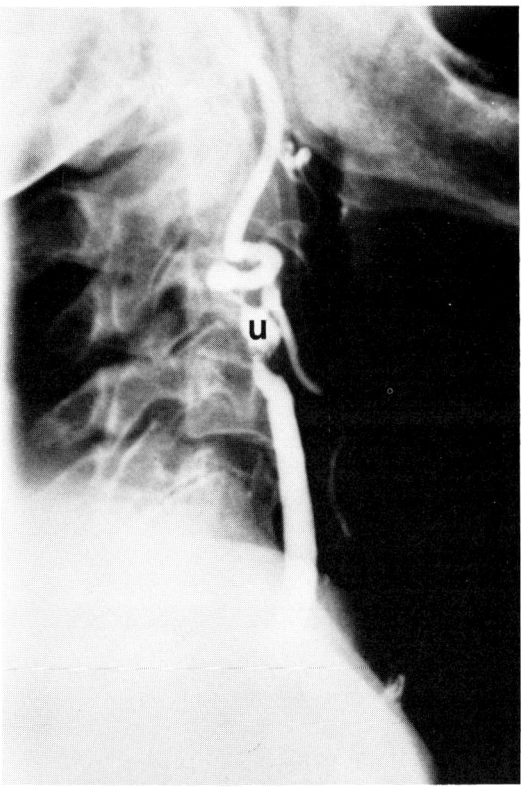

FIG. 7–3. Ulcerated carotid plaque with stenosis. The ulcer cavity (u) appears as a superimposed collection of contrast material. The proximal portions of both the internal and external carotid arteries are stenosed.

Ulcerated Atherosclerotic Plaques. Ulceration of atherosclerotic plaques most commonly occurs at the carotid bifurcation, usually along the posterior wall[14] (Fig. 7–3). The angiographic criteria for diagnosis of ulcerated atherosclerotic plaques are as follows: (1) a penetrating niche; (2) irregularity of the vessel outline; (3) delayed washout of contrast agent in a segment of artery between areas of stenosis; and (4) a well-circumscribed double density of contrast medium superimposed on the artery.[15] In practice, these criteria are difficult to apply and result in a large percentage of false-positive (34%) and false-negative (40%) angiographic diagnoses of carotid bifurcation ulceration.[16] Many false-negative results are due to the presence of ulceration in minimally stenotic, angiographically smooth lesions.[16] False-positive angiographic diagnoses are frequently caused by irregularities created by intimal elevation due to intraplaque hematomas rather than intimal ulcerations.[16,17] Noninvasive methods, including high-resolution real-time ultrasound, are currently even less reliable in showing the presence or absence of ulceration at the carotid bifurcation.[18]

Subclavian Steal Phenomenon. This disorder results from an occlusion of the subclavian or innominate artery proximal to the origin of the vertebral artery.[19] Blood supplied by the contralateral vertebral artery flows in a retrograde direction down the ipsilateral vertebral artery to supply the distal subclavian artery. When the origin of the innominate artery is occluded, retrograde flow down the right vertebral artery may supply not only the right brachial artery, but also the right common carotid artery. Arteriographically, the subclavian or innominate arterial occlusion is usually seen on the aortic arch study, and the retrograde vertebral arterial flow is shown during the later films.

Tumors. The group of vascular tumors of the head and neck that includes the chemodectomas (glomus jugulare tumors, carotid body tumors, and nonchromaffin paragangliomas) and the nasopharyngeal angiofibromas requires angiography for full evaluation.[20] Glomus jugulare tumors arise in the bulb of the jugular vein and are primarily supplied by the external carotid arterial circulation. Carotid body tumors are supplied by the external carotid artery, often with some branches from the internal carotid artery as well. The nasopharyngeal angiofibromas of children and adolescents are usually vascular tumors deriving most blood supply from the internal maxillary branch of the external carotid artery, often with some supply from small branches of the internal carotid artery. Percutaneous embolization has been used to decrease the vascularity of glomus jugulare tumors and nasopharyngeal angiofibromas preoperatively.[21]

Spinal Angiography

Spinal angiography with transfemoral catheterization is used in the diagnosis and preoperative evaluation of spinal vascular malformations. The technique involves selective bilateral catheterization of the vessels that supply feeder vessels to the anterior spinal artery, such as the vertebral, costocervical trunk, intercostal, or lumbar arteries, depending on the level. Because selective spinal arteriography involves the additional risk of spinal cord damage, with consequent quadriplegia or paraplegia, it should only be performed on carefully selected patients by angiographers skilled in the technique.[22]

Cerebral Angiography

PROCEDURE. The cerebral angiogram is usually divided into arterial, capillary, and venous phases for purposes of interpretation. The angiographer looks for normal features in each of these phases and for a normal circulation time of about 5 to 7 sec between the appearance of contrast medium in the internal carotid artery and its disappearance from the veins of the brain. The main indications for cerebral angiography are vascular disorders and tumors. The arteries and veins are examined for evidence of intrinsic disease, such as arteriosclerotic narrowing or widening, aneurysm, or thrombosis, for vessel displacement or distortion by a mass, and for abnormalities, such as those associated with neoplasm, inflammation, or vascular malformation.[23]

ANEURYSMS AND VASCULAR MALFORMATIONS. Angiography is the definitive diagnostic procedure for cerebral aneurysms and vascular malformations. Computed tomography (CT) should be performed prior to angiography and may show subarachnoid hemorrhage, abnormal enhancement with contrast medium, or abnormal calcification suggesting an aneurysm or vascular malformation.[24,25] The goals of arteriography are the definition of the location, origin, size, and type of the lesion and the identification of any additional aneurysms or vascular malformations. Precise visualization of the origin and size of the neck of an aneurysm is desirable and may require special projections.[26] At present, the resolution obtainable by DSA is sufficient for the diagnosis of intracranial aneurysms, but not for detailed preoperative evaluation.[27,28] On the other hand, DSA is adequate for the postoperative evaluation of cerebral aneurysms and vascular malformations.[27]

Aneurysms. Intracranial aneurysms may be classified as congenital (berry), arteriosclerotic, mycotic, or post-traumatic. Most congenital aneurysms occur at points of vessel branching, particularly around the circle of Willis; the most common sites are the anterior communicating artery (Fig. 7–4), the origin of the posterior communicating artery, and the first branching of the middle cerebral artery.[29] Mycotic and post-traumatic aneurysms are usually more pe-

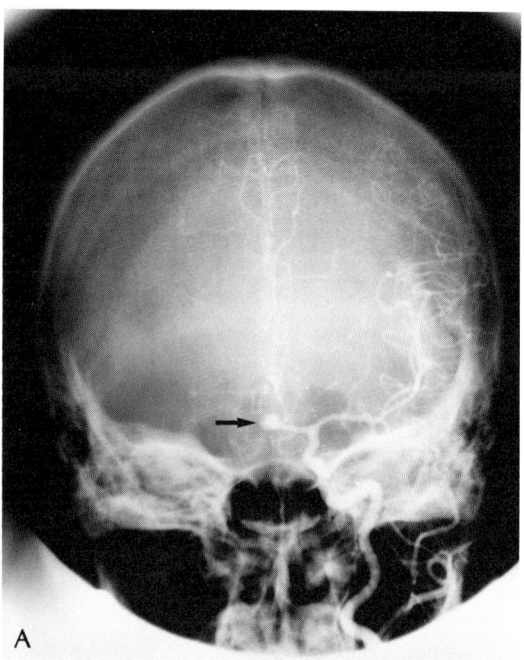

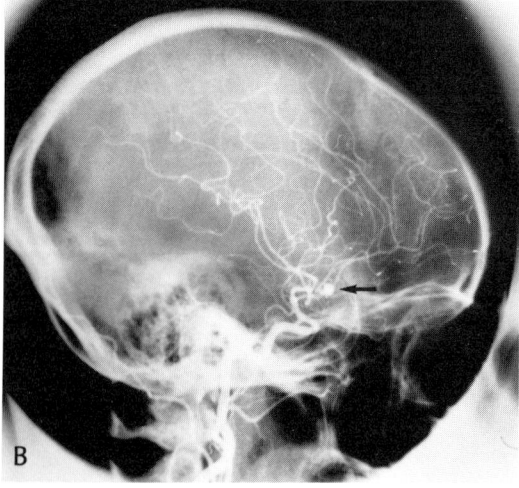

FIG. 7–4. Anterior communicating artery aneurysm (arrow) shown in frontal *(A)* and lateral *(B)* views made during a selective left common carotid injection. One sees narrowing of the anterior cerebral artery due to associated spasm.

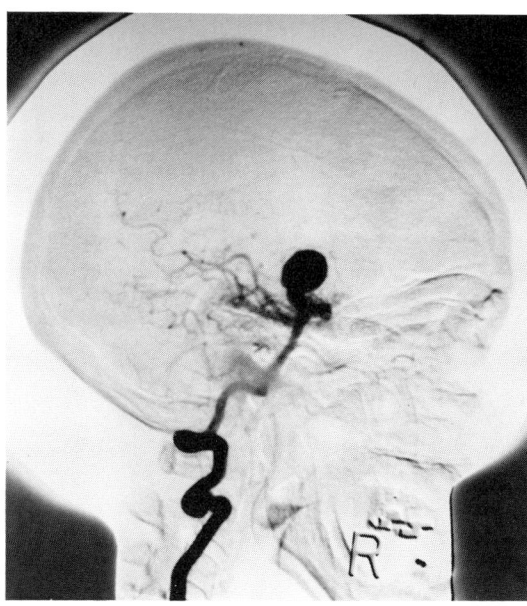

FIG. 7–5. Basilar artery aneurysm shown by selective vertebral angiography.

ripherally located, particularly in the middle cerebral arterial distribution.[30,31] Fusiform arteriosclerotic aneurysms are most common in the basilar artery and the cavernous portion of the internal carotid artery (Fig. 7–5). Cavernous carotid aneurysms may become large and may cause cranial nerve compression, or they may rupture to produce a carotid-cavernous fistula rather than subarachnoid hemorrhage.

If multiple aneurysms are present in a patient with subarachnoid hemorrhage, angiographic features such as larger size, local arterial spasm, and excrescence (punctum) from the dome of the aneurysm are used to determine which aneurysm has bled.[32] If no aneurysm is visualized, but if arterial spasm due to subarachnoid hemorrhage is present, an angiographic study done several days later, or when the patient's condition improves, may show an aneurysm that previously did not fill because of the spasm.[26] A giant aneurysm may appear smaller than its true size on an angiogram as a result of filling of the sac with thrombus. As with other types of aneurysms, CT is an invaluable complementary study. Correlation between CT and angiographic findings is useful in identifying hematoma, infarction, and herniation as complications of aneurysmal rupture.

Vascular Malformations. The most common congenital cerebral vascular malformation is the arteriovenous malformation (Fig. 7–6). Angiography usually shows multiple arteries feeding directly into multiple veins, although direct communication between a single artery and a single vein can occur. Selective carotid and vertebral angiography is usually necessary to define all feeding and draining vessels and to identify any additional malformations. The draining veins of an arteriovenous malformation characteristically fill during the early arterial phase, owing to the rapid flow and direct arteriovenous connections. High-volume shunting through an arteriovenous malformation may result in an aneurysmal dilation of the vein of Galen. Small arteriovenous malformations that have ruptured and then clotted may occasionally escape arteriographic detection. Venous angiomas, consisting entirely of veins, show a normal arterial phase; abnormal veins appear in the venous phase. Successful treatment of cerebral arteriovenous malformations by transcatheter embolotherapy has been reported, although the rate of recurrence of the lesion is high.[33] Occlusion of the nidus of the malformation with tissue adhesives applied through the catheter may become the treatment of choice in the future.[33,34]

ARTERIAL OCCLUSIVE DISEASE. Intracranial arteriosclerotic disease may be seen angiographically as irregularity, narrowing, widening, or occlusion of arteries. Arteriosclerotic plaques causing irregularity and luminal narrowing or widening are common in the cavernous internal carotid and basilar arteries. Other common intracranial sites are the middle and posterior cerebral arteries and their branches and the internal carotid artery as it crosses the dura mater. The cerebral angiogram may also show collateral circulation as a manifestation of arteriosclerotic or other occlusive disease. The circle of Willis connects the internal carotid and basilar arterial systems and usually allows filling of the anterior cerebral from the anterior communicating artery, and of the middle cerebral through the posterior communicating artery, in cases of internal carotid arterial occlusion in the neck. Collateral circulation from external to internal carotid systems, by retrograde flow through the ophthalmic artery or through anastamoses with the middle meningeal artery, is also common in patients with internal carotid arterial occlusion.

VASCULITIS. Inflammatory involvement of cerebral blood vessels may be seen in patients with many conditions, including infections, drug abuse, and vasculitides such as giant cell arteritis and periarteritis nodosa, and systemic lupus erythematosus. The most common angiographic findings are irregularity and narrowing or occlusion of the lumen of the vessel. Tuberculous or fungal meningitis may cause narrowing of the large vessels at the base of the brain.[35,36] Methamphetamine abuse causes arterial changes including beading, stenosis, and occlusion.[37] The brachiocephalic arteries are primarily involved in Takayasu's arteritis, which usually

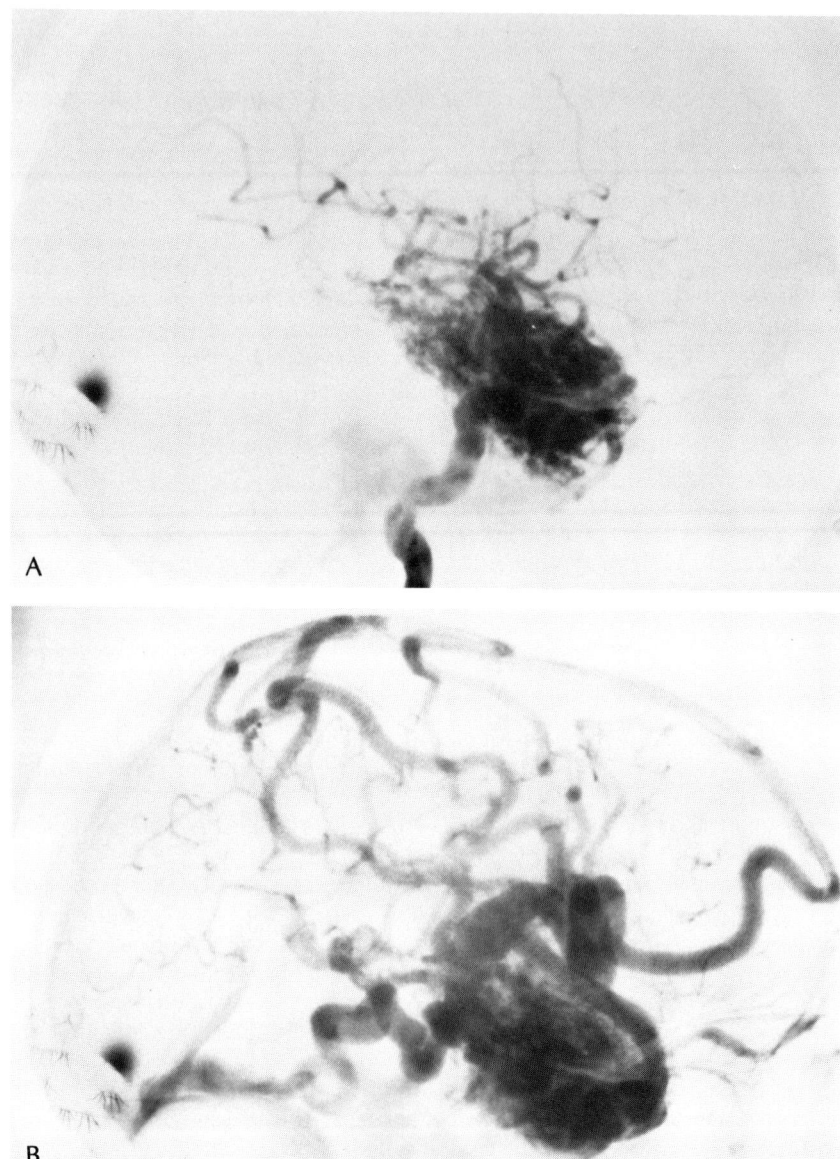

FIG. 7-6. Arteriovenous malformation. *A*, Large tangle of abnormal vessels is supplied by an enlarged internal carotid artery. *B*, Because of the rapid flow through the malformation, large draining veins are seen while normal arteries are still filled.

spares cranial vessels, but may involve the carotid arteries in the neck.[38]

TUMORS. Most brain tumors are initially visualized and localized on CT scans. Angiography can provide further information about the localization and blood supply of tumors that is useful if surgical intervention is contemplated. The number, size, and type of vessels and the circulation dynamics seen angiographically may also assist one in the diagnostic classification of a tumor.[39] Meningiomas, for example, typically show a blood supply from hypertrophied meningeal vessels and a homogeneous tumor stain that persists into the late venous phase (Fig. 7-7). Low-grade gliomas are usually avascular. Glioblastomas and vascular metastases typically show rapid circulation with early draining veins (Fig. 7-8). Hemangioblastomas of the cerebellum usually appear as a small, hypervascular nodule. Although such angiographic features are helpful in characterizing tumors when correlated with CT findings,

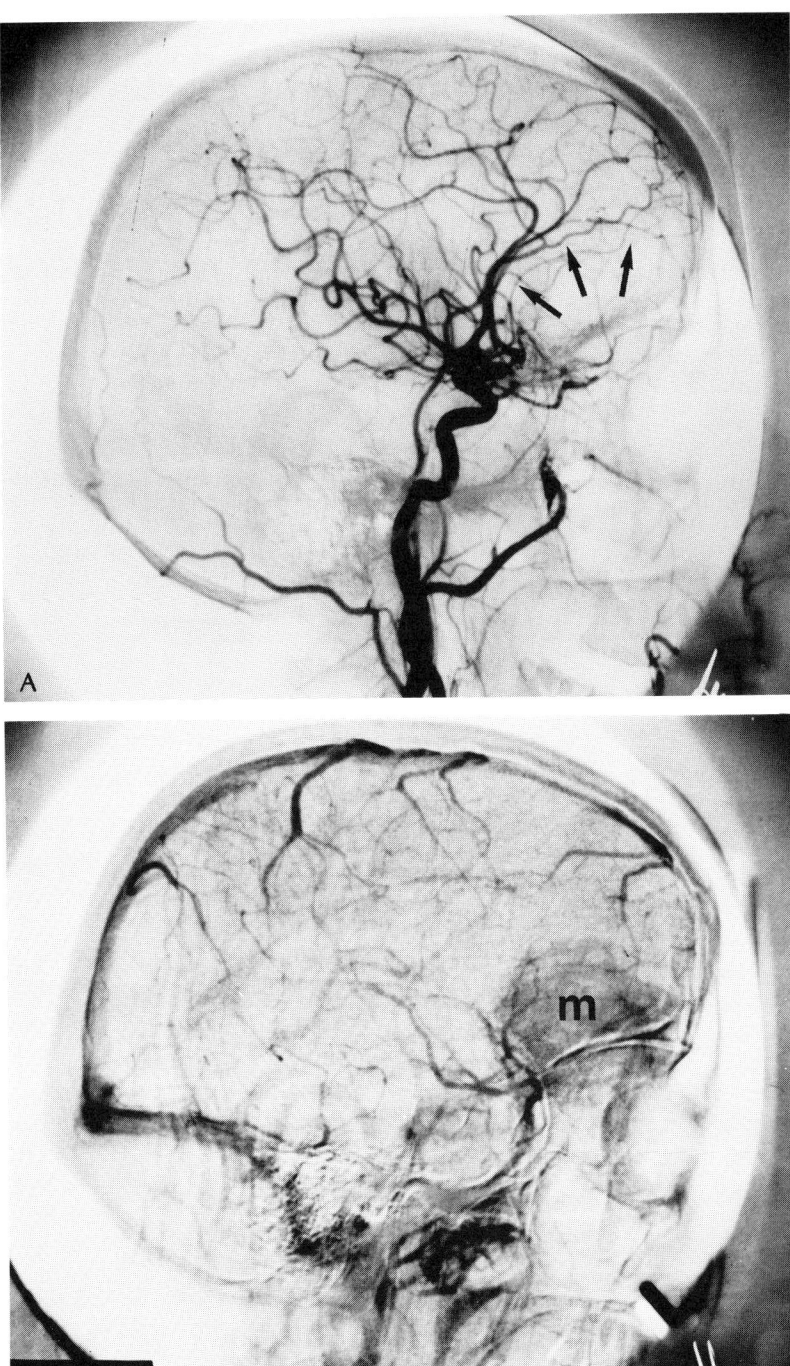

FIG. 7-7. Subfrontal meningioma. *A*, In the arterial phase, displacement of vessels away from the skull (arrows) indicates the extracerebral origin of the mass. *B*, Dense staining of the meningioma (m) is seen in the venous phase.

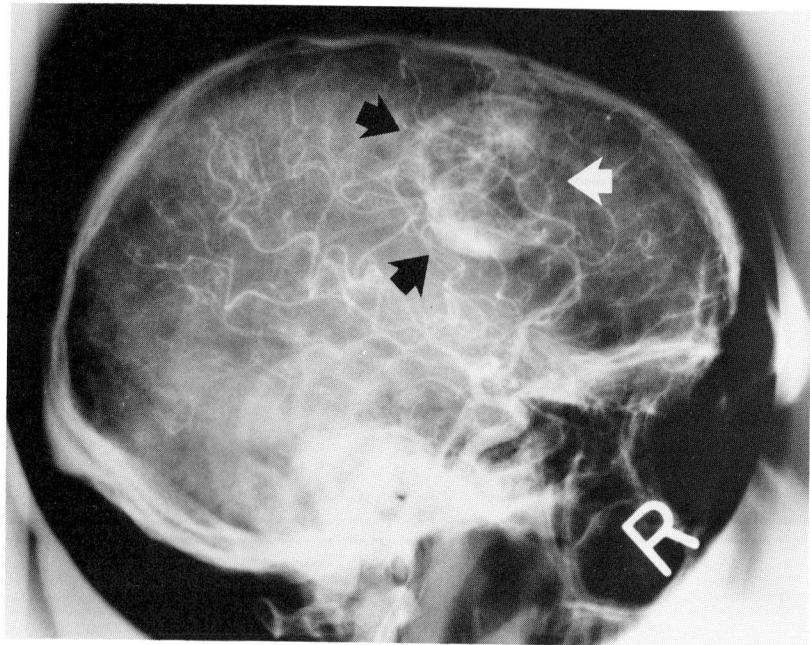

FIG. 7–8. Glioblastoma multiforme. Arterial phase of a carotid angiogram shows a hypervascular mass with marked tumor blush (arrows).

the primary role of angiography is in planning a surgical approach, not in arriving at the pathologic diagnosis.

THORACIC STUDIES
Thoracic Aortography

The preferred method for thoracic aortography is retrograde catheterization from a femoral approach.[40] An axillary approach is used when iliac or aortic occlusive disease prevents access from the femoral arteries. Usually, 50 to 60 ml of contrast material are used in adult patients. Simultaneous biplane filming enables one to obtain both oblique views with a single injection. The right posterior oblique view or its equivalent, the left anterior oblique view, usually provides the most information, by showing the aortic arch and the origins of the brachiocephalic arteries without superimposition.

DSA of the thoracic aorta may be performed by intravenous or intra-arterial injection. Both methods are less informative than conventional aortography, but they have certain advantages. The technique for intra-arterial DSA is similar to that for conventional aortography, except a smaller catheter and less-concentrated contrast media are required. Intravenous DSA is less invasive and avoids the potential neurologic complications of aortic arch injection.

CONGENITAL ANOMALIES OF THE AORTIC ARCH. Congenital anomalies of the aortic arch and its branches may produce symptoms by compression of the esophagus or trachea, or they may appear as mediastinal masses on chest radiographs.[41] Initial detection and evaluation of these anomalies is usually accomplished by chest radiography and barium studies, but final diagnosis is usually made by angiography or contrast-enhanced CT. DSA is often the procedure of choice for documenting anomalies that do not require operative correction (Fig. 7–9). When a vascular ring requiring surgical treatment is suspected, angiography in axial projections is the diagnostic method of choice.[42]

An aberrant right subclavian artery is the most common anomaly of the thoracic aorta. It arises as the last branch of an otherwise normal aortic arch and passes posterior to the esophagus, to produce a characteristic esophagographic indentation as it passes from left to right.

A right-sided aortic arch may occur either with mirror-image branching of the brachiocephalic vessels or with an aberrant left subclavian artery crossing from right to left posterior to the esophagus. The mirror-image type of right aortic arch is almost always associated with congenital heart defects.

The two most common causes of a vascular ring are double aortic arch and right-sided aorta with both an aberrant left subclavian artery and an encircling ductus arteriosus or ligamentum arteriosum. Vascular rings frequently produce symptoms by compression of the esophagus and trachea. The presence on chest radiographs of an aortic arch on the right side, with localized indentation of the tra-

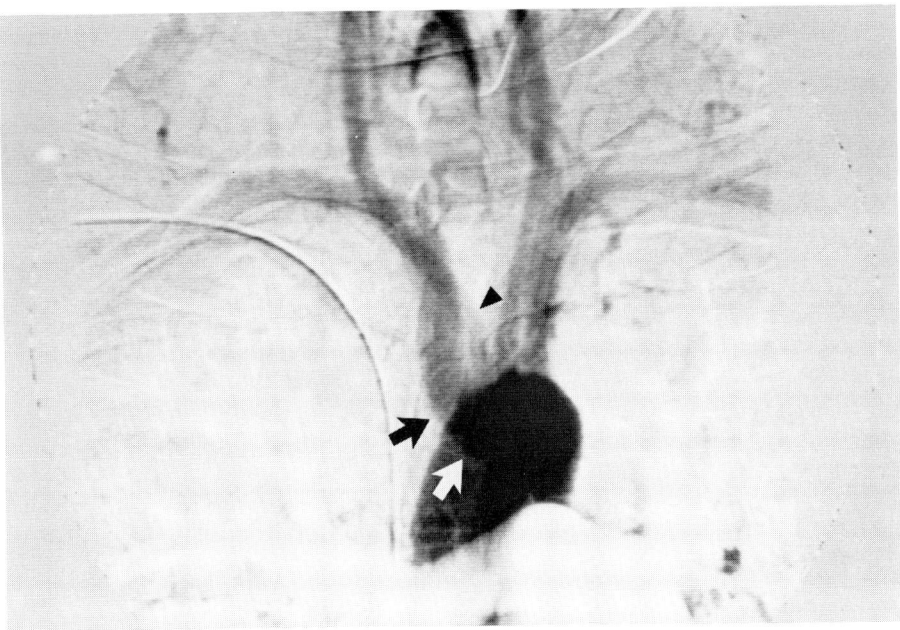

FIG. 7–9. Aberrant right subclavian artery. Intravenous digital subtraction angiogram shows the right subclavian artery (arrows) arising distal to the other aortic arch branches. The right common carotid artery (arrowhead) is the first branch of the aorta in this patient.

chea, suggests one of these entities, and angiography is confirmatory.

The pulmonary sling or "aberrant left pulmonary artery" also compresses the trachea and esophagus and is usually symptomatic. The aberrant artery passes around the right side of the trachea and then crosses to the left between the trachea and the esophagus, to produce right-sided and posterior indentation on the trachea and anterior indentation of the esophagus visible on a barium study. Conventional or digital pulmonary angiography with craniocaudal tube angulation is the most precise means of diagnosis.

COARCTATION AND PSEUDOCOARCTATION. Thoracic aortography is the definitive diagnostic procedure in patients with coarctation of the aorta.[43] Angiography usually shows a localized narrowing at or adjacent to the ligamentum arteriosum, with poststenotic dilation of the aorta distal to the narrowed segment. Collateral circulation and enlargement of the left subclavian artery are frequently visible. Associated malformations, such as bicuspid aortic valve and patent ductus arteriosus, should be sought. Aortic regurgitation or aortic stenosis at a valvular or subvalvular level may also be present.[43]

Pseudocoarctation is a congenital kinking of the thoracic aorta that most often becomes apparent in elderly patients when the kink is exaggerated by arteriosclerotic widening and elongation of the aorta. Usually, no pressure gradient is present across the kink, and no collateral circulation exists.[44] Digital or conventional aortography may be necessary to differentiate this lesion from a nonvascular mass.

THORACIC AORTIC ANEURYSMS. Aortic aneurysms are localized dilations due to disease affecting the aortic wall. Aneurysms may be classified as true or false. The wall of a true aortic aneurysm contains all three layers of the wall: intima, media, and adventitia. A false aneurysm (pseudoaneurysm) represents a contained rupture of the aorta with a wall consisting of adventitia and surrounding connective tissue, along with organized blood clot.

The most common thoracic aortic aneurysm is the true aneurysm caused by arteriosclerosis. The second most common is the post-traumatic false aneurysm (aortic rupture), usually caused by a rapid-deceleration injury. Mycotic, syphilitic, and Valsalva sinus aneurysms are rare. Aneurysms also occur in the brachiocephalic branches of the thoracic aorta.

Aortography is the most definitive and also the most invasive means of evaluating thoracic aortic aneurysms. Aortography is usually indicated to confirm a mediastinal mass as an aneurysm and to evaluate a known aneurysm preoperatively. The goals of aortography include assessment of the following: (1) the size and extent of the aneurysm and the site of any rupture; (2) the presence or absence of involvement of branch vessels such as the coronary or carotid arteries; (3) the involvement of other mediastinal structures such as the trachea or esophagus; (4) the presence or absence of aortic valve regurgitation; and (5) the presence of any additional aneurysms.[45]

Arteriosclerotic Aneurysms. The majority of thoracic aortic aneurysms are arteriosclerotic in origin.[46] The incidence is higher in males, and the lesion is associated with hypertension, coronary artery and cerebrovascular disease, and abdominal aortic aneurysms. Arteriosclerotic aneurysms most often involve the distal aortic arch and the descending aorta. The ascending aorta is rarely involved primarily; aneurysmal widening of the ascending aorta from arteriosclerosis is usually seen in continuity with involvement of the aortic arch and descending aorta.[47] Arteriosclerotic thoracic aneurysm may be either fusiform or saccular in configuration; the former is more common.

Traumatic Aneurysms. Such lesions of the thoracic aorta are pseudoaneurysms resulting from localized aortic rupture. The most common cause is tearing of the aorta by rapid, forceful deceleration or blunt trauma, or both. The most common site is the aortic isthmus just distal to the left subclavian artery, at the site of the ligamentum arteriosum[48] (Fig. 7–10). The wall of the ascending aorta or distal descending aorta may also tear. When the periaortic hematoma produced by the tear is contained by the surrounding mediastinal connective tissues, a false aneurysm is formed. If untreated, secondary rupture of the pseudoaneurysm within hours or days is the rule, although chronic false aneurysm may result.[48]

On plain chest radiographs, aortic rupture may be suspected because of widening of the mediastinal shadow due to mediastinal hematoma. Other signs of mediastinal hematoma include irregularity of the aortic knob, widening of the paraspinal lines, deviation of the trachea or nasogastric tube to the right, depression of the left main bronchus, and evidence of fluid in the left apical pleural space.[49] If chest radiographic findings or the clinical status of the patient suggest aortic rupture, immediate aortography will be necessary to establish or to exclude the diagnosis. The transfemoral approach is usually used because of its speed, safety, and versatility.[50]

Angiographically, an aortic laceration is typically seen as an area of irregularity or interruption of the aortic wall. A saccular false aneurysm is usually present.[51] A small percentage of patients have associated laceration of one or more of the brachiocephalic arteries.[50]

The role of intravenous DSA in the patient with possible thoracic aortic rupture has not been established. The advantages of DSA are speed and avoidance of catheterization of the traumatized aorta. The resolution of DSA is sufficient to detect all but the smallest pseudoaneurysm of the thoracic aorta. With further experience, DSA may become the procedure of choice for confirming or excluding traumatic aortic rupture in patients with a definite abnormality on chest radiographs. Patients with small intimal tears will probably continue to require aortography for diagnosis.

Mycotic and Syphilitic Aneurysms. Mycotic aneurysms of the thoracic aorta are most often true aneurysms and are typically saccular in configuration.[52] The most common sites are the ascending aorta and the sinuses of Valsalva. Unlike syphilitic aneurysms, mycotic lesions are rarely calcified. Conventional or digital aortographic techniques are used to establish the diagnosis and the extent of aortic involvement.

Syphilitic aortitis is usually manifested radiographically as calcification in the ascending aorta, with or without an aneurysm. Syphilitic aneurysms usually occur in the ascending aorta or aortic arch and contain calcium in the ascending aorta, but not in the aortic arch. Typically, the ascending aorta is dilated, and a saccular aneurysm is present.

Congenital Aneurysms. Aortography is the most precise means for diagnosis of congenital aneu-

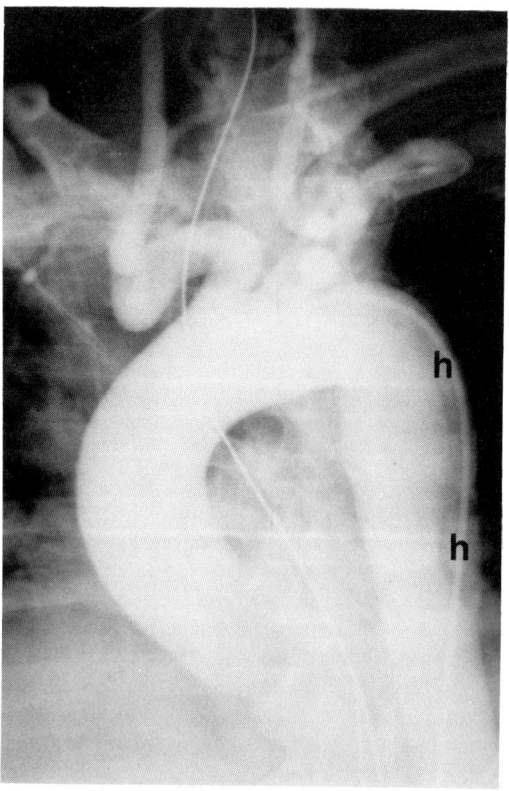

FIG. 7–10. Traumatic aortic transection (pseudoaneurysm). A resulting periaortic hematoma (h) compresses the proximal descending aorta in the region distal to the left subclavian artery.

rysms of the sinus of Valsalva. Such aneurysms usually involve a single sinus, most often the right. Acquired sinus of Valsalva aneurysms may be mycotic (bacterial endocarditis) or syphilitic in origin.[53]

Innominate and Subclavian Artery Aneurysms. The thoracic aortic branch vessels most likely to develop aneurysms are the innominate and left subclavian arteries. The most common causes are arteriosclerosis and trauma.[54] Such aneurysms may appear as a superior mediastinal or apical pulmonary mass on chest radiographs. Similar masses may be due to marked arterial tortuosity. Dynamic, contrast-enhanced CT may differentiate a vascular structure from other masses. DSA or aortography is used to differentiate among arterial tortuosity, ectasia, and aneurysm. Ultrasound may be useful in characterizing a palpable, pulsatile mass as either arterial or nonvascular and may enable one to differentiate aneurysms from tortuous vessels.[55]

AORTIC DISSECTION. This lesion results when a tear in the intima leads to a hematoma dissecting into the media for a variable distance along the aorta. Predisposing factors include hypertension, familial tendency, Marfan's syndrome, congenital conditions such as coarctation of the aorta and bicuspid aortic valve, and pregnancy.[56]

A chest radiograph should be obtained as soon as possible in any patient with suspected acute aortic dissection. Plain radiographic findings in aortic dissection include the signs of thoracic aneurysms. The most important signs are widening of the aortic arch, a change in the aortic configuration on successive radiographs, and a localized bulge or irregularity in the aortic contour.[57]

The goal of aortography in aortic dissection is the accurate identification of the type of dissection and of its extent. The angiographer attempts to show the proximal and distal extents of the lesion, the presence or absence of involvement of aortic branches such as the renal or iliac arteries, and aortic insufficiency, if present.

CLASSIFICATION. In DeBakey's classification, Type I aortic dissection begins at the aortic root or ascending aorta and involves the arch and descending aorta.[58] Type II dissection involves only the ascending aorta. Type III aortic dissection begins just distal to the left subclavian artery and involves the descending thoracic aorta, with a tendency to continue into the abdominal aorta (Fig. 7–11). In the treatment-oriented classification of Miller and colleagues, those dissections involving the ascending aorta (DeBakey Types I and II) are classified as Type A and those involving the descending aorta only (DeBakey Type III) are classified as Type B.[59]

Intravenous DSA does not at present give sufficient detail to allow identification of many of these features in the initial evaluation of aortic dissection,

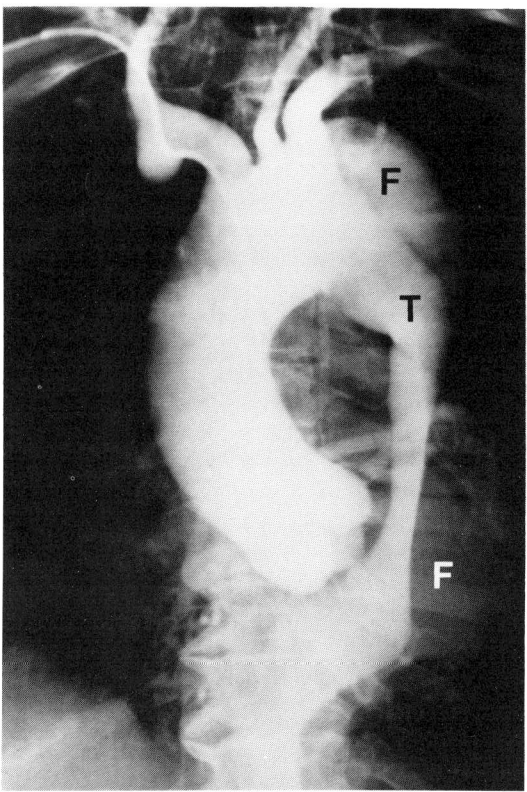

FIG. 7–11. Type III aortic dissection. The true lumen of the descending thoracic aorta (T) is compressed and is distorted by the false lumen. A small amount of contrast material has entered the proximal false lumen (F). The right and left coronary arteries are visible.

but the procedure may be useful in following patients after treatment.[60]

Characteristics. The most specific angiographic finding in aortic dissection is opacification of both true and false lumens with a linear lucency, representing the intimal flap, between them ("double-barreled" aorta). The false lumen may show delayed filling and slow washout of contrast material. If only the true lumen fills during aortography, widening of the outer border of the aorta or compression of the true lumen by the hematoma may be seen. Constriction of the true lumen by the hematoma may result in a "twisted-tape" appearance. Injection into the false lumen may occur, especially in the ascending aorta. In such a patient, filling of a blind channel showing delayed washout, without filling of the sinuses of Valsalva, allows recognition of the situation.[56] Aortic regurgitation may be seen when the aortic root is involved. In a few patients, the aortogram may be either normal or confusing, because of unusual findings.[61]

Dissections in peripheral arteries that have not

extended from the aorta are unusual.[62] Dissection may also be limited to the abdominal aorta.

Because of the potential for both false-negative and false-positive examinations by CT, we currently prefer aortography for the initial diagnosis of aortic dissection. CT is useful in the evaluation of mediastinal masses when aortic dissection has been excluded angiographically.

TAKAYASU'S ARTERITIS. Arteriographically, Takayasu's arteritis is suspected when smooth areas of stenosis or dilation are seen in the aorta and the brachiocephalic, visceral, or renal arteries with abrupt transition from normal to abnormal.[38] Various combinations of aortic narrowing and aneurysm formation may be seen.

Bronchial Arteriography

Bronchial arteriography may be useful in the diagnosis and treatment of hemoptysis in selected patients. Therapeutic bronchial artery embolization is indicated in patients with severe hemoptysis when medical treatment has failed and when surgical treatment is contraindicated (Fig. 7–12). Unfortunately, both bronchial artery embolization and arteriography are hazardous because of the risk of serious spinal cord complications such as paraplegia. Therapeutic embolization is contraindicated when the bronchial arteriogram shows that the vessel serving as the source of hemoptysis also supplies a branch to the spinal cord.[63]

Pulmonary Angiography

PULMONARY EMBOLISM. The most common indication for pulmonary angiography is suspicion of pulmonary embolism. Although a normal radionuclide perfusion lung scan is accurate in excluding a diagnosis of pulmonary embolism,[64] pulmonary angiography is often necessary because of the low specificity of a positive scan.[65] Accurate angiographic diagnosis or exclusion of pulmonary embolism allows appropriate therapy of a potentially fatal disorder or avoidance of the risk of unnecessary anticoagulant therapy. The price paid for accurate diagnosis is the risk of the angiogram itself, which has a mortality rate of up to 0.7% and a morbidity rate of up to 5%.[66]

The major risks of pulmonary angiography are cardiac arrhythmias, acute pulmonary hypertension, and cardiac perforation, any of which can be fatal.[66] The patients at greatest risk of death are those with marked pulmonary arterial hypertension.[66] Patients with left bundle branch block are at increased risk of cardiac arrest during catheter movements. Digitalis toxicity is also a relative contraindication to transcardiac catheterization.

Preliminary Studies. Chest radiographs are not usually helpful in the diagnosis of pulmonary em-

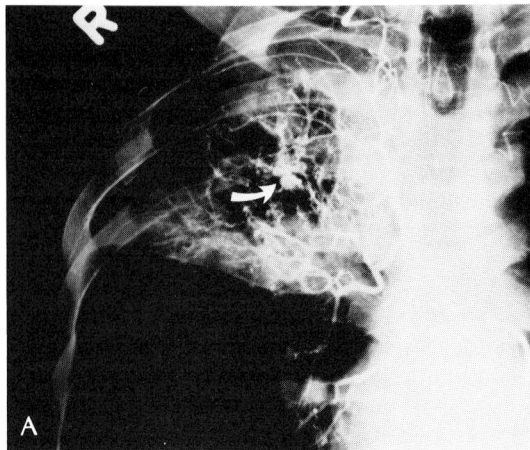

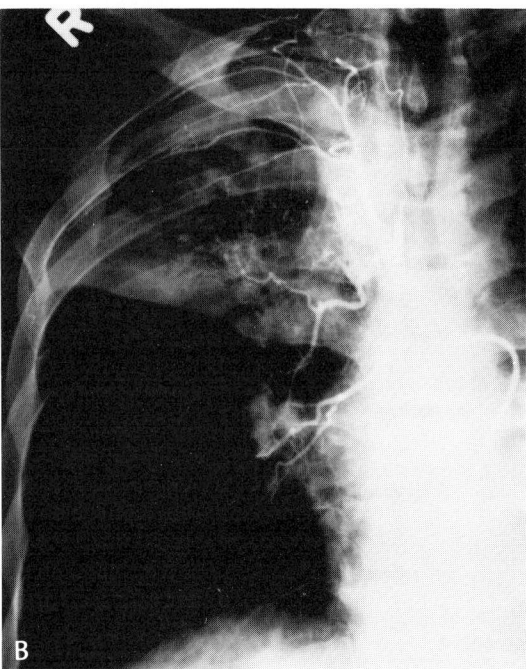

FIG. 7–12. Medically intractable hemoptysis due to bronchiectasis. *A*, Selective bronchial arteriogram showing abnormal vessels and contrast extravasation at the bleeding site (arrow). *B*, After transcatheter embolization, the hemoptysis is controlled.

bolism. A wedge-shaped, pleural-based density associated with effusion and elevation of the hemidiaphragm is characteristic, but not specific, for pulmonary embolism with infarction. Other signs, such as localized pulmonary oligemia (Westermark's sign) or enlargement of the pulmonary arteries, may suggest the diagnosis, but they are rare and are nonspecific.[67]

Whenever possible, radionuclide lung scanning should precede pulmonary angiography if pulmonary embolism is suspected because a normal pulmonary perfusion scan virtually rules out pulmonary embolism and eliminates the need for angiography.[65] An abnormal perfusion scan guides the angiographer in selecting pulmonary vessels for injection and appropriate projections.[68] Selective injections increase the detection rate of pulmonary emboli and decrease the incidence of complications such as arrhythmias.

Procedure. Conventional pulmonary angiography involves passage of a catheter from either a femoral or antecubital vein, through the right atrium and ventricle, and into the main pulmonary artery beyond the pulmonary valve. Selective catheterization of the right or left pulmonary arteries or their branches is usually possible, if necessary. The electrocardiogram is carefully monitored for arrhythmias as the catheter is passed through the right ventricle, the time of greatest risk of cardiac arrest from catheter manipulation. Monitoring of the intracardiac pressure helps one to determine the location of the catheter tip and to identify patients with pulmonary arterial hypertension. If elevated pulmonary artery and right ventricular pressures are identified, small selective injections are used to decrease the risk of cardiac arrest.

Digital Subtraction Angiography. The role of DSA in the diagnosis of pulmonary embolism has not been established, but it appears to be of great potential value. Intravenous DSA allows nonselective visualization of the pulmonary arteries without transcardiac catheterization. A sensitivity rate of up to 90% in the detection of pulmonary embolism has been reported.[69,70] This technique appears to be most useful when used in conjunction with a prior radionuclide perfusion lung scan. Arterial DSA may permit smaller injections associated with fewer complications. Patients suspected of having multiple small emboli require conventional pulmonary angiography with selective injections.

Characteristics. Pulmonary embolism is characterized by the appearance of the emboli as intraluminal filling defects or the abrupt "cutoff" of a branch of the pulmonary artery due to an occluding embolus (Fig. 7–13). The shorter the interval between the onset of symptoms of pulmonary embolism and the obtaining of a pulmonary angiogram, the greater the chance of seeing one of these diagnostic features. Because pulmonary emboli usually fragment and migrate distally over time, angiographic abnormalities may disappear or may be limited to nonspecific findings, such as localized decreased vascular markings, a few days after the embolic event.[71]

OTHER DISORDERS. Pulmonary angiography is also used to assess congenital abnormalities such as pulmonary sling, anomalous pulmonary venous return, pulmonary dysgenesis, pulmonary sequestration, and arteriovenous malformations. Conventional pulmonary angiography, possibly including magnification, is necessary for maximum sensitivity in detecting pulmonary arteriovenous malformations, which are associated with hereditary hemorrhagic telangiectasia and are frequently multiple.[72] Angiographically, these lesions may be classified as solitary, multiple, or diffuse,[73] and as either simple or complex.[74] Simple pulmonary arteriovenous malformations have a single supplying artery and a single draining vein, whereas complex malformations have multiple feeding arteries and draining veins.[74] Unlike systemic congenital arteriovenous malformations, pulmonary malformations may be cured by percutaneous embolotherapy.[75,76] A risk of paradoxic embolization of the therapeutic occlusive material into the systemic arterial system exists, particularly in patients with the simple type of pulmonary arteriovenous malformation.

Intravenous pulmonary DSA may be sufficient for evaluating other congenital pulmonary abnormalities in many patients. This technique is probably also adequate in the preoperative evaluation of patients with chronic obstructive pulmonary disease in whom bullectomy is considered.

ABDOMINAL AND RETROPERITONEAL STUDIES

Angiography of the Liver and Portal Circulation

NEOPLASMS AND METASTASES. CT scanning, radionuclide liver scanning, and ultrasound are now the primary means of evaluating liver masses. Hepatic arteriography remains an important secondary means of evaluating liver masses because it allows one to determine the extent and resectability of hepatic neoplasms and may provide a specific diagnosis. When surgical treatment is not possible, hepatic angiography may be a prelude to an intraarterial therapeutic procedure.

Primary hepatic neoplasms require angiography for diagnosis and staging. Hemangioma, the most common benign liver neoplasm, may be small or large, solitary or multifocal. Most such lesions are asymptomatic. The angiographic appearance is characteristic, with normal-sized hepatic arteries and dilated vascular spaces in which prolonged pooling of contrast medium is seen[77] (Fig. 7–14). Focal nodular hyperplasia and liver cell adenoma have similar angiographic features, and it is not usually possible to differentiate between the two or to rule out malignant disease by angiographic means alone. Angiographic features suggesting focal nodular hyperplasia are discrete margination, arrangement of small tumor arteries in a radial, spoke-wheel pattern, and central lucency corresponding to the

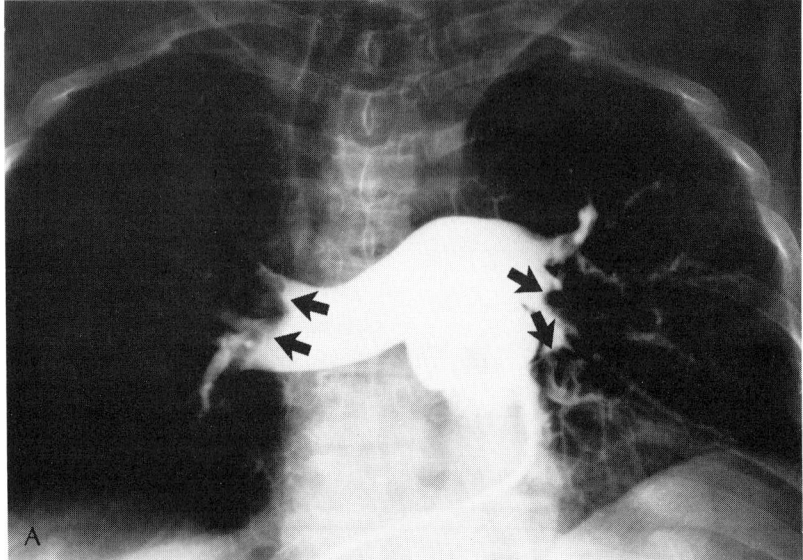

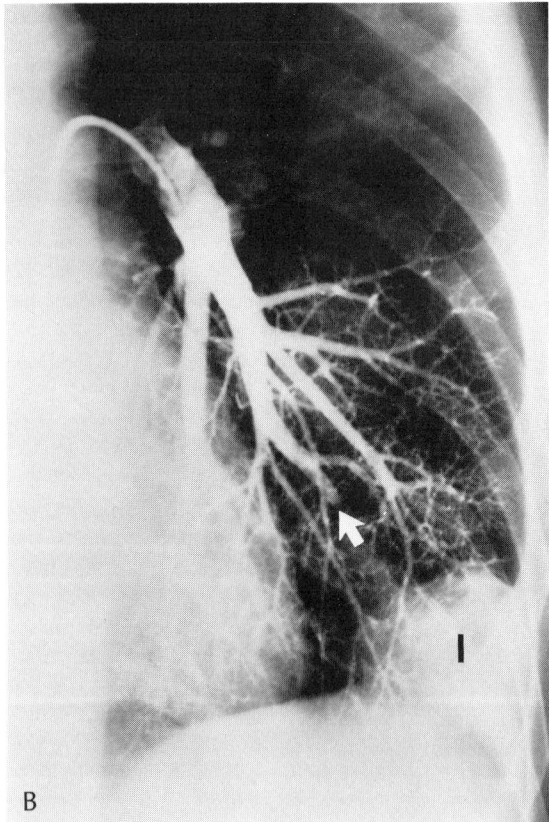

FIG. 7–13. *A*, Pulmonary embolism; multiple filling defects due to emboli are present in the branches of the right and left main pulmonary arteries (arrows). *B*, Pulmonary embolism with infarction; the occluding embolus cuts off a lower lobe artery (arrow). The resulting pulmonary infarct creates a rounded opacity in the peripheral lung (I).

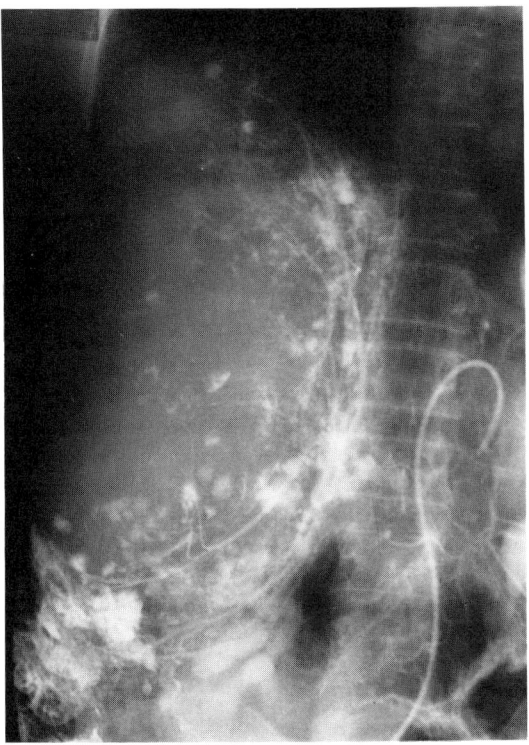

FIG. 7-14. Large hemangioma of the liver. Dilated vascular spaces showing slow and prolonged contrast opacification are the angiographic hallmark of this tumor. The hepatic arteries are stretched by the mass, but they are otherwise normal.

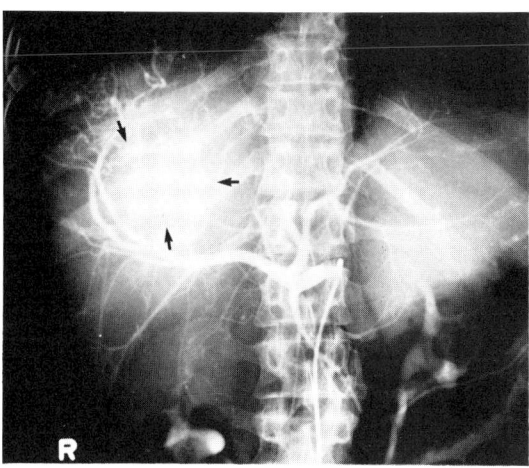

FIG. 7-15. Hepatoma. Obviously abnormal tumor vessels (arrows) are supplied by a large hepatic artery.

central scar.[78] Liver cell adenoma is usually hypervascular and may mimic focal nodular hyperplasia and hepatocellular carcinoma.

Hepatocellular carcinoma may be either hypervascular or hypovascular (Fig. 7-15). Dilation of the feeding arteries, obviously abnormal tumor vessels, and arteriovenous shunting are suggestive angiographic features.[79] Angiography is useful in assessing resectability and in defining the vascular anatomic structures of the liver.[80] Invasion of hepatic or portal veins is an important indication of unresectability of neoplasms.

Liver metastases may be hypervascular, hypovascular, or avascular, usually corresponding to the vascularity of the primary tumor. Hepatic arteriography is indicated in the evaluation of the single liver metastasis, to exclude additional metastases prior to resection and to define the vascular anatomic features. Evaluation of the extent and blood supply of hepatic metastases is also useful when transcatheter tumor embolization or chemotherapy infusion is considered.[81]

HEPATIC ARTERY ANEURYSMS. Angiography may be necessary for evaluation of hepatic artery aneurysms. These lesions are most often traumatic or mycotic in origin; arteriosclerotic hepatic artery aneurysms are rare. Clinically, hepatic artery aneurysms may manifest as hemobilia, and therapeutic transcatheter embolization may be considered after diagnostic arteriography.[81] Multiple angiomas of the liver can be seen in patients with hereditary hemorrhagic telangiectasia.[82]

DISORDERS OF PORTAL CIRCULATION. Angiography of the liver is used to demonstrate the hemodynamics of portal hypertension prior to shunt operations. The usual studies are hepatic wedge pressure measurements, hepatic venography, hepatic arteriography, and indirect (venous-phase) portography by means of splenic or superior mesenteric arterial injection. The angiographic goal is to define the level of obstruction causing portal hypertension, the anatomic features of the arterial and venous flow, and the location of collateral vessels.[83,84]

Hepatic venous manometry and venography are performed by selective catheterization of the hepatic veins. Hepatic venous wedge pressure measurements accurately reflect the elevated portal venous pressure in patients with sinusoidal and postsinusoidal portal hypertension. In presinusoidal hypertension, caused by extrahepatic portal vein obstruction, hepatic wedge pressure is normal, a feature that permits the diagnosis of this type of portal hypertension.

The portal vein and collateral vessels such as esophageal varices are studied on the venous phase of a prolonged selective splenic or superior mesenteric arterial injection. This method may also be used to evaluate shunt patency in the postoperative patient. Hepatic arteriography in patients with cirrhosis may show enlarged hepatic arteries, increased arterial flow, and "corkscrew" tortuosity of the intrahepatic arteries. Occasionally, one detects hepatocellular carcinoma as a complication of cirrhosis.

When bleeding from gastroesophageal varices is not controlled by vasopressin, percutaneous transcatheter occlusion of varices is possible in some patients.[85] A transhepatic or umbilical vein (cutdown) approach to the portal system may be used.[86] In patients with a patent portocaval shunt, access to the bleeding varices may be possible by maneuvering the catheter through the shunt.

Pancreatic Angiography

Angiography contributes little to the diagnosis of inflammatory diseases of the pancreas, with the notable exception of the vascular complications of pancreatitis: hemorrhage, pseudoaneurysms, and arterial stenoses or occlusions.[87,88] Angiography no longer plays a role in the diagnosis and staging of most patients with pancreatic ductal carcinoma.[89] Angiographic studies may be indicated in difficult cases, however, when the diagnosis of carcinoma is uncertain or when assessing the resectability of smaller tumors.[89] The angiographic criteria of unresectability are encasement and invasion of major extrapancreatic arteries or veins.[91]

ISLET CELL TUMORS. Pancreatic islet cell tumors are frequently too small to be localized by sonography or CT scanning.[92] One should conduct these tests, however, because of the possibility of detecting the pancreatic tumor or evidence of metastases. If the results of noninvasive studies offer insufficient information, angiography should be performed for tumor localization prior to surgical treatment (Fig. 7–16). Arteriographic localization is based on the hypervascularity of most islet cell tumors. The reported accuracy of arteriography is highest for insulinomas (75 to 80%), which are usually hypervascular, and lowest for gastrinomas (15 to 85%), which are more often small and hypovascular.[93] Transhepatic portal vein catheterization for selective pancreatic venous sampling with radioimmunoassay for the appropriate islet cell hormone is an accurate means of tumor localization.[94] This method appears to be important when arteriographic localization is unsuccessful.

Hormonally inactive islet cell tumors may mimic pancreatic ductal carcinoma clinically. Angiography is an important complementary study to CT because pancreatic ductal carcinomas are hypovascular, whereas nonsecreting islet cell tumors are almost always hypervascular.[93] Other hypervascular pancreatic neoplasms are mucinous cystadenoma, mucinous cystadenocarcinoma, and microcystic adenoma, all of which have similar angiographic features. These cystic pancreatic neoplasms usually show characteristic CT features of cysts and calcifications that allow one to distinguish them from islet cell tumors.[95]

Gastrointestinal Tract Angiography

Gastrointestinal hemorrhage often poses a diagnostic problem. Several diagnostic techniques such as endoscopy, isotope scanning, angiography, and exploratory celiotomy may be used in an attempt to localize and to treat the bleeding. A major goal during the early period is to distinguish between upper and lower gastrointestinal bleeding. Hematemesis or the presence of blood in a nasogastric tube almost invariably localizes the hemorrhage proximal to the ligament of Treitz. Endoscopic examination is preferred for upper gastrointestinal bleeding because most lesions can be reached by the endoscope. Angiographic study should be reserved for patients in whom results of endoscopy are inconclusive, for those in whom endoscopy is contraindicated, and for those in whom transcatheter control of the bleeding is contemplated.

LOCALIZATION OF HEMORRHAGE. For successful angiographic localization of the site, the patient should be actively bleeding during the procedure at a rate of at least 0.5 ml/min.[96] Diagnostic angiography for upper gastrointestinal bleeding should include celiac and superior mesenteric arteriograms and occasional superselective arteriograms of the left gastric and gastroduodenal arteries. Lesions frequently responsible for acute upper gastrointestinal hemorrhage include peptic ulcers, gastritis, Mallory-Weiss lacerations, and esophageal or gastric varices (Fig. 7–17).

In patients with acute lower gastrointestinal bleeding, radionuclide imaging with either ^{99m}technetium (^{99m}Tc)-sulfur colloid or ^{99m}Tc-labeled red cells is commonly used to time the arteriographic procedure.[97,98] The patients should be followed with repeated radionuclide scans to detect intermittent bleeding.[99] ^{99m}Tc-pertechnetate may also demonstrate Meckel's diverticulum if acid-secreting gastric cells are present. In patients with acute bleeding, barium studies are of little value, and colonoscopic examinations are often inconclusive.

The angiographic evaluation usually begins with a superior mesenteric arteriogram because most sources of bleeding are found within the territory supplied by this artery.[99] Subsequently, inferior mesenteric and celiac arteriograms are performed if warranted. If a rectosigmoid lesion is suspected, the study should begin with an inferior mesenteric arteriogram, to visualize that area before the bladder is filled with contrast material. Lesions frequently responsible for acute lower gastrointestinal hemorrhage include colonic diverticula, angiodysplasias, tumors, ulcers, and Meckel's diverticula (Figs. 7–18 and 7–19).

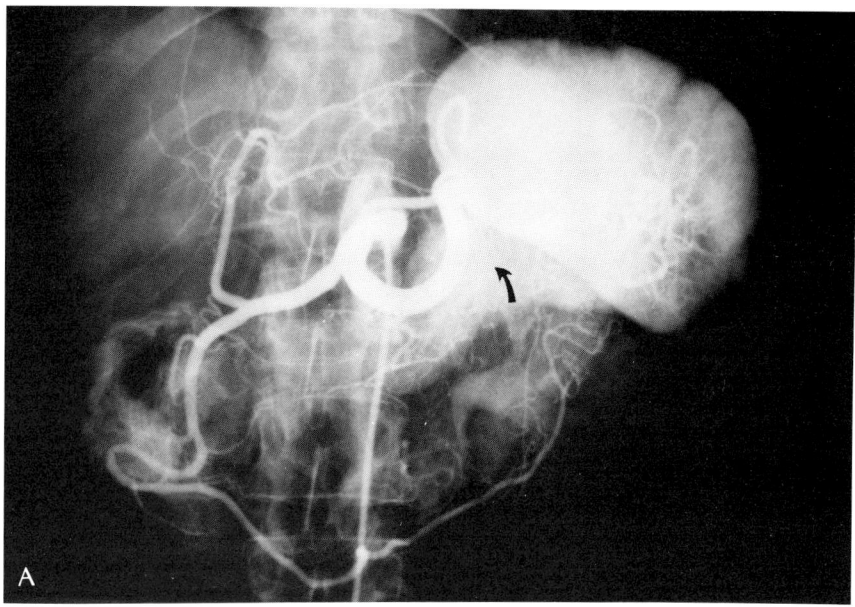
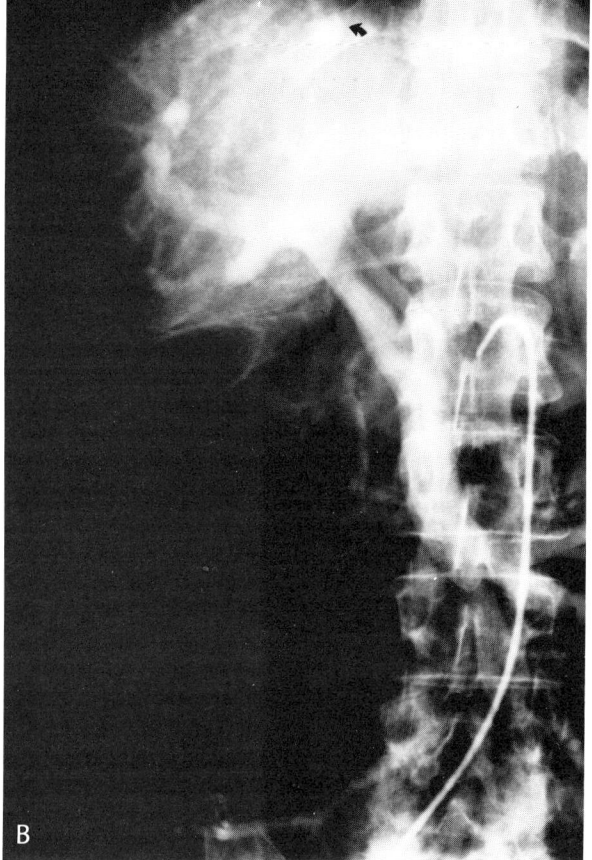

FIG. 7–16. Insulinoma. A, Small hypervascular tumor (arrow). B, Liver metastasis (arrow).

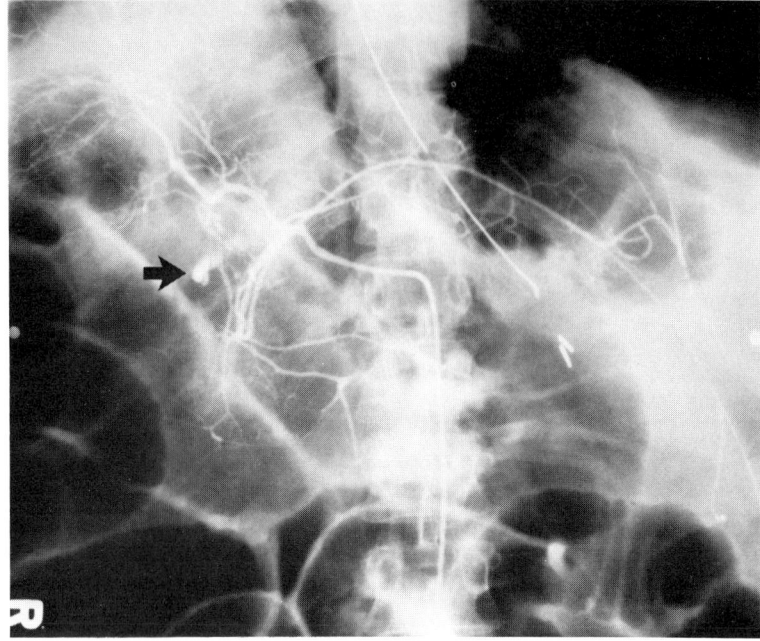

FIG. 7–17. Upper gastrointestinal bleeding. Common hepatic arteriography shows a bleeding site (arrow) in the descending duodenum, supplied by branches of the gastroduodenal artery.

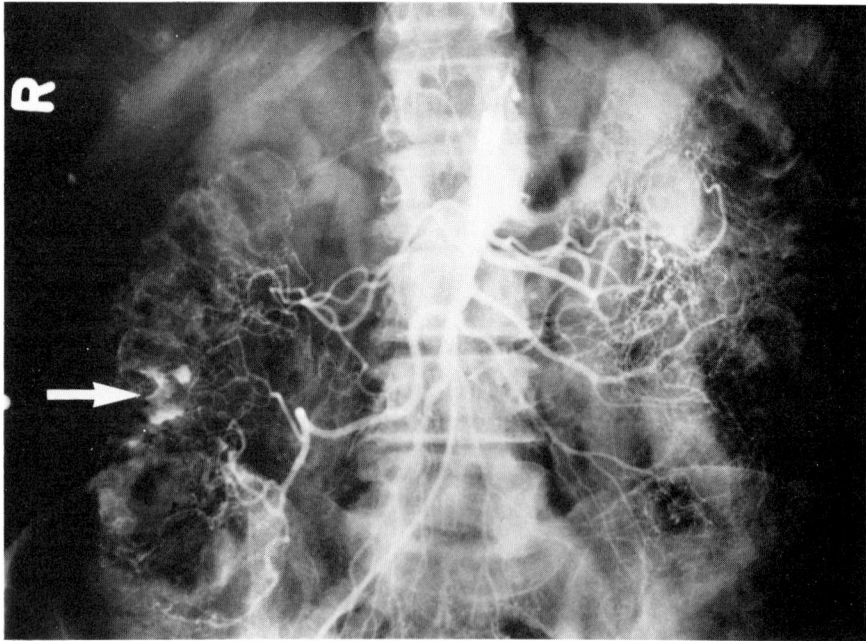

FIG. 7–18. Contrast extravasation in the right colon (arrow) because of an actively bleeding diverticulum.

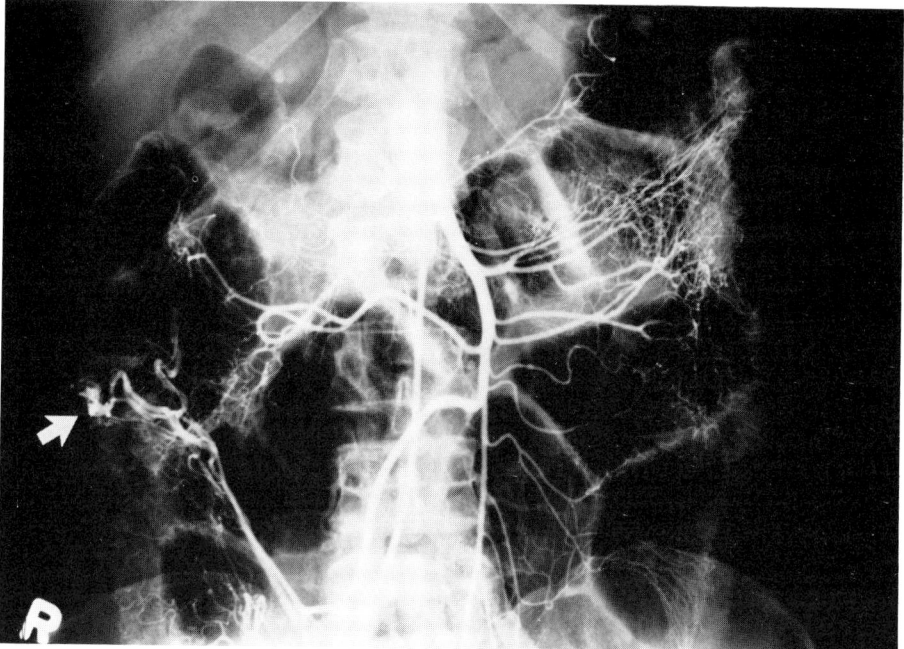

FIG. 7–19. Angiodysplasia of the right colon (arrow). The location and the early-draining veins, which are much larger than the adjacent arterial branches, are characteristic of this disorder.

In patients with chronic recurrent gastrointestinal hemorrhage, barium studies in conjunction with endoscopic examinations are used in the initial evaluation. Angiographic examination is reserved for patients in whom results of these studies are inconclusive. The lesions most frequently encountered are colonic angiodysplasias, tumors of the bowel, and Meckel's diverticula.

Renal Angiography

The indications for renal angiography have been reduced by the advent of accurate noninvasive methods. Currently, the major indications for renal angiography are evaluation of pathologic processes involving the renal vessels, evaluation prior to renal surgical procedures, and planning of interventional radiologic procedures.

RENAL VASCULAR DISORDERS. Diagnostic renal arteriography is most often performed from a femoral approach. An aortogram usually precedes selective renal artery injection because of the information obtained on possible variations in size, number, and origin of the renal arteries. Aortography is necessary in patients with renovascular hypertension, to avoid mistaking spasm of the renal artery for a fixed stenosis and to detect stenosis of the renal orifice by aortic plaque (Fig. 7–20). A normal aortogram also helps one to distinguish renal artery stenosis due to fibromuscular dysplasia from that due to arteriosclerosis.[100] When severe atheromatous disease involves the origin of the renal artery, selective renal arteriography may be hazardous. Approximate contrast agent requirements are 40 ml for the aortogram and 8 to 12 ml for each selective renal artery injection. When necessary, magnification arteriography, transcatheter infusion of vasodilators or vasoconstrictors, and renal venography are used to amplify the arteriographic findings.

CYSTS AND TUMORS. Angiography is not necessary when a renal mass fits strict criteria for definition as a simple cyst by ultrasound and CT.[101] When a cystic mass cannot be defined as a simple cyst by noninvasive means, percutaneous cyst puncture can be performed if the cyst is safely accessible.[102] If the results of cyst puncture suggest a cyst associated with neoplasm, or if the cyst is not safely accessible to percutaneous puncture, then selective renal angiography should be performed.

Renal Cell Carcinoma. Angiography is an accurate means of diagnosis of renal cell carcinoma and is therefore useful whenever the benign or malignant nature of a renal mass is not clearly established by other means.[103,104]

Angiography remains a mainstay of diagnosis and preoperative evaluation in patients with renal cell carcinoma because of its accuracy and its precise definition of vascular anatomic features for surgical planning. CT is superior to arteriography in preoperative staging of renal carcinoma, however, by enabling one to evaluate perinephric extension and metastases more accurately.[105] Because CT is less accurate in showing the status of the renal vein and

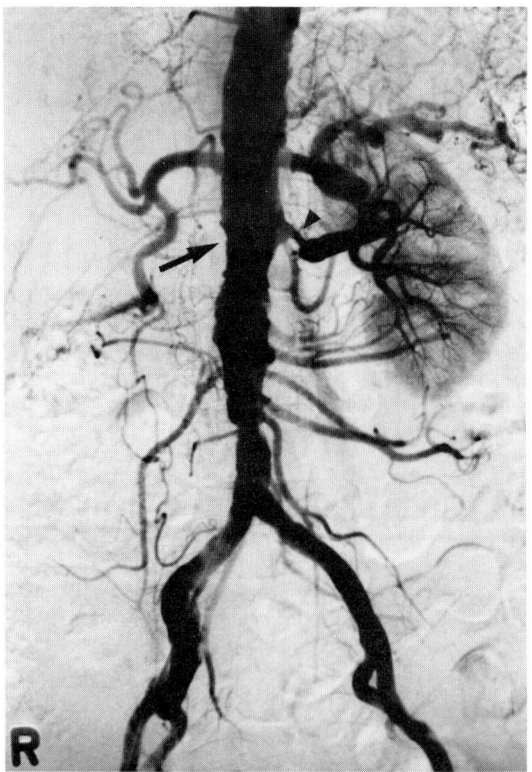

FIG. 7-20. Renovascular hypertension. One sees extensive atherosclerotic irregularity of the aorta, complete occlusion of the right renal artery (arrow), and stenosis of the left renal artery (arrowhead) with poststenotic dilation.

inferior vena cava, inferior vena cavography and, occasionally, renal venography should be used when the question of tumor extension into the venous system is not clearly established during staging of renal carcinoma by CT.

Most renal cell carcinomas are angiographically hypervascular and typically show distorted and irregular vessels, areas of pooling of contrast medium, and arteriovenous connections[103] (Fig. 7-21). An important minority of renal carcinomas are avascular or poorly vascular and may resemble benign cysts angiographically. A cystic renal mass with a wall thickness greater than paper may well be malignant.[101,103]

INDICATIONS FOR VENOGRAPHY. Renal venography can be a useful adjunct to arteriography in patients with renal carcinoma, although with selective renal arteriography, it is usually possible to visualize the renal vein adequately enough to determine tumor invasion. Renal venography is also used in patients with suspected renal vein thrombosis and may be helpful in the identification of varicosities of submucosal veins as a cause of unilateral hematuria.[106,107] Occasionally, renal venography may help one to differentiate a congenitally absent kidney

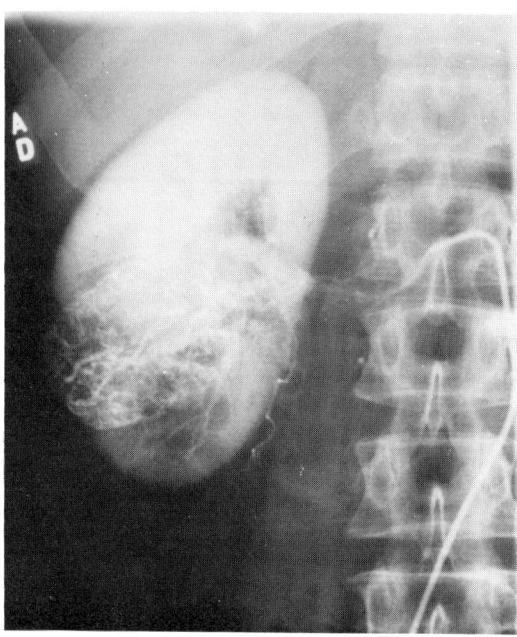

FIG. 7-21. Renal cell carcinoma with arteriographic features of hypervascularity and abnormal tumor vessels.

from a small, contracted kidney.[108] Selective renal vein catheterization for venous sampling is an important means of documenting renovascular hypertension in patients with renal artery stenosis.[106,107]

TRAUMA. Renal injuries may be classified as either penetrating or blunt.[109] Most penetrating injuries are surgically explored. Blunt renal trauma presents a more complex and controversial diagnostic problem, the goal of which is to differentiate minor parenchymal injuries requiring no surgical treatment from major parenchymal and vascular pedicle injuries requiring surgical intervention.[109–111] Most patients with renal trauma are initially evaluated with excretory urography with tomography. When the type of injury is not clearly defined by excretory urography, either CT or arteriography can be then performed.[112,113] CT is useful in differentiating among minor lacerations, major lacerations without extravasation, and major lacerations with extravasation.[112] Arteriography should be performed if a renal pedicle injury or an arteriovenous fistula is considered likely or if a major renal parenchymal injury is suspected clinically, but is not confirmed by noninvasive methods.[109]

Arteriographic findings in patients with renal trauma and their contribution to the classification of renal trauma have been described.[113,114] The arteriogram may show a prolonged arterial phase as a temporary hemodynamic disturbance due to renal contusion. The integrity of the renal parenchyma is assessed on the nephrographic phase of the arteriogram. Vascular injuries such as transections, thrombotic occlusions, and arteriovenous fistulas are identified by examining the arterial and venous phases of the study.

Angiography in Abdominal Trauma

In patients with significant blunt abdominal trauma, angiography has been largely replaced by CT scanning, both in screening for injury and in evaluation of injuries to specific organs.[115] The advantages of CT include its safety and its ability to show all organs of both the peritoneal and retroperitoneal compartments in a single, easily performed study, as well as its ability to show and to quantitate hemoperitoneum. Angiography is limited by the need for selective catheterization of the vessels supplying each organ. Nonetheless, angiography is useful when specific injuries to the blood vessels, such as aneurysms, pseudoaneurysms, or traumatic arteriovenous fistulas, are suspected after trauma.

Angiography of the Adrenal Glands

Computed tomography has become the primary method of imaging the adrenal glands. If a hormonally active adrenal lesion has been documented biochemically, but is not visualized by noninvasive methods, selective adrenal venography with sampling for hormonal assays may help in localization of the lesion.[116] Although CT has become the method of choice for imaging pheochromocytomas,[117] these tumors are hypervascular and may be localized arteriographically when necessary. Pheochromocytomas are multicentric in 10% of cases, extra-adrenal in 10%, bilateral in 5%, and malignant in 13%.[117] Ectopic pheochromocytomas are most often located in the retroperitoneum, either in the area of the aortic bifurcation or medial to the kidneys. If accurate localization is not possible with CT alone, as is possible in patients with recurrent or ectopic tumors, the use of adrenal venography with venous sampling or adrenal arteriography in combination with CT may be useful.[116,118] Arteriography is generally the next study performed if no mass is identified by CT, and adrenal venography is used when results of arteriography are negative or confusing because of previous surgical procedures.[116]

STUDIES OF THE PELVIS AND EXTREMITIES

Most mass lesions of the pelvis are now diagnosed by ultrasound and CT. As in other anatomic areas, angiography is useful for evaluation of unusually large or vascular pelvic lesions prior to surgical or transcatheter interventional procedures.

Angiography in Pelvic Trauma

Blunt pelvic trauma resulting in pelvic fracture has a high incidence of intractable retroperitoneal hemorrhage.[119] With angiography, one can usually identify the source of bleeding, and it is the procedure of choice in investigating the possibility of vascular injury after blunt pelvic trauma.[120] The most common arteriographic finding is arterial bleeding due to laceration or transection, with extravasation of contrast material.[120,121]

Angiography in Musculoskeletal Trauma

Penetrating trauma to the extremities results in vascular injury in 25 to 35% of patients.[122] Vascular injury is usually suspected because of large amounts of bleeding, expanding hematoma, decreased or absent distal pulses, or a penetrating wound in close proximity to a major vessel (Fig. 7–22). If the patient's condition is stable, then angiographic evaluation of the vascular injury is usually possible.[122]

Vascular injuries due to blunt trauma to the extremities are often associated with fractures or dislocations[122] (Fig. 7–23). The arteries most commonly injured are those fixed in close proximity to bones: the proximal third of the brachial artery, the femoral artery in the adductor canal, and the popliteal artery.[123]

In the patient who has sustained either blunt or penetrating trauma to the extremities, the goal of arteriography is to establish precisely the location of the vascular injury, the type of injury, the presence or absence of effective collateral flow, and the route of collateral flow. These factors are important in planning surgical procedures. When the patient whose condition is stable has absent or diminished pulses, arteriography should be performed immediately.[124] When a penetrating wound or fracture is located near a major vessel, but the patient's condition is stable and has normal, symmetric pulses, arteriography can be performed electively.[124]

Arteriography in Peripheral Vascular Disease

In the patient with arterial occlusive disease of the lower extremities, a combination of clinical history, physical examination, and the noninvasive techniques of Doppler-derived pressures with ankle-arm

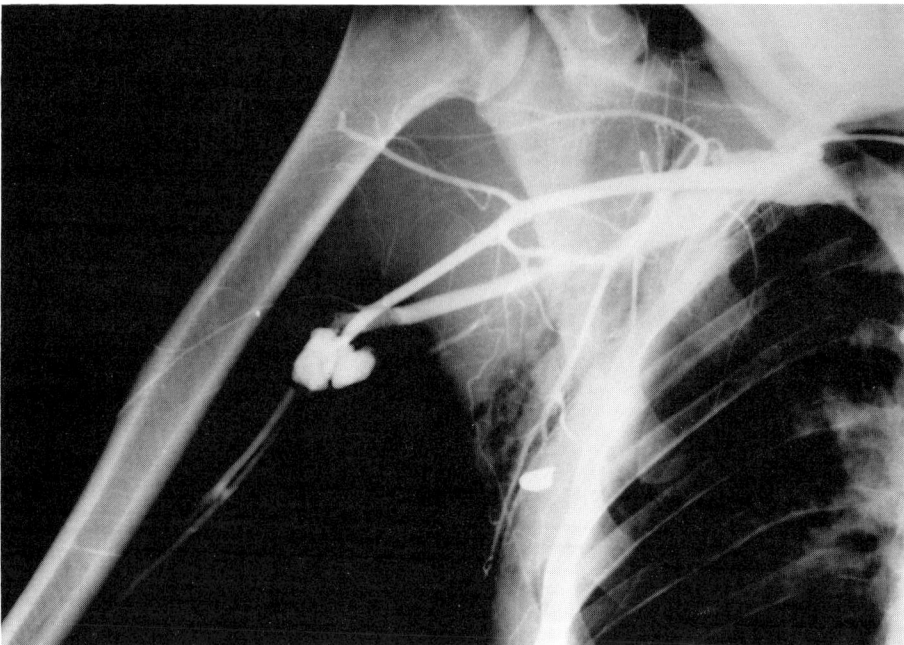

FIG. 7–22. Traumatic arteriovenous fistula. Selective axillary arteriogram shows contrast material entering a pseudoaneurysm and draining directly into the axillary vein. The bullet responsible is seen adjacent to the ribs.

index can enable one to localize stenotic lesions accurately. Consequently, arteriography is usually performed once the decision to proceed surgically has been made. Arteriography is necessary for detailed preoperative assessment of vascular anatomic features and for identification of ulcerated plaques or aneurysms that may be sources of emboli without creating measurable hemodynamic disturbances.

The arteriographic examination of patients with peripheral vascular disease usually includes biplane views of the abdominal aorta, to assess the "inflow" to the lower extremities, to identify possible sources of emboli, and to evaluate the suitability of the lower aorta as a bypass graft site. Biplane oblique views are used to assess the pelvic arteries because these views show stenotic and ulcerated lesions more clearly than the straight anteroposterior projection. Arteriography of the femoral and popliteal vessels is usually accomplished with serial views from the pelvis to the toes, made with incremental motions of the table and patient during a prolonged injection of contrast medium[125] (Fig. 7–24). These studies are usually performed by a retrograde femoral technique, with an axillary approach when necessary in patients with iliac occlusive disease. Complete arteriography as described requires a large dose of contrast agent, between 140 and 200 ml.

When occlusive disease is seen arteriographically, it is also important to visualize the patency of the vessels distal to an occlusion, to assess the feasibility of bypass grafting. Balloon occlusion arteriography,[126] or intra-arterial DSA, may be helpful in showing smaller vessels in the lower leg or foot, by achieving a higher concentration of contrast agent in the vessel lumen or by computer enhancement of contrast resolution, respectively (Fig. 7–25).

Arteriography of Bone

Arteriography can be useful in differentiating benign from malignant bone tumors when the study is interpreted in conjunction with standard radiographs and CT scans.[127,128] Angiographic features of malignancy indicate a high probability of malignancy, but the lack of angiographic features of malignancy does not exclude the presence of a malignant lesion. Angiography may be useful in showing soft tissue extension of bone tumors,[129] particularly in conjunction with CT scanning. Arteriography prior to biopsy allows selection of vascular and more probably malignant portions of the tumor for biopsy and avoidance of avascular, necrotic areas. Because the

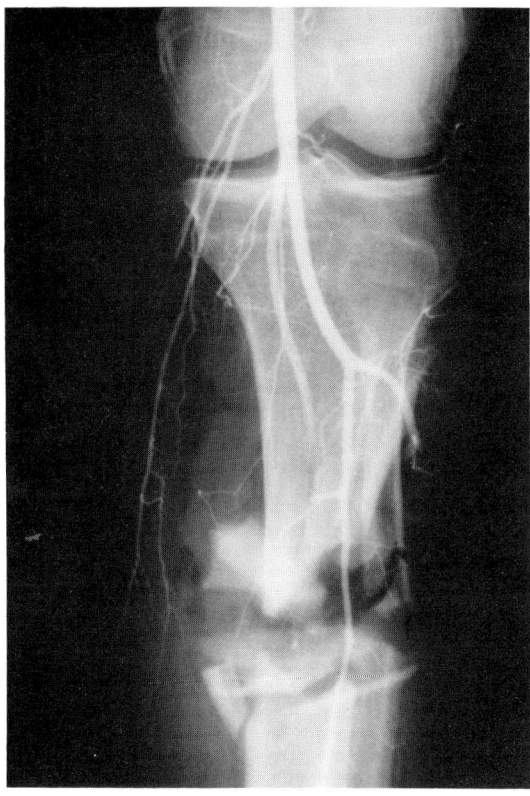

FIG. 7-23. Arterial compromise due to bone fracture. The anterior and posterior tibial arteries do not fill. The peroneal artery remains patent.

nidus of an osteoid osteoma is vascular, it may be accurately localized by properative angiography when it cannot be identified by conventional tomography or CT.[130]

VENOGRAPHY

Lower Extremity Venography

The veins of the lower extremities are best evaluated by ascending or descending venography. The ascending venogram is more frequently used.

ASCENDING VENOGRAPHY. Depending on the patient's condition and the suspected disorder, ascending venography is performed with or without ankle tourniquets. A common technique is for the patient to be in a semierect or supine position, with one tourniquet at the ankle and another above the knee.[131-133] Most ascending venograms are performed by percutaneous puncture of a small vein on the dorsum of the foot with a 20- to 22-gauge needle and manual injection of 50 to 100 ml meglumine diatrizoate, 60%. The flow of the contrast agent is observed fluoroscopically, and pertinent radiographs are taken of the leg in frontal and lateral projections and of the thigh, groin, and pelvis in the frontal projection. When percutaneous venipuncture is not possible because of severe pedal edema, a cutdown on the dorsum of the foot almost always provides an appropriate vein. A rarely used alternative is intraosseous venography if superficial veins are not available for study.

Most ascending venograms are performed to confirm a clinical suspicion of thrombophlebitis. Accurate diagnosis and treatment of deep venous thrombosis of the lower extremities are essential because of the risk of pulmonary embolism,[134] but the diagnosis is often difficult when clinical criteria alone are used. Venography is about 95% accurate in showing deep venous thrombosis.[135] Superficial thrombophlebitis is always diagnosed clinically, however. The three most important venographic findings in deep venous thrombosis are: (1) constant filling defects; (2) abrupt termination of the contrast column; and (3) nonfilling of the deep venous system with diversion of flow (Fig. 7-26).

Other indications for ascending venography include the evaluation of the postphlebitic syndrome, venous malformations, varicose veins, and trauma.

DESCENDING VENOGRAPHY. This study requires the percutaneous insertion of a catheter into the common femoral vein. The patient is in a semierect position and breathes normally.[136] This technique can usually distinguish competent from incompetent venous valves. In patients with severe valvular incompetence, one sees retrograde passage of contrast material inferiorly through the valves with little or no central flow.

Although venography of the lower extremities is generally simple, reliable and safe, complications such as skin necrosis, gangrene, and venous thrombosis have been reported.[137-139] These complications can usually be prevented with the use of small plastic intravenous catheters instead of steel needles for the contrast injection and with the use of more dilute contrast media. DSA has the potential for high-quality venography, using diluted contrast material with an osmolality approaching that of plasma.[140]

Vena Cavography

INFERIOR VENA CAVOGRAPHY. This vessel can be studied by placing a catheter in either the leg or the arm. If one wishes to visualize the pelvic veins as well, one uses simultaneous injection of catheters placed in both femoral veins. Inferior vena cavography may be helpful in evaluating involvement of the vena cava by primary neoplasms such as leio-

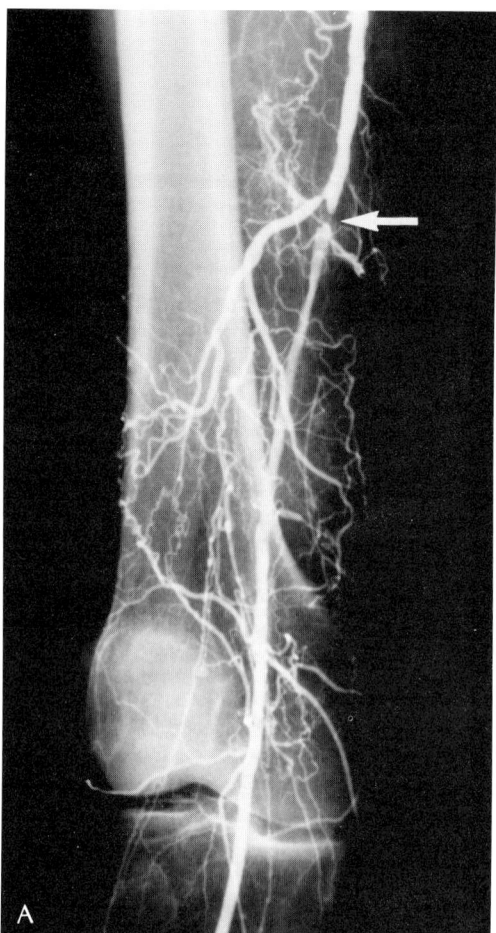 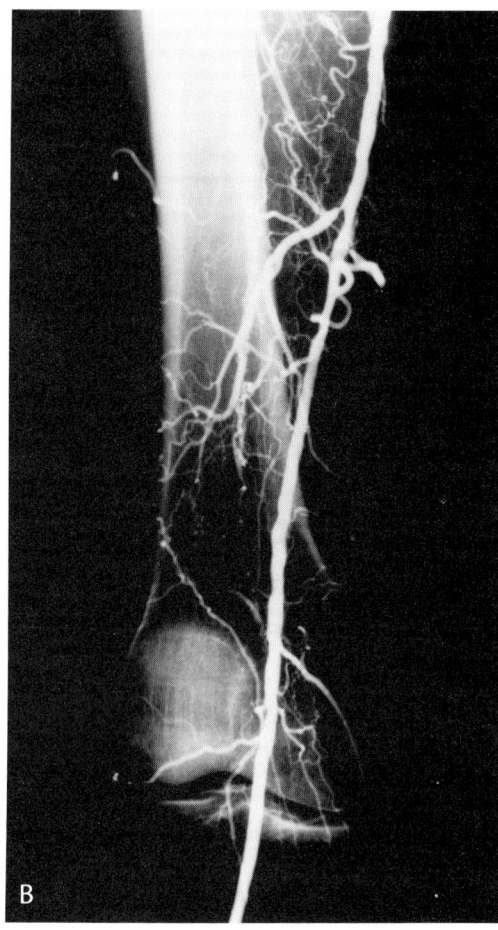

FIG. 7–24. Atherosclerotic stenosis of the superficial femoral artery (arrow). *A,* Severe stenosis (99%) at the level of the adductor canal with numerous collateral vessels. *B,* Favorable result following percutaneous transluminal angioplasty.

myosarcoma or secondary involvement of the vena cava by tumors such as renal carcinoma. Inferior vena cavography is useful when one suspects extension of thrombosis from the pelvic, renal, or hepatic veins into the vena cava. Injection of contrast material into the femoral vein at the time of puncture is performed in patients with possible ileofemoral or inferior vena cava thrombosis to avoid dislodgement of clots by passage of a catheter.[141] Trauma to the vena cava is another indication for inferior vena cavography. Vena cavography may also enable one to identify thrombosis, external compression, or congenital anomalies of the iliac veins or inferior vena cava as a cause of difficult femoral insertion of filter devices.[142]

SUPERIOR VENA CAVOGRAPHY. This study is usually performed through the basilic vein, although a femoral approach can also be used. The indications for superior vena cavography are similar to those for study of the inferior vena cava and include evaluation of involvement by neoplasm or thrombosis and assessment of trauma. The superior vena cava may be occluded by tumor or by thrombosis secondary to indwelling catheters or pacemakers. An unusual cause of obstruction of the superior vena cava is sclerosing mediastinitis, which may be a complication of histoplasmosis. When one wishes to document obstruction of the superior vena cava in a patient with marked clinical signs of occlusion of that vessel, radionuclide venography or DSA venography are less traumatic and more comfortable alternatives to conventional phlebography.[143]

The angiographic signs of phlebothrombosis in cavography are similar to the leg venographic signs.

Severe local complications of catheterization through the femoral and basilic veins for venography or DSA are uncommon. Although thrombosis and venous intimal dissection occur, the consequences are usually minor, when compared with local complications of arterial punctures. A severe, acute thrombosis causing pain and swelling severe enough to produce arterial compromise in the affected limb is a rare complication.[141]

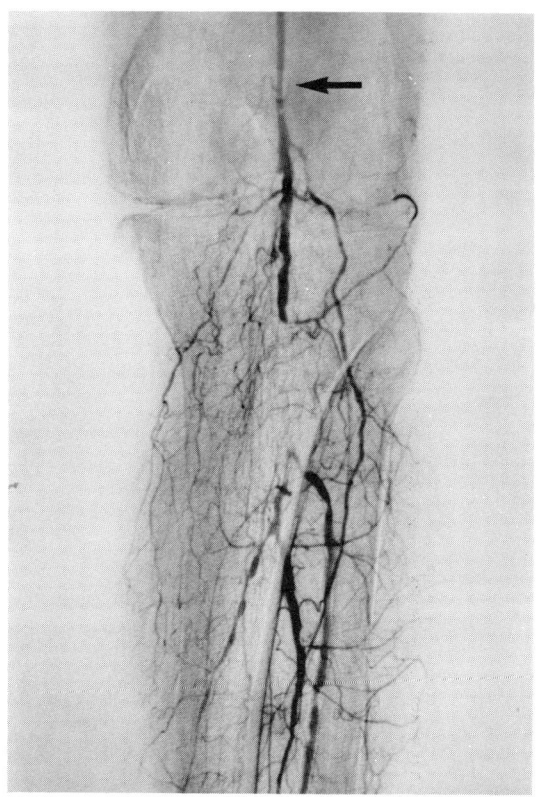

FIG. 7–25. Balloon-occlusion arteriography. The catheter and inflated balloon (arrow) are visible in the popliteal artery. Filling of the distal branches of the occluded popliteal artery is satisfactory.

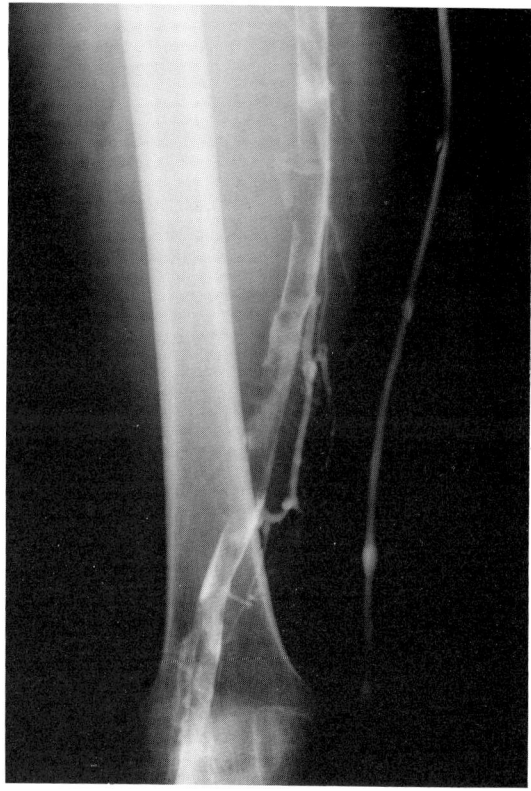

FIG. 7–26. Deep venous thrombosis. Contrast material outlines a thrombus (filling defect) in the popliteal and superficial femoral veins.

REFERENCES

1. Hessel, S.J., Adams, D.F., and Abrams, H.L.: Complications of angiography. Radiology, 138(2):273, 1981.
2. Rose, J.S.: Invasive Radiology: Risks and Patient Care. Chicago, Year Book, 1983, p. 3.
3. American College of Radiology: Prevention and Management of Adverse Reactions to Intravascular Contrast Media. Chicago, Committee on Drugs, Commission on Public Health and Radiation Protection, 1977.
4. Pomeranc, M.M.: Acute renal failure in association with administration of radiographic contrast agents. JAMA, 239:125, 1978.
5. Shehadi, W.H.: Contrast media adverse reactions: occurrence, recurrence and distribution patterns. Radiology, 143:11, 1982.
6. Kelly, J.F., et al.: Radiographic contrast media studies in high risk patients. J. Allergy Clin. Immunol., 62(3):181, 1978.
7. Eisenberg, R.L., and Mani, R.L.: Pressure dressing and postangiographic care of the femoral puncture site. Radiology, 122:677, 1977.
8. Seldinger, S.I.: Catheter replacement of the needle in percutaneous angiography: a new technique. Acta Radiol., 39:368, 1953.
9. Spigos, D.G., Tan, W.S., and Jonasson, O.: Arterial embolizations, indications, contraindications, and techniques. Surg. Annu., 18:361, 1981.
10. Bradac, G.B., et al.: Angiographic aspects of extra-intracranial bypass (EIAB) for cerebral arterial occlusive disease. Neuroradiology, 20:111, 1980.
11. Thiele, B.L., and Strandness, D.E.: Ultrasound imaging in the detection of carotid disease. In Practical Noninvasive Vascular Diagnosis. Edited by R.F. Kempozinski and J.S.T. Yao. Chicago, Year Book, 1982, p. 239.
12. Wood, G.W., et al.: Digital subtraction angiography with intravenous injection: assessment of 1,000 carotid bifurcations. AJR, 140:855, 1983.
13. Hass, W.K., et al.: Joint study of extracranial arterial occlusion. JAMA, 203:961, 1968.
14. Wood, E.H., and Cornell, J.W.: Atheromatous ulceration in major neck vessels as a cause of cerebral embolization. Acta Radiol. (Diagn.), 9:520, 1969.
15. Blaisdell, F.W., Glickman, M., and Trunkey, D.D.: Ulcerated atheroma of the carotid artery. Arch. Surg., 108:491, 1974.
16. Edwards, J.H., et al.: Angiographically undetected ulceration of the carotid bifurcation as a cause of embolic stroke. Radiology, 132:369, 1979.
17. Lusby, R.J., et al.: Carotid plaque hemorrhage. Arch. Surg., 117:1479, 1982.
18. Wolverson, M.K., et al.: Carotid atherosclerosis: high resolution real-time sonography correlated with angiography. AJR, 140:355, 1983.
19. Killen, D.A., et al.: The subclavian steal syndrome. J. Thorac. Cardiovasc. Surg., 51:539, 1966.
20. Medellin, H., and Wallace, S.: Angiography in neo-

plasms of the head and neck. Radiol. Clin. North Am., 8:307, 1970.
21. Hilal, S.K., and Michelson, J.W.: Therapeutic percutaneous embolization for extra-axial vascular lesions of the head, neck, and spine. J. Neurosurg., 43:275, 1975.
22. Doppman, J.L., DiChiro, G., and Ommaya, A.K.: Selective Angiography of the Spinal Cord. St. Louis, Wm. Green, 51, 1969.
23. Taveras, J.M., and Wood, E.H.: Diagnostic Neuroradiology. 2nd Ed. Vol. 2. Baltimore, Williams & Wilkins, 1976, p. 576.
24. van Gijn, J., and van Dongen, K.J.: Computerized tomography in subarachnoid hemorrhage: difference between patients with and without an aneurysm on angiography. Neurology, 30:538, 1980.
25. Schubiger, O., Valvanis, A., and Hayek, J.: Computed tomography in cerebral aneurysms with special emphasis on giant intracranial aneurysms. J. Comput. Assist. Tomogr., 4:24, 1980.
26. Lin, J.P., and Kricheff, I.I.: Angiographic investigation of cerebral aneurysm: technical aspects. Radiology, 105:69, 1972.
27. Modic, M.T., et al.: Digital subtraction angiography of the intracranial vascular system: comparative study in 55 patients. AJR, 138:299, 1982.
28. Enzmann, D.R., et al.: Intracranial intravenous digital subtraction angiography. Neuroradiology, 23:241, 1982.
29. Locksley, H.B.: Natural history of subarachnoid hemorrhage, intracranial aneurysms, and arteriovenous malformations. Report on the Cooperative Study of Intracranial Aneurysms and Subarachnoid Hemorrhage: section V, Part I. J. Neurosurg., 25:219, 1966.
30. Olmsted, W.W., and McGee, T.P.: The pathogenesis of peripheral aneurysms of the central nervous system: a subject review from the AFIP. Radiology, 123:661, 1977.
31. Frazee, J.G., Cahan, L.D., and Winter, J.: Bacterial intracranial aneurysms. J. Neurosurg., 53:633, 1980.
32. Wood, E.H.: Intracranial aneurysms. Radiol. Clin. North Am., 4:217, 1966.
33. Wolpert, S.M., Barnett, F.J., and Prager, R.J.: Benefits of embolization without surgery for cerebral arteriovenous malformations. AJR, 138:99, 1982.
34. Debrun, G., et al.: Embolization of cerebral arteriovenous malformations with bucrylate. J. Neurosurg., 56:615, 1982.
35. Greitz, T.: Angiography in tuberculous meningitis. Acta Radiol. (Diagn.), 2:369, 1964.
36. Wickbom, G.I., and Davidson, A.J.: Angiographic findings in intracranial actinomycosis. Radiology, 88:536, 1967.
37. Rumbaugh, C.L., et al.: Cerebral angiographic changes in the drug abuse patient. Radiology, 101:335, 1971.
38. Lande, A., and Rossi, P.: The value of total aortography in the diagnosis of Takayasu's arteritis. Radiology, 114:287, 1975.
39. Taveras, J.M., and Wood, E.H.: Diagnostic Neuroradiology. 2nd Ed. Vol. 2. Baltimore, Williams & Wilkins, 1976.
40. Abrams, H.L.: Techniques, indications, and hazards. In Abrams Angiography, Vascular and Interventional Radiology. 3rd Ed. Vol. 1. Edited by H.L. Abrams. Boston, Little, Brown, 1983, p. 339.
41. Keith, H.H.: Vascular rings and tracheobronchial compression in infants. Pediatr. Ann., 6:540, 1977.
42. Tonkin, I.L., Elliot, L.P., and Bergeron, L.M.: Concomitant axial cineangiography and barium esophagography in the evaluation of vascular rings. Radiology, 135:69, 1980.
43. Abrams, H.L., and Jonasson, G.: Coarctation of the aorta. In Abrams Angiography, Vascular and Interventional Radiology. 3rd Ed. Vol. 1. Edited by H.L. Abrams. Boston, Little, Brown, 1983, p. 383.
44. Abrams, H.L.: Techniques, indications, and hazards. In Abrams Angiography, Vascular and Interventional Radiology. 3rd Ed. Vol. 1. Edited by H.L. Abrams. Boston, Little, Brown, 1983, p. 479.
45. Randall, P.A., and Jarmolowski, C.R.: Aneurysms of the thoracic aorta. In Abrams Angiography, Vascular and Interventional Radiology. 3rd Ed. Vol. 1. Edited by H.L. Abrams. Boston, Little, Brown, 1983, p. 417.
46. Joyce, J.W., et al.: Aneurysms of the thoracic aorta: a clinical study with special reference to prognosis. Circulation, 29:176, 1964.
47. Sprayregen, S.: Radiologic spectrum of arteriosclerotic aneurysms of the aortic arch. N.Y. State J. Med., 78:2198, 1978.
48. Parmley, L.F., et al.: Nonpenetrating traumatic injury of the aorta. Circulation, 17:1086, 1958.
49. Seltzer, S.E., et al.: Traumatic aortic rupture: plain film findings. AJR, 137:1011, 1981.
50. Fisher, R.G., Hadlock, F., and Ben-Menachem, Y.: Laceration of the thoracic aorta and brachiocephalic vessels by blunt trauma. Radiol. Clin. North Am., 19:91, 1981.
51. Fishbone, G., et al.: Trauma to the thoracic aorta and great vessels. Radiol. Clin. North Am., 11:543, 1973.
52. Wientraub, R.A., and Abrams, H.L.: Mycotic aneurysms. AJR, 102:354, 1968.
53. Boutefeu, J.M., et al.: Aneurysms of the sinus of Valsalva: report of seven cases and review of the literature. Am. J. Med., 65:18, 1978.
54. Thomas, T.V.: Intrathoracic aneurysms of the innominate and subclavian arteries. J. Thorac. Cardiovasc. Surg., 63:461, 1972.
55. Yeh, H.C., et al.: Ultrasonography of the brachiocephalic arteries. Radiology, 132:403, 1979.
56. Wheat, M.W., Jr.: Acute dissecting aneurysms of the aorta: diagnosis and treatment—1979. Am. Heart J., 99:373, 1980.
57. Itzchak, Y., et al.: Dissecting aneurysm of the thoracic aorta: reappraisal of radiologic diagnosis. AJR, 125:559, 1975.
58. DeBakey, M.E., et al.: Surgical management of dissecting aneurysms of the aorta. J. Thorac. Cardiovasc. Surg., 49:130, 1965.
59. Miller, D.C., et al.: Operative treatment of aortic dissections: experience with 125 patients over a sixteen year period. J. Thorac. Cardiovasc. Surg., 78:365, 1979.
60. Guthaner, D.F., Brody, W.R., and Miller, D.C.: Intravenous aortography after aortic dissection repair. AJR, 137:1019, 1981.
61. Smith, D.C., and Jang, G.C.: Radiologic diagnosis of aortic dissection. In Aortic Dissection. Edited by R.M. Poroghazi and E.E. Slater. New York, McGraw-Hill, 1983, p. 71.
62. Sutton, D.: A Textbook of Radiology and Imaging. 3rd Ed. London, Churchill Livingstone, 1980, p. 610.
63. Remy, J., et al.: Treatment of hemoptysis by embolization of bronchial arteries. Radiology, 122:33, 1977.
64. McNeil, B.J.: A diagnostic strategy using ventilation-perfusion studies in patients suspected for pulmonary embolism. J. Nucl. Med., 17:613, 1976.
65. Robin, E.D.: Overdiagnosis and overtreatment of pul-

monary embolism: the emperor may have no clothes. Ann. Intern. Med., 87:775, 1977.
66. Mills, S.R., et al.: The incidence, etiologies, and avoidance of complications of pulmonary angiography in a large series. Radiology, 136:295, 1980.
67. Fraser, R.G., and Pare, J.A.P.: Diagnosis of Diseases of the Chest. 2nd Ed. Vol. II. Philadelphia, W.B. Saunders, 1978, p. 1143.
68. Johnson, B.A., James, A.E., and White, R.I.: Oblique and selective pulmonary angiography in diagnosis of pulmonary embolism. AJR, 118:801, 1973.
69. Pond, G.D., Ovitt, T.W., and Capp, M.P.: Comparison of conventional pulmonary angiography with intravenous digital subtraction angiography for pulmonary embolic disease. Radiology, 147:345, 1983.
70. Ludwig, J.W., et al.: Digital subtraction angiography of the pulmonary arteries for the diagnosis of pulmonary embolism. Radiology, 147:639, 1983.
71. Novelline, R.A., et al.: The clinical course of patients with suspected pulmonary embolism and a negative pulmonary angiogram. Radiology, 126:561, 1978.
72. Dines, D.E., et al.: Pulmonary arteriovenous fistulas. Mayo Clin. Proc., 49:460, 1974.
73. Higgins, C.B., and Wexler, L.: Clinical and angiographic features of pulmonary arteriovenous malformations in children. Radiology, 119:171, 1976.
74. White, R.I., et al.: Angioarchitecture of pulmonary arteriovenous malformations: an important consideration before embolotherapy. AJR, 140:681, 1983.
75. Kaufman, S.L., et al.: Transcatheter embolization in the management of congenital arteriovenous malformations. Radiology, 137:21, 1980.
76. Gomes, A.B., Mali, W.P., and Oppenheim, W.L.: Embolization therapy in the management of congenital arteriovenous malformations. Radiology, 144:41, 1982.
77. Goldstein, H.M., et al.: Angiographic findings in benign liver cell tumors. Radiology, 110:339, 1974.
78. Reuter, S.R., Redman, H.C., and Siders, D.B.: The spectrum of angiographic findings in hepatoma. Radiology, 94:89, 1970.
79. Marks, W.M., et al.: Hepatocellular carcinoma: clinical and angiographic findings and predictability for surgical resection. AJR, 132:7, 1979.
80. Chuang, V.P.: Hepatic tumor angiography: a subject review. Radiology, 148:633, 1983.
81. Kadir, S., et al.: Transcatheter embolization of intrahepatic arterial aneurysms. Radiology, 134:335, 1980.
82. Halpern, M., Turner, A.F., and Criton, B.P.: Hereditary hemorrhagic telangectasia. Radiology, 90:1143, 1968.
83. Warren, W.D., et al.: Preoperative assessment of portal hypertension. Ann. Surg., 165:999, 1967.
84. Fuchs, W.A., et al.: Hepatic arteriography in cirrhosis of the liver and portal hypertension. Invest. Radiol., 7:369, 1972.
85. Lunderquist, A., and Vang, J.: Transhepatic catheterization of the coronary vein in patients with portal hypertension and esophageal varices. N. Engl. J. Med., 291:646, 1974.
86. Spigos, D.G., et al.: Umbilical venous cannulation: a new approach for embolization of esophageal varices. Radiology, 146:53, 1983.
87. Levin, D.C., Wilson, R., and Abrams, H.L.: The changing role of pancreatic arteriography in the era of computed tomography. Radiology, 136:245, 1980.
88. Freeny, P.C., Ball, T.J., and Ryan, J.: Impact of new diagnostic imaging methods on pancreatic angiography. AJR, 133:619, 1979.
89. Freeny, P.C., and Lawson, T.L.: Radiology of the Pancreas. New York, Springer, 1982, p. 465.
90. This reference has been deleted.
91. Freeny, P.C., and Lawson, T.L.: Radiology of the Pancreas. New York, Springer, 1982, p. 471.
92. Dunnick, N.R., et al.: Computed tomographic detection of nonbeta pancreatic islet cell tumors. Radiology, 135:117, 1980.
93. Freeny, P.C., and Lawson, T.L.: Radiology of the Pancreas. New York, Springer, 1982, p. 540.
94. Lunderquist, A., et al.: Selective pancreatic vein catheterization for hormone assay in endocrine tumors of the pancreas. Cardiovasc. Radiol., 1:117, 1978.
95. Wolfman, N.T., et al.: Cystic neoplasms of the pancreas: CT and sonography. AJR, 138:37, 1982.
96. Nusbaum, M., and Baum, S.: Radiographic demonstration of unknown sites of gastrointestinal bleeding. Surg. Forum, 14:374, 1963.
97. Alavi, A.: Detection of gastrointestinal bleeding with Tc^{99m} sulfur-colloid. Semin. Nucl. Med., 12:126, 1982.
98. Winzelberg, G.G., et al.: Detection of gastrointestinal bleeding with ^{99m}Tc-labeled red blood cells. Semin. Nucl. Med., 12:139, 1982.
99. Casarella, W.J.: Lower gastrointestinal tract hemorrhage: new concepts based on arteriography. AJR, 121:357, 1974.
100. Scott, J.A., et al.: Angiographic assessment of renal artery pathology: how reliable? AJR, 141:1299, 1983.
101. McClennan, B.L., et al.: CT of the renal cyst. Is cyst aspiration necessary? AJR, 133:671, 1979.
102. Lang, E.K.: Roentgenographic approach to the diagnosis and management of the cystic lesion of the kidney: is cyst exploration mandatory? Urol. Clin. North Am., 7:677, 1980.
103. Watson, R.C., Fleming, R.J., and Evans, J.A.: Arteriography in the diagnosis of renal carcinoma. Radiology, 91:888, 1968.
104. Lang, E.K.: The accuracy of roentgenographic techniques in the diagnosis of renal mass lesions. Radiology, 98:119, 1971.
105. Weyman, P.J., et al.: Comparison of computed tomography and angiography in the evaluation of renal cell carcinoma. Radiology, 137:417, 1980.
106. Beckman, C.F., and Abrams, H.L.: Renal venography: anatomy, technique, applications, analysis of 132 venograms, and review of the literature. Cardiovasc. Intervent. Radiol., 3:45, 1980.
107. Oleaga, J.A., et al.: Renal venography. Urology, 12:609, 1978.
108. Athanasoulis, C.A., Brown, B., and Baum, S.: Selective renal venography in differentiating between congenitally absent and small contracted kidney. Radiology, 108:301, 1973.
109. Guerriero, W.G.: Trauma to the kidneys, ureters, bladder, and urethra. Surg. Clin. North Am., 62:1047, 1982.
110. Peters, P.C., and Bright, T.C.: Blunt renal injuries. Urol. Clin. North Am., 4:17, 1977.
111. Mendez, R.: Renal trauma. J. Urol., 118:698, 1977.
112. McAninch, J.W., and Federle, M.P.: Evaluation of renal injuries with computed tomography. J. Urol., 128:456, 1982.
113. Lang, E.K.: Arteriography in the assessment of renal trauma: the impact of arteriographic diagnosis on preservation of renal function and parenchyma. J. Trauma, 15:553, 1975.

114. Halpern, M.: Angiography in renal trauma. Surg. Clin. North Am., 48:1221, 1968.
115. Federle, M.P.: Computed tomography of blunt abdominal trauma. Radiol. Clin. North Am., 21:461, 1983.
116. Dunnick, N.R., et al.: Localization of functional adrenal tumors by computed tomography and venous sampling. Radiology, 148:501, 1983.
117. Welch, T.J., Sheedy, P.F., II, and vanHeerdin, J.A.: Pheochromocytoma: value of computed tomography. Radiology, 148:501, 1983.
118. Kadir, S., and Robinette, C.: Accuracy of angiography in the localization of pheochromocytoma. J. Urol., 126:789, 1981.
119. Rothenberger, D.A., et al.: The mortality associated with pelvic fractures. Surgery, 84:356, 1978.
120. Kam, J., Jackson, H., and Ben-Menachem, Y.: Vascular injuries in blunt pelvic trauma. Radiol. Clin. North Am., 19:171, 1981.
121. Matalon, T.S., et al.: Hemorrhage with pelvic fractures: efficacy of transcatheter embolization. AJR, 133:859, 1979.
122. Lim, R.C., and Miller, S.E.: Management of acute civilian vascular injuries. Surg. Clin. North Am., 62:113, 1982.
123. Pradham, D.J., et al.: Arterial injuries of the extremities associated with fractures. Arch. Surg., 105:582, 1972.
124. Smith, P.L., et al.: Emergency arteriography in extremity trauma: assessment of indications. AJR, 137:803, 1981.
125. Agee, O.: Arteriography of the pelvis and lower extremities with moving table top technique. AJR, 106:400, 1969.
126. Spigos, D.G., et al.: Occlusive iliofemoral arteriography. Paper presented at the sixty-eighth Annual Meeting and Scientific Assembly of the Radiologic Society of North America, Chicago, 1982.
127. Strickland, B.: The value of arteriography in the diagnosis of bone tumors. Br. J. Radiol., 32:705, 1959.
128. Voegeli, E., and Uehelinger, E.: Arteriography in bone tumors. Skeletal Radiol., 1:3, 1976.
129. Yaghmai, I., et al.: Value of arteriography in the diagnosis of benign and malignant bone lesions. Cancer, 27:1134, 1971.
130. Swee, R.G., McLeod, R.A., and Beabout, J.W.: Osteoid osteoma: detection diagnosis, and localization. Radiology, 130:117, 1979.
131. DeWeese, J.A., and Rogoff, S.M.: Functional ascending phlebography of the lower extremity by serial long film technique: evaluation of anatomic and functional detail in 62 extremities. Am. J. Roentgenol., 81:841, 1959.
132. Rabinev, K., and Paulin, S.: Roentgen diagnosis of venous thrombosis of the leg. Arch. Surg., 104:134, 1972.
133. Thomas, M.L.: Phlebography. Arch. Surg., 104:145, 1972.
134. Kakkar, V.V., et al.: Natural history of postoperative keep vein thrombosis. Lancet, 2:230, 1969.
135. Browse, N.L.: Diagnosis of deep vein thrombosis. Br. Med. Bull., 34:163, 1978.
136. Kistner, R.L.: Surgical repair of the incompetent femoral vein valve. Arch. Surg., 110:1336, 1975.
137. Spigos, D.G., Thane, T., and Capek, V.: Skin necrosis following extravasation of contrast medium during peripheral phlebography of the leg. Radiology, 123:605, 1977.
138. Thomas, M.L.: Gangrene following peripheral phlebography of the legs. Br. J. Radiol., 43:528, 1970.
139. Homans, J.: Thrombosis as a complication of venography. JAMA, 119:136, 1942.
140. Spigos, D.G.: Unpublished data.
141. White, R.I., Jr.: Fundamentals of Vascular Radiology. Philadelphia, Lea & Febiger, 1976, p. 122.
142. Stewart, J.R., and Greenfield, L.J.: Transvenous vena cava filtration and pulmonary embolectomy. Surg. Clin. North Am., 62:411, 1982.
143. Maxfield, W.S., and Meckstroth, G.R.: Technetium-99m superior vena cavography. Radiology, 92:913, 1969.

8

Luminal Contrast Studies of the Bile and Pancreatic Ducts

Luminal contrast studies of the biliary tree and pancreas have developed rapidly in recent years. For this reason, the subject material is divided into two sections. The first section deals with the older techniques of oral cholecystography and intravenous cholangiography. The second section describes the newer procedures of percutaneous transhepatic cholangiography and endoscopic retrograde cholangiopancreatography.

SECTION 1
ORAL CHOLECYSTOGRAPHY AND INTRAVENOUS CHOLANGIOGRAPHY
JOSEPH M. BECKER ■ GEORGE N. STEIN

ORAL CHOLECYSTOGRAPHY

Until the mid-1970s, the oral cholecystogram was the gold standard for the evaluation of the gallbladder[1-6] (Figs. 8–1 to 8–5). Since that time, the study has been replaced to a significant extent by ultrasound for assessment of size and position of the gallbladder and for determining the presence of stones, other filling defects, pericholecystic fluid collections, and thickness of the wall.[7] Since the late 1970s, hepatobiliary cholescintigraphy with one of the ^{99m}technetium (^{99m}Tc)-iminodiacetic acid congeners has all but replaced the oral cholecystogram in the evaluation of acute and chronic cholecystitis.[8] With this isotopic study, one can assess the patency of the cystic and common ducts, the rate of emptying of the common duct, and the size, position, and contractility of the gallbladder when the cystic duct is patent; one can obtain incidental information about the anatomic features of the liver; and one can see spontaneous or postoperative bile leaks. Ultrasound and hepatobiliary cholescintigraphy do not require the patient to fast and are not dependent on bilirubin levels. Both studies give images far more promptly than the minimum overnight wait required by oral cholecystography. When ultrasound and hepatobiliary cholescintigraphy are available, the principal indication for oral cholecystography is to provide additional information when the results of the other studies are equivocal or enigmatic.

Diagnostic opacification of the gallbladder after oral administration of the cholecystographic agent depends on many variables,[9-12] including retention of the agent in the gut long enough to permit intestinal absorption. Vomiting, gastric outlet obstruction, abdominal ileus, or intestinal hypermotility may interfere with this process. Absorption within the intestine depends on the hydrogen ion concentration and the level of bile salts. After intestinal absorption, these agents travel in the portal venous flow to the liver bound to albumin. There they enter the hepatocytes and are excreted in the bile. Once the bile enters the gallbladder, that is, when the cystic duct and the common ducts proximal to the cystic duct are unobstructed, the bile is concentrated by resorption of water and permits opacification after a given length of time.[13,14] Nephrotoxicity is seen in patients with depressed hepatic excretion and in those who receive high doses or a combination of two or more oral agents or oral and intravenous agents.

Technique

Although one should ideally obtain a scout film of the abdomen prior to oral cholecystography, this is rarely done, even in inpatients, and the incidence of incorrect diagnosis is low.[15-17] The administration of a fatty meal the night before the study can increase the percentage of visualization of the gallbladder from 47 to 70% with iopanoic acid (Telepaque)[18] (see Fig. 8–4). The patient should then fast, and films should be obtained 10 hours after the administration of tyropanoate sodium (Bilopaque) and 14 to 19 hours after the administration of iopanoic acid.[13,14] Unlike that with iopanoic acid, hepatic excretion of tyropanoate sodium and of ipodate (Orografin) does not depend on bile salts and does

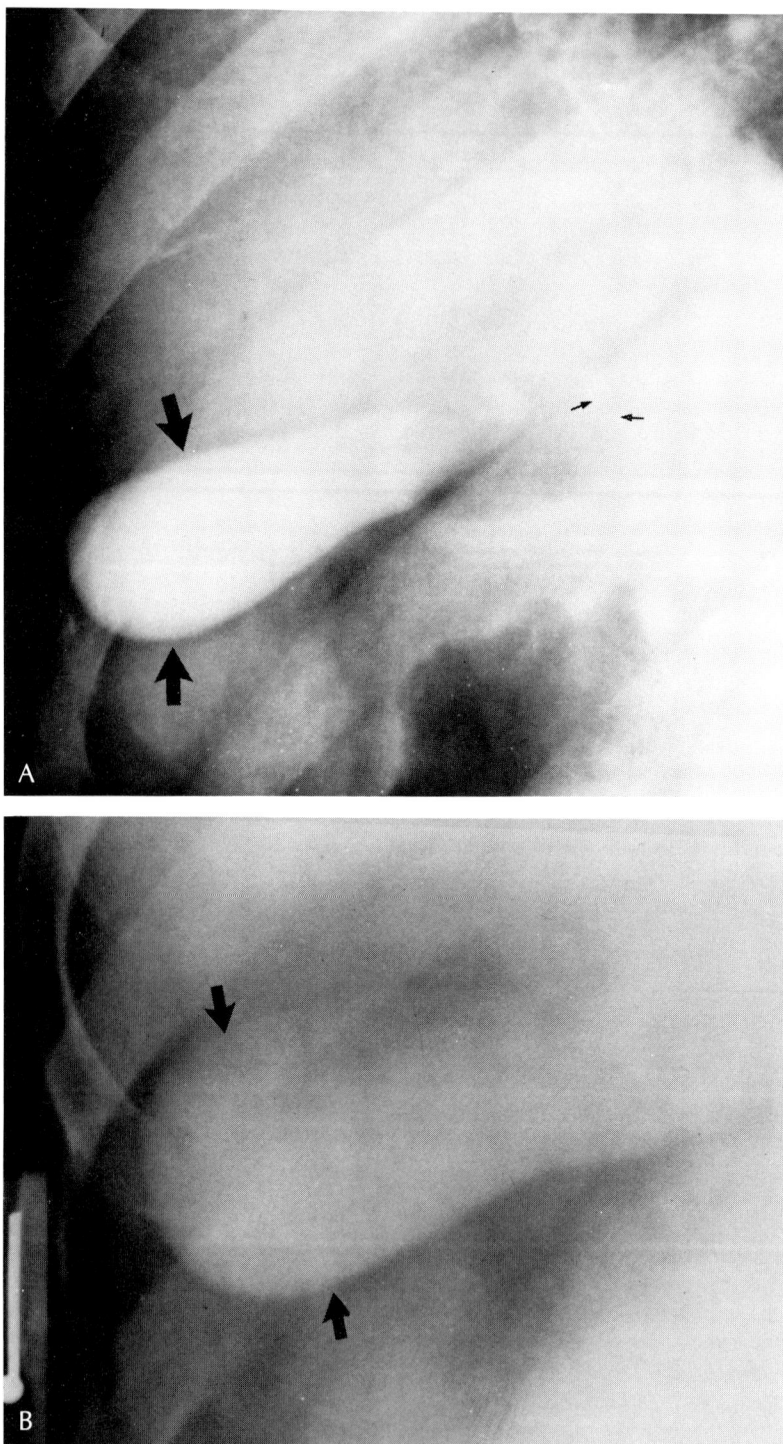

FIG. 8–1. Normal oral cholecystogram. Prone oblique overhead *(A)* and erect *(B)* fluoroscopic spot films show adequate opacification of the gallbladder (large arrows), as well as faint visualization of the common bile duct (small arrows).

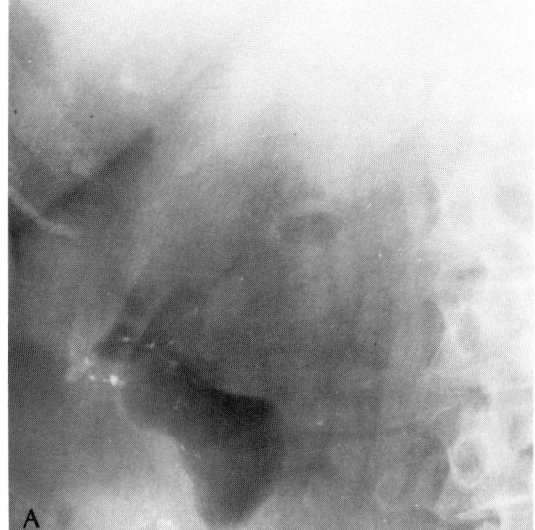

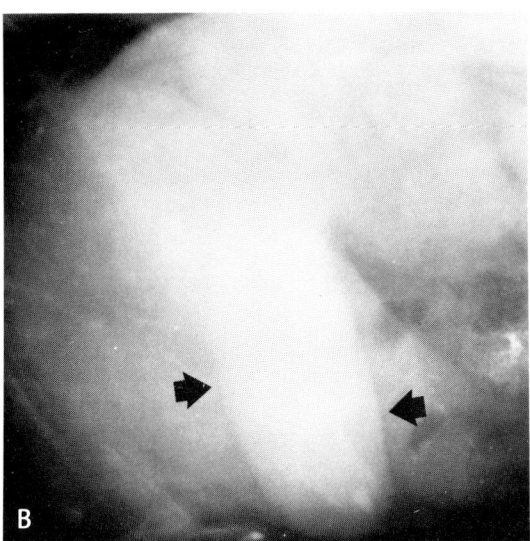

FIG. 8-2. Failure to visualize the gallbladder in first-dose study, in the absence of disease. No opacification of the gallbladder is noted after a single dose of contrast material (A), but adequate diagnostic opacification is observed a day later (B, arrows), after a second dose.

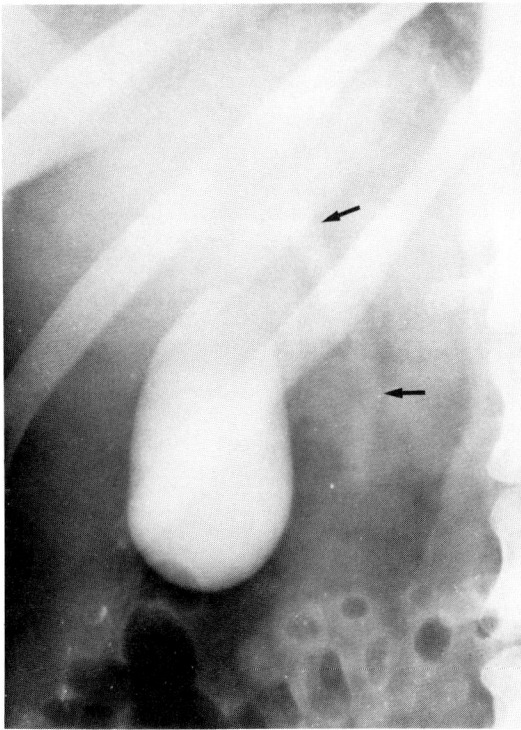

FIG. 8-3. Visualization of the common duct in a normal oral cholecystogram. A normal common bile duct (arrows) is visualized during the course of a normal oral cholecystogram.

not require the ingestion of a fatty meal at the time of their administration.[19,20]

If the initial prone or left anterior oblique overhead radiographs of the abdomen fail to show calculi in the opacified gallbladder, one must obtain right-side-down decubitus and/or erect fluoroscopic spot films with compression (Figs. 8-6 and 8-7). An enema may be used if the patient's gallbladder is obscured by feces in the hepatic flexure of the colon (Fig. 8-8). If the initial overhead film suggests the presence of calculi, an examination in some other projection should usually be obtained, to ensure that the filling abnormality really lies within the gallbladder.

Depending on the series, a repeat-dose oral cholecystogram is required in up to 50% of patients[21,22] (Figs. 8-2 and 8-9). Nonbiliary causes of nonvisualization or poor visualization include fasting (see Fig. 8-4), inadequate retention of contrast material in the gastrointestinal tract prior to absorption, hepatic dysfunction, recent surgical intervention, pancreatitis, peptic ulcer disease, and peritonitis, as well as other, less-common entities. Burhenne and Obata have recommended a double dose (two consecutive daily doses) before radiography of outpatients[23] (see Fig. 8-2), as well as a single-day combination of iopanoic acid and ipodate for inpatients[24] (Fig. 8-9). Nonvisualization of the gallbladder after an intensified study is indicative of gallbladder disease if no other cause is present. Visualization of the common duct but not of the gallbladder, even on an initial study, indicates cystic duct obstruction (Figs. 8-10 to 8-13), as does nonvisualization of the gallbladder in the face of conjugated bile in the bowel. Because of these variables, only 80% of patients with a nonvisualized gallbladder after a second dose of contrast material have provable gallbladder disease.[7] One may see

186 IMAGING

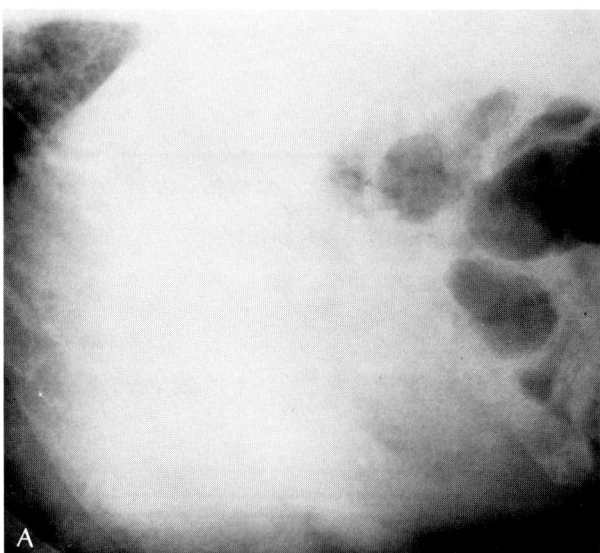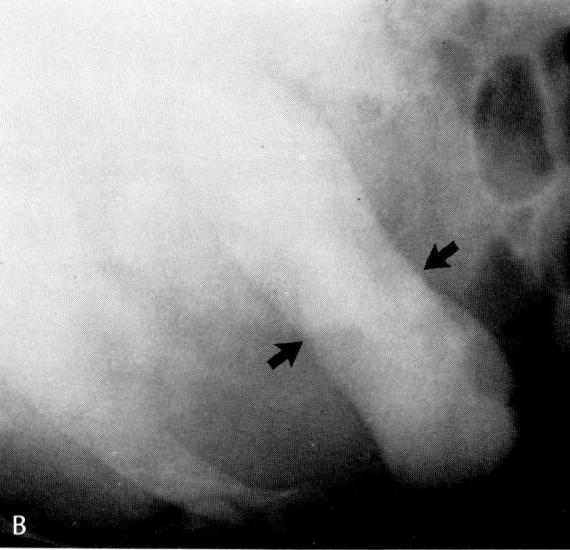

FIG. 8–4. Initial failure to visualize the gallbladder due to fasting. Initial examination in this patient not receiving food showed no opacification of the gallbladder (A). A repeat examination (B), when the patient was no longer fasting, other than overnight prior to the study, showed adequate opacification of the gallbladder (arrows).

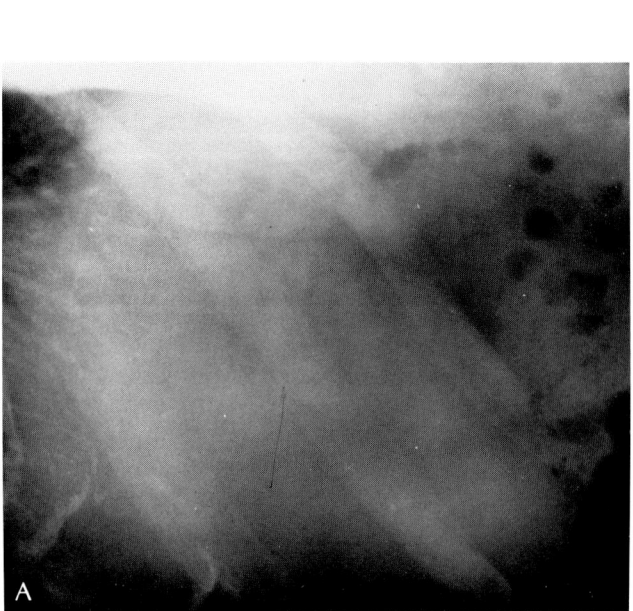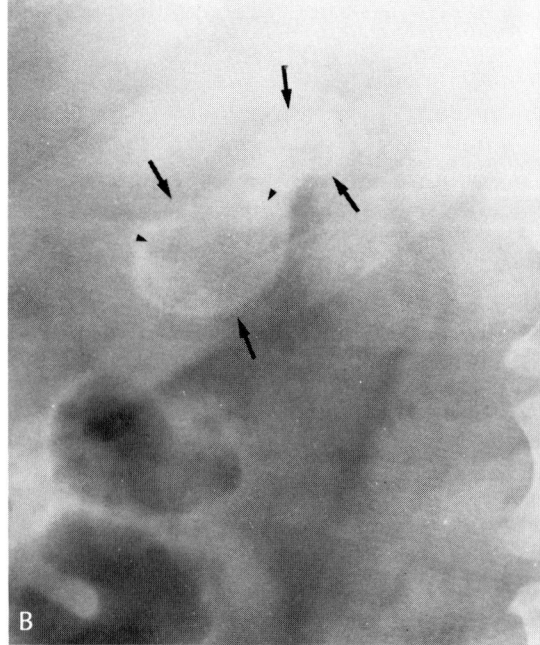

FIG. 8–5. Poor opacification due to cholelithiasis. The gallbladder was not visualized in the single-dose study (A). After a repeat dose (B), the gallbladder (arrows), which contains a large, nonopaque calculus (arrowheads), is faintly seen.

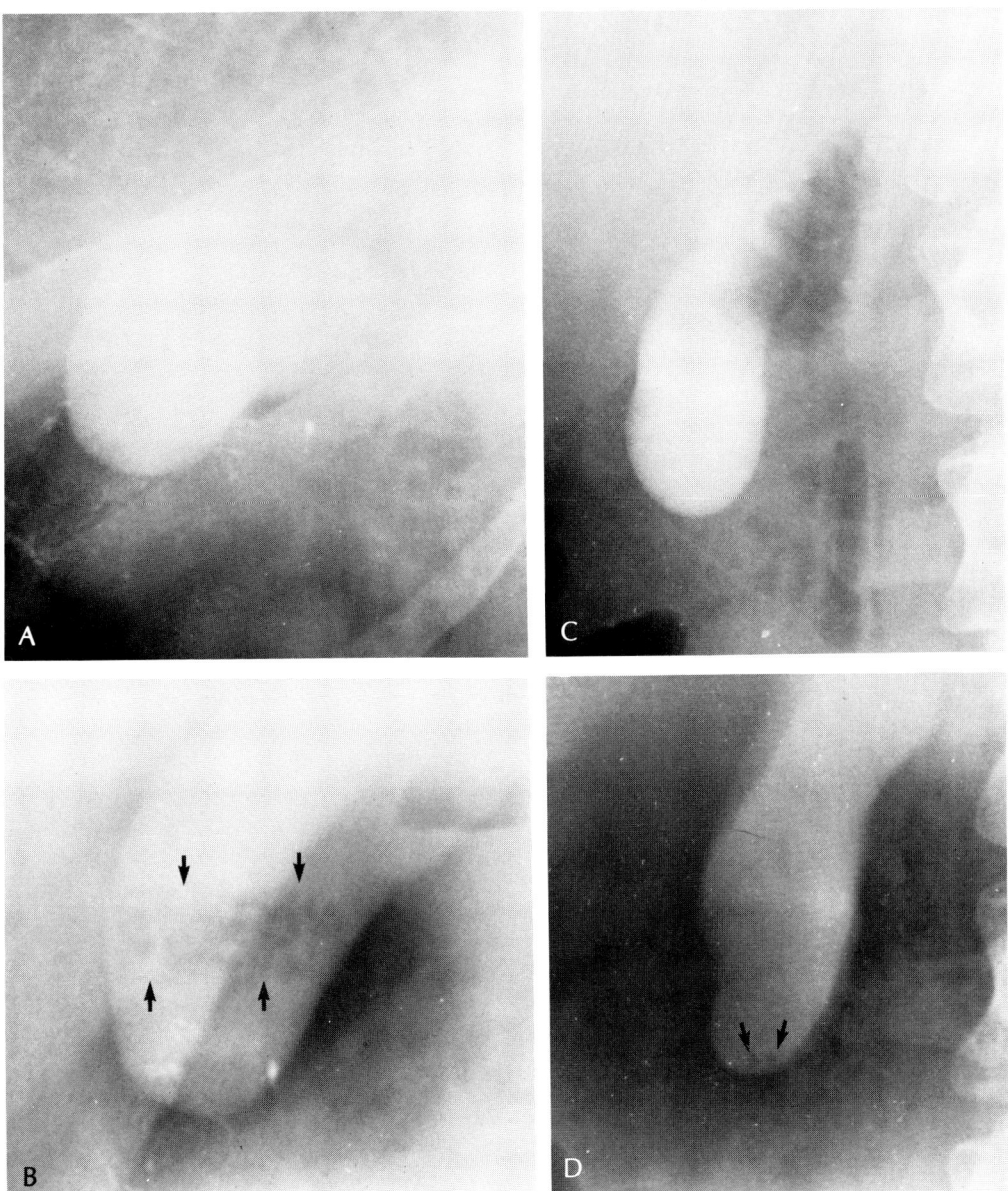

FIG. 8–6. Value of erect films with compression. Prone films (A,C) suggest the possibility of calculi in two patients, but such entities are best seen in erect spot films with compression (B,D, arrows).

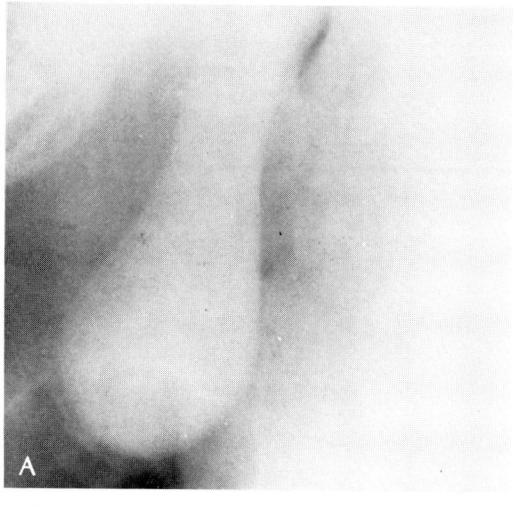

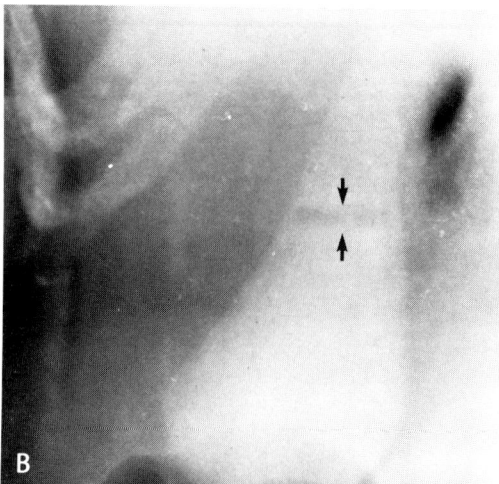

FIG. 8–7. Delayed erect spot films. The initial erect spot film (A) shows no evidence of calculi. A repeat study (B), taken after the patient stood erect for 5 minutes, shows layering of calculi (arrows).

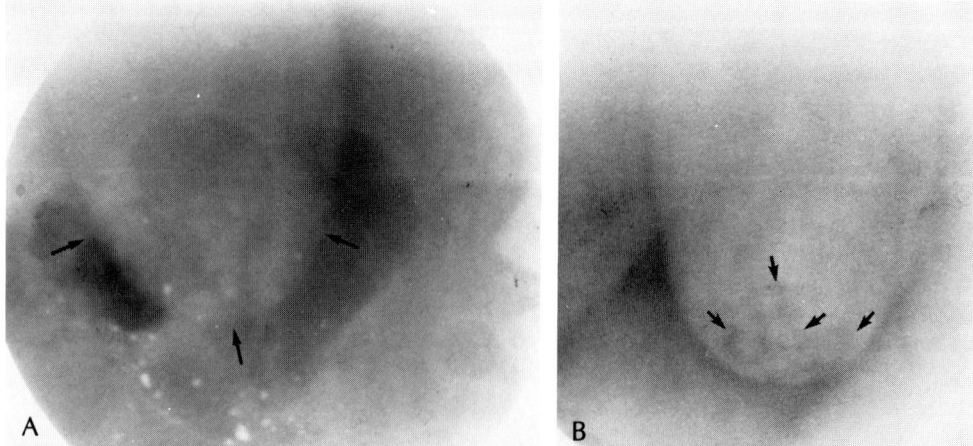

FIG. 8–8. Fundal calculi obscured by bowel contents. In the erect spot film (A), the fundus of the gallbladder (arrows) is obscured by the contents of the hepatic flexure. Re-examination (B), after a cleansing enema the same morning, allows clear visualization of this area and shows the presence of calculi (arrows).

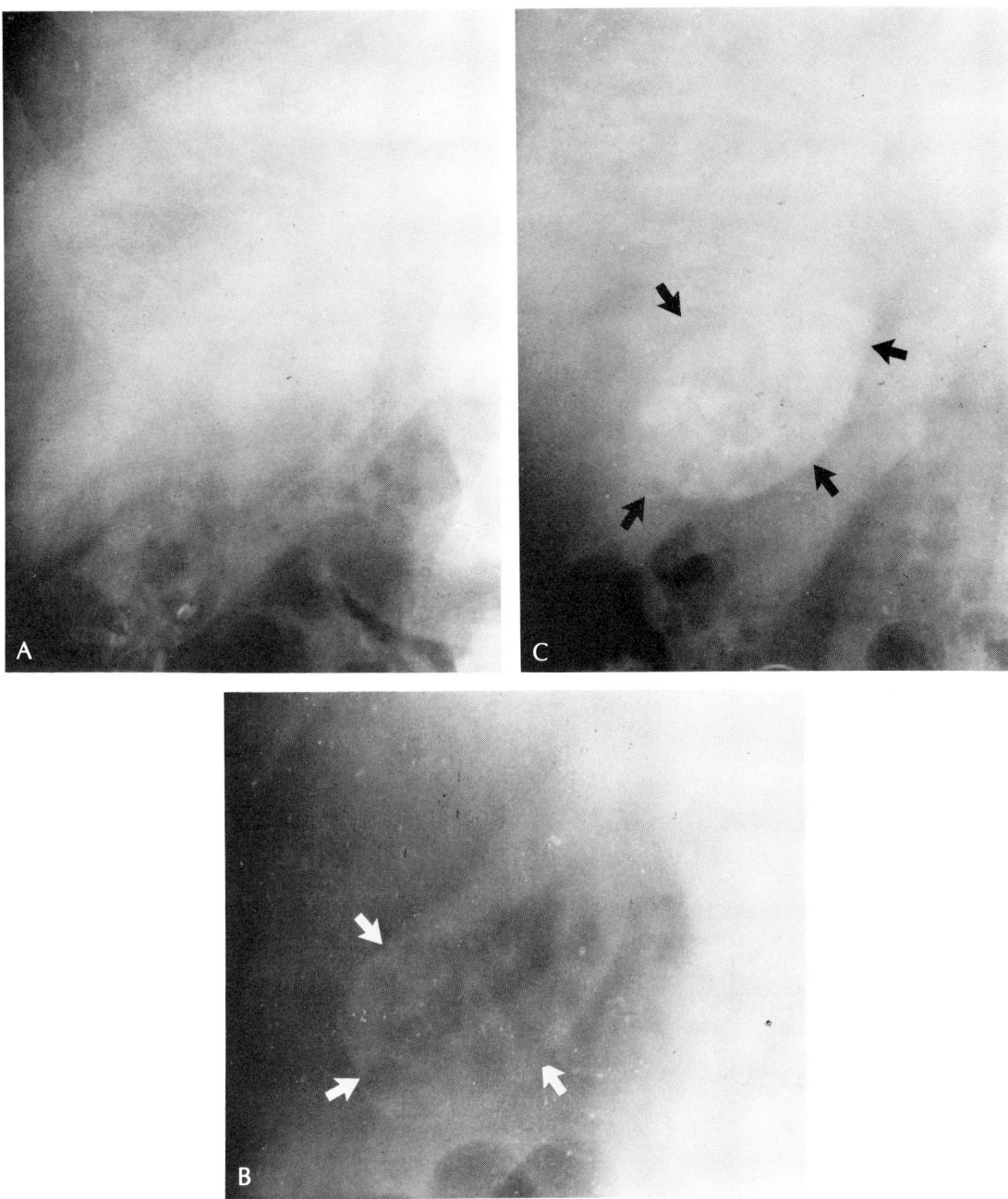

FIG. 8–9. Repeat single-day examination. *A,* Failure to visualize the gallbladder after a single dose of iopanoic acid (Telepaque). *B,* Faint visualization of the gallbladder (arrows) and multiple calculi 8 hours after a dose of ipodate (Orografin), administered immediately following *A*. *C,* Slight further opacification of the gallbladder (arrows) the next day, after a second dose of iopanoic acid the night before.

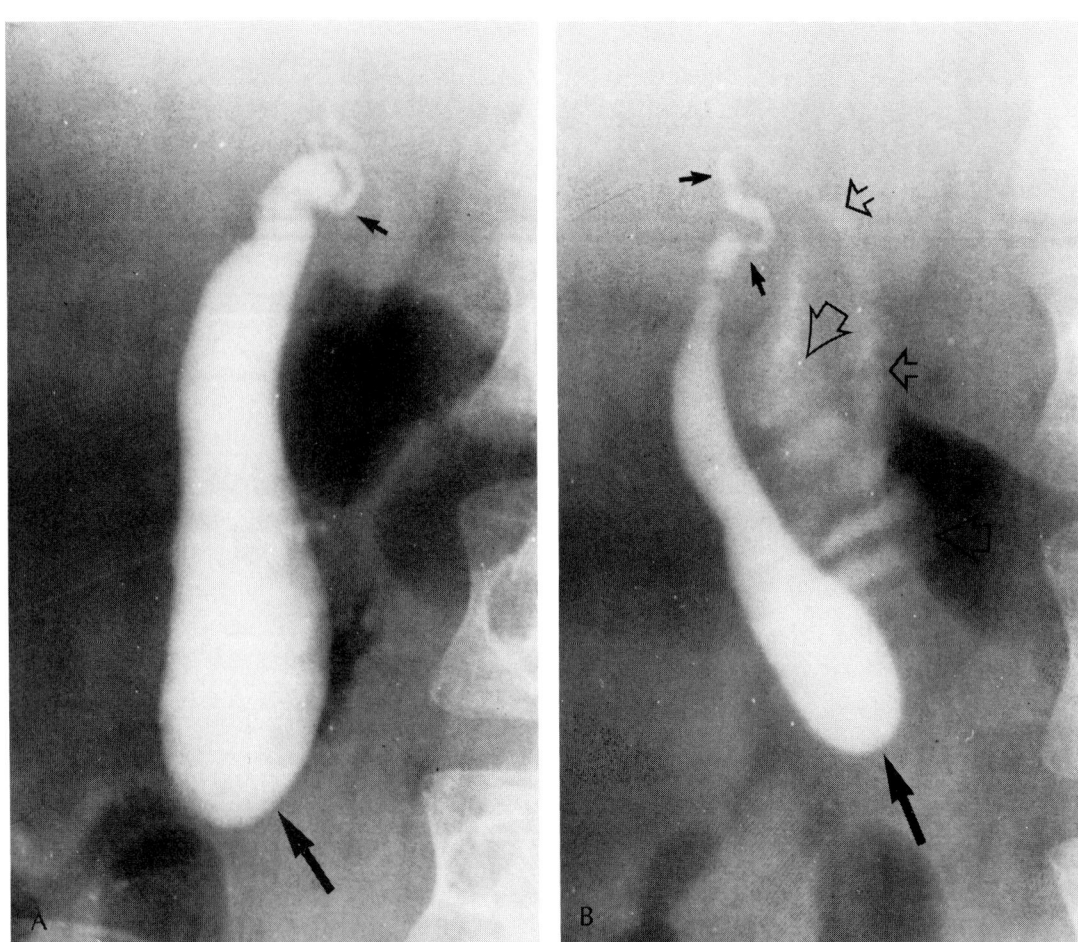

FIG. 8–10. Normal fatty-meal examination. *A*, Initial examination shows the gallbladder (large arrow) and the cystic duct (small arrow). *B*, After a fatty meal one sees marked contraction of the gallbladder (large arrow), with visualization of the cystic duct (small arrows) and spiral valves of Heister and a normal common duct (small open arrows), with drainage of contrast material into the duodenum (large open arrows).

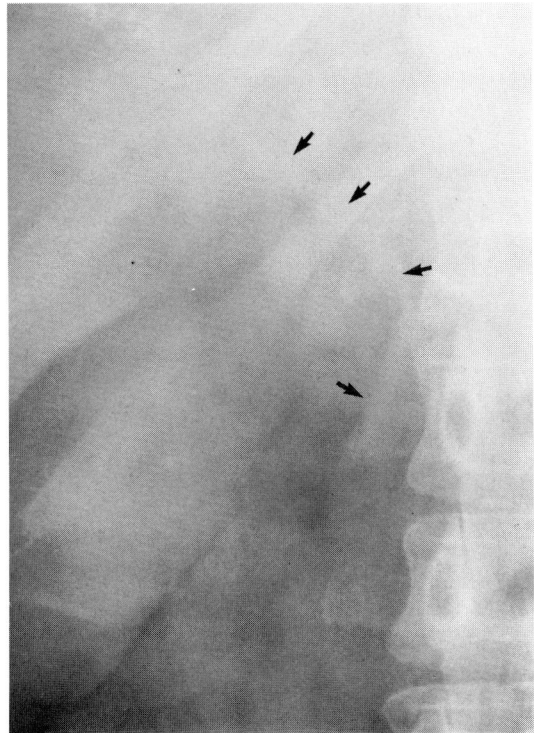

FIG. 8-11. Normal oral cholangiogram with obstructed cystic duct. Double-dose oral cholecystogram shows a faintly visualized common duct (arrows), but no opacification of the gallbladder; this pattern is consistent with cystic duct obstruction.

layering of opacified bile secondary to poor mixing of the cholecystographic agent in the gallbladder. The examination should be repeated several hours later, when the patient is ambulatory (Fig. 8-14).

The administration of a fatty meal plays little part in oral cholecystography, although it may be valuable in confirming the diagnosis of hyperplastic cholecystoses and in better demonstrating the bile ducts.[18,25,26,27] (Figs. 8-10 and 8-15 to 8-17). Intravenous administration of the polypeptide cholecystokinin has been used in the evaluation of biliary dyskinesia and acalculous cholecystitis, to produce gall bladder contraction.[28,29] Administration of a fatty meal or cholecystokinin can help one to delineate the common bile duct and may enable one to see stones within that duct (see Figs. 8-10 and 8-13).

Interpretation

The normal gallbladder can vary in size, position, and mobility.[30,31] In the absence of inflammatory or neoplastic obstruction of the cystic duct, enlargement of the gallbladder is seen in patients with diabetes and after vagotomy.[32,33] A small gallbladder may be a normal variant, or it may represent a contracted viscus resulting from fasting, chronic inflam-

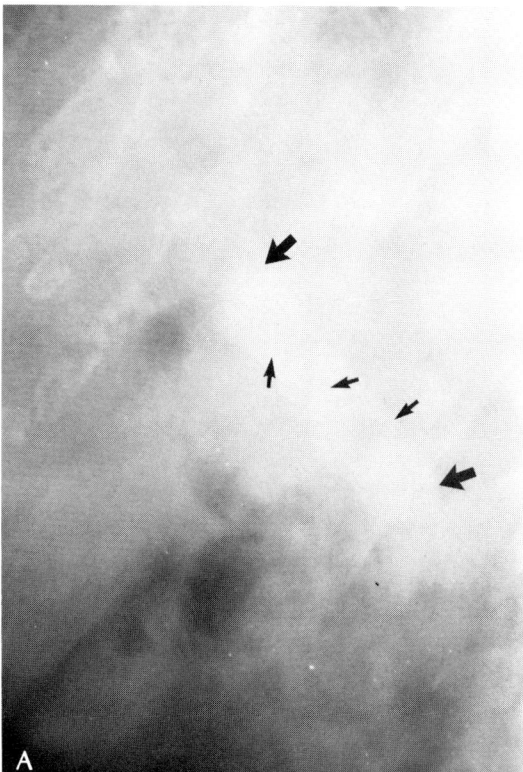

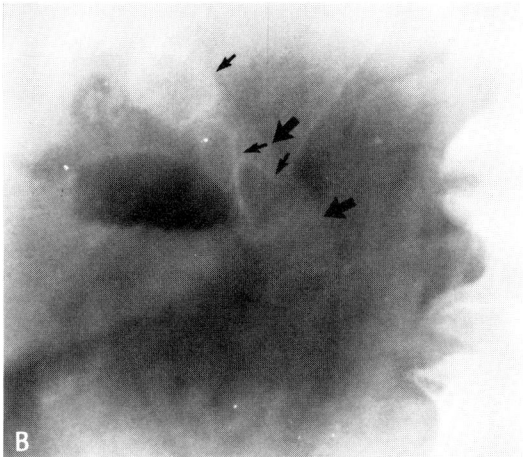

FIG. 8-12. Abnormal oral cholangiogram with obstructed cystic duct. Prone (A) and erect (B) films show contrast material in the common duct (large arrows) outlining three calculi (small arrows). The gallbladder failed to opacify because a calculus obstructed the cystic duct.

mation, or mucoviscidosis.[1,2,4-6,34] The phrygian cap (Fig. 8-18), postural kink, and multiseptate gallbladder must not be confused with the septation(s) that can occur in patients with adenomyomatosis.[26,27,35] Developmental variations in gallbladder position include situs inversus (Fig. 8-19), long gallbladder mesentery, and intrahepatic location, as

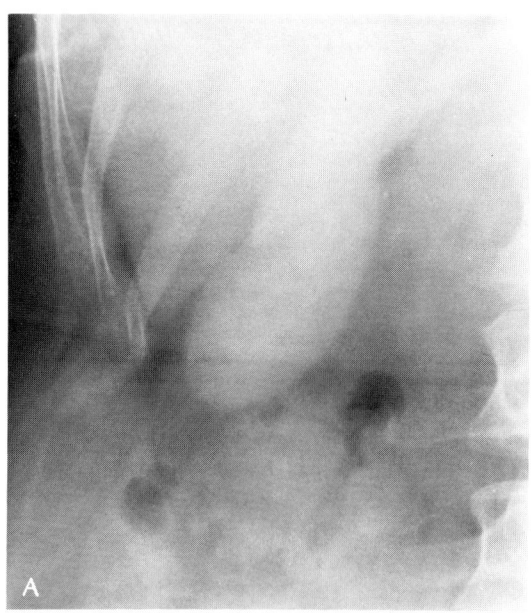

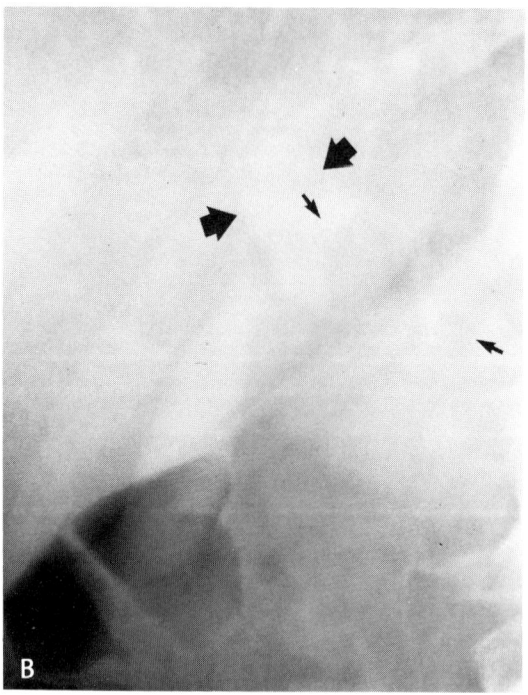

FIG. 8–13. Normal oral cholecystogram with abnormal oral cholangiogram. *A,* Routine prone film shows normal gallbladder. *B,* After a fatty meal, one sees strong contraction of the gallbladder with opacification of a dilated common duct (large arrows) containing multiple calculi (small arrows).

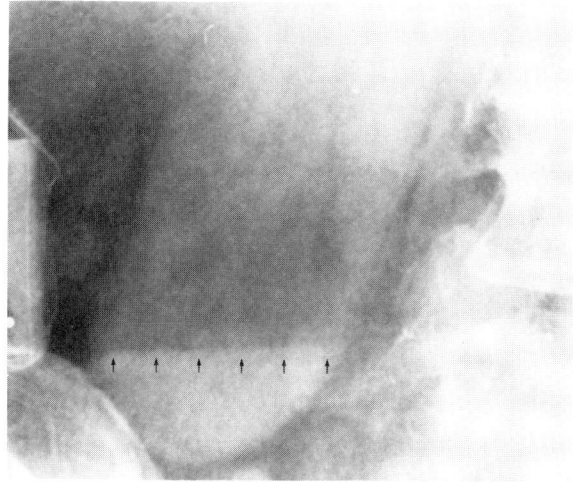

FIG. 8–14. Incomplete mixing of opacified bile. Erect spot film shows layering (arrows) of opacified bile in the gallbladder representing poor mixing in a patient who did not receive fat at the time of administration of iopanoic acid (Telepaque).

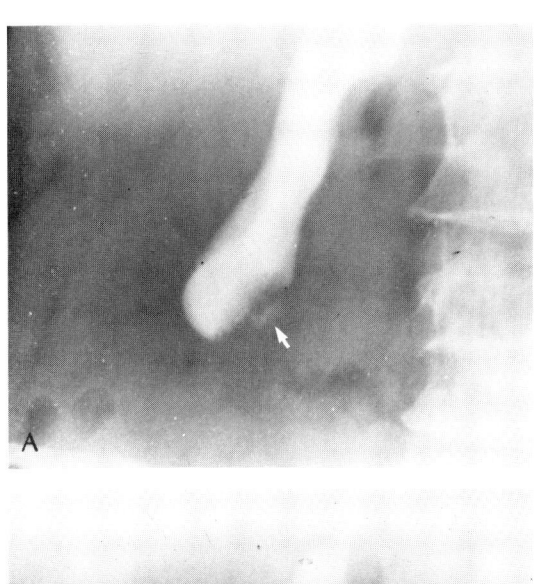

FIG. 8–15. Adenomyomatosis. Segmental, intramural adenomyomatosis (arrows) before *(A)* and after *(B)* administration of a fatty meal.

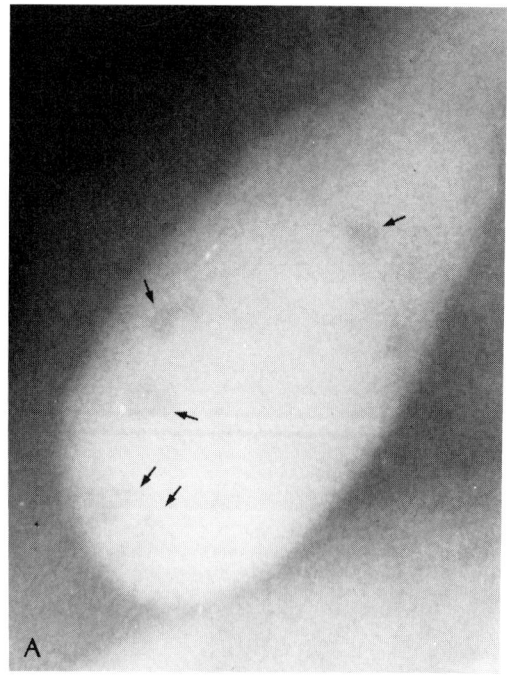

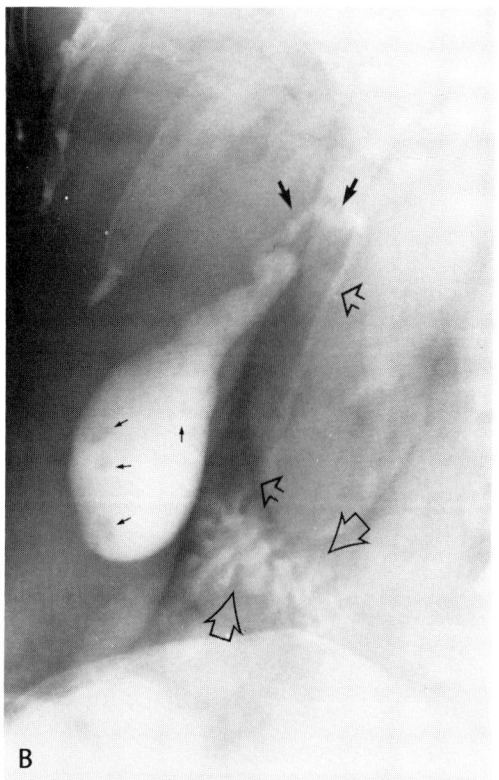

FIG. 8–16. Cholesterolosis. Examination before *(A)* and after *(B)* administration of a fatty meal shows the presence of multiple fixed filling defects (such as shown by small arrows), subsequently proved to be cholesterol polyps. The nonspecific radiographic findings are similar to those seen in patients with multiple papillomas or adherent calculi. Cystic duct, large arrows; common duct, small open arrows; duodenum, large open arrows.

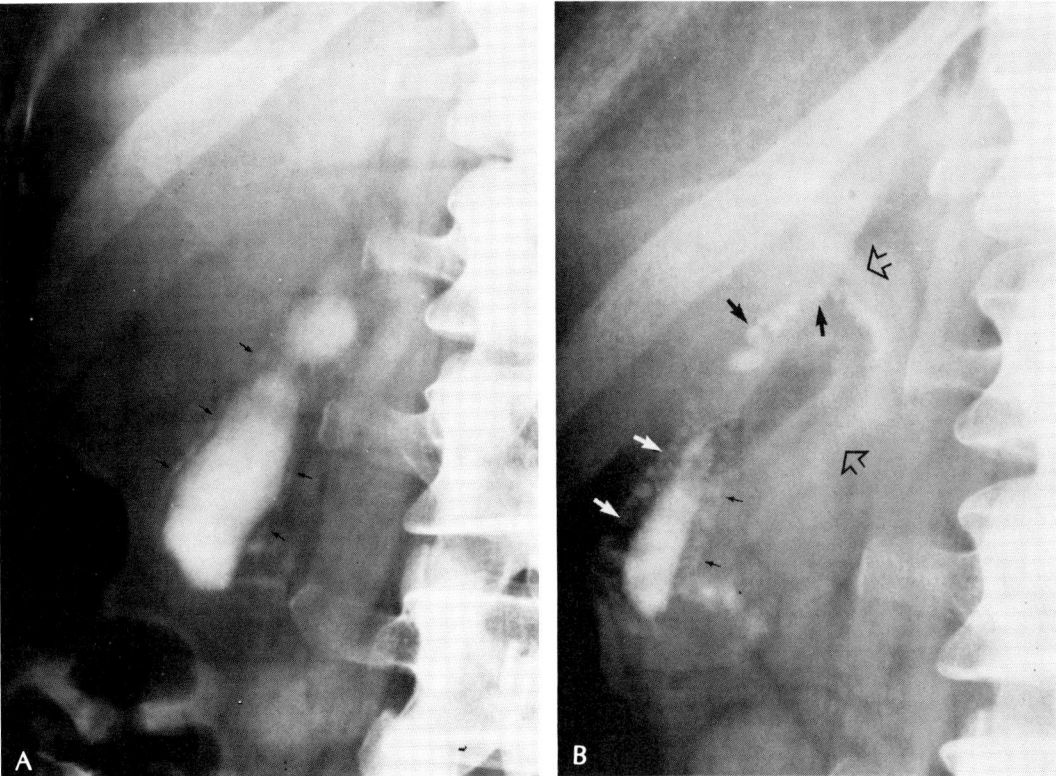

FIG. 8–17. Aschoff-Rokitansky sinuses. Examination before *(A)* and after *(B)* administration of a fatty meal shows extensive filling of the Aschoff-Rokitansky sinuses (small arrows), the cystic duct (large arrows), and the common duct (open arrows).

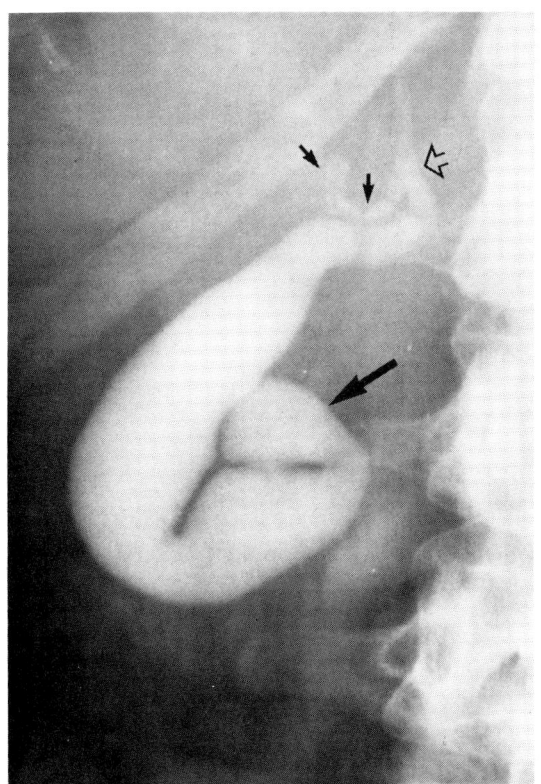

FIG. 8–18. Phrygian cap. Prone film shows a phrygian cap (large arrow), a redundant cystic duct (small arrows), and the common duct (open arrow).

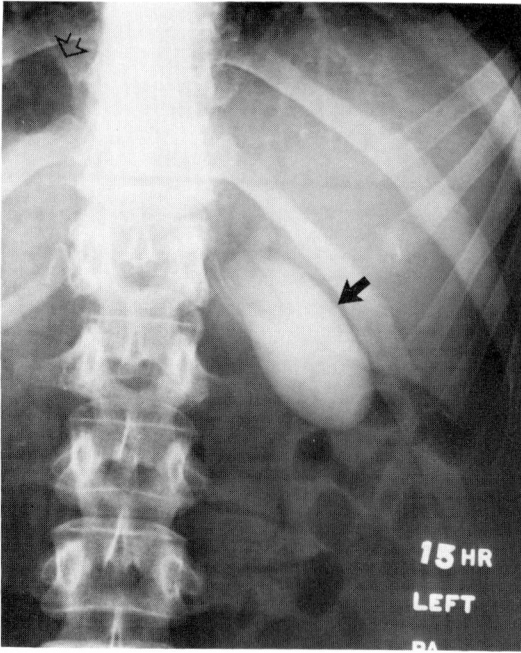

FIG. 8–19. Situs inversus. Prone film shows the gallbladder (arrow) in the left upper quadrant and the gastric air bubble (open arrow) in the right upper quadrant.

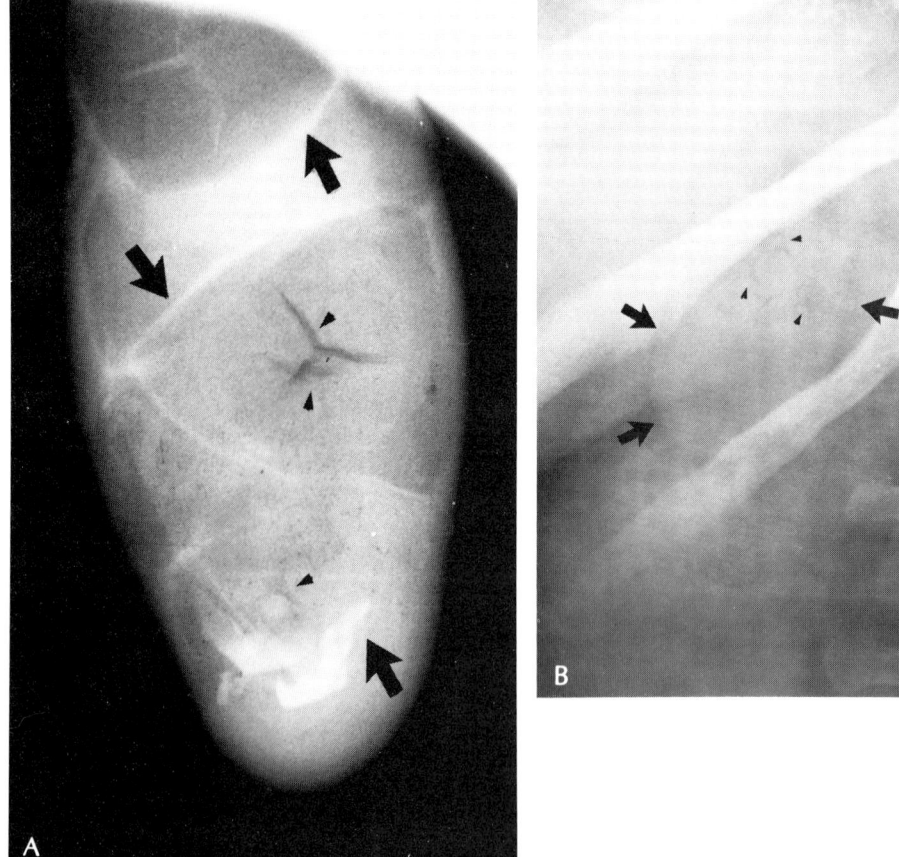

FIG. 8–20. Mercedes-Benz sign. *A*, Postoperative radiographic specimen shows several fissured gallstones (arrows) containing gas (arrowheads). *B*, Faintly opacified gallbladder (arrows) in another patient shows fissured gallstones with gas (arrowheads).

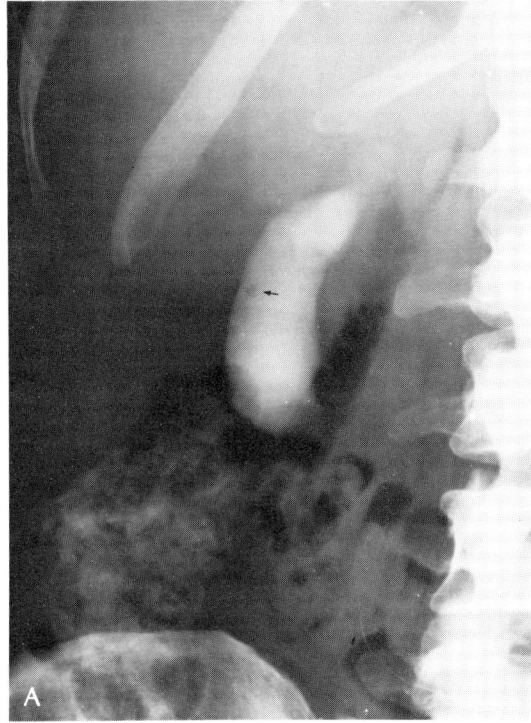

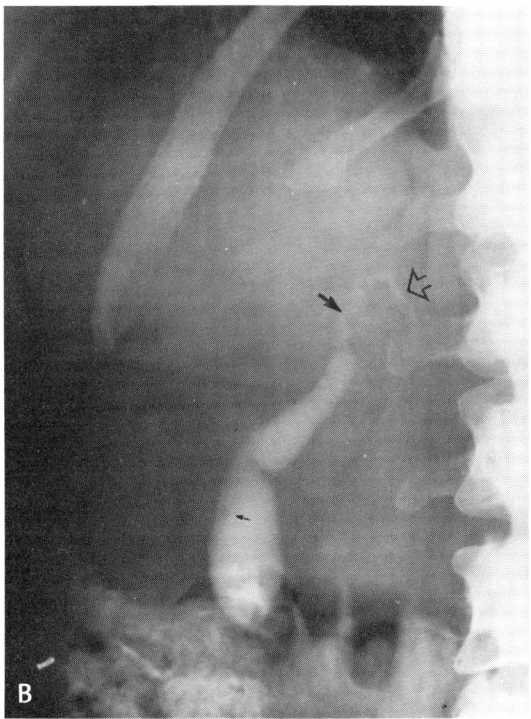

FIG. 8–21. Papilloma. Examination before *(A)* and after *(B)* a fatty meal shows a solitary, fixed radiolucency (small arrow) surgically proved to be a papilloma. The radiographic appearance is nonspecific and could be that of a cholesterol polyp or adherent calculus. Cystic duct, large arrow; common duct, open arrow.

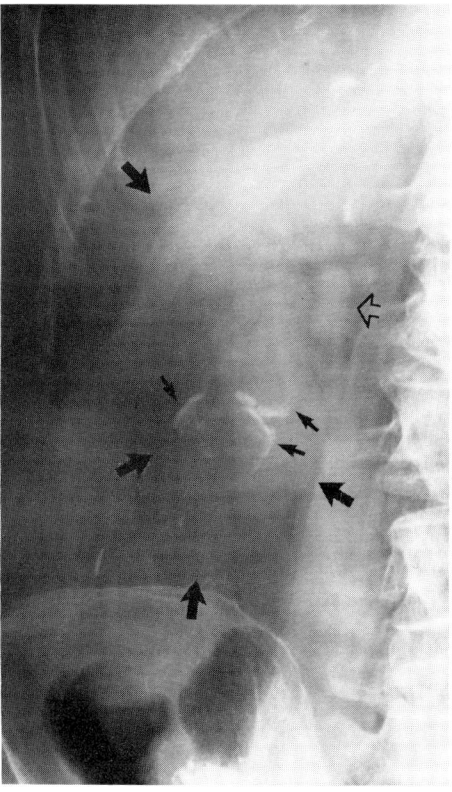

FIG. 8–22. Carcinoma of the gallbladder. Examination after a repeat dose of contrast material shows a large, nonopacified soft tissue mass (large arrows) representing a dilated, nonfunctioning gallbladder containing opaque calculi (small arrows). The opacification of the common duct (open arrow) is consistent with cystic duct obstruction. The patient had noted the appearance of this mass of the right upper quadrant 2 years previously. During the surgical procedure, the patient underwent extensive local excision of carcinoma of the gallbladder, as well as excision of a metastatic nodule in the left hepatic lobe.

well as other, less-common intra-abdominal sites.[36] Abnormal position of the gallbladder may be due to hepatomegaly, hepatic masses, other abdominal masses, or dilatation of an adjacent bowel loop. Agenesis of the gallbladder is rarely an isolated anomaly.[37,38] Duplication and triplication of the gallbladder can occur.

Hyperplastic cholecystoses consist of cholesterolosis and adenomyomatosis[26,27] (see Figs. 8–15 to 8–17). These disorders may occur together, with or without calculus formation. Both disorders are characterized by a marked contractile response to fat or cholecystokinin. In cholesterolosis, the cholesterol deposit may be restricted to the lamina propria, or it may extend into the lumen in a polypoid fashion. In adenomyomatosis, the Aschoff-Rokitansky sinuses represent diverticulum-like mucosal extensions through the muscular layer (see Fig. 8–17). Septations are frequently present.

The radiopacity, size, shape, and quantity of stones in a gallbladder may also vary[1,2,4–6,21,34,39,40] (see Figs. 8–5 to 8–9). It is sometimes possible to diagnose opaque calculi on plain films or other abdominal radiographs.[15–17] Most gallstones are composed of cholesterol; the remainder are composed of bilirubin. Small calculi may be visible only by layering in decubitus or erect radiographs (see Figs. 8–6 and 8–7). Small and medium-sized stones may layer in the opacified bile. In contrast to polyps, gallstones, unless adherent, change in position when the patient changes position (Figs. 8–16 and 8–21). The "Mercedes-Benz sign" represents gas within a gallstone[41] (Fig. 8–20).

Oral cholecystography may not enable one to differentiate nonmobile filling defects from one another or cholesterol polyps from other benign neoplastic and inflammatory lesions[42,43] (Figs. 8–16 and 8–21). Carcinoma of the gallbladder detectable on an oral cholecystogram is usually far advanced. In the majority of such patients, the gallbladder is not opacified, because of duct obstruction; many patients with carcinoma of the gallbladder also have stones, probably as a result of duct obstruction[44–46] (Fig. 8–22).

INTRAVENOUS CHOLANGIOGRAPHY

The death knell for intravenous cholangiography was sounded in the 1970s with the advent and proliferation of the newer imaging techniques of percutaneous transhepatic cholangiography, endoscopic retrograde cholangiopancreatography, ultrasound, hepatobiliary cholescintigraphy, and computed tomography. This study is rarely performed and now is almost only of historical interest.[47–49]

REFERENCES

1. Berk, R.N.: Oral cholecystography. In Radiology of the Gallbladder and Bile Ducts: Diagnosis and Intervention. Edited by R.N. Berk, J.T. Ferrucci, Jr., and G.R. Leopold. Philadelphia, W.B. Saunders, 1983, p. 83.
2. Hatfield, P.H., and Wise, R.E.: Radiology of the Gallbladder and Bile Ducts. Baltimore, Williams & Wilkins, 1976.
3. Cole, W.H.: Historical features of cholecystography. Radiology, 76:354, 1961.
4. Berk, R.N.: Radiology of the gallbladder. In Alimentary Tract Radiology. 3rd Ed. Edited by A.R. Margulis and H.J. Burhenne. St. Louis, C.V. Mosby, 1983, p. 1434.
5. Spiro, H.M.: Clinical Gastroenterology. 2nd Ed. New York, Macmillan, 1977, p. 890.
6. Amberg, J.: Radiography of the biliary tract. In Gastrointestinal Disease: Pathophysiology, Diagnosis, Management. 2nd Ed. Edited by M.H. Sleisinger and J.S. Fordtran. Philadelphia, W.B. Saunders, 1978, p. 1265.
7. Leopold, G.R.: Biliary ultrasonography. In Radiology of the Gallbladder and Bile Ducts: Diagnosis and Intervention. Edited by R.N. Berk, J.T. Ferrucci, Jr., and G.R. Leopold. Philadelphia, W.B. Saunders, 1983, p. 201.
8. Weissmann, H.: Cholescintigraphy. In Radiology of the Gallbladder and Bile Ducts: Diagnosis and Intervention. Edited by R.N. Berk, J.T. Ferrucci, Jr., and G.R. Leopold. Philadelphia, W.B. Saunders, 1983, p. 261.
9. Berk, R.N., and Loeb, P.M.: Biliary contrast materials. In Radiology of the Gallbladder and Bile Ducts: Diagnosis and Intervention. Edited by R.N. Berk, J.T. Ferrucci, Jr., and G.R. Leopold. Philadelphia, W.B. Saunders, 1983, p. 55.
10. Berk, R.N., and Loeb, P.M.: Pharmacology and physiology of the biliary radiographic contrast materials. Semin. Roentgenol., 11:147, 1976.
11. Reinke, R.T., and Berk, R.N.: The mode of Telepaque absorption from the intestine. AJR, 113:578, 1971.
12. Lasser, E.C.: Pharmacodynamics of biliary contrast media. Radiol. Clin. North Am., 4:511, 1966.
13. Whalen, J.P., Rizzuti, R.J., and Evans, J.A.: Time of optimal gallbladder opacification with Telepaque (iopanoic acid). Radiology, 105:523, 1972.
14. Oliphant, M., Whalen, J.P., and Evans, J.A.: Time of optimal gallbladder opacification with Bilopaque (tyropanoate sodium). Radiology, 112:531, 1974.
15. Harned, R.K., and LaVeen, R.T.: Preliminary abdominal films in oral cholecystography: are they necessary? AJR, 130:477, 1978.
16. Anderson, J.F., and Madsen, P.E.: Value of the plain abdominal radiograph prior to oral cholecystography. Radiology, 133:309, 1979.
17. Shehadi, W.H.: Radiologic examination of the biliary tract. Plain film of the abdomen: oral Cholecystography. Radiol. Clin. North Am., 4:463, 1966.
18. Stanley, R.J., et al.: A comparison of three cholecystographic agents: a double blind study with and without a prior fatty meal. Radiology, 112:513, 1974.
19. Loeb, P.M., et al.: The effect of fasting on gallbladder opacification during oral cholecystography: a controlled study in normal volunteers. Radiology, 126:395, 1978.
20. Parks, R.E.: Double blind study of four oral cholecystographic preparations. Radiology, 112:525, 1974.
21. Lorman, J.G., and Rosenbaum, H.D.: How to do an oral cholecystogram. Semin. Roentgenol., 11:165, 1976.
22. Berk, R.N.: The consecutive dose phenomenon in oral cholecystography. AJR, 110:230, 1970.
23. Burhenne, H.J., and Obata, W.G.: Single visit oral cholecystography. N. Engl. J. Med., 292:627, 1975.
24. Burhenne, H.J., Morris, D.C., and Graeb, D.A.: Single visit oral cholecystography for inpatients. Radiology, 140:505, 1981.
25. Laufer, I., and Gledhill, L.: The value of the fatty meal in oral cholecystography. Radiology, 114:525, 1975.
26. Jutras, J.A.: Hyperplastic cholecystoses. AJR, 83:795, 1960.
27. Jutras, J.A., and Lévesque, H.P.: Adenomyoma and adenomyomatosis of the gallbladder: radiologic and pathologic correlations. Radiol. Clin. North Am., 4:483, 1966.
28. Goldberg, H.I.: Cholecystokinin cholecystography. Semin. Roentgenol., 11:175, 1976.
29. Nathan, M.H., et al.: Cholecystokinin cholecystography: a four year evaluation. AJR, 110:250, 1970.
30. Hatfield, P.M., and Wise, R.E.: Anatomic variation in the gallbladder and bile ducts. Semin. Roentgenol., 11:157, 1976.
31. Hatfield, P.M., Scholz, F.J., and Wise, R.E.: Congen-

ital diseases of the gallbladder and bile ducts. Semin. Roentgenol., 11:235, 1976.
32. Bloom, A.A., and Stachenfeld, R.: Diabetic cholecystomegaly. JAMA, 208:357, 1969.
33. Fegerberg, S., et al.: Vagotomy and gallbladder function. GT, 11:789, 1970.
34. Palayew, M.J.: Chronic cholecystitis and cholelithiasis. Semin. Roentgenol., 11:249, 1976.
35. Simon, M., and Tandon, B.N.: Multiseptate gallbladder: a case report. Radiology, 80:84, 1963.
36. Blanton, D.E., Bream, C.A., and Mandel, S.R.: Gallbladder ectopia. AJR, 121:396, 1974.
37. Bartone, N.F., and Grieco, R.V.: Absent gallbladder and cystic duct. AJR, 110:252, 1970.
38. Haughton, V., and Lewicki, A.W.: Agenesis of the gallbladder: is preoperative diagnosis possible? Radiology, 106:305, 1973.
39. Wheeler, H.O.: Pathogenesis of gallstones. In Gastrointestinal Disease: Pathophysiology, Diagnosis, Management. 2nd Ed. Edited by M.H. Sleisinger and J.S. Fordtran. Philadelphia, W.B. Saunders, 1978, p. 1284.
40. Way, L.W., and Sleisenger, M.H.: Cholelithiasis and chronic cholecystitis. In Gastrointestinal Disease: Pathophysiology, Diagnosis, Management. 2nd Ed. Edited by M.H. Sleisinger and J.S. Fordtran. Philadelphia, W.B. Saunders, 1978, p. 1294.
41. Meyers, M.A., and O'Donohue, N.: The Mercedes Benz sign: an insight into the dynamics of formation and disappearance of gallstones. AJR, 119:63, 1973.
42. Ochsner, S.F.: Solitary polypoid lesions of the gallbladder. Radiol. Clin. North Am., 4:501, 1966.
43. Grieco, R.V., Bartone, N.F., and Vasilas, A.: A study of fixed filling defects in the well opacified gallbladder and their opacification. AJR, 90:844, 1963.
44. Way, L.W., and Sleisenger, M.H.: Neoplasms of the gallbladder and bile duct. In Gastrointestinal Disease: Pathophysiology, Diagnosis, Management. 2nd Ed. Edited by M.H. Sleisinger and J.S. Fordtran. Philadelphia, W.B. Saunders, 1978, p. 1327.
45. Melson, G.L., Reiter, F., and Evens, R.G.: Tumorous conditions of the gallbladder. Semin. Roentgenol., 11:269, 1976.
46. Beltz, W.R., and Condon, R.E.: Primary carcinoma of the gallbladder. Ann. Surg., 180:180, 1974.
47. Hatfield, P.M., and Wise, R.E.: Radiology of the Gallbladder and Bile Ducts. Baltimore, Williams & Wilkins, 1976.
48. Berk, R.N.: Intravenous Cholangiography. In Radiology of the Gallbladder and Bile Ducts: Diagnosis and Intervention. Edited by R.N. Berk, J.T. Ferruci, Jr., and G.R. Leopold. Philadelphia, W.B. Saunders, 1983, p. 163.
49. Berk, R.N., et al.: The radiological diagnosis of gallbladder disease: an imaging symposium. Radiology, 141:49, 1981.

SECTION 2
PERCUTANEOUS TRANSHEPATIC CHOLANGIOGRAPHY AND ENDOSCOPIC RETROGRADE CHOLANGIOPANCREATOGRAPHY

GERALD M. KLEIN ■ GEORGE N. STEIN

PERCUTANEOUS TRANSHEPATIC CHOLANGIOGRAPHY

Huard and Do-Xylan-Hop first described the technique of percutaneous transhepatic cholangiography in 1937.[1] The procedure was used only sparingly for the following 30 years because of associated morbidity. Until the introduction of the "skinny needle" in the early 1970s, the procedure was performed with an 18-gauge, Teflon-sheathed needle by an anterior or, more recently, a lateral approach. The procedure was associated with a high incidence of intraperitoneal hemorrhage and bile leakage and was thus performed by or with surgeons and was often followed by laparotomy. Use of the "skinny needle," which is small in caliber (22 gauge) and is thin walled, in combination with the lateral approach, has reduced potential complications and is now the method of choice for diagnostic percutaneous transhepatic cholangiography.[2]

Technique

The object of the procedure is to opacify the biliary tree. The punctured duct should be well within the liver, to lessen the chance of intraperitoneal bile leakage. One should avoid puncturing the gallbladder and extrahepatic ducts, particularly in a patient with extrahepatic biliary obstruction, for the same reason.

When one has prepared and draped the surgical site, the patient should be asked to suspend respiration, and the needle should be quickly inserted parallel to the table. The needle should be inserted laterally, slightly anterior to the midaxillary line, usually in the eighth or ninth intercostal space, high enough to avoid the gallbladder and low enough to avoid the right lung base. The highest safe puncture site on the skin should be chosen. In the majority of cases, aiming the needle toward the T11 to T12 disc space enables one to puncture a duct 1 to 2 cm superior to the confluence of the left and right hepatic ducts.[3] Other authors suggest aiming the needle toward a point midway between the diaphragm and the apex of the duodenal bulb, if visualized.[4] Still others suggest directing the needle toward T12.[5,6] The tip of the needle should lie adjacent to the patient's vertebral column after insertion. The stylet should then be removed, and the patient should be instructed to breathe quietly. A syringe tube system filled with contrast material should be attached to the needle. Care must be taken not to inject any air bubbles, which might be mistaken for stones. Under fluoroscopic guidance, the needle should be slowly withdrawn while one continuously injects small amounts of contrast material.

During the procedure, the needle may traverse hepatic arterial or venous branches, portal venous branches, or lymphatic vessels. All have a characteristic fluoroscopic appearance; contrast material injected into a blood vessel flows away from the needle rapidly. Opacification of lymphatic vessels shows a network of channels flowing toward the porta with a beaded appearance. As soon as a tubular structure is visualized, one should stop withdrawing the needle until that structure has been identified. The biliary tree is usually easy to identify because contrast material flows through the ducts slowly, and the flow is hepatofugal. As the needle traverses these different structures during the procedure, one may observe the formation of many small biliary-vascular fistulas. In a patient with biliary sepsis secondary to obstruction, this process often represents a source of septicemia resulting from the procedure.

Failure to enter the biliary tree is common, particularly if the ducts are not dilated. Virtually all dilated ducts are opacified during this procedure.[5,7] The success rate is related to the number of passes made; the rate is 99% if more than 6 passes are made (average 10 to 14). The incidence of serious complications is not related to the number of passes, however.[8] The success rate for visualizing nondilated ducts is reported to range from 50% to 76.5%.[9,10] The overall success rate ranges between 80 and 85%.[6] Again, the rate rises with the number of passes attempted.[11]

Indications

Primary indications for percutaneous transhepatic cholangiography include the need for visualization of the biliary tree in an attempt to localize the site, nature, and extent of an obstructing lesion. Screening studies such as ultrasound or computed tomography (CT) often show dilated ducts in a jaundiced patient, but the exact site and cause of the obstruction may not be identified. If screening procedures fail to show dilated ducts in a patient with clinical evidence of biliary obstruction, percutaneous transhepatic cholangiography should be performed. Many cases of intermittent or partial obstruction associated with nondilated ducts have been reported in the literature.[12]

Contraindications and Preventive Measures

Contraindications to the procedure include significant coagulopathy from any cause, uncooperativeness of the patient, more than minimal ascites, a history of allergy to contrast media, a suspected large abscess of the right lobe of the liver, or hydatid disease. Patients should have any clotting disturbances corrected prior to the procedure, either with vitamin K or with fresh-frozen plasma. All patients in whom biliary obstruction or cholangitis is suspected should be treated with broad-spectrum antibiotics, both before and after the study.

Complications

The major complications of percutaneous transhepatic cholangiography include sepsis, bile leakage, hemorrhage, and death. The most frequent complication is sepsis (1.4 to 3.6%).[3] Sepsis presumably results from the biliary vascular fistulas created during needle positioning and admixing of blood with infected bile. This complication occurs most frequently in patients with mechanical biliary obstruction. Another postulated cause is distention of the biliary tree during opacification, which allows infected bile to leak out of the ducts and into the circulatory system. To lessen the risk, bile should be aspirated in an amount equal to the amount of contrast material instilled. It is difficult to aspirate bile from a 22-gauge needle, however. Many radiologists therefore inject contrast material in an amount sufficient only to visualize major biliary radicles and move the contrast material around in the biliary tree by changing the position of the patient, either by rotation or by standing the patient erect. A thin, stiff wire may then be inserted into the biliary tree through the 22-gauge needle, and the needle may be removed. A larger sheath can be passed over the wire into the originally punctured bile duct. Alternatively, once the major bile ducts have been opacified through the 22-gauge needle cholangiogram, a second puncture may be made with a larger-sheathed needle under fluoroscopic control, to catheterize one of the larger central ducts. When the larger sheath is in place, thick bile may be easily aspirated, and a biliary drainage catheter may be inserted by this route at the end of the diagnostic procedure.

Bile leakage has been reported in 1.45 to 3.6% of cases.[6] It invariably occurs in patients with mechanical biliary obstruction. Most authors suggest that, in patients with an obstructed biliary system, aspiration or drainage of bile should be performed after the procedure, to decrease the likelihood of later intraperitoneal bile leakage.[3,6] The chances of bile leakage are diminished if a central intrahepatic duct is punctured for the study, whereas the chances are increased if an extrahepatic or peripheral duct is punctured.

Significant hemorrhage is rare (0.2 to 0.64%).[3] Hemobilia may occur following percutaneous trans-

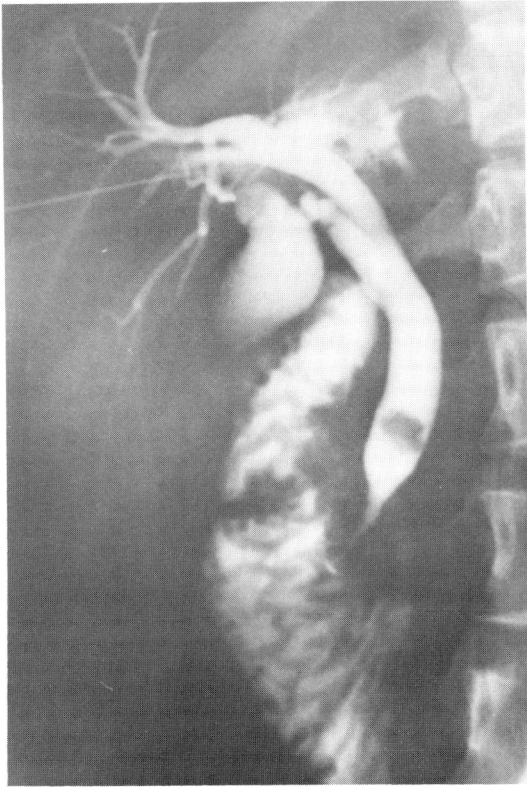

FIG. 8-23. Anteroposterior film from a percutaneous transhepatic cholangiogram. Note the round filling defect in the distal common bile duct secondary to a calculus within that duct. The common bile duct is dilated, but the flow of contrast material into the duodenum is not obstructed. The common hepatic duct and the intrahepatic biliary radicles are normal in size. The gallbladder is also visualized.

hepatic cholangiography, but is much more common following biliary drainage in which larger catheters and multiple guidewires are introduced into the bile ducts. Other infrequent complications include pneumothorax, if the skin is punctured superior to the costophrenic angle, allergic reactions to contrast material, vasovagal reactions, formation of small arteriovenous fistulas in the liver, and formation of bile cysts.[13] Death has been reported to occur rarely (0 to 0.9%).[3]

Interpretation

In a normal study, both right and left hepatic duct systems should fill, as well as the common hepatic and common bile ducts. The cystic duct and gallbladder may or may not be visualized in the normal patient. Although failure to visualize the gallbladder does not necessarily indicate cystic duct obstruction, in patients with obstruction distal to the entrance of the cystic duct into the common bile duct, an inability to visualize the gallbladder indicates either cystic

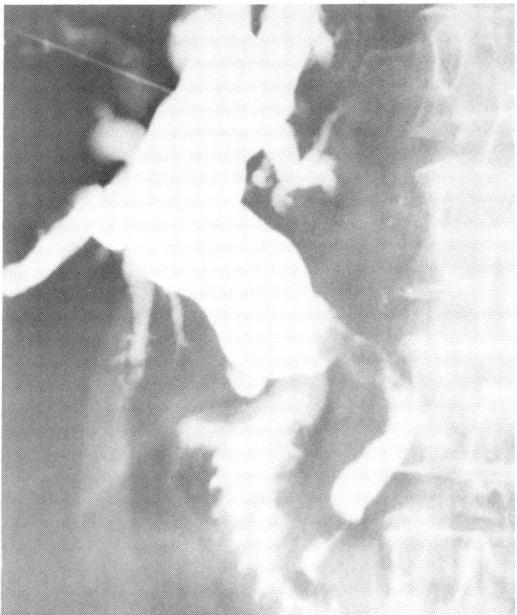

FIG. 8-24. Film from a transhepatic cholangiogram showing intraluminal filling defects at the level of the proximal common bile duct. Note the marked dilatation of the biliary radicles proximal to the filling defects, as well as the normal-caliber common bile duct distal to the filling defects. These filling defects do not appear to be free-floating within the common bile duct, and, in fact, represent primary carcinoma of the bile duct.

duct obstruction or absence of the gallbladder. In patients with left hepatic duct obstruction, an anterior subcostal puncture of the left duct may be required for visualization.

The site of obstruction can almost always be identified. The cause of the obstruction cannot always be determined with certainty, but it may be suggested. Once the site of obstruction has been identified, however, one may begin biopsy procedures in an attempt to obtain a definitive diagnosis, either percutaneously under fluoroscopic guidance or through a drainage catheter with a brush. The commonest extrahepatic causes of obstruction are pancreatic carcinoma, chronic pancreatitis, periampullary neoplasm, and gallstones. Filling defects in a duct usually represent gallstones (Figs. 8-23 and 8-24), although clot and intraductal tumor may present a similar picture. Owen evaluated different appearances of the bile duct at the point of complete obstruction visible by percutaneous transhepatic cholangiography and found the most specific sign to be an upward-pointing convexity, which always indicated an impacted gallstone[14] (Fig. 8-25). In this study, a downward-pointing convexity or a smooth-edge cutoff was seen in 75% of patients with pancreatic carcinoma (Figs. 8-26 and 8-27). In his series of 146 patients who underwent percutaneous

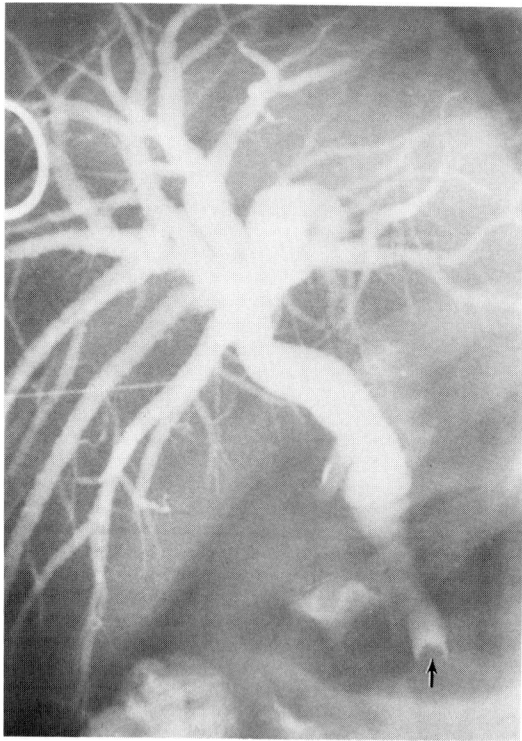

FIG. 8–25. Transhepatic cholangiogram showing moderate dilatation of the intrahepatic biliary radicles and the visualized extrahepatic biliary tree. No contrast material is seen to enter the duodenum. A superiorly oriented convexity (arrow) is noted at the distal end of the visualized common bile duct. This feature represents an impacted stone.

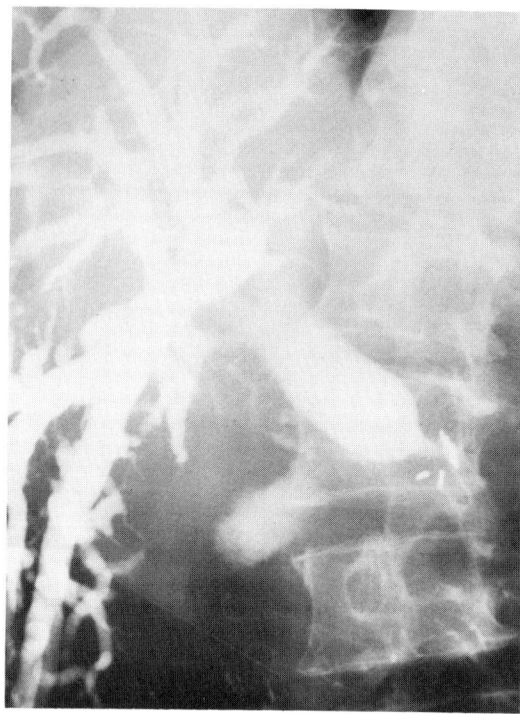

FIG. 8–26. Representative film from a transhepatic cholangiogram showing complete obstruction of the common bile duct in the area of the head of the pancreas due to pancreatic carcinoma. Note the sudden rat-tail tapering of the common duct.

transhepatic cholangiography, Owen found that 89% of these studies accurately showed the site of the obstruction and 71% accurately showed the cause. Freeny and Ball found that percutaneous transhepatic cholangiography had a sensitivity of 100% and specificity of 96% in the diagnosis of pancreatic carcinoma.[15]

In patients with incomplete obstructing lesions, neoplastic lesions are shorter and of a higher grade, and the duct has a less regular appearance at the area of narrowing (Figs. 8–28 and 8–29). Inflammatory lesions are often longer, and the duct appears smoothly narrowed (Figs. 8–30 to 8–32). Extrinsic displacement or compression of the duct by malignant lesions may mimic a benign disorder. Moreover, because any of the foregoing features may be seen with either neoplastic or inflammatory lesions, such findings are usually suggestive, but not pathognomonic, of a specific diagnosis (Fig. 8–33).

Percutaneous transhepatic cholangiography is simple, safe, and only minimally uncomfortable for the patient. The only required equipment is a tilting radiographic table with fluoroscopic capability. The skill required to perform the procedure is on a level with that needed for safe percutaneous needle biopsy of the liver. The study should be interpreted by a radiologist experienced in biliary tract radiography. Theoretically, percutaneous transhepatic cholangiography could be performed during a single day of hospitalization. In practice, however, most patients who undergo this procedure are ill and are already hospitalized for other reasons. The time required to do the study may vary from 20 min to several hours, depending on whether one attempts biliary drainage. A diagnostic percutaneous transhepatic cholangiogram takes about 20 to 30 min to perform; an average biliary drainage procedure requires about 1.5 hours.

ENDOSCOPIC RETROGRADE CHOLANGIOPANCREATOGRAPHY

Endoscopic retrograde cholangiopancreatography (ERCP) was developed in the early 1970s and provides another method for evaluating the biliary tree, as well as the pancreatic ductal system.

Technique

An experienced operator cannulates the common bile duct or pancreatic duct through the papilla using

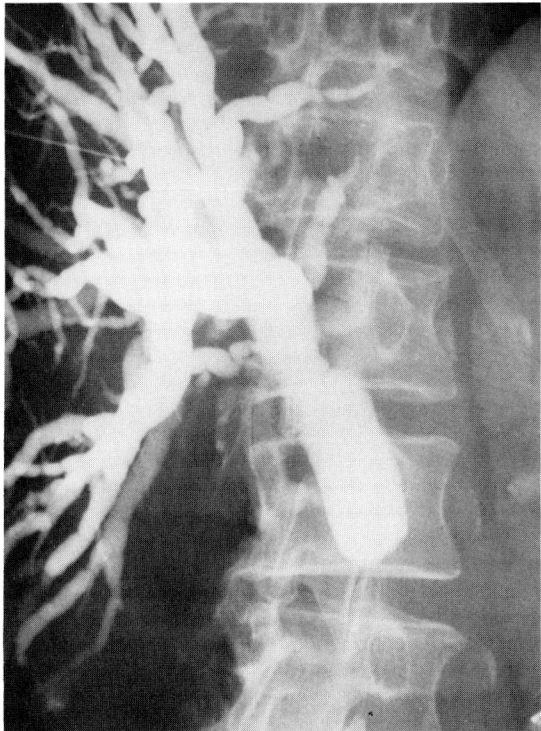

FIG. 8–27. Transhepatic cholangiogram showing complete obstruction of the common bile duct in the area of the head of the pancreas. Note the flat occlusion of the distal common duct due to carcinoma of the pancreas and resultant biliary obstruction.

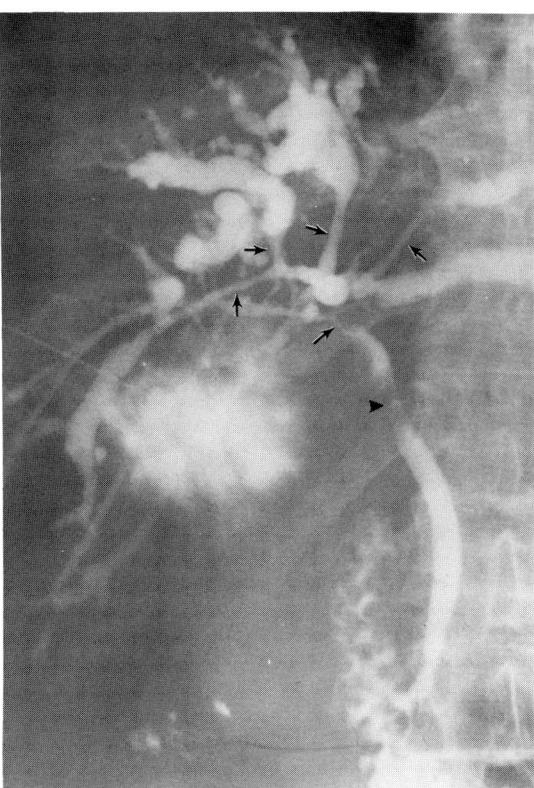

FIG. 8–29. Transhepatic cholangiography showing encasement of the ducts in the area of the porta (arrows), as well as actual invasion of the common hepatic duct (arrowhead). These findings are secondary to metastatic carcinoma from the colon to the liver and periportal lymph nodes.

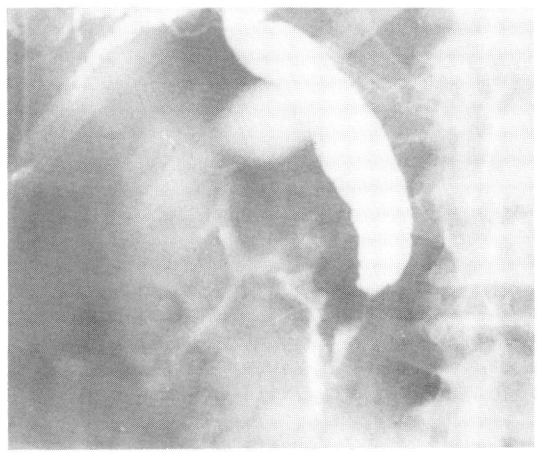

FIG. 8–28. A short, high-grade obstruction with irregular, overhanging edges at the distal end of the common bile duct. These radiographic findings indicate a carcinoma of the pancreas.

a special side-viewing duodenoscope. During the procedure, a standard endoscopic examination with direct visualization of the gastrointestinal tract may also be performed. If a lesion is visualized, a biopsy specimen may be taken through the endoscope. The patient must be adequately sedated prior to the study. Once the duodenoscope enters the duodenum, atony is produced by intravenous administration of small amounts of glucagon, as needed. After cannulation of the common or pancreatic duct, diluted contrast material is injected, and films are obtained. Interventional procedures performed following ERCP include decompression of an obstructed biliary tree by insertion of a catheter through the endoscope,[16] sphincterotomy, and endoscopic removal of retained common duct stones.

Many studies have shown that the success rate of ERCP is directly proportional to the endoscopist's skill and experience, and the complication rate inversely proportional to the same.[17,18] When ERCP is performed by experienced endoscopists, success rates range from 70 to 85%.[18–20] Much lower success

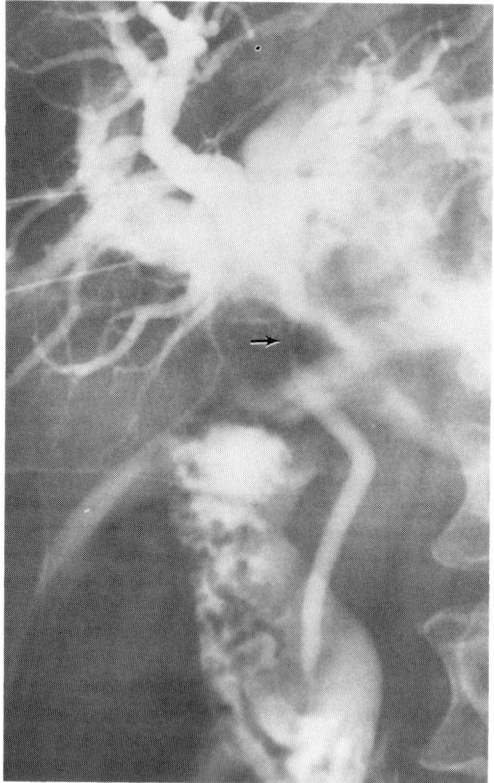

FIG. 8–30. The intrahepatic biliary radicles are distended. A smooth stricture is noted in the area of the common hepatic duct (arrow). The common bile duct distally is normal. This disorder is secondary to cholecystectomy and common bile duct exploration, performed 2 years prior to this study.

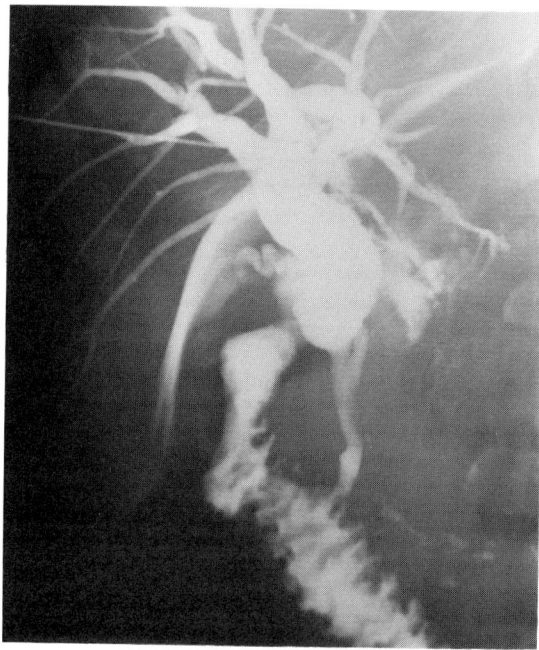

FIG. 8–31. A long, smooth stricture of the common bile duct in the area of the head of the pancreas associated with dilatation of the bile ducts proximal to the stricture. The radiographic appearance indicates a benign stricture secondary to chronic pancreatitis.

rates are reported by endoscopists who have performed few of these studies.

Indications

The primary purpose of ERCP is to distinguish surgical from nonsurgical disease in the biliary tree and the pancreas (Fig. 8–34). In the biliary system, the procedure allows direct visualization of the papilla. Lesions in this area may undergo biopsy directly. Pressure measurements at the sphincter of Oddi may be obtained to exclude sphincteric stenosis; delayed common bile duct emptying can be assessed. These findings are often associated with the postcholecystectomy syndrome[21] (Figs. 8–35 and 8–36). In fact, that symptoms may actually be reproduced during the injection into the common bile duct suggests that increased pressure in the duct may be responsible for such symptoms.[22] In these patients, endoscopic sphincterotomy often relieves the symptoms.

In the normal endoscopic cholangiogram, the common bile duct is of uniform caliber, ranging in

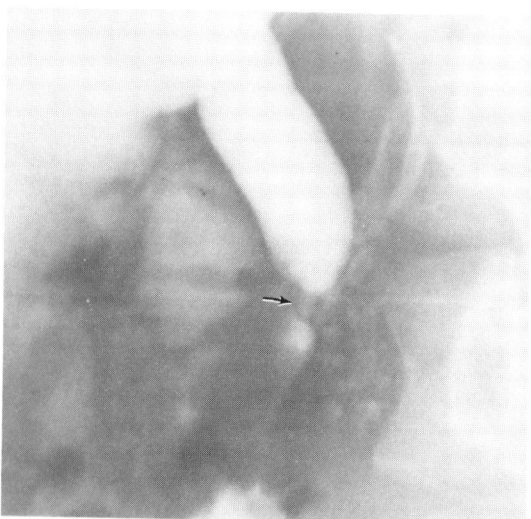

FIG. 8–32. A short, smooth stricture (arrow) of the distal common bile duct in the area of the head of the pancreas. Note the calcifications within the pancreas. This pattern represents a benign stricture of the common bile duct secondary to chronic pancreatitis.

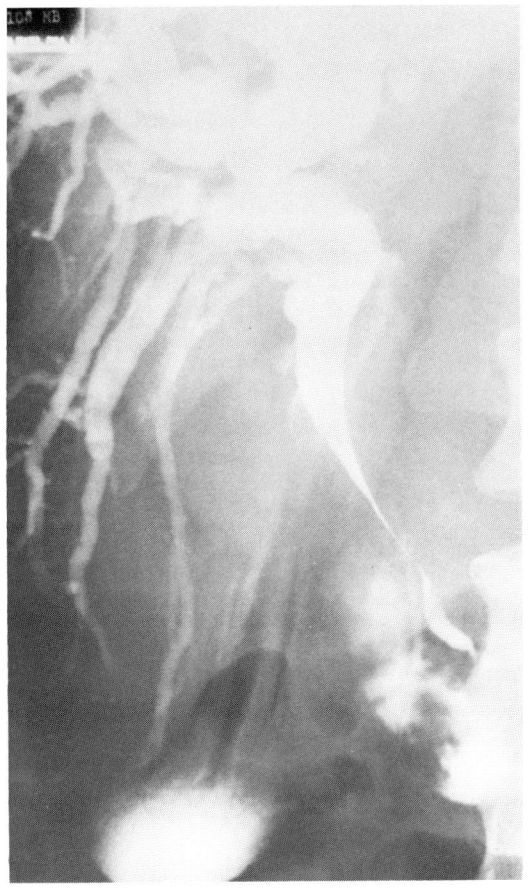

FIG. 8-33. Marked compression and lateral displacement of the common bile duct in the area of the pancreas. This disorder was secondary to a large pancreatic pseudocyst, which compressed the common bile duct. Following drainage of the pseudocyst, the patient's bilirubin level returned to normal.

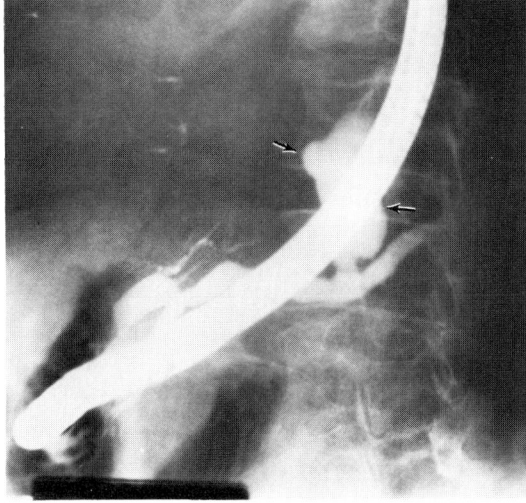

FIG. 8-34. Endoscopic retrograde cholangiopancreatogram showing filling of a pancreatic pseudocyst (arrows) during catheterization and injection of the pancreatic duct. Filling of the pseudocyst resulted in no additional symptoms in this patient. (Courtesy of William Long, M.D., Department of Gastroenterology, Hospital of the University of Pennsylvania, Philadelphia.)

size from 4.6 to 9 mm.[17] The intrahepatic ducts are clearly seen, and filling of the gallbladder should be noted. In the absence of prior cholecystectomy, failure to fill the gallbladder with contrast material suggests cystic duct obstruction. The common bile duct does not dilate after cholecystectomy; dilatation suggests obstruction. Moreover, one should obtain delayed films, to evaluate drainage of contrast material. After cholecystectomy, the normal common bile duct should drain completely of contrast material within 45 min.

In patients with biliary obstruction and dilated ducts detected during screening tests, percutaneous transhepatic cholangiography should be the procedure of choice unless contraindicated because it is safe and simple to perform. ERCP, however, is generally safe in patients with bleeding diatheses, ascites, or allergy to iodinated contrast agents. In patients with nondilated bile ducts, the success rate

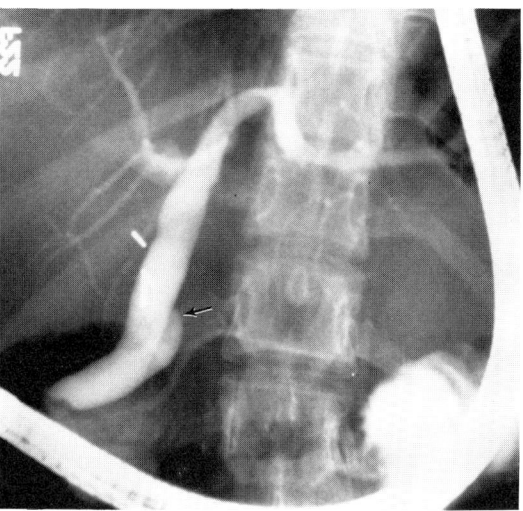

FIG. 8-35. Endoscopic retrograde cholangiopancreatogram showing a common bile duct that drains slowly and a long cystic duct remnant (arrow). Sphincter pressures were elevated on manometry. This study shows a case of postcholecystectomy syndrome secondary to sphincteric stenosis; the patient was treated satisfactorily by sphincterotomy. (Courtesy of William Long, M.D., Department of Gastroenterology, Hospital of the University of Pennsylvania, Philadelphia.)

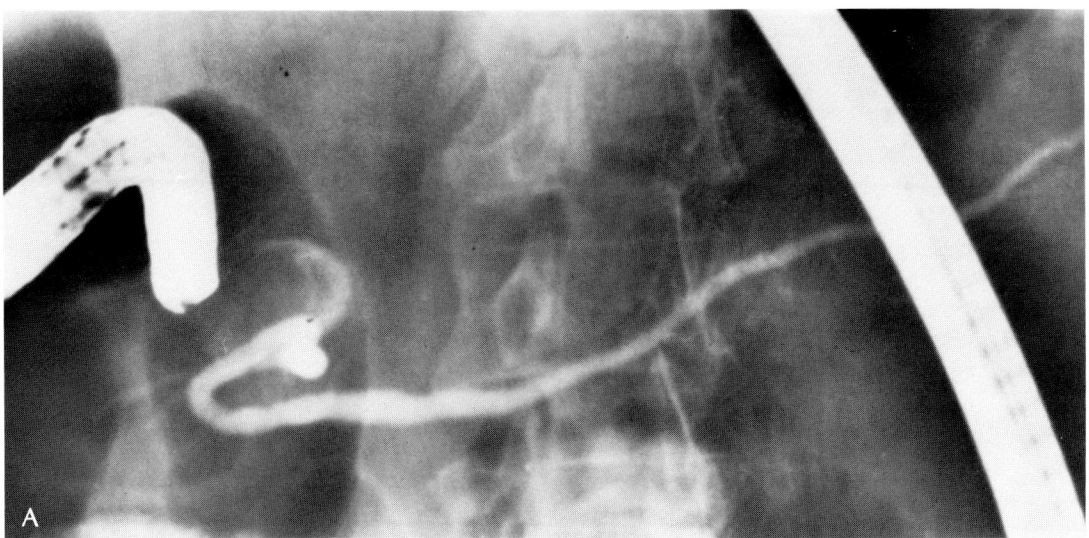

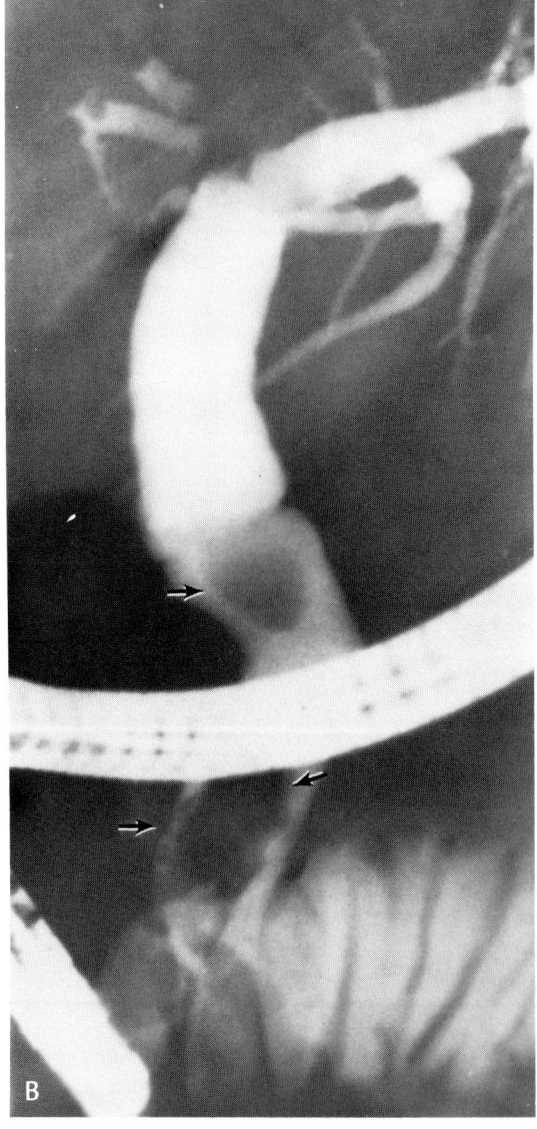

FIG. 8–36. *A,* Endoscopic retrograde cholangiopancreatographic examination of the pancreatic duct, which is normal. *B,* A similar examination of the common bile duct of the same patient shows several large filling defects within the common bile duct (arrows) caused by calculi. This patient had pain in the right upper quadrant following cholecystectomy; the pain was due to these retained common duct stones. Such calculi may cause postcholecystectomy syndrome. (Courtesy of William Long, M.D., Department of Gastroenterology, Hospital of the University of Pennsylvania, Philadelphia.)

FIG. 8-37. Endoscopic retrograde cholangiopancreatogram showing poor filling of the common bile duct and intrahepatic biliary radicles. Multiple areas of narrowing separated by areas of normal-caliber ducts are noted. This patient had longstanding sclerosing cholangitis. (Courtesy of William Long, M.D., Department of Gastroenterology, Hospital of the University of Pennsylvania, Philadelphia.)

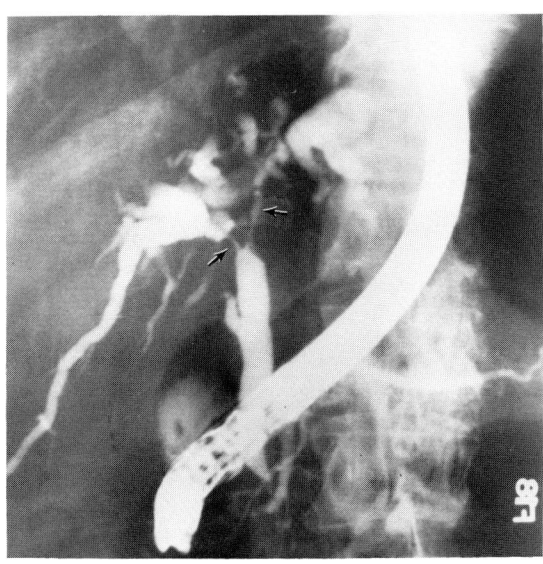

FIG. 8-38. Endoscopic retrograde cholangiopancreatogram of the common bile duct showing a stenotic lesion at the bifurcation of the common hepatic duct secondary to cholangiocarcinoma (Klatskin tumor) (arrows). (Courtesy of William Long, M.D., Department of Gastroenterology, Hospital of the University of Pennsylvania, Philadelphia.)

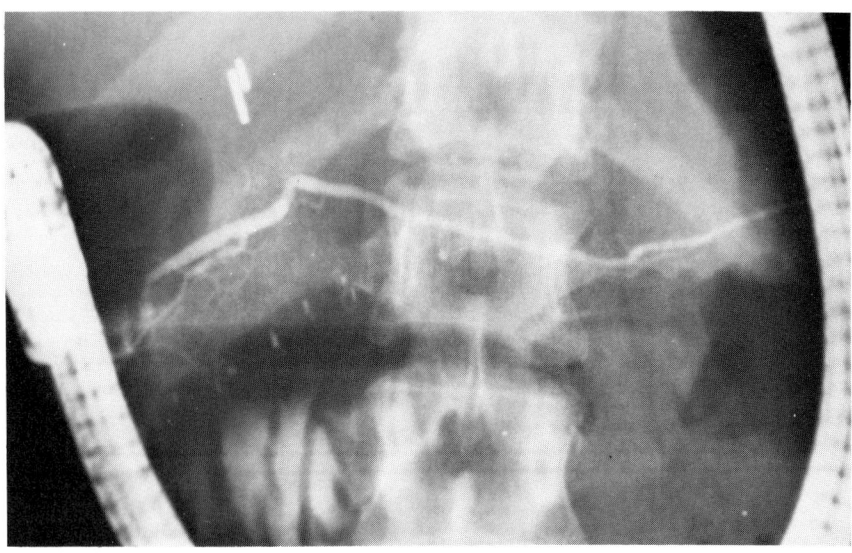

FIG. 8–39. Normal pancreatic ductogram. Note the smooth caliber of the pancreatic duct and the small branches throughout the entire gland. (Courtesy of William Long, M.D., Department of Gastroenterology, Hospital of the University of Pennsylvania, Philadelphia.)

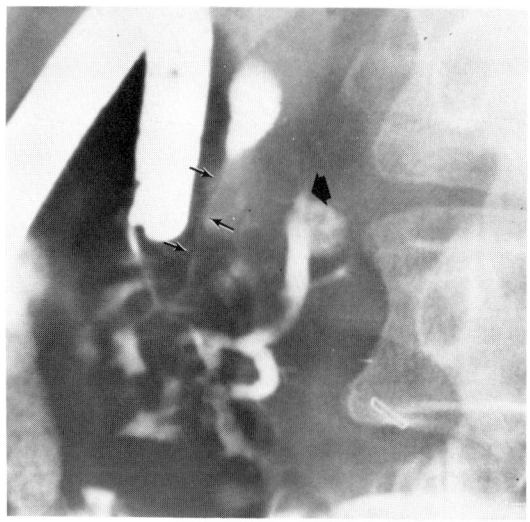

FIG. 8–40. Carcinoma of the pancreas. Note the stricture of the distal common bile duct (small arrows), as well as complete occlusion of the pancreatic duct (large arrow) near the area of the common bile duct stricture. These associated findings suggest carcinoma of the pancreas. (Courtesy of William Long, M.D., Department of Gastroenterology, Hospital of the University of Pennsylvania, Philadelphia.)

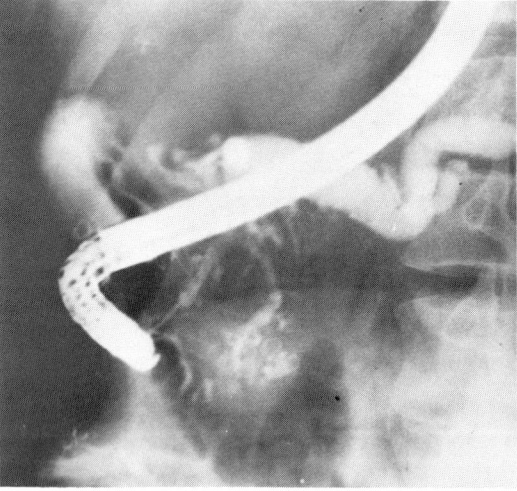

FIG. 8–41. Endoscopic retrograde cholangiopancreatogram showing marked dilatation of the pancreatic duct without associated proximal stricture. This finding indicates chronic pancreatitis. (Courtesy of William Long, M.D., Department of Gastroenterology, Hospital of the University of Pennsylvania, Philadelphia.)

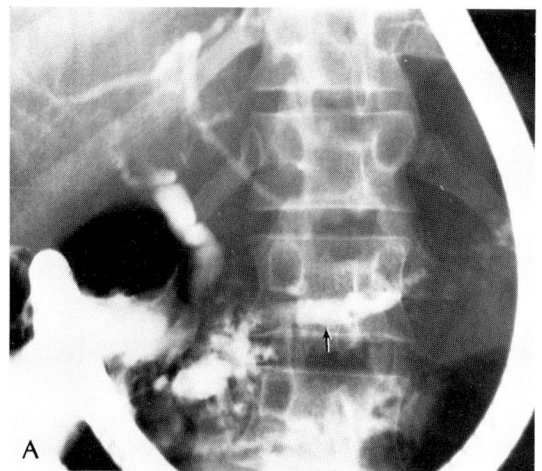

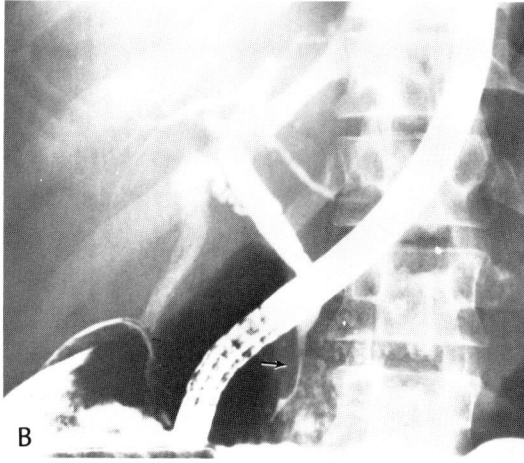

FIG. 8-42. A, Endoscopic retrograde pancreatogram shows significant dilatation of the pancreatic duct (arrow) without evidence of a proximal stricture. B, Cholangiographic portion of the examination shows a smooth stricture (arrow) in the distal common bile duct. Also note the multiple calcifications within the body of the pancreas. These changes represent a benign stricture of the common bile duct secondary to chronic calcific pancreatitis. (Courtesy of William Long, M.D., Department of Gastroenterology, Hospital of the University of Pennsylvania, Philadelphia.)

of percutaneous transhepatic cholangiography is lower than in patients with dilated ducts. With ERCP, one can visualize the ductal system of up to 85% of patients, regardless of whether the bile ducts are dilated or not. ERCP may be used in patients with nondilated biliary trees as the test of first choice, depending on the availability of the procedure and of experienced personnel to perform the test. Because it provides information about the pancreatic duct, ERCP is useful in evaluating diseases of the pancreas.

Contraindications

Contraindications to the procedure include an uncooperative patient, who may harm himself or the endoscopist or may damage the duodenoscope. A recent history of acute pancreatitis is a relative contraindication, unless one is looking for a surgically correctable lesion. Allergy to iodinated contrast material is not a contraindication because no contrast material should be introduced intravascularly during the procedure. Anaphylaxis has not been reported.[18]

Complications

The rate of complications is inversely proportional to the experience of the endoscopist. It may be as low as 1 to 3%, with a mortality rate of 0.1%.[17] Complications include pancreatitis, sepsis, injury to the gastrointestinal tract, and side effects of medication.[23] As many as 75% of patients develop significant hyperamylasemia and increased urinary amylase excretion after the procedure. This complication is usually asymptomatic and resolves in 1 to 4 days. Clinically apparent acute pancreatitis develops in 0.7 to 7.4% of patients.[23] Such patients are usually under study to determine the cause of a previous bout of acute pancreatitis. The cause of pancreatitis following ERCP is unknown, but several factors, including rate, pressure, and volume of injections, type of contrast material, and number of injections, have been implicated.[18] The mortality rate in patients with pancreatitis induced by ERCP is lower than that in patients with other forms of pancreatitis. Generally, this complication is mild and is not fatal.

Cholangitic sepsis and pancreatic sepsis are serious complications of ERCP. Cholangitic sepsis occurs in about 0.8% of patients and has a mortality rate of 0.1%.[18] It rarely occurs unless mechanical obstruction of the biliary tree is present. The administration of systemic antibiotics prior to the procedure may decrease the risk of this complication. Pancreatic sepsis occurs in 0.3% of patients and has a mortality rate of 0.06%.[18] Most cases are associated with pseudocysts or partial pancreatic duct obstruction. When a pseudocyst fills during ERCP (Fig. 8-34), close observation of the patient is required, and early surgical drainage of cysts that retain contrast material is recommended. Generally, ERCP is not needed in a patient with a known pseudocyst. The risk of bacteremia during the procedure is negligible, and prophylactic antibiotics are not necessary unless bile duct obstruction is present.[25]

Perforation of the duodenum with the cannulation catheter is another potential but rare complication. It usually occurs in patients with duodenal anatomic features distorted as a result of previous surgical procedures, inflammatory disease, or neoplasms.

Because ERCP takes an average of 2 to 4 hours to perform,[26] large amounts of medication must be used to keep the patient sedated and to cause duodenal ileus. Thus, the likelihood of drug reactions is higher than with ordinary endoscopy. Bilbao reported an incidence of 0.6% in her series.[18]

Interpretation

Radiographically, gallstones can be detected as filling defects in the ducts, and benign and malignant strictures may also be identified. The criteria for distinguishing strictures are similar to those discussed under percutaneous transhepatic cholangiography.

The pancreatic ductogram may give helpful information not provided by percutaneous transhepatic cholangiography. If results suggest chronic pancreatitis, then a stricture of the distal common bile duct will probably be benign. If results suggest pancreatic carcinoma, then the stricture will be more likely to be malignant. Strictures in the mid-duct region must be presumed to be malignant unless the patient has a history of previous biliary tract operation or trauma; previous surgical procedures or trauma may cause such strictures. The degree of duct dilatation with obstruction bears no relation to the degree or duration of the obstruction.

Intrahepatic biliary disease may be evaluated by ERCP. Sclerosing cholangitis can occur in a primary form or in association with inflammatory bowel disease.[27] Although the common bile duct is usually involved, localized intrahepatic disease can be seen. Radiographically, irregular beading of the ducts is the result of multiple, noncontinuous strictures (Fig. 8-37). Tumors of the liver, either primary or metastatic, may displace, may encase, or may invade biliary radicles. Cholangiocarcinoma usually causes bile duct stricture, often at the bifurcation of the common hepatic duct (Fig. 8-38), but the tumor may also appear as an intraluminal filling defect.

In the pancreas, both benign and malignant lesions manifest themselves most commonly as obstruction or strictures of the main pancreatic duct. Complete obstruction of the main pancreatic duct, especially when associated with stricture of the common bile duct, suggests a malignant tumor (double-duct sign) (Figs. 8-39 and 8-40). Strictures of the pancreatic duct occur in both benign and malignant disease. Frequently, the length and characteristics of the stricture suggest its most likely cause. Long strictures that are irregular and beaded are more often malignant, whereas short, smooth strictures are more often benign. Ductal dilatation without a predilatation stricture is indicative of chronic pancreatitis (Figs. 8-41 and 8-42). The combination of multiple, discrete stenoses and areas of ductal dilatation, intraductal calculi, and irregularities of the contour of the main pancreatic duct suggests pancreatic inflammatory disease. Areas that do not fill with contrast material usually represent carcinoma when the duct is sufficiently injected to produce a diffuse acinar pattern in the ductal tree of the gland. Freeny and Ball believe that ERCP has a sensitivity rate of 94% and specificity rate of 97% in the diagnosis of pancreatic carcinoma.[15] Other authors believe that the differentiation of primary from secondary pancreatic malignant tumors is difficult, particularly if one relies on the radiographic appearance alone.[28] Difficulty in differentiating benign from malignant disease may also be encountered.

In summary, ERCP is a complex procedure requiring the skills of an experienced endoscopist. Aside from high-quality x-ray equipment with fluoroscopic capabilities, a special side-viewing endoscope must be used. The procedure takes longer than percutaneous transhepatic cholangiography and is more uncomfortable for the patient. The cost of the procedure is also higher.[26] ERCP may be safer than percutaneous transhepatic cholangiography when the latter is contraindicated. Percutaneous transhepatic cholangiography probably should be the initial procedure of choice in differentiating obstructive from parenchymal jaundice. ERCP may be used primarily to evaluate biliary and pancreatic disease in the absence of jaundice, after cholecystectomy, and when percutaneous transhepatic cholangiography is contraindicated or has failed.

REFERENCES

1. Huard, P., and Do-Xylan-Hop: La ponction transhépatique des canaux biliaires. Bull. Soc. Med. Chir. Indochine, 15:1090, 1937.
2. Okuda, K., et al.: Nonsurgical percutaneous transhepatic cholangiography—diagnostic significance in medical problems of the liver. Am. J. Dig. Dis., 19:21, 1974.
3. Jüttner, H.U., and Redeker, A.G.: Fine needle transhepatic colangiography: current status and critical review of the technic. Am. J. Gastroenterol., 75:454, 1981.
4. Pereiras, R., Jr., et al.: Percutaneous transhepatic cholangiography with the skinny needle: a rapid, simple and accurate method in the diagnosis of cholestasis. Ann. Intern. Med., 86:562, 1977.
5. Choi, S.H., Pralzer, F.A., and Park, H.C.: Percutaneous transhepatic cholangiography with thin needle: recent update. J. Med., 12:147, 1981.
6. Schiff, E.R.: Diagnostic percutaneous transhepatic cholangiography. Semin. Liver Dis., 2:49, 1982.
7. Harbin, W.P., Mueller, P.R., and Ferrucci, J.T., Jr.: Transhepatic cholangiography. Complication and use patterns of the fine needle technique: a multi-institutional survey. Radiology, 135:15, 1980.
8. Ariyama, J., et al.: Experience with percutaneous transhepatic cholangiography using the Japanese needle. Gastrointest. Radiol., 2:359, 1978.
9. Kreek, M.J., and Balint, J.A.: "Skinny needle" cholangiography—results of a pilot study of a voluntary prospective method for gathering risk data on new procedures. Gastroenterology, 78:598, 1980.
10. Dilawari, J.B., et al.: Endoscopic retrograde cholan-

giopancreatography and percutaneous transhepatic cholangiography in obstructive jaundice. Indian J. Med. Res., 75:287, 1982.
11. Jaques, P.F., Mauro, M.A., and Scatliff, J.H.: The failed transhepatic cholangiogram. Radiology, 134:33, 1980.
12. Muhletaler, C.A., et al.: Diagnosis of obstructive jaundice with nondilated bile ducts. AJR, 134:1149, 1980.
13. Vujic, I., Meredith, H.C., and Anderson, M.C.: A huge bile cyst—an unusual complication of percutaneous transhepatic cholangiography. Australas. Radiol., 23:113, 1979.
14. Owen, J.P.: Analyis of the signs of common bile duct obstruction at percutaneous transhepatic cholangiography. Clin. Radiol., 31:271, 1980.
15. Freeny, P.C., and Ball, T.J.: Endoscopic retrograde cholangiopancreatography and percutaneous transhepatic cholangiography in the evaluation of suspected pancreatic carcinoma: diagnostic limitations and contemporary roles. Cancer, 47:1666, 1981.
16. Siegel, J.H., Harding, G.T., and Chateau, F.: Endoscopic decompression and drainage of benign and malignant biliary obstruction. Gastrointest. Endosc., 28:79, 1982.
17. Shapiro, H.A.: Endoscopic diagnosis and treatment of biliary tract disease. Surg. Clin. North Am., 61:843, 1981.
18. Bilbao, M.K., et al.: Complications of endoscopic retrograde cholangiopancreatography (ERCP): a study of 10,000 cases. Gastroenterology, 70:314, 1976.
19. Beazley, R.M., and Cohn, I., Jr.: Decisions in pancreatic carcinoma. Semin. Oncol., 7:435, 1980.
20. Satake, K., et al.: Evaluation of cholangiographic procedures in diagnosis of obstructive jaundice. Am. Surg., 47:387, 1981.
21. Cooperman, M., et al.: Endoscopic retrograde cholangiopancreatography: its use in the evaluation of nonjaundiced patients with the postcholecystectomy syndrome. Arch. Surg., 116:606, 1981.
22. Whiteside, C., Frieman, J.M., and Connon, J.J.: Retrograde cholangiography in the postcholecystectomy syndrome. Can. Med. Assoc. J., 125:597, 1981.
23. Shahmir, M., and Schuman, B.M.: Complications of fibreoptic endoscopy. Gastrointest Endosc., 26:86, 1980.
24. Nebel, O.T., et al.: Complications associated with endoscopic retrograde cholangiopancreatography: results of the 1974 ASGE survey. Gastrointest. Endosc., 22:34, 1975.
25. Dutta, S.K., et al.: Prospective evaluation of the risk of bacteremia during ERCP. (Abstract.) Gastrointest. Endosc., 25:37, 1979.
26. Jander, H.P., Galbraith, J., and Aldrete, J.S.: Percutaneous transhepatic cholangiography using the Chiba needle: comparison with retrograde pancreatocholecystography. South. Med. J., 73:415, 1980.
27. Sivak, M.V., Farmer, R.G., and Lalli, A.F.: Sclerosing cholangitis: its increasing frequency of recognition and association with inflammatory bowel disease. J. Clin. Gastroenterol., 3:261, 1981.
28. Swensen, T., Osnes, M., and Serck-Hanssen, A.: Endoscopic retrograde cholangiopancreatography in primary and secondary tumours of the pancreas. Br. J. Radiol., 53:760, 1980.

9

Luminal Contrast Studies of the Gastrointestinal Tract

David J. Ott

Luminal contrast studies are the traditional means of examining the gastrointestinal tract. Although fiberoptic endoscopy has challenged the role of radiology in the initial evaluation of gastrointestinal disease, the volume of radiographic examinations of the gastrointestinal tract has declined only modestly in recent years.[1]

This chapter begins with a general discussion of the equipment, cost, radiation risk, contrast agents, and interpretative principles of the radiographic examination of the gastrointestinal tract. Subsequent sections of the chapter are devoted to the pharynx and esophagus, stomach and duodenum, small bowel, and large bowel. In each of these organ-related sections, the indications, preparation, methods, technical problems, interpretation, and efficacy of the applicable radiographic examinations are discussed.

GENERAL CONSIDERATIONS

Such considerations include apparatus, cost, risk of ionizing radiation, contrast agents in current use, and general guidelines for interpreting radiographs.

Equipment, Cost, and Radiation Risk

EQUIPMENT. Radiographic examination of the gastrointestinal tract involves the use of modern fluoroscopic equipment. Image intensifiers, three-phase x-ray generators, better x-ray tubes, automatic exposure devices, and improved film-cassette combinations have all improved the quality of gastrointestinal radiographs. Two types of fluoroscopic-study rooms can also be used for these examinations. In the conventional room, the radiologist is near the fluoroscope and must wear a protective apron because of exposure to scattered radiation. More recently, however, remote-control rooms have become available, and the advantage over the conventional room includes elimination of radiation exposure to the radiologist and improved quality of the radiographic films.

COST. The cost of installing a room for fluoroscopic study is major, but variable, depending on the type of equipment and the choice of optional devices such as a spot-film camera or video recording system. The actual costs of individual radiographic examinations of the gastrointestinal tract vary throughout the United States. The absolute costs of these examinations also depend on the type of study. The double-contrast barium enema is the most expensive examination because the materials used are costly and because the amount of time spent in the fluoroscopic study room is greater.[2]

RISK OF RADIATION. Exposure to ionizing radiation for diagnostic evaluation of the gastrointestinal tract is associated with a low risk of deleterious effects on the genetic pool. This consideration is important in patients during their procreative years, however. The amount of radiation exposure depends on the equipment used, the time taken to perform a fluoroscopic study, the number of films exposed, and the type of examination. In general, during an upper gastrointestinal series of radiographs, the patient receives a gonad dose comparable to that obtained during a plain abdominal series, whereas the gonad dose received during a barium enema examination is several times higher and is similar to that received during a lumbar spine series or an intravenous urogram.[3]

Luminal Contrast Agents

BARIUM SULFATE. Barium sulfate is almost totally inert, with little physiologic effect on the gastrointestinal tract other than responses to volume and fluidity. The many commercially available barium products vary widely in their physical properties of density, viscosity, and coating ability. Many products have a wide application throughout the gastrointestinal tract, whereas others are specifically formulated for more limited use, such as for double-contrast examination of the stomach.[4]

Barium sulfate is the contrast agent preferred in the examination of the gastrointestinal tract. Its ability to coat and define the mucosal surface and to resist dilution is superior to that of the water-soluble contrast media. Furthermore, modern barium suspensions are resistant to inspissation and impaction because they contain excellent suspending agents.

Complications. Complications of barium sulfate administration are rare.[5] The risks of oral ingestion of the agent include perforation, obstruction, impaction, and aspiration and are related primarily to the disease process in the individual patient under study. Extravasation of barium sulfate, particularly into the peritoneal cavity, is potentially the most serious complication and occurs most commonly in conjunction with peptic ulcer perforation. This complication is avoidable by communication with the clinician regarding the patient's medical history, by the use of appropriate plain radiographs of the abdomen, and by the administration of water-soluble contrast agents when perforation is suspected.

Obstruction and impaction from orally administered barium sulfate occur only rarely in the upper gastrointestinal tract or small bowel. Even in the presence of gastric or small-bowel obstruction, the fluidity of the barium suspension is maintained. As a result, barium sulfate is the contrast agent preferred for oral examination of a patient with an obstruction proximal to the colon.[6]

Aspiration of barium sulfate into the tracheobronchial tree in small amounts is nearly always inconsequential. Indeed, its innocuous effects in this area have led some radiologists to advocate the use of barium sulfate as a bronchographic contrast agent. On the other hand, aspiration of the iodinated water-soluble agents is potentially dangerous. The hyperosmolarity of these agents may cause acute pulmonary edema and even death. Thus, if it is likely that contrast material will enter a patient's airway by aspiration or by a fistulous tract with the esophagus, one should use barium sulfate for the examination.

Perforation is the most frequent serious complication of the barium enema examination. The reported incidence varies from 0.008 to 0.04%.[5] Depending on the site and the extent of colonic injury, the perforation may be intramural, retroperitoneal, or intraperitoneal. The most common causes of perforation are the improper insertion of enema tips and the use of balloon devices to facilitate retention of the barium. Perforation does not appear to be related to the type of barium enema examination because the intraluminal pressures generated with either the single-contrast or the double-contrast method are of similar amplitude.[7]

In the colon, obstruction and impaction are more important considerations than in the upper gastrointestinal tract because of the progressive dehydration of retained barium by the colonic mucosa. The most serious outcome of swallowed barium is impaction of barium proximal to a complete or even incomplete obstruction of the colon, with subsequent perforation. This complication is less likely with the newer and better-suspended bariums; the presence of a modest amount of such an agent proximal to an incomplete colonic obstruction is of little consequence.[8] To avoid this potential complication, however, a barium enema should be performed initially when an obstructing lesion in the colon is suspected.

Other complications of barium enema examination are rare, but they are often serious. The most lethal complication is intravasation of barium into the venous system. Inadvertent insertion of the enema tip into the vagina is possible and may lead to venous intravasation, to vaginal rupture, and to extraperitoneal or intraperitoneal contamination with barium sulfate.

WATER-SOLUBLE CONTRAST AGENTS. A number of iodinated contrast agents can be used to examine the gastrointestinal tract. Several of these are flavored and are more palatable when given orally, but they are also more expensive than their unflavored counterparts. The less-costly agents should be used for other than oral administration.

That the water-soluble contrast agents are hyperosmolar solutions has important implications regarding potential complications. These agents are inferior to barium sulfate as diagnostic contrast materials. The major indication for their use is in evaluating patients with possible perforations of the gastrointestinal lumen, particularly if free peritoneal communication is likely. Under most other circumstances, barium sulfate is preferred.[9]

Complications. The use of water-soluble contrast agents may have complications. Oral ingestion may be contraindicated if the patient is likely to aspirate the contrast material or if a fistulous communication with the tracheobronchial tree is suspected. Because of their tendency to draw fluid into the bowel, these agents must be used with caution in hypovolemic or dehydrated patients, especially young and elderly patients. Indeed, intestinal perforation has resulted from rapid fluid distention of the obstructed bowel. Stasis of these agents in the stomach or colon has also led to severe hemorrhage, presumably because of a direct irritant effect on the gastrointestinal mucosa.[10] Finally, these materials may be absorbed systemically, and contrast reactions similar to those occurring during intravenous urography are theoretically possible.[11]

General Interpretative Principles

Pathologic alterations affecting the gastrointestinal tract fall into six general categories: (1) caliber changes; (2) projecting lesions; (3) filling defects;

(4) extrinsic effects; (5) altered connections; and (6) functional changes. Extrinsic effects and altered connections related to fistulization or to surgical anastomoses are straightforward. Although functional disorders can presumably affect any organ of the gastrointestinal tract, radiographic assessment of such disorders is clearly understood only in the esophagus.

CALIBER CHANGES. Changes in luminal caliber include narrowing and dilatation, which may be either focal or diffuse. Occasionally, a combination of these changes is seen, as in patients with achalasia with functional narrowing at the esophagogastric junction combined with diffuse dilatation of the esophageal body, as well as in patients with annular carcinoma of the colon associated with colonic obstruction.

PROJECTING LESIONS. The two most common lesions that project from the gastrointestinal lumen are ulcers and diverticula. Their appearance depends on the organ affected and on the causative disease. In the upper gastrointestinal tract, ulcers are usually single or few in number and are of peptic origin, whereas in the colon, diffuse ulceration from inflammatory bowel disease is more typical. Diverticula may be seen throughout the gastrointestinal tract, but they are most numerous in the sigmoid colon.

FILLING DEFECTS. Such defects can vary from subtle mucosal abnormalities, such as the exudates seen in patients with esophagitis, through polypoid lesions of various sizes, to fungating masses occupying most of the lumen of the bowel. Obviously, the radiographic detection and differentiation of these types of lesions depend on their size and appearance. Distinguishing benign from malignant filling defects is often impossible radiographically, particularly smaller polypoid lesions of the colon.

PHARYNX AND ESOPHAGUS

Indications and Preparation

Radiographic examination of the pharynx and esophagus is performed to assess swallowing and esophageal motor disorders, esophageal obstruction, esophageal perforation, inflammatory or neoplastic lesions, esophageal varices, postoperative complications, and extrinsic effects. The most common indications, however, are in patients with pyrosis and dysphagia in whom reflux esophagitis and focal narrowing from peptic stricture, carcinoma, or mucosal ring are suspected.

Preparation of the patient for examination of the pharynx and esophagus usually requires an overnight fast. In an emergency, however, the examination can be performed if the patient has eaten, provided one does not need to study the stomach and duodenum. If esophageal retention is known to be present, as in patients with severe achalasia, thorough preliminary aspiration of the esophagus will improve the quality of the subsequent radiographic examination. This principle also applies to examination of the stomach, if gastric outlet obstruction is present.

Types of Examination

Multiple radiographic techniques are available for examining the pharynx and esophagus.[12] The single-contrast method includes full-column views of the barium-distended esophagus and mucosal relief views of the collapsed organ (Fig. 9–1). In the double-contrast method, the esophagus is coated with barium and is distended with air, to permit evaluation of both its caliber and its mucosal surface (Fig. 9–1). Motion-recording methods, such as videotape, are useful for the evaluation of pharyngeal and esophageal motility disorders.

Esophageal varices are best detected using mucosal relief films.[13] The collapsed lower esophagus is coated with dense barium, and the patient is prohibited from swallowing. Varices, if present, usually become distended in 5 to 10 minutes. Anticholinergic agents may be helpful, to relax the esophagus further and to promote variceal distention (Fig. 9–2). Moreover, these drugs, along with glucagon, are sometimes used to dislodge meat impactions at the lower end of the esophagus.

Water-soluble contrast agents are used in examining the esophagus when perforation into the mediastinum is suspected. These agents are especially helpful when one evaluates the lower esophagus for spontaneous perforation or traumatic perforation following penetrating injuries, surgical procedures, or pneumatic dilatation for achalasia. Under these circumstances, a negative water-soluble contrast examination should be followed by a barium study, which may show small leaks not shown on the previous examination.[14]

Technical Problems

Radiographic examination of the pharynx and esophagus is easily performed and is well tolerated by the patient. Swallowing difficulties that misdirect the barium into the nasopharynx or trachea and regurgitation due to retching or esophageal obstruction limit the performance of the examination. Some of these problems may be prevented by injection of barium through a nasogastric tube situated in the esophagus.

Obtaining high-quality films for each method used to examine the esophagus is crucial. Careful fluoroscopic observation is necessary to detect transient abnormalities, such as small Zenker's diverticula, and to identify esophageal motor disorders. Fully distended barium-filled or double-contrast views are

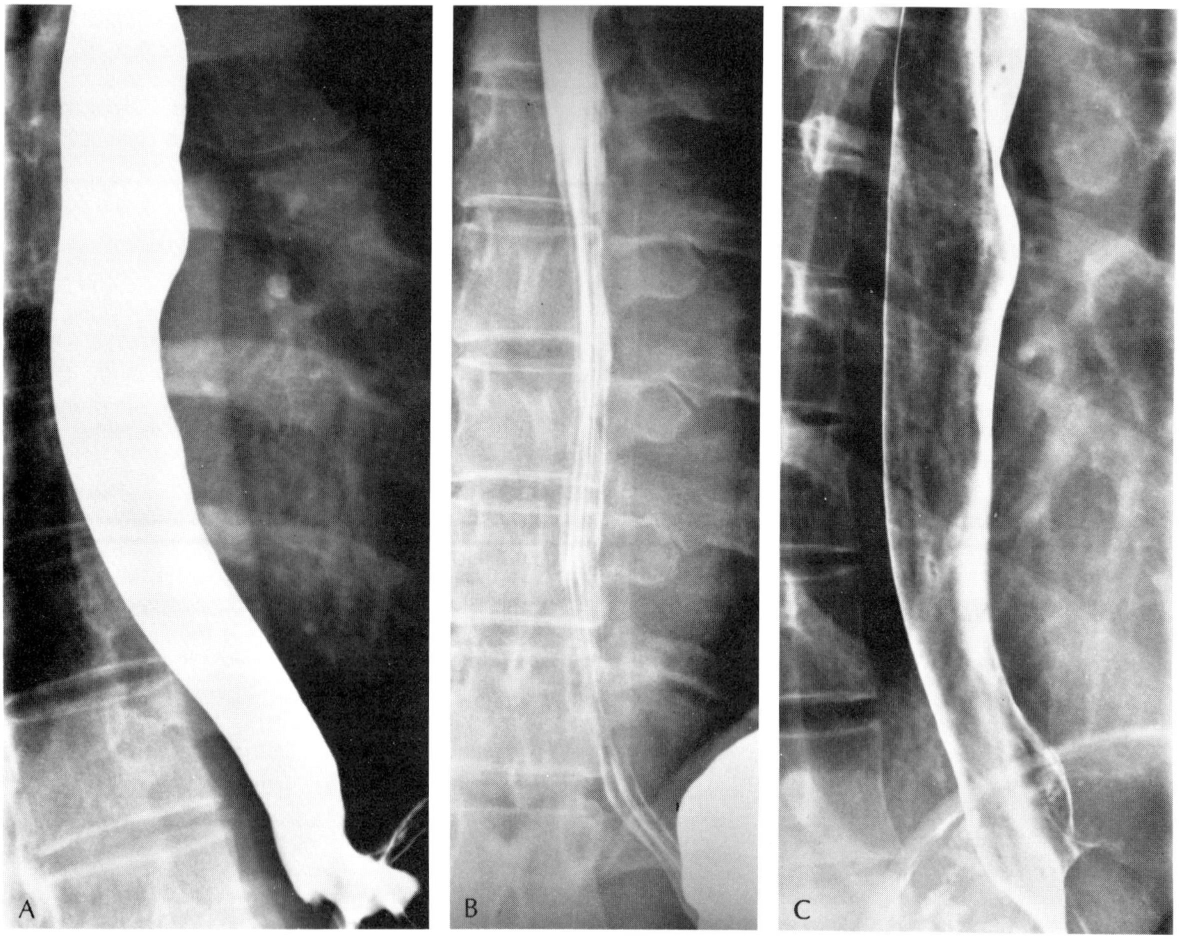

FIG. 9-1. *A,* Full-column view of the barium-distended esophagus. *B,* Mucosal relief view of the collapsed normal esophagus, showing the thin, longitudinal folds. *C,* Double-contrast view of the distended esophagus, showing homogeneous coating of the mucosal surface.

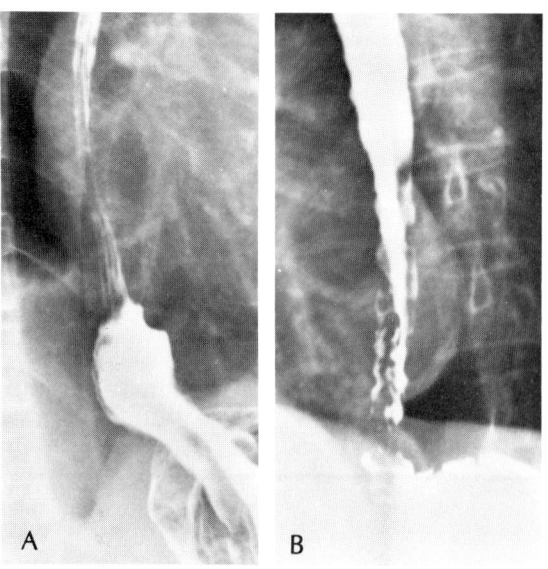

FIG. 9-2. *A,* Standard mucosal relief view of the inferior portion of the esophagus, showing no evidence of varices in a patient with cirrhosis. *B,* Repeat examination following administration of 30 mg parenteral probantheline bromide showing serpiginous esophageal varices.

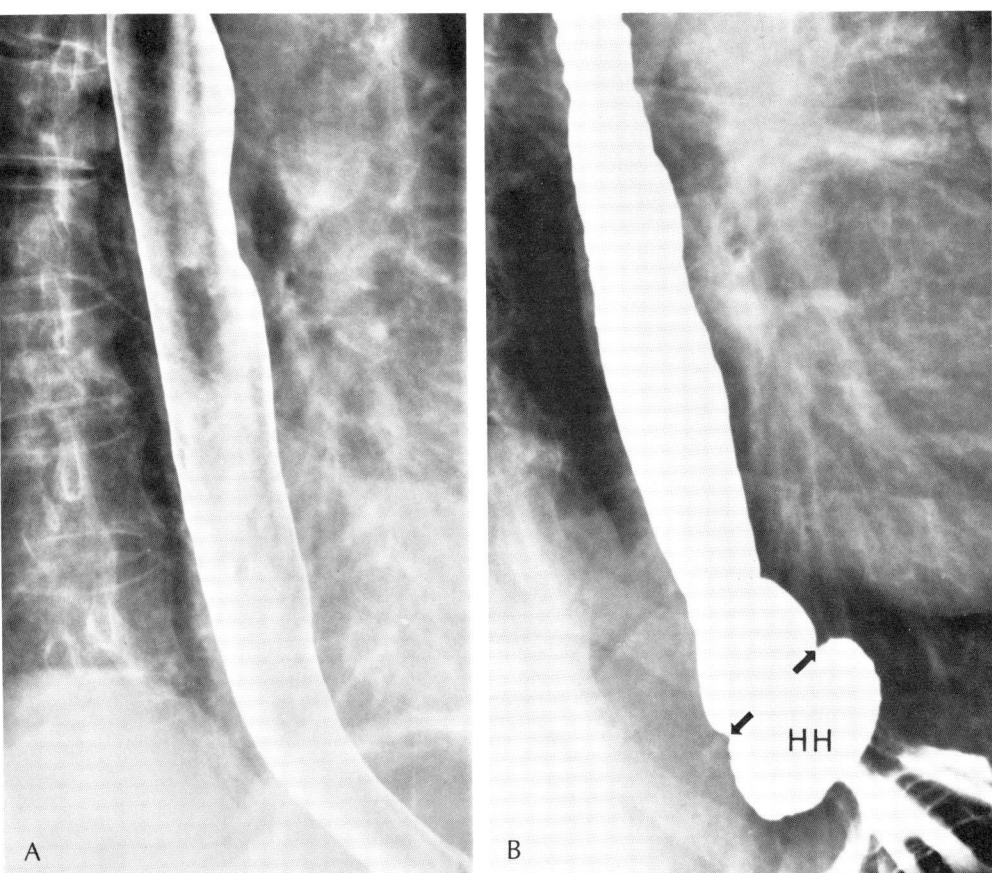

FIG. 9-3. *A,* Upright double-contrast view showing no abnormalities. Hiatal hernia and narrowing of the inferior portion of the esophagus are easily missed in this position. *B,* Examination of the same patient in the prone position, to promote better distention of the esophagogastric region. A lower esophageal mucosal ring (arrows) and hiatal hernia (HH) are visible.

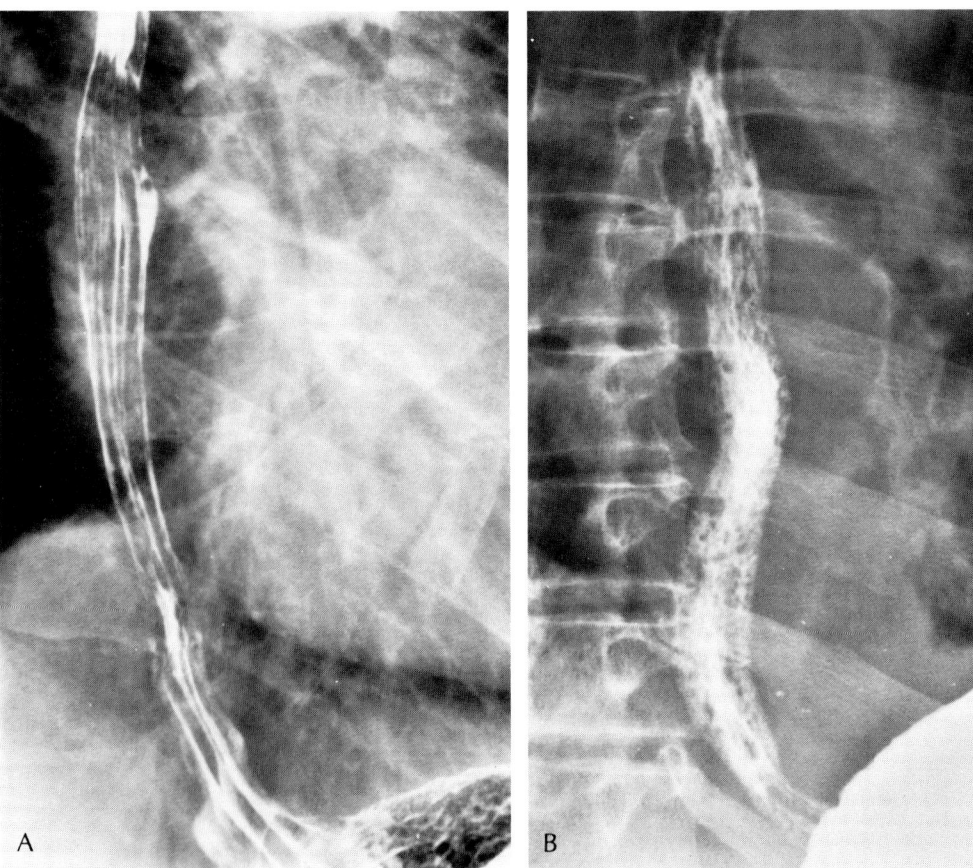

FIG. 9–4. *A,* Mucosal relief view in a patient with moderate endoscopic esophagitis, showing thickening of the esophageal folds. *B,* Mucosal relief view in an immunosuppressed patient with dysphagia, showing diffuse nodularity of the esophageal surface due to candida-induced esophagitis.

needed for the diagnosis of esophageal strictures and rings (Fig. 9-3). Detailed mucosal views are important to detect small neoplasms and subtle inflammatory changes (Fig. 9-4).

Basics of Interpretation

In the esophagus, the most common category of pathologic alteration includes caliber changes and filling defects. Smooth and focal narrowing of the esophagus usually represents benign disease. Peptic stricture is most likely if the narrowing is tapered, whereas a thin, annular narrowing suggests a lower esophageal mucosal ring (Fig. 9-5). Esophageal rings smaller than 12 to 13 mm in caliber are invariably associated with dysphagia. If the narrowing is irregular, esophagitis or carcinoma must be considered (Fig. 9-6).

Lesions protruding into the lumen of the esophagus may be either benign or malignant. A smooth contour and gradual transition to the normal esophageal margin suggests a nonepithelial process, such as a leiomyoma. Surface irregularity and an abrupt transition suggest a malignant tumor, although focal inflammatory disease may have a similar appearance (Fig. 9-6).

Diagnostic Efficacy

The efficacy of the radiologic examination of the esophagus depends on the technical quality and thoroughness of the study and on the specific types of disorders to be detected.[15] Data pertaining to esophageal carcinoma and reflux esophagitis, two important entities, are more complete than for other esophageal disorders. Although the radiographic detection rates for esophageal varices and infectious esophagitis are less thoroughly documented, they are 75% or better; most lower esophageal mucosal rings are accurately diagnosed.[15]

The radiographic detection of esophageal carcinoma in part depends on the size of the lesion. Large, circumferential tumors are easily diagnosed, whereas detection of smaller neoplasms necessitates the use of multiple radiographic techniques, particularly double-contrast and mucosal relief views. When properly performed, radiographic examination of the esophagus enables one to detect virtually all symptomatic esophageal carcinomas.

The ability to diagnose reflux esophagitis radiographically predominantly depends on the severity of the disorder.[16-18] In patients with mild esophagitis, the radiographic examination is generally normal. In those with moderate or severe esophagitis, however, which is manifested endoscopically by marked exudation, erosions, ulceration, or stricture formation, the reported combined rate of radiographic sensitivity is 77 to 91%. In the specific category of peptic esophageal stricture, radiologic reports have detection rates of 95 to 100%.[19]

STOMACH AND DUODENUM

Indications and Preparation

The upper gastrointestinal radiographic series is routinely used to examine the esophagus, stomach, and duodenum. The indications for esophageal examination have been previously discussed. In the stomach and duodenum, radiography is used most commonly to evaluate patients with neoplastic and inflammatory disorders, particularly peptic ulcer disease. Functional disorders of the stomach that cause gastric stasis are best studied with radionuclide imaging methods. Extrinsic processes that may secondarily affect the stomach or duodenum, such as inflammatory and neoplastic disease of the pancreas, are better evaluated with abdominal ultrasound and computed tomography.

Preparation of the patient for the upper gastrointestinal series consists of an overnight fast. The presence of any food or liquid in the stomach adversely affects the quality of the examination. The scheduling of the upper gastrointestinal examination must also be closely co-ordinated with that of other abdominal imaging procedures. The stomach is often filled with water for ultrasonic examination of the pancreas, whereas an aqueous solution containing an iodinated contrast agent is frequently used to opacify the gastrointestinal tract during computed tomography of the abdomen. Consequently, an upper gastrointestinal or small bowel series cannot be performed immediately after these other procedures if fluid has been given to the patient.

Types of Examination

The two primary methods of examining the upper gastrointestinal tract are the single-contrast and the double-contrast examinations. The traditional single-contrast method uses a combination of techniques,[20] including compression and mucosal relief films of the stomach containing only a small amount of barium, views of the stomach and duodenum after further distention with barium, and limited double-contrast filming using the air that is naturally present (Fig. 9-7). A barium sulfate suspension of moderate density is used. If necessary, a peroral examination of the small bowel can easily follow a single-contrast upper gastrointestinal series because the density of the barium used for these two examinations is usually identical.

The double-contrast examination of the upper gastrointestinal tract differs from the single-contrast study.[21,22] A specifically formulated high-density barium suspension is used, along with a gas-producing substance that generates a large volume of carbon

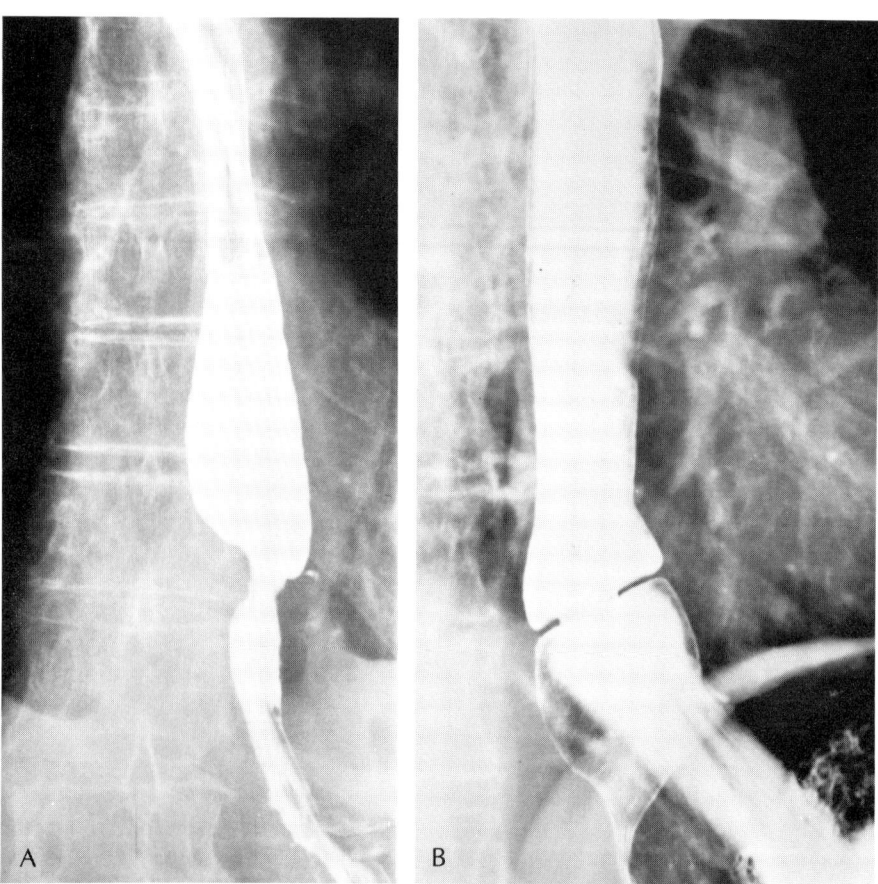

FIG. 9–5. *A,* Smooth, tapered narrowing at the inferior end of the esophagus caused by a peptic stricture. *B,* Thin, annular mucosal ring at the esophagogastric junction in a patient with dysphagia.

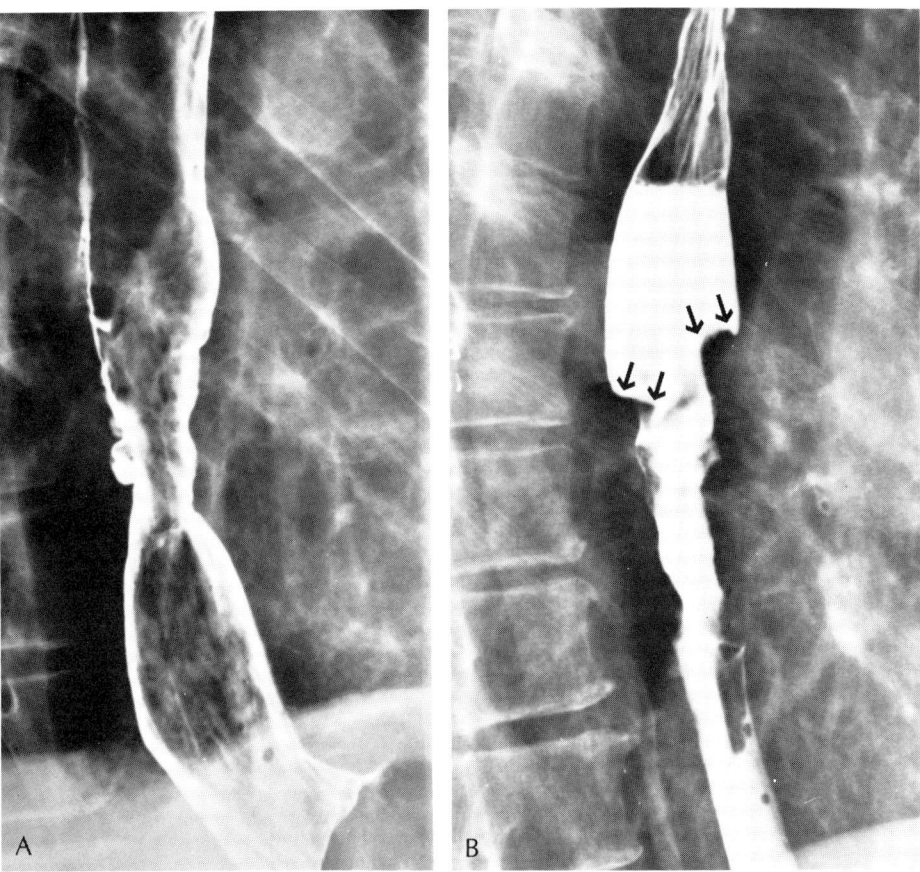

FIG. 9–6. *A,* Peptic esophageal stricture with irregularity from ulceration and pseudodiverticular formation. *B,* Annular carcinoma of the esophagus, showing abrupt margins (arrows) and surface irregularity due to mucosal destruction.

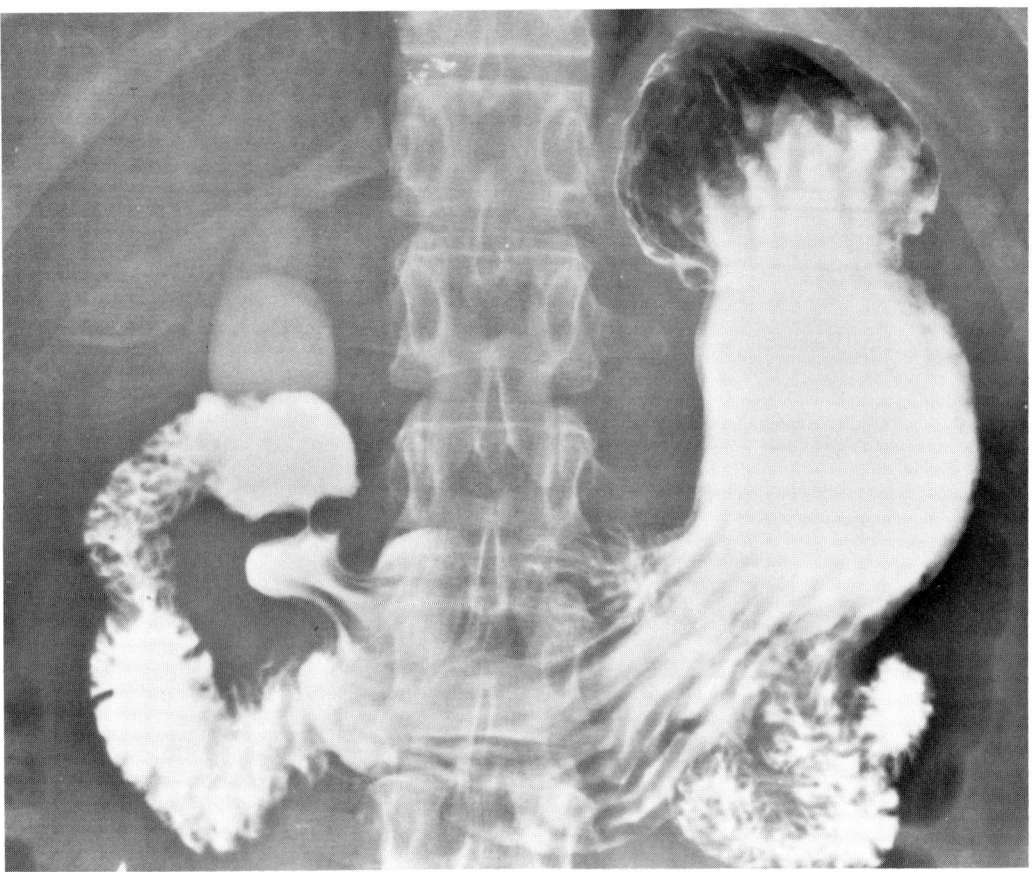

FIG. 9–7. Prone view of the stomach and duodenum from a single-contrast examination. Only a small amount of air is present in the fundus of the stomach. The gallbladder is also opacified.

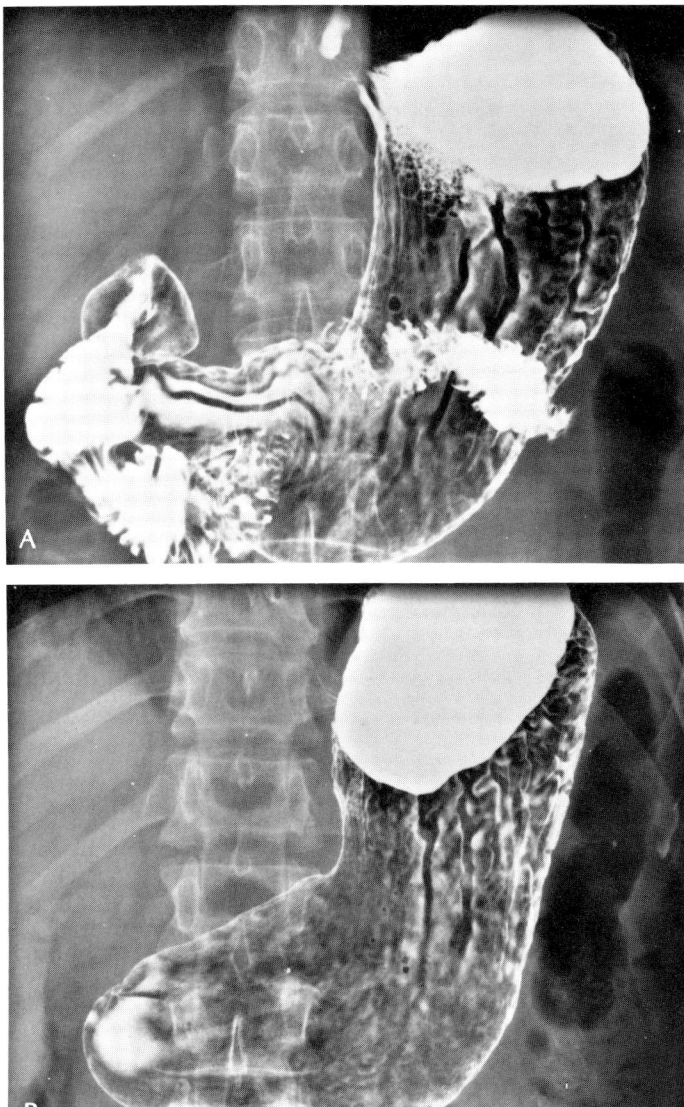

FIG. 9–8. *A*, Supine view of the stomach and duodenum from a double-contrast examination. A hypotonic agent was not used, and portions of the stomach are obscured by barium in the duodenum. *B*, Similar double-contrast view in another patient who received 0.2 mg glucagon intravenously. The stomach is clearly visualized because filling of the duodenum has been delayed by the gastric hypotonia.

dioxide. A hypotonic agent, such as glucagon, is often given intravenously, to promote relaxation and further gaseous distention (Fig. 9–8). Each segment of the stomach and duodenum must be filmed in double-contrast relief because the high density of the barium used in this study otherwise obscures lesions. Compression filming of the stomach and duodenum has been incorporated into the double-contrast method. This combination has become known as the "multiphasic" or "biphasic" examination of the upper gastrointestinal tract.

Examination of the postoperative stomach can be performed by any of the previously described methods. In recent years, however, the hypotonic double-contrast examination has been advocated because of better distention of the gastric remnant and improved delineation of the surgical anastomosis (Fig. 9–9).

Technical Problems

The upper gastrointestinal series is well tolerated by most patients. The examination is more difficult to perform in debilitated and immobile patients and in those unable to retain the barium or the generated gas. Under these circumstances, the single-contrast examination is recommended because it is more easily performed and is less subject to degradation of quality if conditions are not optimal.

Before allowing the patient to leave the fluoroscopic area, one should review each film from the examination. Films of poor quality should be repeated, and questionable abnormalities should be confirmed by additional fluoroscopic observation and filming. Technical difficulties arise more often during the double-contrast examination than during the single-contrast study. If coating with the high-density barium is suboptimal, as occurs in the presence of excessive gastric secretions, or if much of the gas is eructated, the quality of the double-contrast examination will be compromised.

Basics of Interpretation

In the stomach and duodenum, pathologic alterations are most frequently either projecting lesions or filling defects. Although extrinsic disorders may secondarily involve either organ, the observed changes are often nonspecific. Pancreatic inflammatory and neoplastic diseases are the most common extrinsic processes that secondarily involve the stomach and duodenum. The radiographic manifestations of functional disorders of the gastroduodenal segment are poorly understood.

Gastric erosions may appear as punctate collections of barium (Fig. 9–10), whereas peptic ulcers appear as larger collections. A gastric ulcer is most likely to be benign if it projects from the gastric lumen, if it has a thin collar of edema at its neck, and if it is surrounded by normal-appearing gastric mucosa (Fig. 9–11). The absence of one or more of these signs increases the likelihood of malignant gastric ulceration. The radiographic diagnosis of duodenal peptic ulcer is based on the visualization of a constant, reproducible barium collection seen as a crater en face or as a niche in profile (Fig. 9–12). Diverticula are rare in the stomach, but they are common in the duodenum, particularly along the medial aspect of the descending portion. Their changeable size and shape and the presence of mucosal folds within the diverticula distinguish them from ulcerations.

Benign gastric polyps are usually hyperplastic or adenomatous in origin[23] (Fig. 9–13). Polyps in the stomach that are under 2 cm in size are nearly always benign.[24] Adenocarcinoma accounts for 95% of all primary malignant gastric tumors, whereas lymphoma and leiomyosarcoma comprise most of the remainder. The morphologic spectrum of adenocarcinoma includes ulcerative, polypoid (Fig. 9–14), fungating, and infiltrative forms. Each form must be differentiated from other benign or malignant gastric processes. For example, an ulcerative carcinoma may resemble a benign gastric ulcer; a polypoid carcinoma may be indistinguishable from

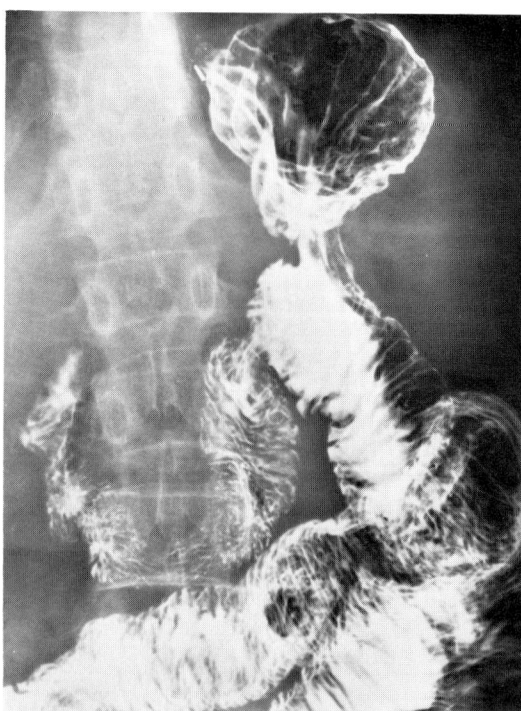

FIG. 9–9. Double-contrast postoperative examination of the stomach showing excellent distention of the gastric remnant and visualization of the afferent and efferent limbs of the gastrojejunostomy.

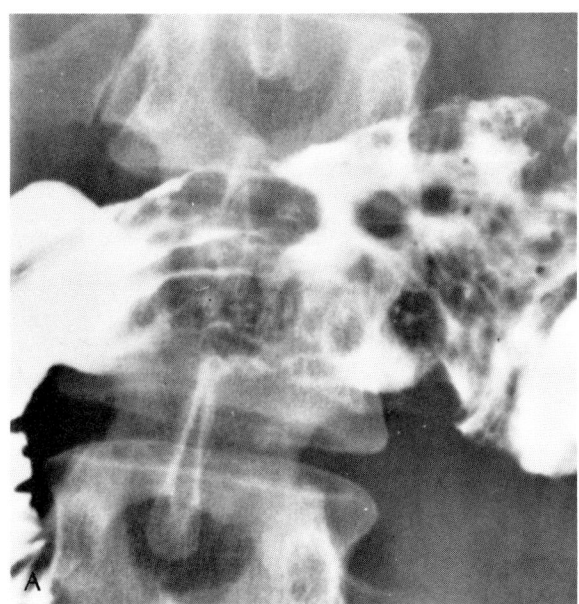
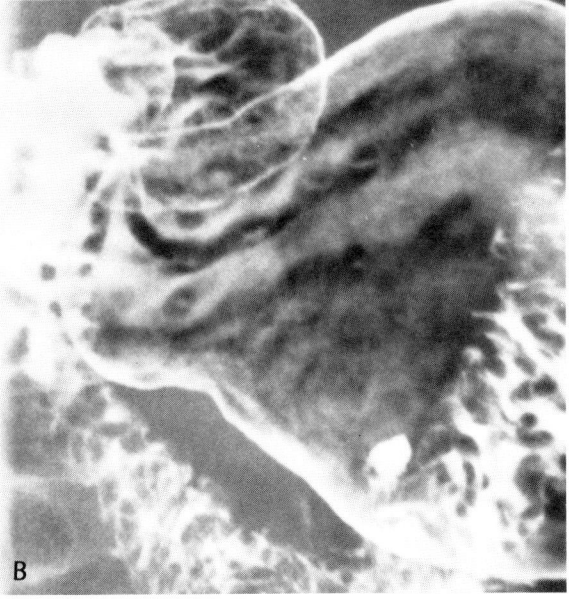

FIG. 9-10. Gastric erosions may be seen as nodular defects, particularly on compression films *(A)*, or as punctate collections of barium *(B)*. (From Ott, D.J., et al.: Sensitivity of single- vs. double-contrast radiology in erosive gastritis. AJR, *138*:263, 1982.)

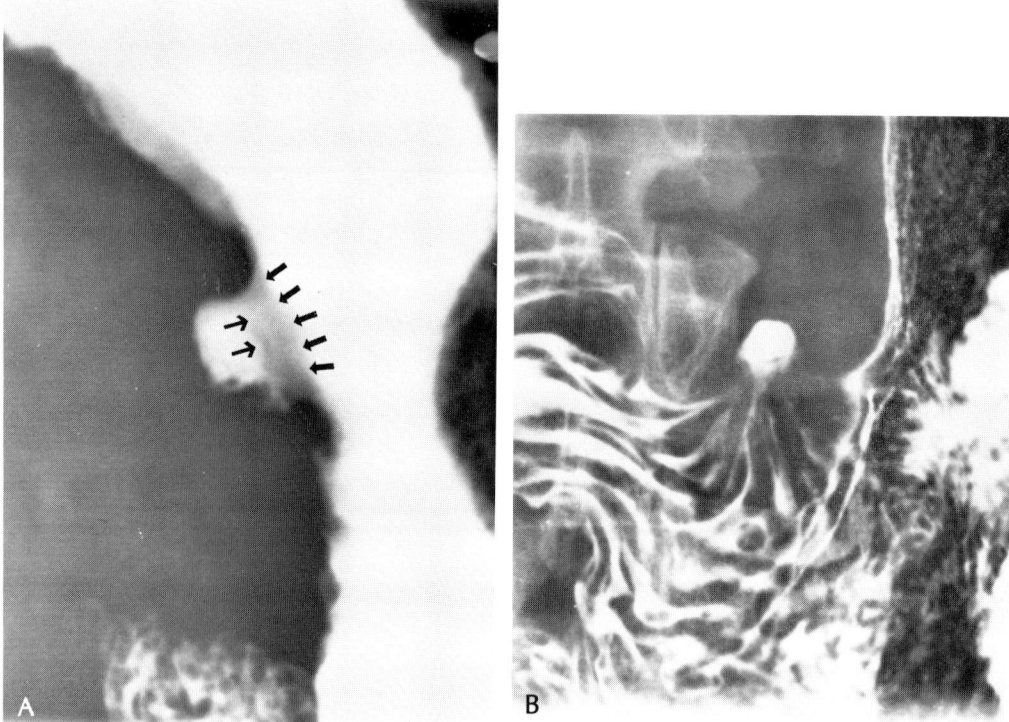

FIG. 9–11. *A,* Close-up view of the lesser curvature of the stomach, showing a penetrating gastric ulcer with a lucent edematous collar (arrows). *B,* Penetrating gastric ulcer along the lesser curvature of the antrum. The adjacent rugal folds are smooth and symmetric, and they radiate to the edge of the ulcer.

a benign adenoma or leiomyoma. Polypoid lesions of the duodenum are rare, and those arising in the duodenal bulb are benign. Carcinoma of the duodenum typically occurs at or distal to the periampullary region and usually appears as a polypoid, fungating, or annular lesion.

Diagnostic Efficacy

The efficacy of the upper gastrointestinal series depends on many factors, including equipment and materials, quality control and careful reading of the study, expertise of the examiner, type of examination, and type of disease. The patient's physical condition and ability to co-operate are also important factors. In debilitated and immobile individuals, the upper gastrointestinal series is often limited, and the propensity for error is greater than in other patients.

Careful fluoroscopic observation of the patient and meticulous review of the study are necessary to ensure that films are of optimal quality. Regardless of the method, each film must be closely scrutinized, and portions of the study should be repeated if needed. Any areas of abnormality should be clarified before the patient is allowed to leave the examining area. Meticulous interpretation of films of optimal quality is necessary to avoid radiologic errors.[25]

Other determinants of diagnostic efficacy of the upper gastrointestinal series are the type of examination and the particular disease. Quantitative data on the radiographic detection of erosive gastritis, gastric ulcer, gastric carcinoma, and duodenal ulcer are sufficient to warrant discussion. Erosive gastritis is poorly visualized with any type of radiographic method. Although the double-contrast examination may be more reliable, its reported rate of sensitivity is still no better than 57%.[26]

The reported sensitivity rate in the detection of gastric ulcer averages 85% for single-contrast radiography, as compared to 76% for double-contrast radiography.[27] The size of a gastric ulcer appears to be a more important determinant of radiographic visualization than the specific technique. In one series, only 48% of gastric ulcers under 5 mm in size were detected, whereas 81% of those over 5 mm were diagnosed; the detection rates were independent of the method used.[28]

Gastric carcinoma is usually detectable during any properly performed examination of the stomach. The reported rate of sensitivity for the single-contrast method averages 92%, as compared to 89% for double-contrast radiography.[27] Thus, these data suggest that the double-contrast examination has no substantial advantage over the single-contrast

MESENTERIC SMALL BOWEL

Indications and Preparation

The indications for radiographic examination of the mesenteric small bowel can be categorized as either nonspecific or specific. This distinction is important because the diagnostic yield is related to the reasons for ordering the examination.[30,31] When a patient has no specific signs or symptoms referable to the small bowel, pertinent radiographic abnormalities are seldom found. Such nonspecific signs include nausea, vomiting, diffuse abdominal pain, diarrhea, and constipation. Conversely, a higher diagnostic yield is obtained when the reasons for performing the study include a history of small bowel disease, fistula localization, obstruction, adhesions, trauma, and involvement of the small bowel by mass, metastases, or local tumor invasion.

Preparation for the peroral examination of the small bowel is identical to that for the upper gastrointestinal series. For other types of small bowel examinations, however, colon cleansing may be required, particularly if a retrograde study is performed by refluxing barium from the colon. Moreover, examination of the small bowel by enteroclysis is facilitated by cleansing of the colon.

Types of Examination

The three general types of examination of the small bowel are the peroral, intubated, and retrograde studies. The peroral examination requires the ingestion of 16 to 24 oz of a dense barium suspension.[32] Serial films of the abdomen are obtained at 30-min intervals for 2 hours and then hourly if necessary. Once the barium has reached the colon, compression films of the entire abdomen are taken under fluoroscopic control, to separate and to visualize all the loops of small bowel (Fig. 9–16). Metoclopramide administration is sometimes useful, to accelerate the passage of barium through the small bowel.

Direct injection of barium through an indwelling tube is another method for examining the small bowel. In enteroclysis, a variation of this technique, the patient swallows a special tube, such as a Bilbao-Dotter tube, that can be stiffened with a guidewire.[33] Under fluoroscopic control, the tip of the tube is manipulated into the jejunum. This technique permits controlled instillation of a dilute barium suspension. The study is monitored fluoroscopically, and sequential films are taken as the loops of small bowel fill with barium (Fig. 9–17). With enteroclysis, distention and visualization of the small bowel are better than with the peroral examination.

Finally, various techniques are available for retrograde examination of the small bowel. The barium enema can be used to examine the ileum by the

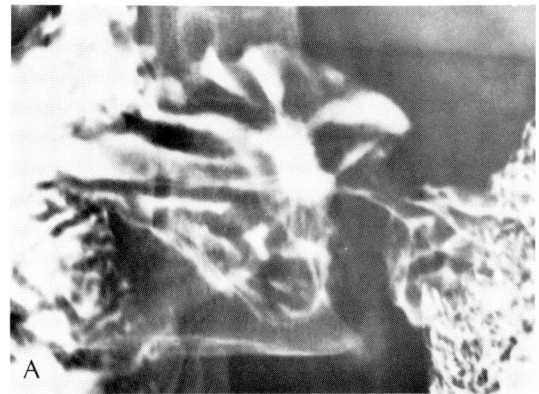

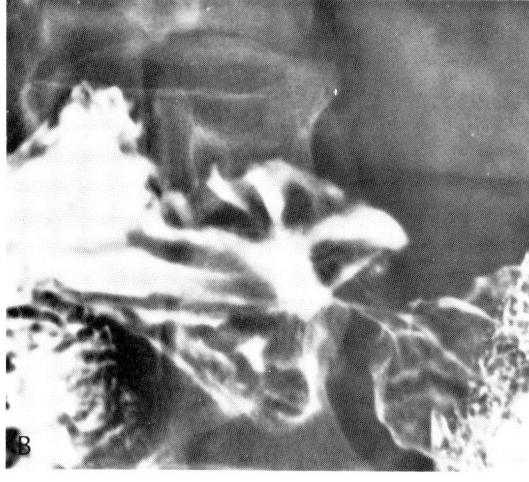

FIG. 9–12. A and B, Two views of the duodenal bulb, showing a constant collection of barium associated with radiating mucosal folds. The unchanging nature of the collection supports the radiographic diagnosis of duodenal ulcer.

method in the diagnosis of gastric ulcer and carcinoma.

Although the double-contrast method has been advocated for examination of the postoperative stomach, few data are available to support its proposed superiority over the single-contrast method. In one comparative study, neither technique had a clear advantage in showing reflux gastritis, recurrent ulceration, and anastomotic obstruction.[29]

The reported rate of sensitivity in the detection of duodenal ulcer averages 79% for the single-contrast method, as compared to 77% for the double-contrast method.[27] This finding suggests that the radiographic detection of duodenal ulcer depends on factors other than the type of examination. Certainly, two important factors are the size of the ulcer and the presence or absence of duodenal deformity. Small duodenal ulcers in deformed duodenal bulbs are poorly shown radiographically, regardless of technique (Fig. 9–15).

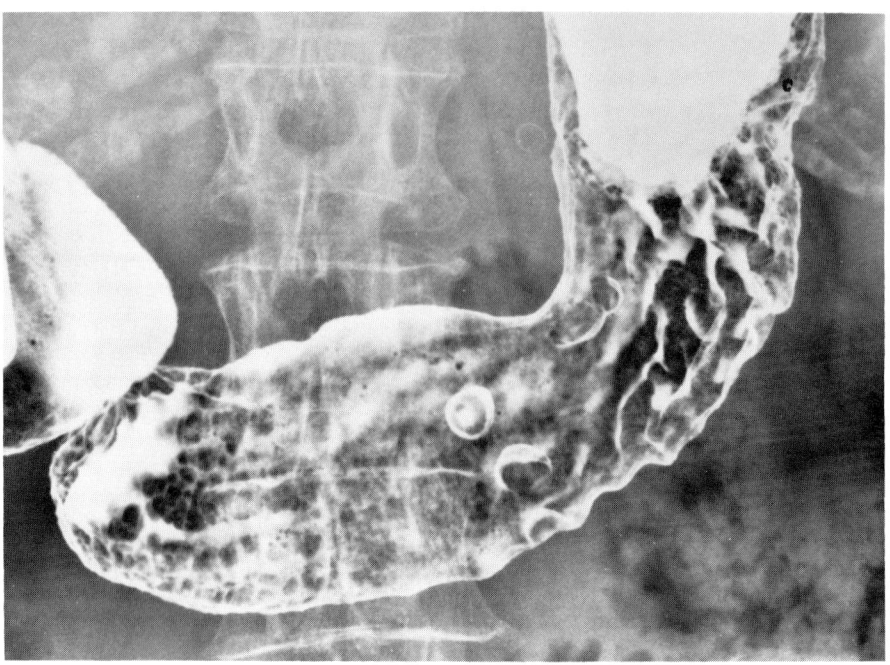

FIG. 9–13. Double-contrast view, showing multiple gastric polyps in the midbody of the stomach. Pathologic examination of several of these polyps showed a hyperplastic origin.

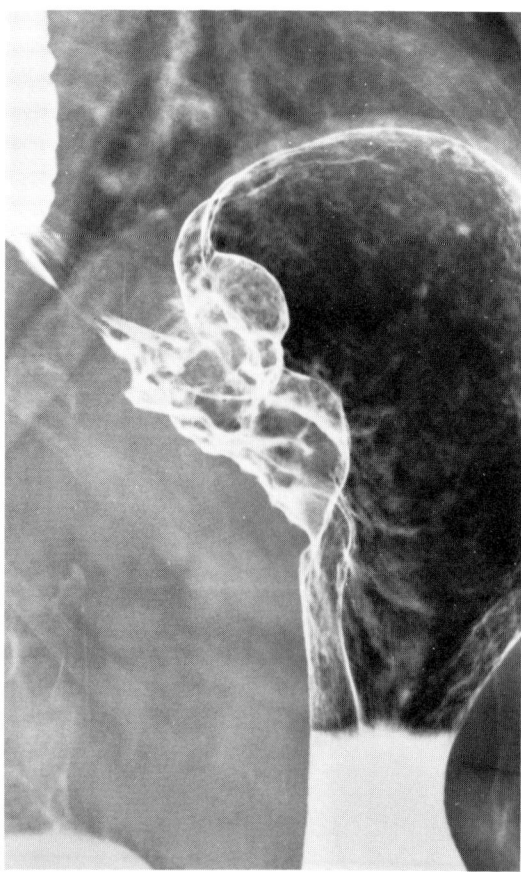

FIG. 9–14. Polypoid carcinoma of the gastric cardia invading the esophagogastric region. The patient's initial complaint was dysphagia, which is common with gastric carcinoma that secondarily involves the esophagus.

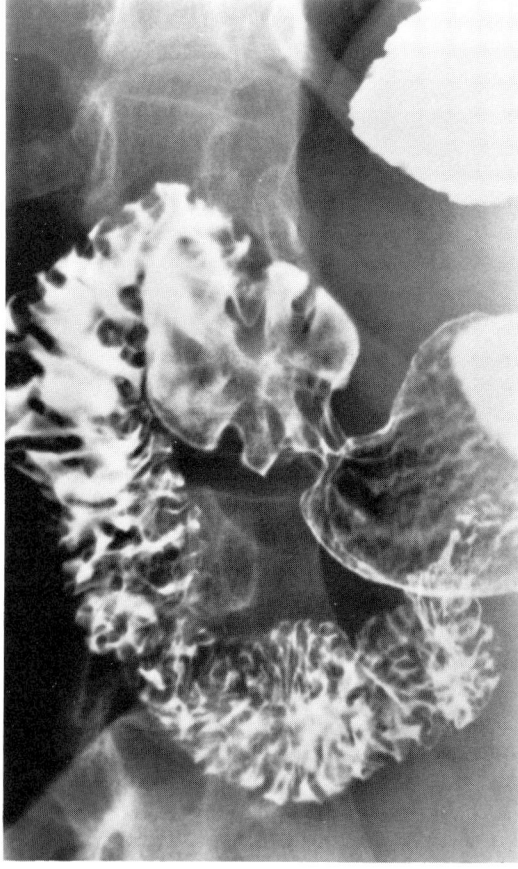

FIG. 9–15. Deformity of the duodenal bulb indicative of chronic peptic ulcer disease. This deformity adversely affects the reliability of the radiographic method for diagnosing or excluding acute ulceration.

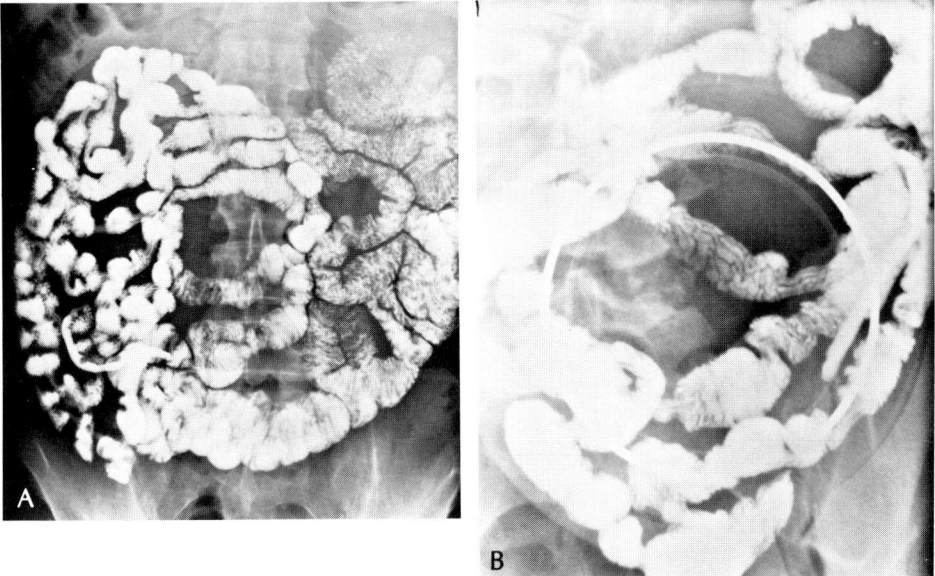

FIG. 9–16. A, Peroral examination of the small bowel at one hour, showing complete filling of the jejunum and ileum. B, Compression film in the same patient, clearly showing several small bowel loops.

reflux of barium through the ileocecal valve. If a colostomy or an ileostomy is present, retrograde filling can be accomplished with any number of commercial devices designed for this purpose.

Radiographic examination of the patient with possible intestinal obstruction warrants special comment. The decision to perform a contrast examination is based primarily on the clinical presentation and on the findings on plain film radiography of the abdomen.[34] If obstruction of the colon or distal small bowel is suspected, a barium enema will be the procedure of choice. This study permits not only examination of the colon, but also, in the absence of colonic obstruction, retrograde filling of the ileum, to assess the distal small bowel for a cause of obstruction (Fig. 9–18). If more proximal obstruction of the small bowel is suspected, and if the clinical and radiographic signs indicate that the colon is not obstructed, barium may be given orally or through an indwelling small bowel tube. The large amounts of fluid present in patients with obstruction of the small bowel prevent inspissation and impaction of barium in that location.[35,36]

Technical Problems

The peroral examination of the small bowel is well tolerated by most patients. Its major disadvantage is the time required to complete the study; the average is 1 to 2 hours. Enteroclysis is often a quicker method of small bowel examination, but it involves the discomfort of intubation. In a minority of patients, enteroclysis is unsuccessful either because of this discomfort or because of difficulty in passing the tube through the pyloric channel. Retrograde examination of the small bowel may cause discomfort similar to that experienced with the barium enema, and glucagon administration may be helpful.

The length of the small bowel and its many overlapping loops are largely responsible for the technical difficulties encountered when examining this organ radiographically. The small bowel must be adequately distended, and each loop must be clearly visualized. The barium suspensions should be stable and should effectively coat the small bowel surface. If flocculation occurs or if the barium coating is poor, the quality and usefulness of the examination will be compromised.

Basics of Interpretation

Diseases of the mesenteric small bowel are rare. Diverticula are occasionally seen and are similar in appearance to those in the duodenum. Polypoid lesions and primary malignant tumors also resemble their counterparts in the stomach and colon. Inflammatory disease and extrinsic involvement of the small bowel are more common.

Crohn's disease and radiation-induced enteritis are two important inflammatory disorders that affect the small bowel (Fig. 9–19). Crohn's disease causes diffuse narrowing associated with transverse and longitudinal ulceration; the ileum is the most common site of involvement. Radiation-induced injury to the small bowel usually occurs in women treated for

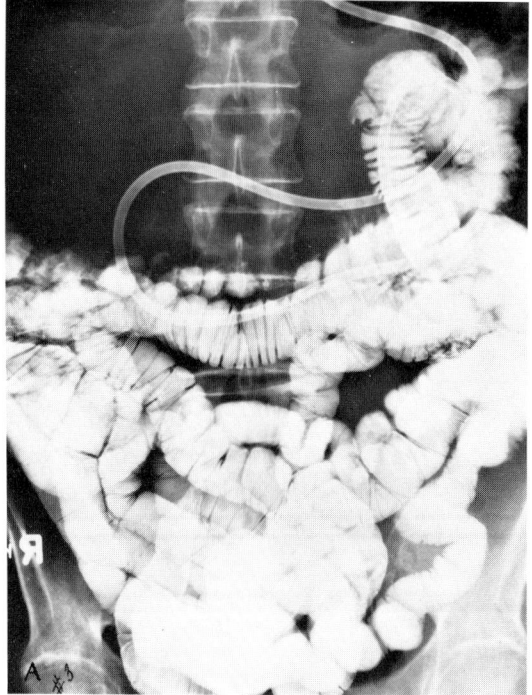

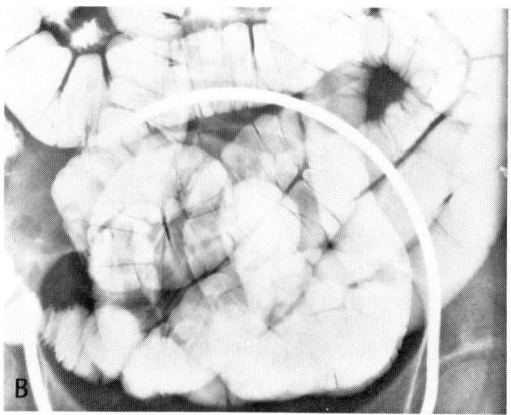

FIG. 9–17. *A*, Enteroclysis examination of the small bowel. The tip of the Bilbao-Dotter tube has been fluoroscopically manipulated into the jejunum. *B*, Compression film during an enteroclysis examination, with excellent distention and visualization of the small loops deep in the pelvis.

malignant pelvic tumors and may mimic Crohn's disease radiographically.

The small bowel is also frequently involved by extrinsic processes. Metastatic disease typically causes multiple polypoid lesions or focal disease with angulation of the bowel lumen (Fig. 9–20). Intraperitoneal spread of tumor or infection may involve the serosal surface of the small bowel. Finally, peritoneal adhesions may be detectable, especially with enteroclysis. The spectrum of appearances of adhesions includes crossing bands narrowing the lumen, angulation of the bowel wall, tented stretching of the mucosal folds, and tacking together of adjacent loops of small bowel (Fig. 9–21).

Diagnostic Efficacy

Few quantitative data are available on the efficacy of radiology of the mesenteric small bowel. The main reasons for this lack of information are the relative rarity of diseases of the small bowel and the inaccessibility of the organ to endoscopic examination. Thus, surgical documentation often determines radiographic efficacy in retrospect.

In recent years, interest has been directed toward the effectiveness of enteroclysis, particularly in comparison to the peroral examination. The efficacy of any examination of the small bowel, however, depends on many factors,[37] as discussed previously with regard to the upper gastrointestinal series of radiographs. Proper barium suspensions must be used, frequent filming is necessary, and compression of the entire small bowel must be thorough.

The type of disease to be detected is also an important consideration. Widespread disorders, such as Crohn's disease or diffuse radiation-induced enteritis, are readily diagnosed during any type of properly performed examination of the small bowel. Conversely, focal diseases, including neoplasms, Meckel's diverticulum, and adhesions, are more difficult to detect. Enteroclysis is more effective than the peroral method in showing Meckel's diverticulum and peritoneal adhesions.[38,39]

LARGE BOWEL

Indications and Preparation

The radiographic examination of the colon can be used to evaluate colonic obstruction, diverticular disease, and neoplastic or inflammatory lesions. The distal small bowel may be evaluated if barium refluxes through the ileocecal valve. Extrinsic diseases secondarily affecting the colon may also be assessed.

Preparation of the patient for the barium enema examination involves thorough colon cleansing.[40,41] Proper preparation of the large bowel necessitates dietary manipulation, the use of one or more cathartic agents, and cleansing enemas preceding the barium examination. If severe colitis or colonic obstruction is suspected, the bowel preparation can be changed or dismissed, as clinically indicated.

Types of Examination

The two primary means of examining the colon are single-contrast and double-contrast studies. The traditional single-contrast method is performed by filling the colon with a dilute barium suspension.[42] Compression films are taken of each segment of the

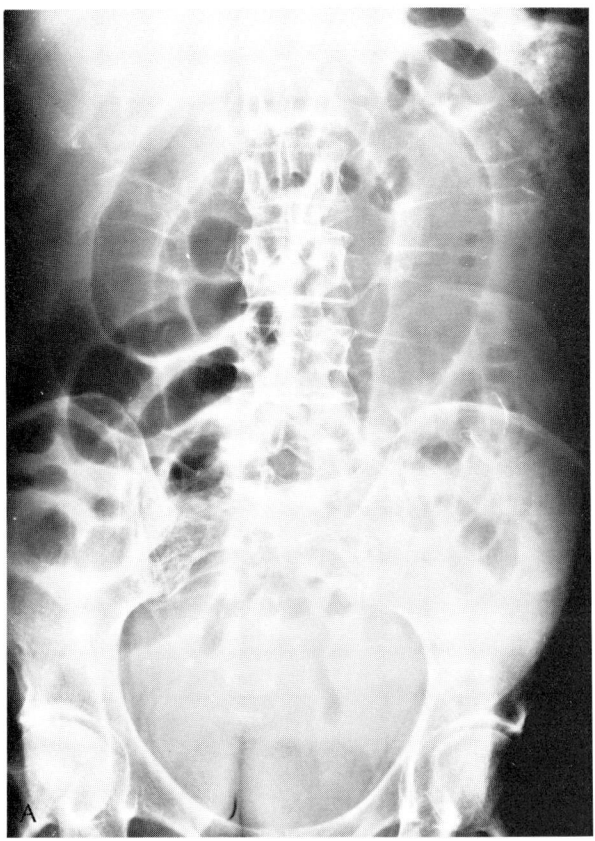 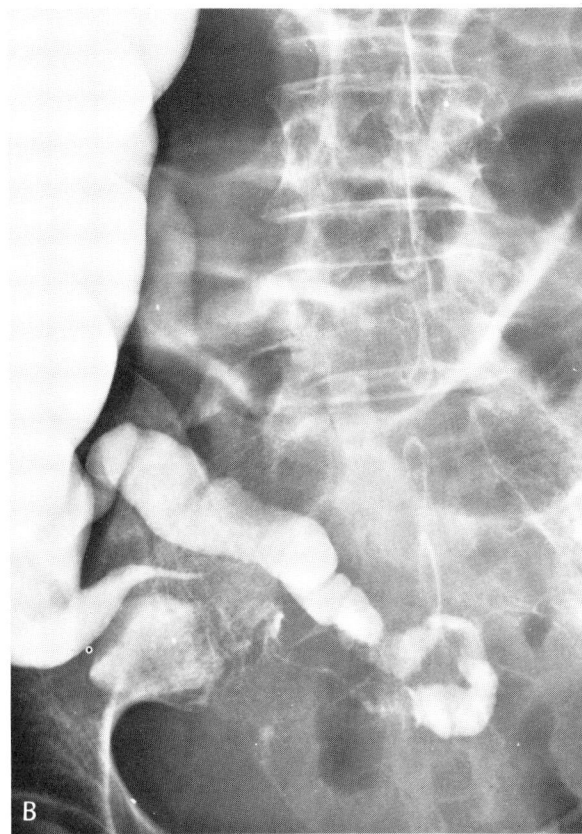

FIG. 9–18. A, Plain abdominal film showing gaseous distention of the small bowel and increased soft tissue density in the pelvis in a patient with advanced ovarian carcinoma. B, Retrograde small bowel examination through a colostomy enema, with angular narrowing of the ileum that represents carcinomatous involvement obstructing the distal small bowel.

colon. The patient must be appropriately turned, to allow clear visualization of any redundant areas, such as the sigmoid colon and the colonic flexures. A routine set of films is obtained with the patient in various positions and should include a lateral view of the rectum (Fig. 9–22).

The double-contrast examination of the colon differs from the single-contrast method.[22] One uses a dense, viscous barium suspension and a specially designed enema tip that permits easy instillation of air and barium into the colon. Glucagon is usually given intravenously, to promote relaxation and distention of the colon. Each segment of the colon must be seen in double-contrast relief because the density of the barium used to perform this examination may obscure lesions (Fig. 9–23). During the double-contrast barium enema, the patient must move frequently, to distribute the barium and air, and must therefore be mobile and co-operative.

The double-contrast examination should be performed in patients with suspected inflammatory or neoplastic disease of the colon. In older and debilitated patients, or when colonic obstruction is likely, a single-contrast examination is usually sufficient. If colonic perforation is suspected, as in patients with diverticulitis, a water-soluble contrast enema can be administered.

Technical Problems

The degree of discomfort from the barium enema varies among patients. Most patients tolerate the procedure with little difficulty, particularly if glucagon has been given. In older patients with poor rectal tone, however, the procedure may be strenuous, and the barium enema may not be adequately retained. Under these circumstances, the single-contrast examination is recommended because it can be more easily and quickly performed.

As with the upper gastrointestinal series, all the films from the barium enema examination need to be reviewed before the patient may be allowed to evacuate the colon. Questionable abnormalities should be confirmed, and poor-quality films should be repeated (Fig. 9–24). The double-contrast examination is more prone to technical difficulties than the single-contrast study. Small polyps and early inflammatory disease can be easily missed on the double-contrast examination if the colon is poorly

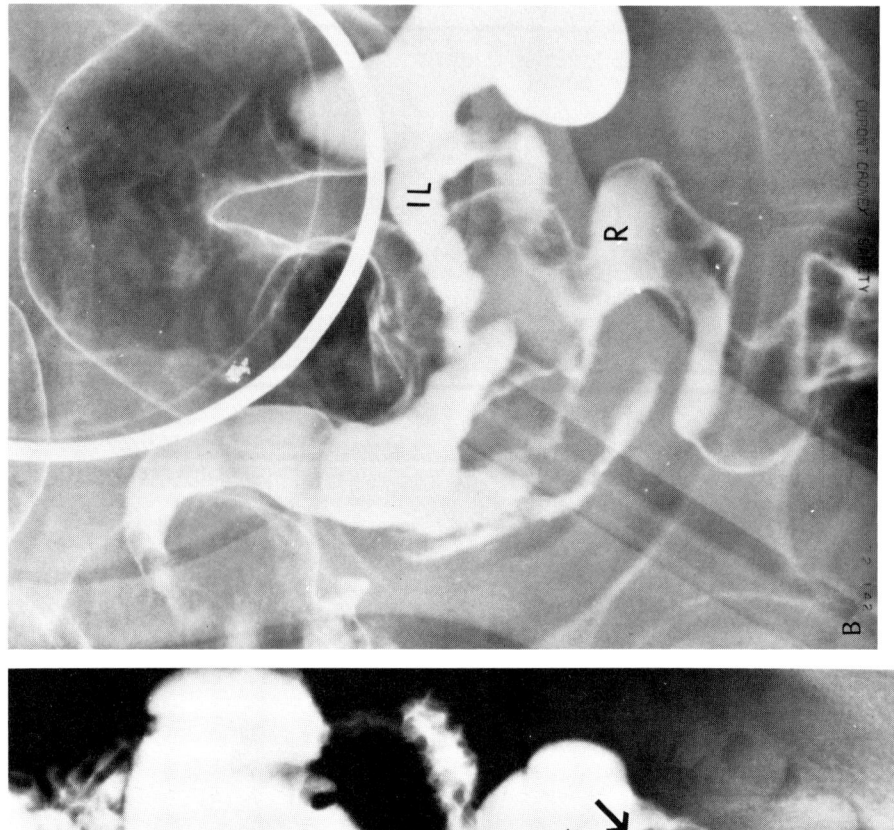
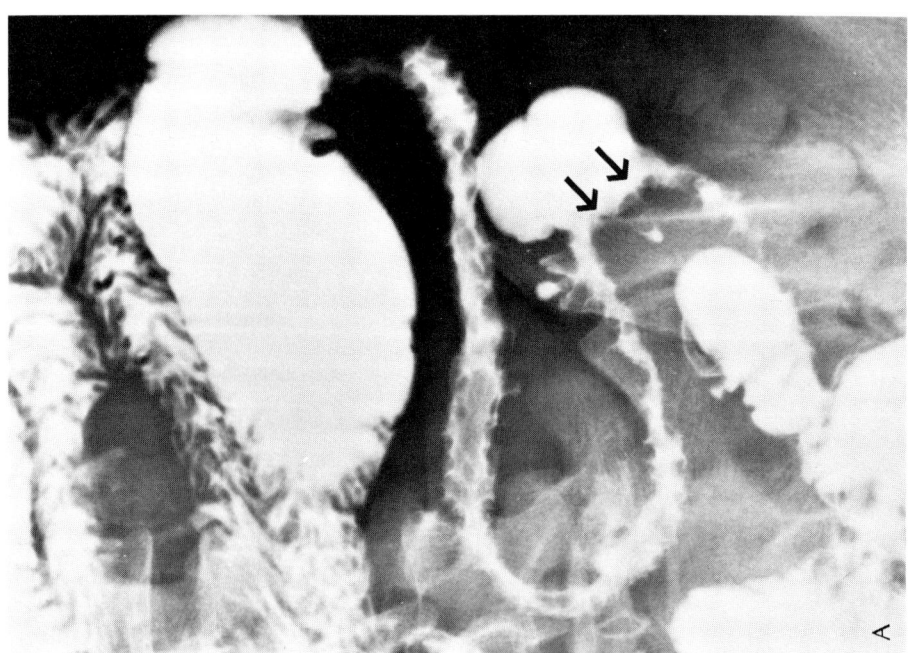

FIG. 9-19. *A*, Crohn's disease of the small bowel manifested by narrowing and nodularity due to transverse and longitudinal ulceration. Eccentric bowel wall involvement (arrows) is also characteristic. *B*, Radiation-induced proctitis (R) and ileitis (IL) shown on a double-contrast barium enema study, with ileal reflux in a patient treated for Stage IIIB carcinoma of the cervix.

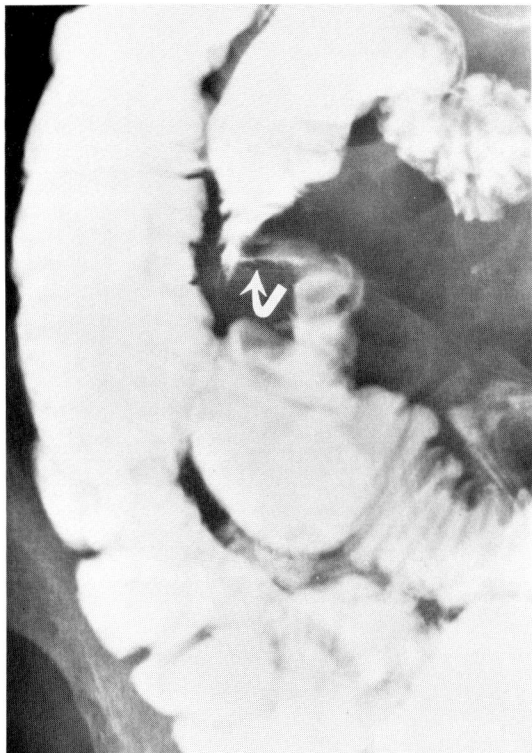

FIG. 9-20. Angular narrowing of the small bowel (arrow) from metastatic carcinoma of the lung.

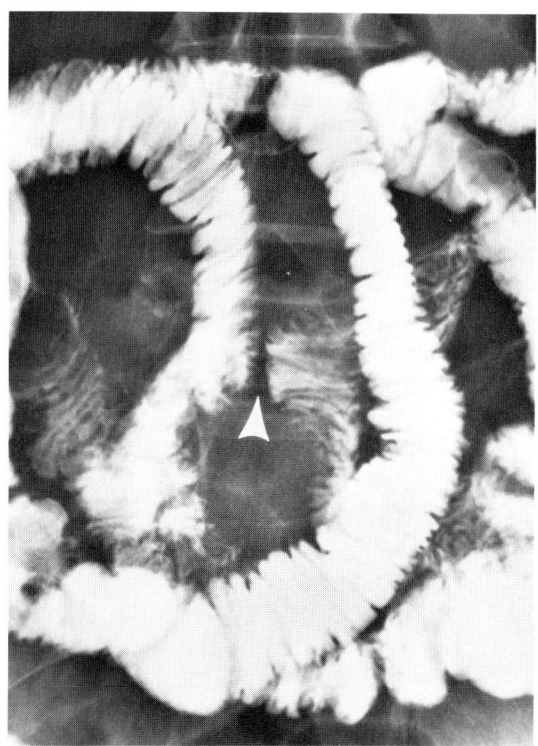

FIG. 9-21. Compression film of the small bowel during an enteroclysis examination. Two adjacent loops of small bowel are tacked together because of peritoneal adhesions (arrowhead).

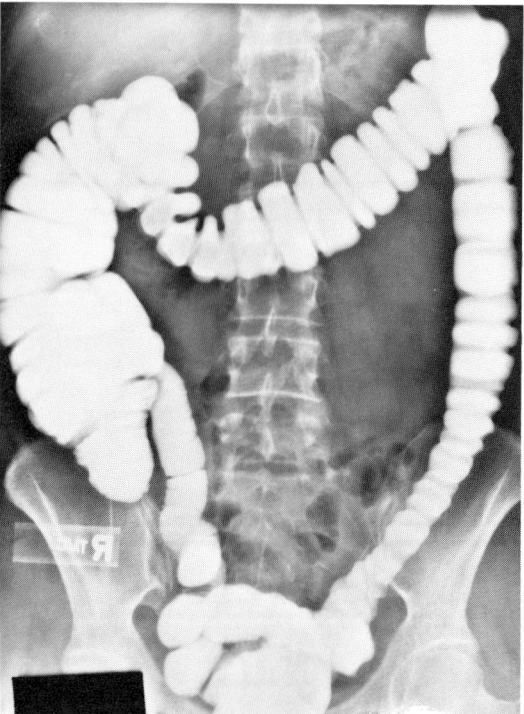

FIG. 9–22. Supine film from a single-contrast examination of the colon with reflux of the terminal ileum.

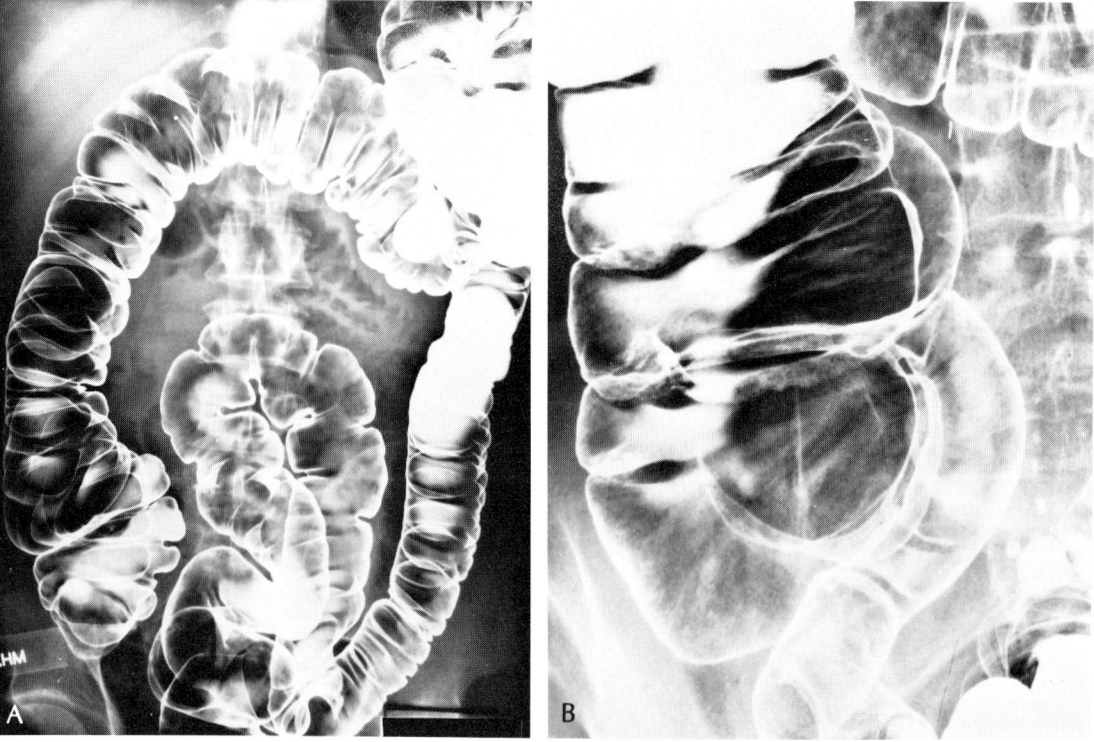

FIG. 9–23. *A*, Supine film from a double-contrast barium enema, showing most of the colon uniformly coated with barium and distended with air. *B*, Double-contrast view of the cecum and ascending colon, with excellent visualization of the terminal ileum.

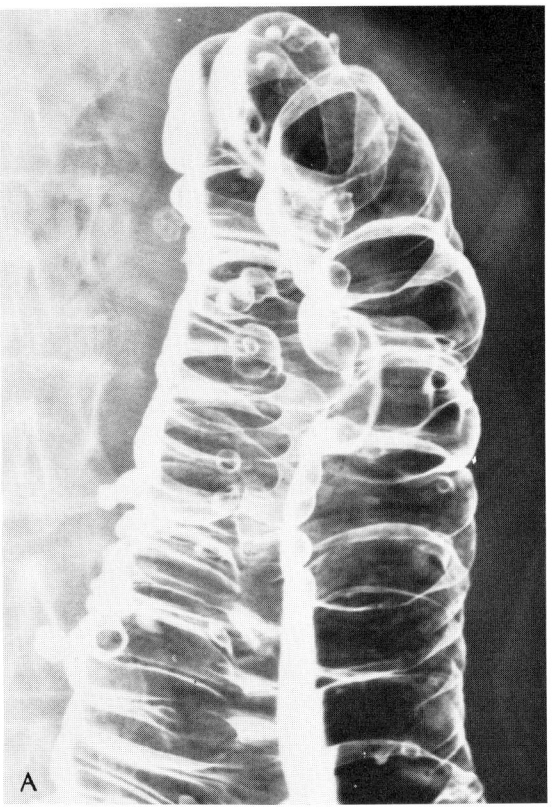 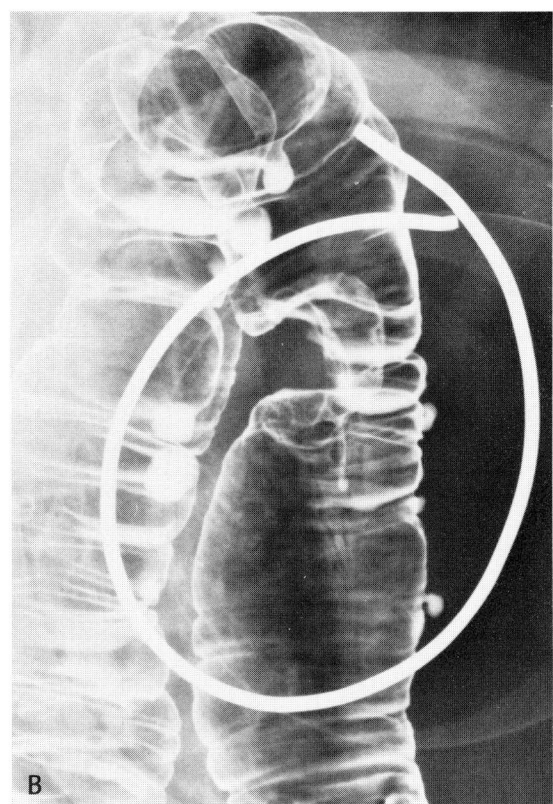

FIG. 9–24. *A*, Double-contrast view of the splenic flexure, showing multiple diverticula. The overlapping segments of colon necessitate further examination, however. *B*, Oblique, compression view of the same area, clearly showing polypoid carcinoma.

coated with barium and is inadequately distended with air.

Basics of Interpretation

Pathologic alterations of the colon most commonly are either projecting lesions or filling defects. The colon may be secondarily affected by extrinsic disorders, and displacement or invasion of the rectum and sigmoid colon by a pelvic mass, such as an ovarian cyst, is most common. Pelvic ultrasound and computed tomography are more useful than radiography in determining the specific nature of a pelvic mass, however.

Diverticular disease most commonly affects the sigmoid colon. Its two pathologic components are muscular thickening and pulsion diverticula that project through the vascular clefts of the colonic wall. The muscle thickening often appears radiographically as lucent bands crossing the colonic lumen and as marginal corrugation. Diverticulitis results from perforation of a diverticulum, with subsequent paracolic abscess formation. The radiographic signs of diverticulitis include contrast extravasation into the abscess, eccentric mass effect (Fig. 9–25), intramural or pelvic fistulization, acute obstruction, and stricture formation.

Inflammatory diseases of the colon most often are idiopathic, infectious, drug related, or induced by radiation. These disorders are usually associated with ulceration and may be indistinguishable from each other. The early radiographic findings in the idiopathic colitides include diffuse granularity in ulcerative colitis (Fig. 9–26) and discrete "aphthoid" ulceration in Crohn's disease (Fig. 9–27). These early changes are well demonstrated and are easily differentiated by examining the results of the double-contrast barium enema. In patients with more severe colitis, the ulcerations are larger and more confluent and are readily shown by either type of radiographic examination of the colon.

Colonic filling defects vary from small, benign, polypoid lesions to larger, malignant masses and annular carcinomas. Nearly all colonic polyps arise from the epithelium and are of hyperplastic or adenomatous origin.[43] The size of the lesion and the presence or absence of pedunculation are the most important radiographic criteria in estimating the risk of malignancy of a colonic polyp.[22,43–46] Polyps under 1 cm in size have only a 1 to 2% chance of harboring

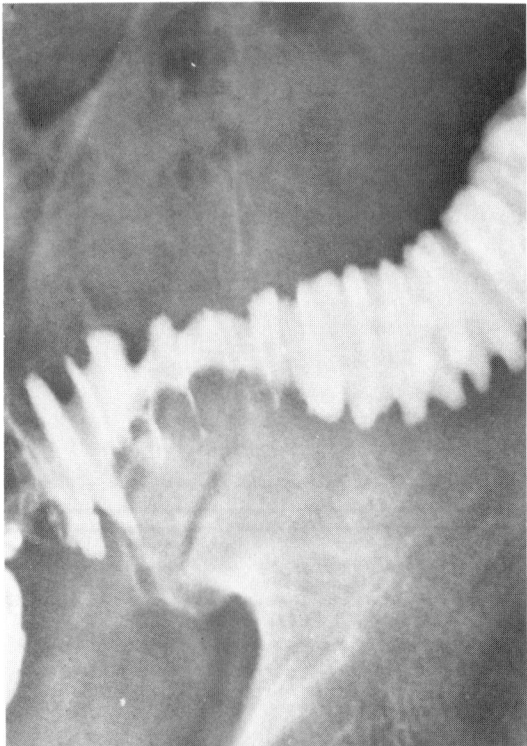

FIG. 9-25. Close-up view of the junction of the sigmoid and descending colon from a single-contrast barium enema study. The eccentric mass effect represents a diverticular abscess in this patient with fever and pain in the left lower quadrant.

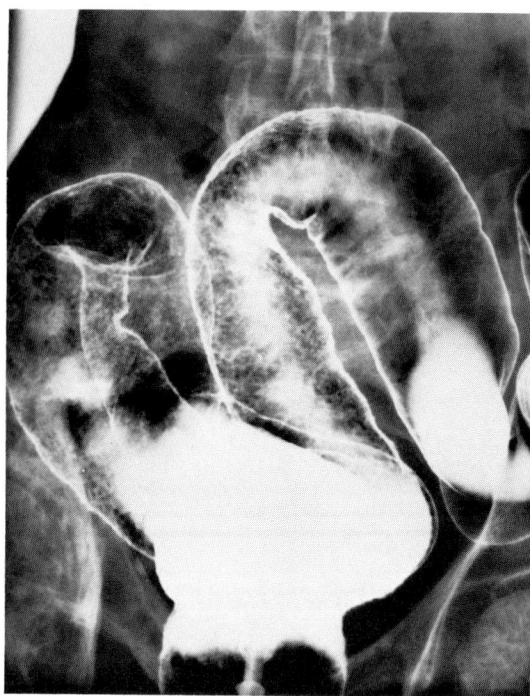

FIG. 9-26. Double-contrast examination of the colon, showing marked granularity of the rectum and much of the sigmoid colon because of idiopathic ulcerative proctosigmoiditis.

invasive malignancy, whereas larger polyps have a higher risk that warrants their routine removal (Fig. 9-28). The presence of a pedicle, a reliable sign of a benign lesion, virtually excludes the presence of malignant invasion into the adjacent colonic wall.

Diagnostic Efficacy

The efficacy of the barium enema depends on thorough colon cleansing, selection of the appropriate technique, careful quality control of the examination, and meticulous interpretation of the study. Thorough colon cleansing is the most important prerequisite for performing any type of barium enema examination.[47] The presence of stool in the colon is the most common cause of errors of interpretation. Up to 20% of colon carcinomas are missed on the initial barium examination, primarily because of poor preparation; the tumor is overlooked or is confused with fecal material.[48,49] Moreover, at least one-third of false-positive radiologic results of studies of the colon are related to the misinterpretation of stool as neoplasm.[50,51]

Selection of the appropriate barium enema technique depends on the age of the patient, the reasons for performing the examination, and the type of disease sought. The double-contrast barium enema is indicated in patients with suspected colonic neoplasia and inflammatory bowel disease, particularly in patients over age 40 because of the increased incidence of colonic neoplasia in that group.

The type of disease to be detected is also important in selecting the method of examination. For idiopathic colitis, the double-contrast barium enema is more sensitive in showing early disease and disease limited to the rectum.[52-56] The reported sensitivity of the double-contrast barium enema in the diagnosis of colitis averages about 90%. Both examinations, however, lead to underestimations of the extent of involvement, when results are compared to those of colonoscopy or histologic examination.[57,58]

The reported sensitivity in the detection of colonic polyps averages 59% for the single-contrast examination and 87% for the double-contrast study.[27] These detection rates partly depend on the size of the polyp. Both examinations enable one to detect polyps over 1 cm in size, whereas only the double-contrast examination reliably enables one to identify polyps of lesser size. Thus, for early inflammatory disease of the colon and for smaller colonic polyps,

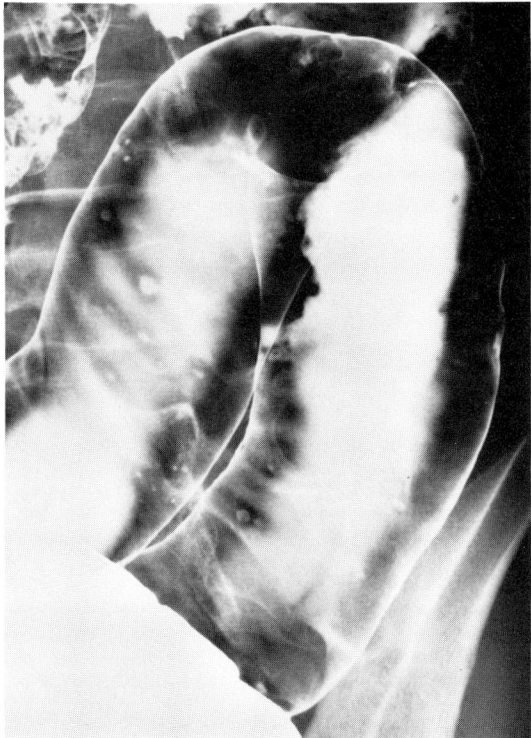

FIG. 9-27. Double-contrast view of a large loop of sigmoid colon with multiple, discrete collections of barium. These lesions represent "aphthoid" ulcers of Crohn's colitis.

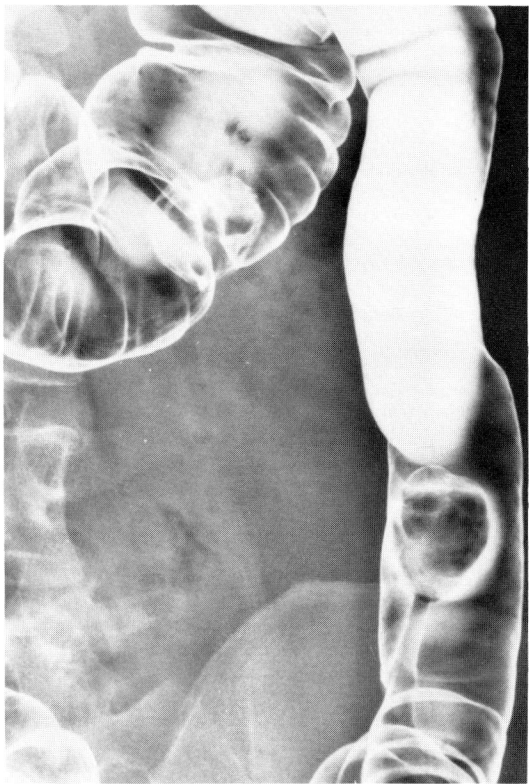

FIG. 9-28. Double-contrast examination showing a 2.5-cm sessile polyp in the transverse colon and a pedunculated polyp of similar size in the descending colon.

the double-contrast barium enema is the more sensitive radiographic method.

The reported sensitivity in the detection of carcinoma of the colon averages 85% for single-contrast radiography and about 95% for double-contrast radiography.[49,59,60-63] Studies on the effectiveness of cancer detection with the single-contrast barium enema have not been published recently, however. If properly performed in patients with a clean colon, both radiographic examinations appear to be equally effective in showing most overt carcinomas of the colon.

As with any radiographic examination of the gastrointestinal tract, careful quality control of the study is important. If the films are of poor quality, then they should be repeated, and questionable abnormalities should be clarified. Finally, meticulous interpretation of the barium enema study is necessary. The radiographs must be closely read because lesions may be seen on only one or a few of the films. Lapses in perception play a significant role in false-negative test results, particularly during interpretation of the double-contrast barium enema. Many colonic polyps and carcinomas that are initially missed on the double-contrast examination are visible in retrospect.[62,64,65] Many of these errors are presumably avoidable by a more thorough reading of the radiographs.

REFERENCES

1. Gelfand, D.W., and Ott, D.J.: Declining volume of gastrointestinal fluoroscopies: a survey of 18 hospitals. Gastrointest. Radiol., 7:227, 1982.
2. Gelfand, D.W., Ott, D.J., and Tritico, R.: Costs of gastrointestinal examinations: a comparative study. Gastrointest. Radiol., 3:135, 1978.
3. Hall, E.J.: Radiobiology for the Radiologist. New York, Harper & Row, 1973.
4. Gelfand, D.W., and Ott, D.J.: Barium sulfate suspensions: an evaluation of available products. AJR, 138:935, 1982.
5. Gelfand, D.W.: Complications of gastrointestinal radiologic procedures: I. Complications of routine fluoroscopic studies. Gastrointest. Radiol., 5:293, 1980.
6. Miller, R.E., and Skucas, J. (Eds.): Radiographic Contrast Agents. Baltimore, University Park Press, 1977.
7. Diner, W.C., et al.: Intraluminal pressure measurements during barium enema: full column vs. air contrast. AJR, 137:217, 1981.
8. Grossman, R.I., Miller, W.T., and Dann, R.W.: Oral barium sulfate in partial large-bowel obstruction. Radiology, 136:327, 1980.
9. Margulis, A.R.: Water-soluble radiographic contrast agents in the gastrointestinal tract. In Radiographic Contrast Agents. Edited by R.E. Miller and J. Skucas. Baltimore, University Park Press, 1977.

10. Lutzger, L.G., and Factor, S.M.: Effects of some water-soluble contrast media on the colonic mucosa. Radiology, 118:545, 1976.
11. Eisenberg, R.L., et al.: Iodine absorption from the gastrointestinal tract during Hypaque-enema examination. Radiology, 133:597, 1979.
12. Gelfand, D.W., and Ott, D.J.: Anatomy and technique in evaluating the esophagus. Semin. Roentgenol., 16:168, 1981.
13. Cockerill, E.M., et al.: Optimal visualization of esophageal varices. AJR, 126:512, 1976.
14. Foley, M.J., Ghahremani, G.G., and Rogers, L.F.: Reappraisal of contrast media used to detect upper gastrointestinal perforations. Radiology, 144:231, 1982.
15. Ott, D.J., Gelfand, D.W., and Wu, W.C.: The sensitivity of single-contrast radiology in esophageal disease: a study of 240 patients with endoscopically verified abnormality. Gastrointest. Radiol., 8:105, 1983.
16. Ott, D.J., Gelfand, D.W., and Wu, W.C.: Reflux esophagitis: radiographic and endoscopic correlation. Radiology, 130:583, 1979.
17. Koehler, R.E., Weyman, P.J., and Oakley, H.F.: Single- and double-contrast techniques in esophagitis. AJR, 135:15, 1980.
18. Ott, D.J., Wu, W.C., and Gelfand, D.W.: Reflux esophagitis revisited: prospective analysis of radiologic accuracy. Gastrointest. Radiol., 6:1, 1981.
19. Ott, D.J., et al.: Radiologic detection and spectrum of appearances of peptic esophageal strictures. J. Clin. Gastroenterol., 4:11, 1982.
20. Burhenne, H.J.: Technique of examination of the stomach and duodenum. In Alimentary Tract Roentgenology. 2nd Ed. Vol. 1. Edited by A.R. Margulis and H.J. Burhenne. St. Louis, C.V. Mosby, 1973.
21. Gelfand, D.W.: The Japanese-style double-contrast examination of the stomach. Gastrointest. Radiol., 1:7, 1976.
22. Laufer, I.: Double Contrast Gastrointestinal Radiology with Endoscopic Correlation. Philadelphia, W.B. Saunders, 1979.
23. Ming, S.C., II: Malignant potential of gastric polyps. Gastrointest. Radiol., 1:121, 1976.
24. Fabry, T.L., Frankel, A., and Waye, J.D.: Gastric polyps. J. Clin. Gastroenterol., 4:23, 1982.
25. Gelfand, D.W., Ott, D.J., and Tritico, R.: Causes of error in gastrointestinal radiology. I. Upper gastrointestinal examination. Gastrointest. Radiol., 5:91, 1980.
26. Ott, D.J., et al.: Sensitivity of single- vs. double-contrast radiology in erosive gastritis. AJR, 138:263, 1982.
27. Gelfand, D.W., and Ott, D.J.: Single- vs. double-contrast gastrointestinal studies: critical analysis of reported statistics. AJR, 137:523, 1981.
28. Ott, D.J., Gelfand, D.W., and Wu, W.C.: Detection of gastric ulcer: comparison of single- and double-contrast examination. AJR, 139:93, 1982.
29. Ott, D.J., et al.: The sensitivity of radiography of the postoperative stomach. Radiology, 144:741, 1982.
30. Fried, A.M., Poulos, A., and Hatfield, D.R.: The effectiveness of the incidental small-bowel series. Radiology, 140:45, 1981.
31. Rabe, F.E., et al.: Efficacy of the small-bowel examination. Radiology, 140:47, 1981.
32. Marshak, R.H., and Lindner, A.E.: Radiology of the small intestine. Philadelphia, W.B. Saunders, 1976.
33. Miller, R.E., and Sellink, J.L.: Enteroclysis: the small bowel enema. How to succeed and how to fail. Gastrointest. Radiol., 4:269, 1979.
34. Goldberg, H.I., and Dodds, W.J.: Roentgen evaluation of small-bowel obstruction. Dig. Dis. Sci., 24:245, 1979.
35. Seltzer, S.E., Jones, B., and McLaughlin, G.C.: Proper choice of contrast agents in emergency gastrointestinal radiology. CRC Crit. Rev. Diagn. Imaging, 12:79, 1979.
36. Han, S.Y., Laws, H.L., and Aldrete, J.S.: How and when to use barium for diagnosis of small bowel obstruction. South. Med. J., 72:1519, 1979.
37. Dodds, W.J., and Goldberg, H.I.: Roentgen examination of the small bowel using intraluminal contrast media. Dig. Dis. Sci., 23:550, 1978.
38. Vallance, R.: An evaluation of the small bowel enema based on an analysis of 350 consecutive examinations. Clin. Radiol., 31:227, 1980.
39. Maglinte, D.D.T., et al.: Meckel diverticulum: radiologic demonstration by enteroclysis. AJR, 134:925, 1980.
40. Dodds, W.J., et al.: An evaluation of colon cleansing regimens. AJR, 128:57, 1977.
41. Irwin, J.P., and Peterson, G.H.: Colon preparation for the barium enema: a guide for the radiologist. Gastrointest. Radiol., 7:75, 1982.
42. Margulis, A.R.: Examination of the colon. In Alimentary Tract Roentgenology. 2nd Ed. Vol. 2. Edited by A.R. Margulis and H.J. Burhenne. St. Louis, C.V. Mosby, 1973.
43. Ott, D.J., and Gelfand, D.W.: Colorectal tumors: pathology and detection. AJR, 131:691, 1978.
44. Youker, J.E., Dodds, W.J., and Welin, S.: Colonic polyps. In Alimentary Tract Roentgenology. 2nd Ed. Vol. 2. Edited by A.R. Margulis and H.J. Burhenne. St. Louis, C.V. Mosby, 1973.
45. Marshak, R.H., Lindner, A.E., and Maklansky, D.: Adenomatous polyps of the colon: a rational approach. JAMA, 235:2856, 1976.
46. Skucas, J., Spataro, R.F., and Cannucciari, D.P.: The radiographic features of small colon cancers. Radiology, 143:335, 1982.
47. Miller, R.E.: The clean colon. Gastroenterology, 70:289, 1976.
48. Saunders, C.G., and MacEwen, D.W.: Delay in diagnosis of colonic cancer—a continuing challenge. Radiology, 101:207, 1971.
49. Clarke, A.M., and Jones, I.S.C.: Diagnostic accuracy and diagnostic delay in carcinoma of the large bowel. N.Z. Med. J., 71:341, 1970.
50. Weyman, P.J., Koehler, R.E., and Zuckerman, G.R.: Resolution of radiographic-endoscopic discrepancies in colon neoplasms. J. Clin. Gastroenterol., 3(Suppl. 1):89, 1981.
51. Ott, D.J., et al.: The predictive value of a diagnosis of colonic polyp on the double-contrast barium enema. Gastrointest. Radiol., 8:75, 1983.
52. Kelvin, F.M., et al.: Double contrast barium enema in Crohn's disease and ulcerative colitis. AJR, 131:207, 1978.
53. Simpkins, K.C., and Stevenson, G.W.: The modified Malmö double-contrast barium enema in colitis: an assessment of its accuracy in reflecting sigmoidoscopic findings. Br. J. Radiol., 45:486, 1972.
54. Laufer, I., Mullens, J.E., and Hamilton, J.: Correlation of endoscopy and double-contrast radiography in the early stages of ulcerative and granulomatous colitis. Radiology, 118:1, 1976.
55. Fraser, G.M., and Findlay, J.M.: The double-contrast enema in ulcerative and Crohn's colitis. Clin. Radiol., 27:103, 1976.
56. Williams, H.J., Jr., Stephens, D.H., and Carlson, H.C.:

Double-contrast radiography: colonic inflammatory disease. AJR, *137*:315, 1981.
57. Bartram, C.I., and Walmsley, K.: A radiological and pathological correlation of the mucosal changes in ulcerative colitis. Clin. Radiol., *29*:323, 1978.
58. Gabrielson, N., et al.: Extent of inflammatory lesions in ulcerative colitis assessed by radiology, colonoscopy, and endoscopic biopsies. Gastrointest. Radiol., *4*:395, 1979.
59. Cooley, R.N., Agnew, C.H., and Rios, G.: Diagnostic accuracy of the barium enema study in carcinoma of the colon and rectum. AJR, *84*:316, 1960.
60. Ott, D.J., et al.: Sensitivity of double-contrast barium enema: emphasis on polyp detection. AJR, *135*:327, 1980.
61. Thorpe, C.D., Grayson, D.J., Jr., and Wingfield, P.B.: Detection of carcinoma of the colon and rectum by air contrast enema. Surg. Gynecol. Obstet., *152*:307, 1981.
62. Kelvin, F.M., et al.: Colorectal carcinoma missed on double contrast barium enema study: a problem of perception. AJR, *137*:307, 1981.
63. Evers, K., et al.: Double-contrast enema examination for detection of rectal carcinoma. Radiology, *140*:635, 1981.
64. Ott, D.J., Gelfand, D.W., and Ramquist, N.A.: Causes of error in gastrointestinal radiology. II. Barium enema examination. Gastrointest. Radiol., *5*:99, 1980.
65. Fork, F.-T.: Double contrast enema and colonoscopy in polyp detection. Gut, *22*:971, 1981.

Part II

ENDOSCOPY, FUNCTION STUDIES, AND MAGNETIC RESONANCE IMAGING

10

Studies of the Urinary Tract

Gerald W. Chodak ■ Harry W. Schoenberg

Current technology has improved our ability to investigate the genitourinary tract and has made it possible to establish a diagnosis preoperatively. Selection of the appropriate study is necessary to minimize the number of studies performed. In this chapter, we shall introduce each of the studies available for investigating the urinary tract, and we shall provide a brief discussion of indications, complications, techniques, and interpretation. Patient studies of the urinary tract involve imaging, endoscopic, and function studies. Some of the imaging procedures are combined with endoscopy.

CYSTOSCOPY

During a cystoscopic examination, the bladder is visualized through a telescopic instrument placed into it. Improved instrumentation has enhanced the diagnostic capability of this technique. The ease of performance increases the attractiveness of this procedure, which enables one to see directly many of the pathologic processes that affect the bladder. It is beyond the scope of this chapter to illustrate each of the abnormalities that may be detected by this procedure; for a comprehensive discussion, the reader is referred elsewhere.[1,2]

Prior to the cystoscopic procedure, one usually obtains an excretory urogram, to identify any abnormalities of the upper tract. The only other requirement of this study is a co-operative patient. The patient's comfort may be enhanced by mild sedation. In the majority of cases, the procedure can be performed on an outpatient basis, with a local anesthetic instilled into the urethra. The procedure usually takes under 10 min. Indications include microscopic or gross hematuria, recurrent infections, a history or urinary tract cancer, or an abnormality noted on a cystogram or excretory urogram. For a satisfactory examination, one must inspect the total bladder wall, the ureteral orifices, and the prostatic urethra. The procedure is better tolerated by women than by men because of the short length and straightness of the female urethra. Although the study enables one to detect gross abnormalities reliably, some lesions may be evident only on microscopic evaluation of the biopsy material.

Technique

The cystoscopic sheaths vary in size, and selection should be based on the procedure planned. For patients who require a simple bladder inspection, the 17-French instrument is sufficient. If a ureteral catheterization or a biopsy is contemplated, however, then a larger instrument must be used, to accommodate the necessary working elements. When performing a cystoscopic examination in a male patient, one usually passes the instrument into the bladder under direct vision because this procedure reduces the chances of creating a false passage in the urethra. When one examines the female bladder, visualization of the urethra during passage of the cystoscope is not usually necessary. Once the cystoscope is in the bladder, the urine is drained prior to instillation of an irrigating fluid, which may be either water, glycine, or saline solution. Complete inspection requires several lenses with different viewing angles. For patients with unexplained hematuria, each ureteral orifice is observed for a bloody efflux that would localize the hematuria to the upper urinary tract on the corresponding side. If a tumor is seen, the patient should be admitted to the hospital for resection under spinal or regional anesthesia.

Complications

The study should not be performed if the patient has a combination of urinary tract infection and obstruction because the possibility of sepsis is increased under these conditions. Currently, the risk of infection in the presence of sterile urine is so low that prophylactic antibiotics are not warranted before or after the procedure. Antibiotics may be of value in patients with a large volume of residual urine.

Another potential complication is trauma to the urethra, which may result in the formation of a stricture. Direct visualization during insertion of the cystoscope minimizes the risk of such trauma.

If a biopsy is performed, the bladder wall may be

perforated, resulting in the extravasation of urine. If the perforation is extraperitoneal, then catheter drainage for several days will be sufficient treatment. When an intraperitoneal rupture occurs, however, surgical exploration may be required to close the bladder defect.

Interpretation

Most abnormalities of the bladder produce consistent changes that are recognizable during cystoscopic examination. For some mucosal abnormalities, a biopsy may be required to establish a diagnosis.

URETEROPYELOSCOPY

Recently developed instrumentation allows endoscopic visualization of the ureter and the renal pelvis. This equipment makes it possible to trap ureteral calculi within a stone basket under direct vision, to fulgurate ureteral tumors, and to dilate ureteral obstructions. The indications include the presence of any filling defect or obstruction in the ureter or pelvis noted by excretory urography or gross hematuria coming from a ureteral orifice. Ureteropyeloscopy offers an attractive alternative to open surgical procedures for ureteral calculi that do not pass spontaneously.

Ureteropyeloscopy is performed under general anesthesia and thus requires hospitalization. The duration of the procedure varies, but it may take up to 5 hours to complete. Even so, it is well tolerated, with only minimal postoperative pain. When colic is expected, one may place an indwelling ureteral catheter for a few days after the procedure, to prevent these symptoms.

Technique

The initial step in performing a ureteropyeloscopic study is dilation of the intramural portion of the ureter. One uses a 25-French cystoscope with special interchangeable metal dilators up to 16 French in diameter. When the ureter has been dilated, an 11 ½-French ureteroscope, 50 cm in length, is gently passed into the ureter. The scope is advanced proximally as long as it is possible to visualize the lumen (Fig. 10–1). This ureteroscope allows passage of a 5-French stone basket, which can then be manipulated under direct vision to engage the calculus (Fig. 10–2). Both the stone basket and the ureteroscope are removed under direct vision simultaneously with the engaged calculus. If the stone is too large to be removed intact, it may be pulverized with a 5-French ultrasonic probe.

In patients with ureteral tumors, one may use an instrument containing a resectoscope loop to fulgurate and to resect small ureteral tumors. Biopsy specimens may also be obtained.

Complications

Several complications can occur as a result of uteropyeloscopy, including injury to the ureter and proximal migration of ureteral calculi. To minimize

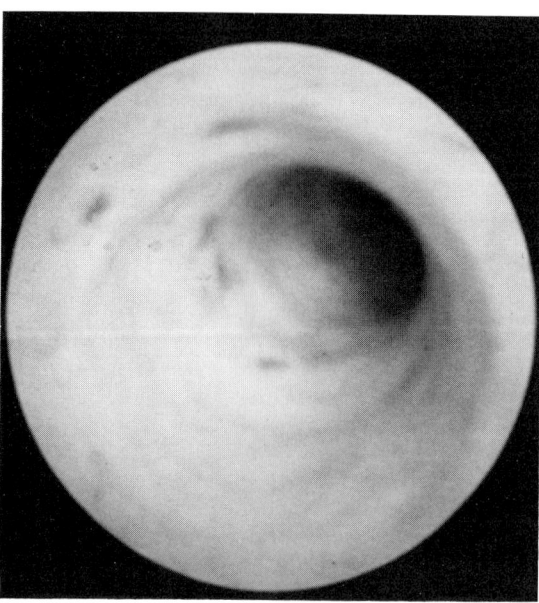

FIG. 10–1. Visualization of midureter through a ureteropyeloscope; no abnormalities seen. (Courtesy of E. Lyon.)

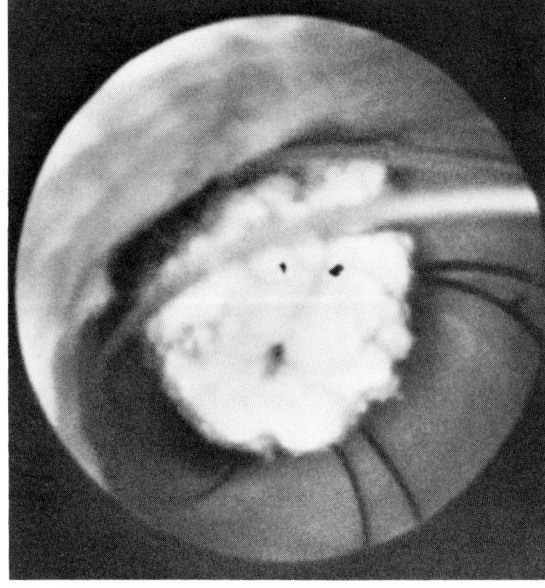

FIG. 10–2. Ureteral calculus trapped in a stone basket under direct vision with a ureteropyeloscope. (Courtesy of E. Lyon.)

the incidence of infection, systemic antibiotics are administered before and for several days after the procedure.

EXCRETORY UROGRAPHY

Excretory urography is the mainstay of the diagnostic investigation of the urinary tract. This study provides information on the renal parenchyma, the collecting system and renal pelvis, the ureters, the bladder, and the prostate gland. Because this study provides so much information about the urinary system and because it has a low rate of complications, it is almost universally performed prior to any other investigation of the urinary system. Urologists usually perform this study before an endoscopic procedure unless certain contraindications exist or unless the problem appears certain to be in the bladder or urethra.

The indications for excretory urography are broad and include the investigation of any suspected abnormality of the urinary tract caused by infection, trauma, neoplasm, or congenital anomaly.

Excretory urography is based on the ability of the kidney to filter a radiopaque substance through the glomeruli. The agents in current use are hypertonic water-soluble salts derived from an iodinated benzoic acid precursor. The compound is administered intravenously, usually by rapid injection, although a drip-infusion method may also be used. The contrast material rapidly equilibrates between the intravascular and the extravascular spaces, and as filtration occurs through the kidney, the extravascular contrast material re-equilibrates with the intravascular space.

The entire study usually takes under 2 hours to complete unless obstruction is present. Obstruction causes a delay in concentration and excretion of the opaque medium on the affected side that requires delayed films for visualization of the entire urinary tract. The study is easily performed on an outpatient basis with a minimum of staff and is generally well tolerated by the patient. Although the procedure is expensive, it usually costs less than most other studies that provide functional and anatomic information about the urinary tract.

Technique and Interpretation

At the beginning of the study, a plain radiograph is obtained to identify any calcifications or other abnormalities. Following rapid intravenous injection of the dye, usually 1 to 1.5 ml/kg, one takes a sequence of films that delineates each portion of the urinary tract. A 30-sec or 1-min film displays a nephrogram that provides information about the kidney itself. This film allows determination of the position, size, orientation, angulation, and shape of each kidney.

Nephrotomography has improved our ability to diagnose renal parenchymal abnormalities not shown on the conventional urogram (Fig. 10-3). One vital requirement for a satisfactory nephrogram is the visualization of the entire renal outline, which is often not possible without nephrotomograms because of the presence of bowel gas.

A 3- to 5-min film shows the collecting system and filling defects or obstructing lesions (Figs. 10-4 and 10-5). The ureter and bladder are shown by the 10- and 30-min films (Figs. 10-6 and 10-7). Normally, because of peristalsis, the ureter is not visualized in its entirety on a single film, unless the patient has a distal obstruction or a full bladder. If a portion of either ureter is not visualized on any film, but a ureteral abnormality exists, then a retrograde ureterogram will be indicated.

As the contrast material fills the bladder, filling defects and abnormalities in the bladder wall may be detected, such as tumors, trabeculation, or diverticulum formation. The final film in the study is taken when the patient has emptied the bladder. For elderly men in particular, this film is important for assessing residual volume related to obstruction either from an enlarged prostate gland or from a urethral stricture. Some confusion may occur, however, because the patient may be sent to the bathroom to urinate but may be unable to void. The technician may fail to question the patient to determine whether voiding was attempted and performed. The result is an incorrect conclusion that a large volume of residual urine has remained in the bladder.

Complications

Performance of excretory urography requires intravenous access and renal function sufficient to allow concentration of the contrast material (creatinine level under 3 to 4 mg/dl). Several relative contraindications exist for this study, although they have been recently modified. They include diabetes with impaired renal function (creatinine level greater than 1.5 mg/dl), acute renal failure, congestive heart failure, and multiple myeloma. Except for congestive heart failure, the other risks are increased by dehydration. Each of these abnormalities is associated with an increased incidence of impaired renal function following the study.

The incidence of allergic reactions is less than 1% and appears to be idiosyncratic. Because anxiety has been suggested as a cause of the reaction, a controversy exists over how much information about side effects should be provided to the patient prior to performing this study.[3] A previous history of an allergic reaction during urography, particularly hives, does not necessarily mean that a reaction will occur during the next examination and is therefore not an absolute contraindication, nor does a relationship

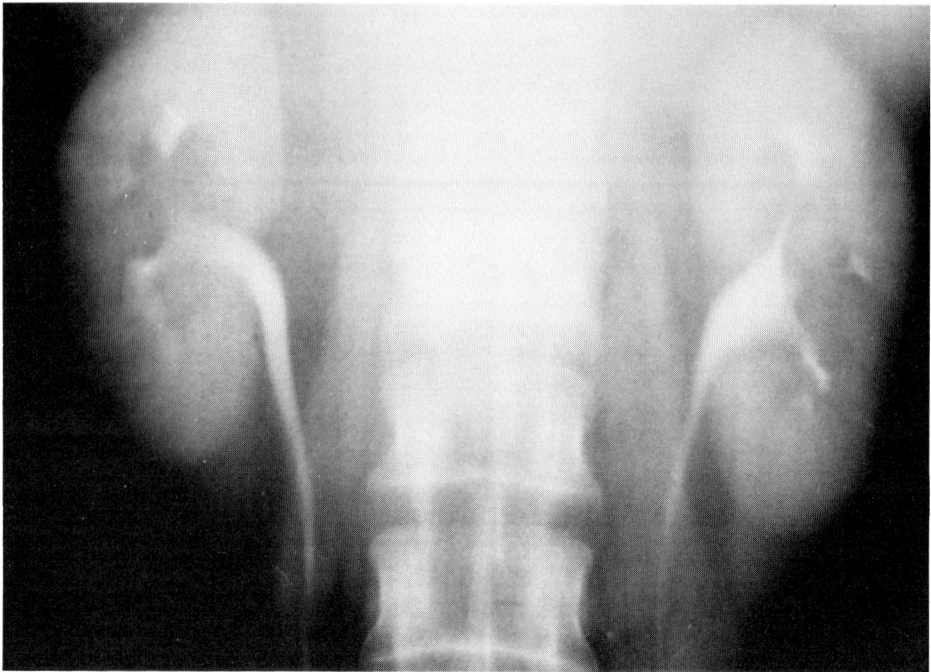

FIG. 10–3. Normal nephrotomogram; symmetric filling of collecting system of both kidneys. The absence of bowel gas makes it possible to visualize the entire outline of each kidney.

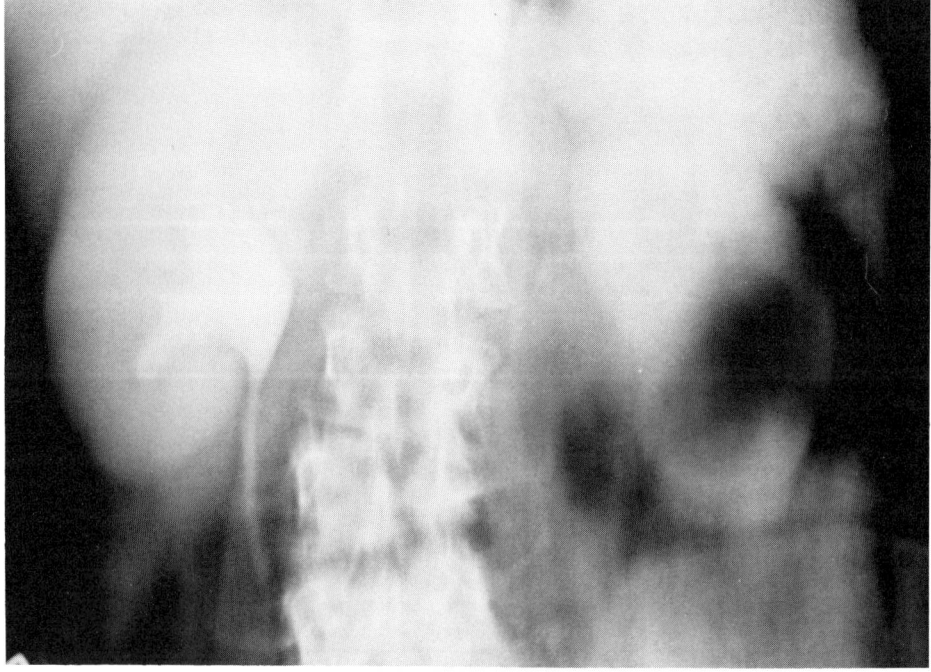

FIG. 10–4. Obstructed left kidney; marked delay in the appearance of contrast media in the collecting system of the left kidney.

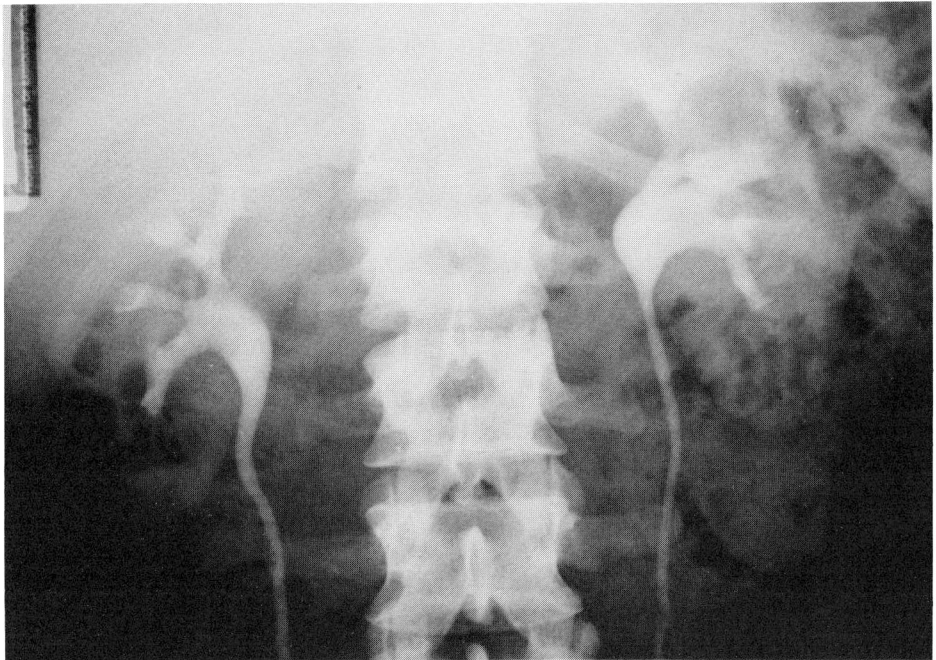

FIG. 10–5. Normal intravenous urogram, 5-min film. Opaque material is present in both collecting systems. The outline of the kidneys is partially visible through overlying bowel gas.

exist between the development of hives during one study and a severe reaction during the next one. Frequently, patients receive corticosteroids prior to the study if they have developed reactions in the past. The use of a test dose of contrast material to determine sensitivity is unjustified.[4] Patients should be told that a frequent but normal response is a metallic taste and a warm flush following injection of the contrast material. The incidence of nausea and vomiting is approximately 5%.

The disadvantages of excretory urography are few. Because the dose of radiation to the uterus is 1 to 2 rads, which might affect a new but unknown pregnancy, information about the patient's latest date of menstruation should be obtained. The technical quality of studies must be assessed. If inadequate studies are accepted, lesions may be missed.

RETROGRADE PYELOGRAPHY

In retrograde pyelography, contrast material is injected into the distal ureter through a cystoscope. Improvements in excretory urographic techniques have reduced the need for this examination. The usual indications are an inadequately visualized ureter on intravenous urography, an obstructed, nonfunctioning kidney of unknown cause, or a severe allergic reaction to contrast media given by the intravenous route.

The study is easy to perform and can usually be completed in 20 to 30 min in uncomplicated cases. It requires a co-operative patient and usually causes only minor discomfort. In apprehensive patients, mild sedation may make the study easier and more comfortable. Retrograde pyelography can usually be performed as an outpatient procedure under local anesthesia. If ureteral obstruction is or may be present, however, the examination should be done on an inpatient basis, and the patient should receive antibiotics. A discovered obstruction should be relieved as soon as it is identified.

Technique

A cystoscope is inserted into the bladder and, under direct vision, a 7- or 8-French cone-tipped catheter is placed 1 to 2 cm into the ureteral orifice. To avoid the formation of air bubbles, which can be confused with a true filling defect, the catheter is filled with contrast medium prior to inserting it into the ureter. The contrast medium is usually the same as for intravenous pyelography, but it can be diluted 1:2 with saline solution. Once the catheter is in the ureter, 5 to 8 ml are injected with a slow, steady pressure. Patients are instructed to hold their breath as a radiograph is taken. Care must be taken to avoid overdistention of the collecting system because extravasation of contrast material may result. Normally, the injection is made under direct vision, to ensure that the dye is not leaking out of the orifice and back into the bladder around the catheter. If the

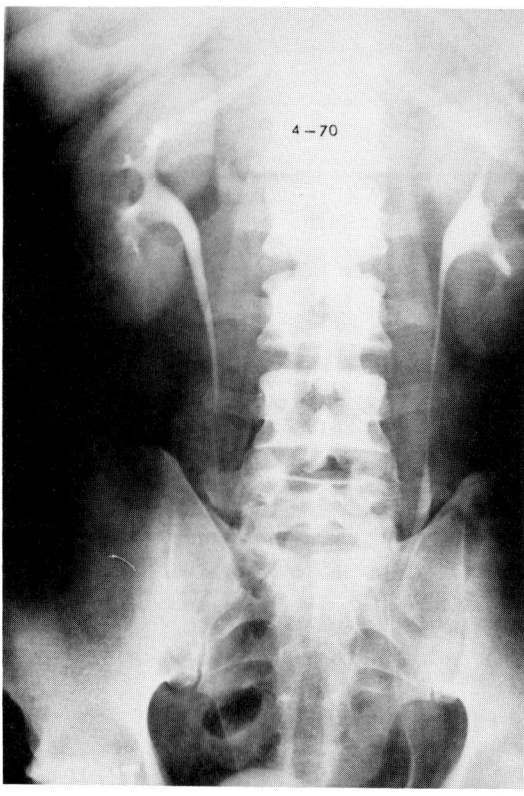

FIG. 10–6. Normal intravenous urogram, 10-min film. A portion of each ureter is visualized in its normal course toward the bladder.

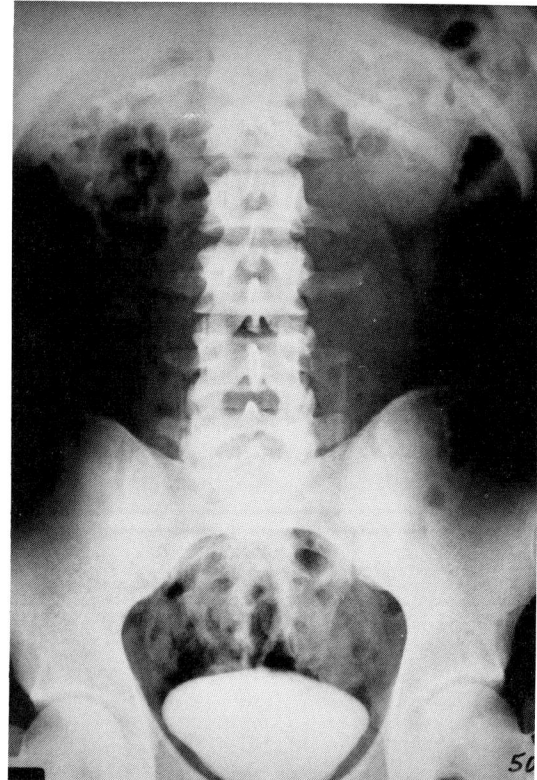

FIG. 10–7. Normal intravenous urogram, 30-min film. Contrast material has filled the bladder, and one sees a smooth wall with no filling defects.

pelvis is not visualized completely, then the study should be repeated with a larger volume of contrast material.

Complications

A retrograde pyelogram is generally not performed in a patient with a urinary infection because of the increased risk of sepsis or pyelonephritis. In the presence of sterile urine, the study has a low incidence of complications, except in patients with urinary obstruction. In such patients, the risk of infection and even of sepsis may be significant if the obstructed kidney is not adequately drained shortly after the procedure. When obstruction is known to exist on the basis of an ultrasonic study, an antibiotic such as a cephalosporin or an aminoglycoside can be mixed with the contrast medium prior to instillation into the catheter. In addition, systemic antibiotics should be administered before and for 24 to 36 hours after the procedure. As a rule, however, any patient with a urinary obstruction evident on a retrograde pyelogram should have it relieved at once because a closed-space infection may result and may be life-threatening. Commercially available indwelling ureteral stents can be placed during the procedure if an obstruction is identified. In some patients, the nature of the obstruction prevents the catheter from bypassing the abnormal area, however. Under these circumstances, a percutaneous nephrostomy may relieve the obstruction on a short-term basis, until a definitive procedure can be undertaken.

RETROGRADE CYSTOGRAPHY

In the retrograde cystogram, contrast material is instilled into the bladder through a urethral catheter (Fig. 10–8). The study is primarily performed to identify bladder rupture after abdominal trauma or pelvic fracture. It is also used to determine whether residual leakage is present following bladder operations. The study causes minimal discomfort to the patient and requires no anesthesia. It is usually completed within 20 to 30 min and is easily performed in a hospital emergency room.

Technique

The study is performed without difficulty as long as a urethral catheter can be passed into the bladder. When a study is indicated in a patient with an impassable or partially transected urethra, then it

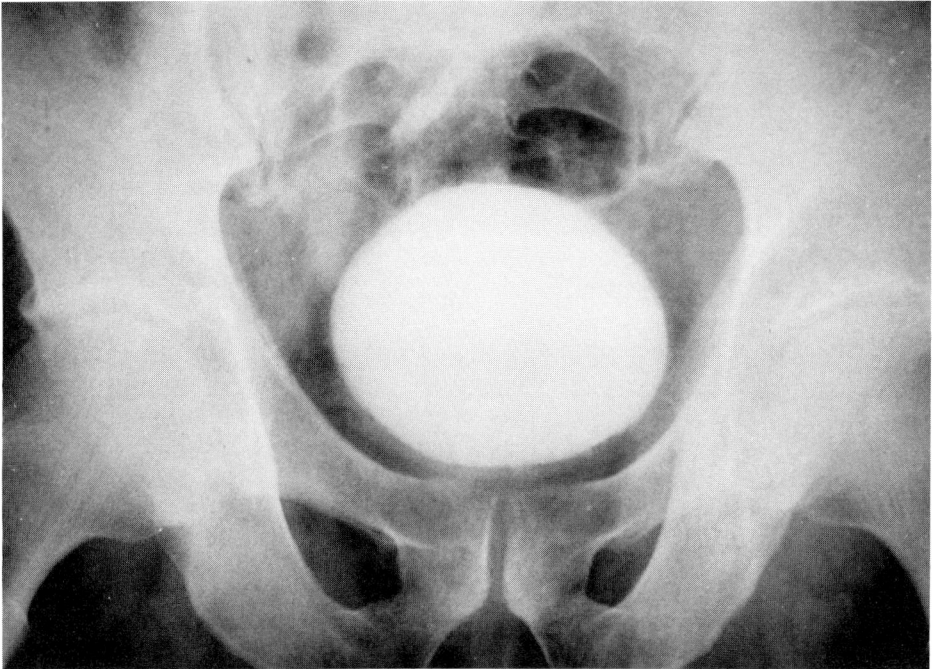

FIG. 10–8. Normal retrograde cystogram; initial film showing a smooth-walled bladder with no abnormalities.

can be performed by percutaneous cystostomy. Once the catheter is in place, all the urine is drained, and 350 ml meglumine diatrizoate (Cystografin) are infused into the bladder. Films are taken prior to instillation of the contrast material, when instillation is complete, and when the bladder has been drained again. The last film allows one to see whether any dye has leaked out of the bladder, as well as whether any contrast material has been retained in a diverticulum. Lateral as well as anteroposterior films are necessary.

Complications

The only serious complications of retrograde cystography are the development of infection and urethral tears. Both complications are infrequent when the procedure is performed by experienced personnel. These complications may be minimized by adequate urethral meatal cleansing and by gentle insertion of the catheter. The primary contraindication to retrograde cystography is a urethral tear because passage of a catheter may render a partial transection complete. Therefore, the urethra must be shown to be intact prior to performing the study. The most common sign of a urethral tear is blood at the meatus. If no blood is seen at the meatus after a traumatic event, such as a pelvic fracture, and if the patient is able to urinate, then it is reasonable to proceed with the study. If the patient cannot urinate or if blood is seen at the meatus, however, then a retrograde urethrogram should be performed first. This principle is most important for emergency room personnel because they are usually involved in the initial management of this problem, before a urologist is consulted.

Interpretation

The management of a bladder perforation depends on the location of the injury: extraperitoneal or intraperitoneal. In patients with an extraperitoneal rupture, the cystogram shows contrast material in reasonable concentration and localized in the soft tissue outside the bladder. This injury can often be managed by catheter drainage alone. If the rupture is intraperitoneal, then the contrast material will be diffusely spread over the entire peritoneal cavity. Patients with this injury usually require surgical repair and suprapubic cystostomy.

RETROGRADE URETHROGRAPHY

A retrograde urethrogram is performed by injecting contrast material directly into the urethral meatus, to visualize the anatomic features of the penile, bulbar, membranous, and prostatic urethra. The principal indications for retrograde urethrography include suspected urethral injury, urethral strictures, urethral tumors, and urethral discharge, to determine the presence of a urethral diverticulum. The study is easy to perform and requires an x-ray technician and someone to inject the contrast material. The examination can be completed in 10 min and is usually well tolerated without any anesthesia.

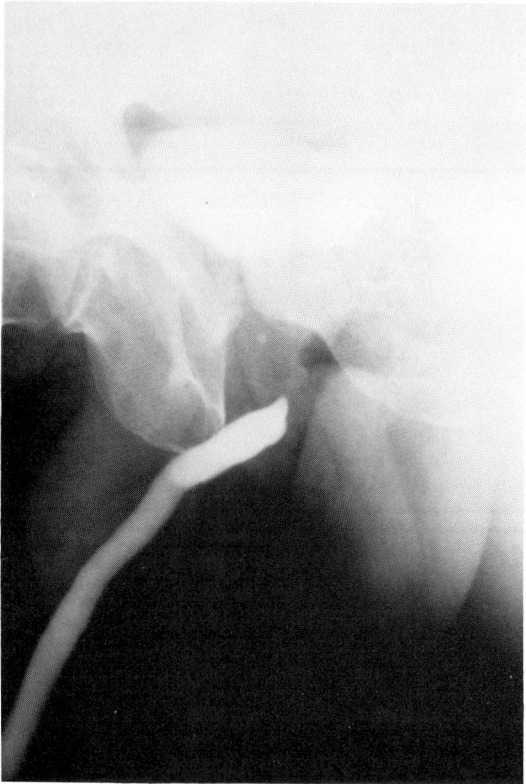

FIG. 10–9. Normal retrograde urethrogram; normal caliber of urethra throughout the entire course, up to the external sphincter. Contrast material passes into the bladder.

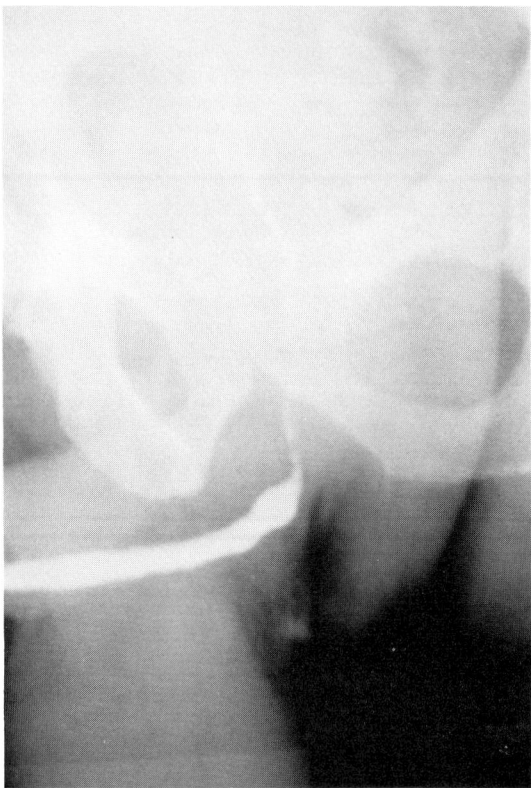

FIG. 10–10. Abnormal retrograde urethrogram; narrow membranous stricture, with dilation of the urethra.

Thus, it can be easily performed without any preparation in a hospital emergency room.

Technique

A retrograde urethrogram is performed in male patients by placing a Foley catheter in the urethra up to the fossa navicularis and by slowly inflating the balloon while exerting gentle traction. The balloon should be inflated just enough to prevent the catheter from slipping out of the urethra. At the start of the procedure, the patient is placed in a right or left oblique position, with the leg of the corresponding side flexed to about 90°. The penis is held along the axis of the flexed leg during injection. Meglumine diatrizoate (Renografin or Cystografin) can be used, after diluting it 1:1 with sterile water. The contrast material is injected slowly, and when approximately 30 ml have been instilled, a film is obtained while the dye instillation is continued. Normally, a narrowed area is seen in the region of the external sphincter (Fig. 10–9). When the study is performed for a urethral stricture, the radiograph shows an additional narrowed area of variable length, with dilatation of the urethra between the stricture and the syringe (Fig. 10–10).

Complications

No real contraindications to this study exist. The only significant complications are infection and venous intravasation, particularly in the presence of strictures, and these complications may be minimized by avoiding high-pressure infusion of the contrast material. In addition, only aqueous contrast solution should be used. If the urine is infected in a patient with a stricture, the risk of bacteremia and sepsis is significant. These patients should receive antibiotics prior to and immediately after the procedure.

Interpretation

Normally, a narrowed area is seen in the region of the external sphincter (Fig. 10–11). When the study is performed for urethral stricture, the radiograph will show another narrowed area of variable length, with dilatation of the urethra between the stricture and the syringe. A voiding cystourethrogram may be more useful than a retrograde urethrogram in the identification of a suspected abnormality in the prostatic urethra.

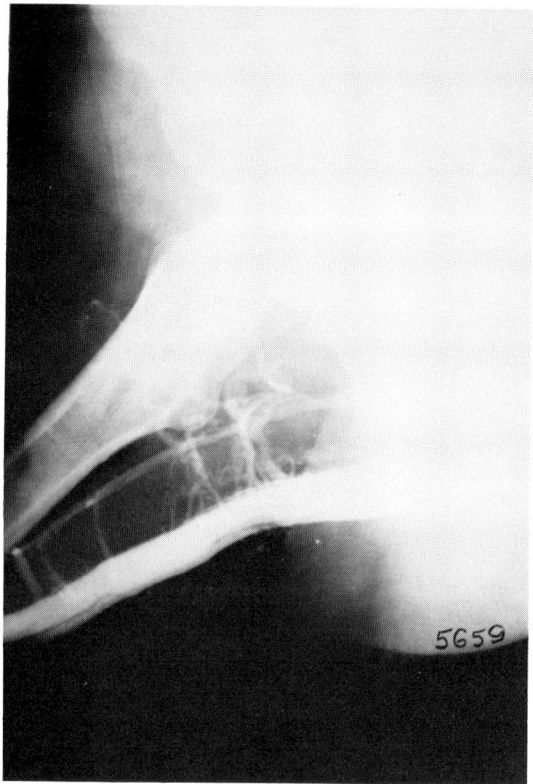

FIG. 10–11. Normal cystogram; smooth-walled bladder and no evidence of extravasation.

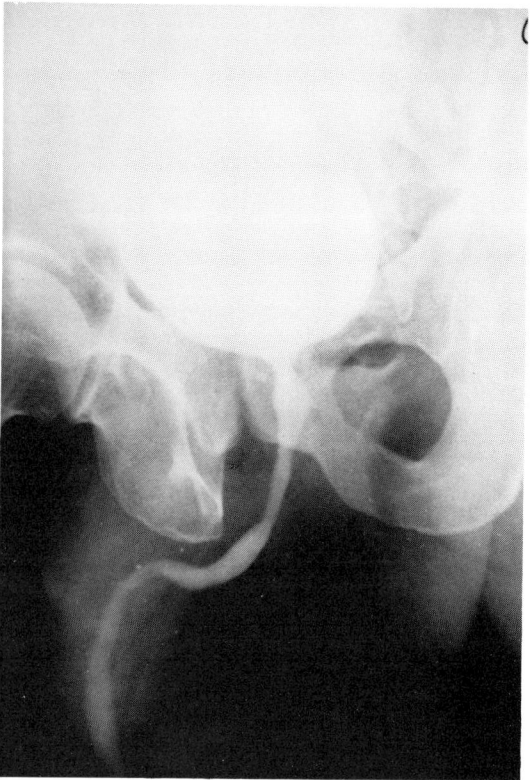

FIG. 10–12. Normal voiding cystourethrogram; normal urethra visualized, and no vesicoureteral reflux evident.

VOIDING CYSTOURETHROGRAPHY

Another means of defining the anatomic features of the proximal and distal urethra is voiding cystourethrography (Fig. 10–12). In this study, radiographs are obtained during urination when the bladder has been filled with contrast material. The technique is useful in the detection of urethral stricture, urethral diverticulum, vesicoureteral reflux, or urethral valve (Fig. 10–13). The study is most often performed in children with recurrent urinary tract infections. Although the study is acceptable for all but the lowest grade of reflux, it has been replaced by the radionuclide cystogram. The radionuclide study is sensitive to lesser degrees of reflux and involves a lower dose of radiation to the patient. The study is well tolerated and requires no hospitalization.

Technique

A voiding cystourethrogram is performed while the patient urinates under fluoroscopic surveillance, with contrast media in the bladder. The procedure is most commonly performed separately from the pyelogram; the dye must therefore first be instilled in the bladder. Usually, one passes a small catheter through the urethra, instills the dye, and removes the catheter prior to asking the patient to void. When information about the urethra is desired, the study may also be performed at the completion of an intravenous urogram if the contrast material in the bladder is sufficiently concentrated. If any difficulty in passing the catheter is encountered, then a suprapubic cystotomy may be used to fill the bladder. In either case, several films are obtained as the patient voids into a container.

Complications

A voiding cystourethrogram is contraindicated in a patient with a urinary tract infection because of the increased risk of sepsis from placement of the catheter or from reflux. In addition, lower urinary tract infection can cause transient reflux, which makes the study difficult to interpret. Normally, no urine enters the ureter during urination. When reflux is present, contrast material can be seen in the ureter or in the collecting system of the kidney. The degree of reflux is graded from 1 to 4+, based on the increasing effect on the ureters and collecting system. In the mildest case, a small amount of dye can be seen part way up the ureter on the involved side, and the ureter is not dilated. In grade 4 reflux, hydroureteronephrosis is present, with marked dil-

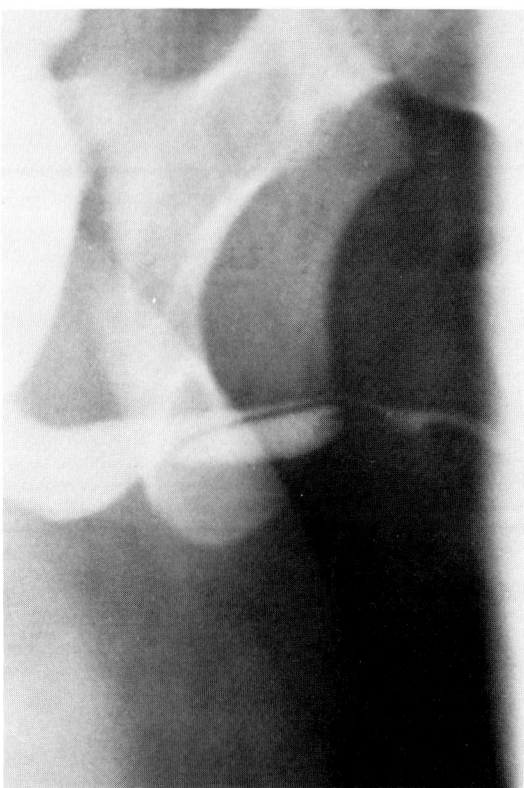

FIG. 10-13. Abnormal voiding cystourethrogram; urethral diverticulum seen in the bulbomembranous urethra.

atation of the ureter. The presence of a urethral diverticulum is seen as a pocket of contrast medium outside the apparent course of the urethra (Fig. 10-13). When urethral valves are present, marked dilatation of the prostatic urethra can be seen, along with a hypertrophied bladder neck. Reflux and hydroureteronephrosis may also be associated with the presence of urethral valves.

UROFLOW STUDIES

As elderly men are prepared for surgical procedures, physicians frequently try to identify patients at risk for postoperative voiding problems. Some of these individuals can be identified by the degree of nocturia and by hesitation, dribbling, and diminished force of the urinary stream. For several years, a simple but useful screening study has provided objective evidence of the presence of significant urinary outlet obstruction and has enabled one to identify patients who warrant further evaluation prior to undergoing other operations. All that is necessary is a co-operative patient and a uroflow meter. This noninvasive test simply requires that a patient urinate into a special apparatus that records the flow rate of urine during the period of urination (Fig. 10-14). The procedure has no complications or contraindications.

Interpretation

Nomograms have been generated that relate uroflow to volume voided.[5,6] Based on the peak and mean flow rates, it is possible to identify patients with significant outlet obstruction. Currently, significant urinary outlet obstruction is thought to be present when the patient's uroflow is more than 2 standard deviations below the mean for that particular volume of urine voided by the patient; the smaller the volume of urine, then the lower the uroflow. In addition, at least 100 ml urine are necessary for a reliable result. Although the study can indicate significant outlet obstruction, it does not determine whether the cause is from an enlarged prostate or from urethral stricture. Once a patient is found to have significant obstruction, then intravenous pyelography and cystoscopy are warranted for further evaluation.

CYSTOMETROGRAPHY

The cystometrogram provides information about the neurologic function of the urinary bladder (Fig. 10-15). It is indicated in patients with voiding dysfunction that may be secondary to endocrine disease such as diabetes, neurologic disease or trauma, major pelvic operations, or urinary obstruction. Special equipment and trained personnel are required. The procedure is usually well tolerated, it takes approximately 30 min to complete, and anesthesia is not required.

Technique

The procedure requires the placement of an indwelling Foley catheter. If the urethra is obstructed, a percutaneous cystostomy may be used. Prior to the procedure, all the urine is drained from the bladder. To quantitate the volume of residual urine, patients are asked to empty their bladder just prior to insertion of the catheter. Once the bladder has been emptied, the distal end of the catheter is connected to the cystometer. Most currently available machines instill carbon dioxide into the catheter. The carbon dioxide is instilled at a constant rate of 30 or 60 ml/min while simultaneously recording the intravesical pressure. The volumes at which the patient first notes bladder filling and at which the patient first feels the desire to void are recorded. The patient is asked to void through the catheter, and the intravesical pressure during vesical contraction is charted.

Complications

Complications are minimal. Although ureteral injury may result from placement of the catheter, this complication is infrequent when the study is per-

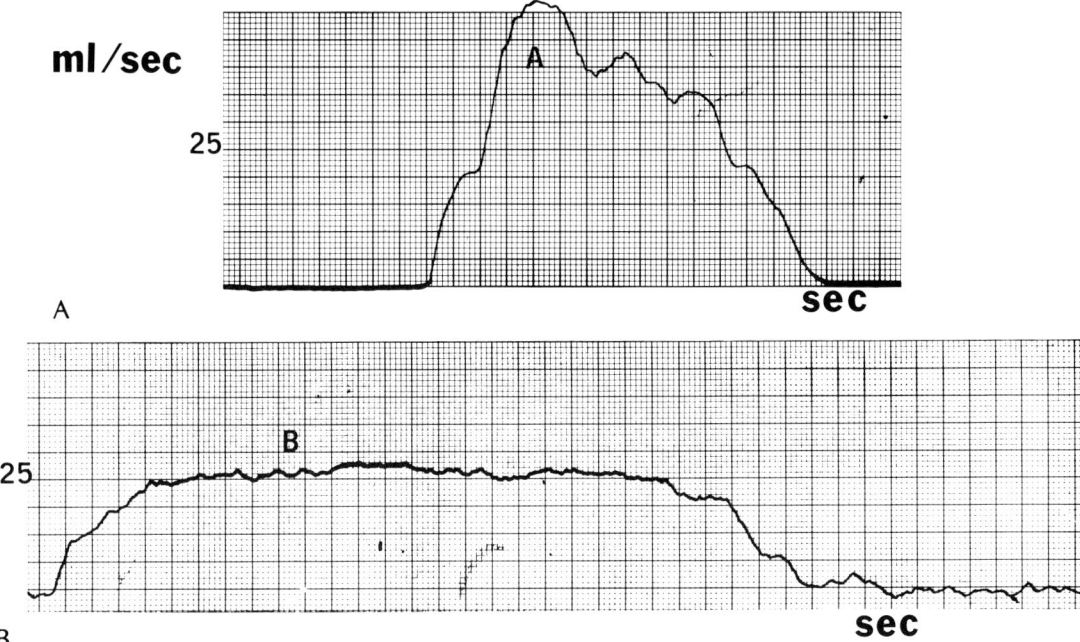

FIG. 10–14. *A,* Normal urinary flow; sharp rise in flow rate, with peak flow of 50 ml/sec (A). *B,* Abnormal urinary flow; prolonged time required to empty the bladder, and a maximum flow rate of only 25 ml/sec (B).

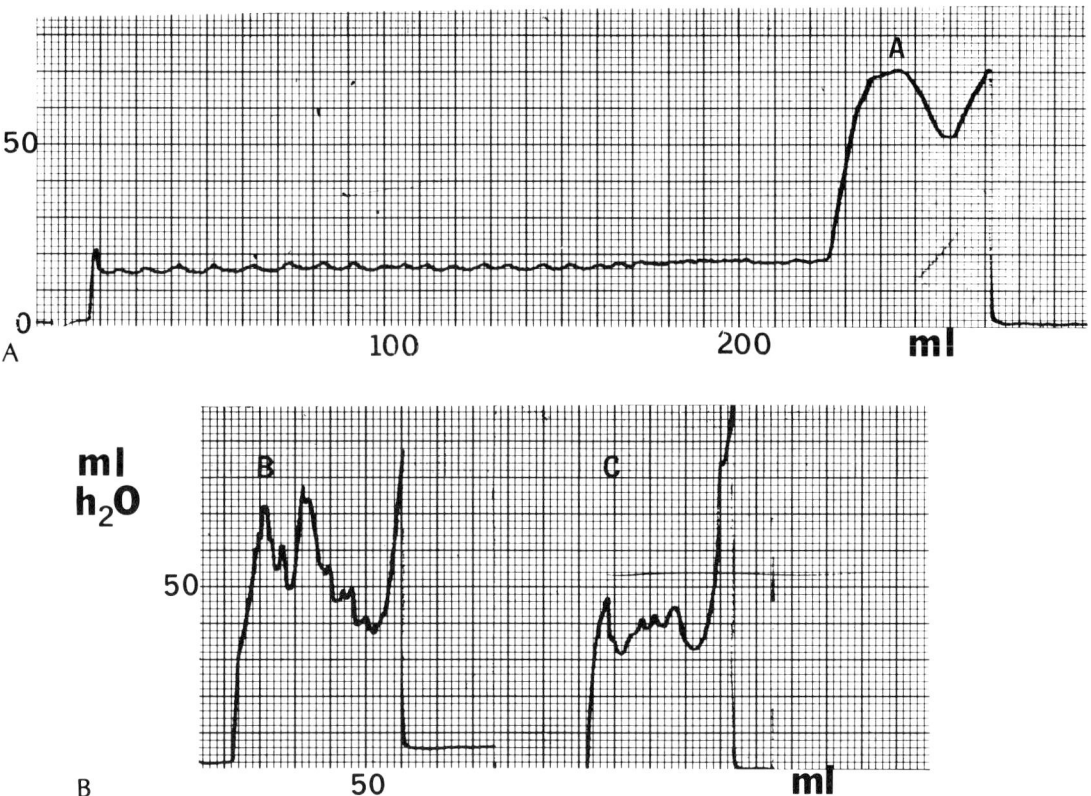

FIG. 10–15. *A,* Normal cystometrogram; no uninhibited contractions noted until voluntary contraction initiated (A) at 240 ml. *B,* Abnormal cystometrogram; involuntary contractions noted at 20 (B) and 110 ml (C).

formed by trained personnel. Another potential complication is the development of infection as a result of catheter placement.

Interpretation

Interpretation of urodynamic studies is a new and complex field and is beyond the scope of this chapter. In the normal patient, the first urge to urinate occurs at approximately 200 ml, and a contraction usually occurs at 450 ml. A multitude of abnormalities produce either no contraction (areflexic bladder), multiple uninhibited contractions (hyperreflexic bladder), or no sensation. Neurourology has evolved into a subspecialty devoted to understanding the neurogenic bladder and the use of pharmacologic agents to treat these abnormalities. The reader is referred elsewhere for a comprehensive discussion on the subject.[7-10]

REFERENCES

1. Barnes, R.W., Bergman, R.T., and Hadley, H.L.: Endoscopy. Berlin, Springer, 1959.
2. Bauer, K.M.: Cystoscopic Diagnosis. Philadelphia, Lea & Febiger, 1969.
3. Lalli, A.F.: Urographic contrast media reactions and anxiety. Radiology, *112*:267, 1974.
4. Fisher, H.W., and Doust, V.L.: An evaluation of pretesting in the problem of serious and fatal reactions to excretory urography. Radiology, *103*:497, 1972.
5. Siroky, M.B., Olsson, C.A., and Krane, R.J.: The flow rate nomogram. I. Development. J. Urol., *122*:665, 1979.
6. Siroky, M.B., Olsson, C.A., and Krane, R.J.: The flow rate nomogram. II. Clinical correlation. J. Urol., *123*:208, 1980.
7. Merrill, D.C., Bradley, W.E., and Markland, C.: Air cystometry. II. A clinical evaluation of normal adults. J. Urol., *106*:678, 1971.
8. Shoukry, I., et al.: Role of uroflowmetry in the assessment of lower urinary tract obstruction in adult males. Br. J. Urol., *47*:559, 1975.
9. Scott, F.B., Quesada, E.M., and Cardus, D.: The use of combined uroflowmetry, cystometry and electromyography in evaluation of neurogenic bladded dysfunction. *In* The Neurogenic Bladder. Edited by S. Boyarsky. Baltimore, Williams & Wilkins, 1967, p. 106.
10. Wear, J.B.: Cystometry. Urol. Clin. North Am., *1*:1, 1974.

SUGGESTED READING LIST

Abrams, H.L., and Adams, D.F.: Radiology of the urinary tract. *In* Campbell's Urology. 4th Ed. Edited by J.H. Harrison, et al. Philadelphia, W.B. Saunders, 1978.

Blaivas, J.G.: A critical appraisal of specific diagnostic techniques. *In* Critical Neuro-Urology. Edited by R.J. Krane and M.B. Sirokey. Boston, Little, Brown and Co., 1979.

Fisher, H.W., and Colgan, F.J.: Causes of contrast media reactions. Radiology, *121*:223, 1976.

Huffman, J.L., Bagley, D.H., and Lyon, E.S.: Treatment of distal ureteral calculi using rigid ureteroscope. Urology, *20*:574, 1982.

Lyon, E.S., Kyker, J.S., and Schoenberg, H.W.: Transurethral ureteroscopy in women: a ready addition to the urological armamentarium. J. Urol., *119*:35, 1978.

Siegle, R.L., and Lieberman, P.: A review of untoward reactions to iodinated contrast material. J. Urol., *119*:581, 1978.

Sussett, J.G., et al.: Critical evaluation of uroflowmeters and analysis of normal curves. J. Urol., *119*:874, 1973.

Wear, J.B.: Cystometry. Urol. Clin. North Am., *1*:1, 1974.

11

Rationale and Selection of Diagnostic Procedures for Airway and Chest Diseases

Paul A. Thomas ■ Donald K. Wood

Complete diagnostic evaluation of patients with disease of the airways, lungs, pleura, or chest wall should include a determination of the cause and an anatomic assessment of the extent of the disease. This information should be acquired efficiently, with minimal morbidity and at minimal cost. Therefore, the selection of appropriate diagnostic procedures, to be conducted in a logical sequence, is essential. The following diagnostic procedures are discussed in this chapter: laryngoscopy, bronchoscopy, bronchography, fine-needle aspiration, thoracentesis, pleural needle biopsy, mediastinoscopy, and thoracoscopy. Also included is an integrated consideration of selected procedures in the diagnosis of such common clinical problems as lung infiltrates and masses, diffuse lung diseases, pleural effusions, and midmediastinal masses.

Sequential selection of diagnostic procedures, from lower-risk interventions to those of greater magnitude and with higher associated morbidity, is an accepted practice.[1] The risk to the patient and potential morbidity are, at times, equated with the anesthetic requirements. Therefore, it may be appropriate to choose a procedure with a recognizably lower diagnostic yield that requires the use of topical or locally administered anesthetic agents before proceeding to a more invasive procedure requiring general anesthesia. Some of the procedures described are used for diagnostic purposes and to establish the extent of disease. For example, mediastinoscopy may be needed to establish a diagnosis of lung cancer, as well as to determine the extent of tumor involvement. The majority of patients who undergo these diagnostic procedures are hospitalized for the period of evaluation. Certainly, in isolated applications, bronchoscopy or thoracentesis may be performed in ambulatory outpatients, but diagnostic and therapeutic considerations usually dictate that most patients be in the hospital.

LARYNGOSCOPY

Indirect laryngoscopy should be an extension of the physical examination in patients who complain of voice change, hoarseness, or breathing limitation and in patients who are to undergo elective neck operations. Direct laryngoscopy is more complete and provides an opportunity to recover biopsy specimens. The examination is helpful in evaluating patients with neck masses, possible foreign-body aspiration, and neck trauma. In addition, assessment of the extent of tumor involvement in patients with oropharyngeal cancer is essential in determining appropriate therapy. Laryngoscopy, indirect or direct, must be preceded by thorough physical examination of the head and neck, including assessment of the quality of dentition, mobility and texture of the tongue, bimanual examination of the oral cavity, and palpation of the neck.

Technique

Indirect laryngoscopy is best accomplished when the patient is sitting upright, with the head extended forward. The patient's tongue is covered with a gauze pad, is grasped gently, and is pulled forward for insertion of a previously warmed mirror into the posterior pharynx. The base of the tongue, epiglottis, pyriform sinuses, and vocal cords are visualized as reverse images of their anatomic positions.

Direct laryngoscopy is possible using topical anesthesia; however, co-operation of the patient is critical. The examination is more complete and more satisfactory when general anesthesia is administered to the patient. When the patient has been properly positioned with the neck extended, the laryngoscope is inserted with pressure on the base of the tongue and epiglottis to visualize the vocal cords. Under direct vision, the function of the vocal cords may be observed, and biopsy specimens may be obtained from areas of pathologic interest. The procedure should be conducted in an appropriate operating room or specially equipped examining room.

Indications

The most frequent indication for laryngoscopy is voice change or hoarseness of worrisome duration. In addition, this examination is essential in evaluating the extent of disease in patients with malignant oropharyngeal tumors and in observing the response to treatment and the recurrence of disease. Diagnostic evaluation of patients with neck masses, dysphagia, and epistaxis is not complete without adequate examination of the pharynx and vocal cords. Other indications are upper airway obstruction, laryngeal nerve paresis, and trauma. Finally, and particularly in children, examination and extraction of foreign bodies may be accomplished laryngoscopically.

Indirect laryngoscopy is within the capability of every physician and should accompany the physical examination in patients with signs or symptoms of pharyngeal or vocal cord disturbance. Direct laryngoscopy should be performed by physicians with expertise in the management of patients with head and neck problems. Recognition of abnormalities is subjective, based on visual inspection and appreciation of normal anatomic variations. Confirmation of a suspected disorder is substantiated by histologic examination of tissue samples obtained for biopsy.

Laryngoscopy is a reliable examination that enables one to make an accurate diagnosis. Patients rarely benefit from a repeat examination. The examiner must recognize the few contraindications, such as trismus, cervical vertebrae fractures, airway stridor, and bleeding, and must be prepared to manage complications, primarily airway obstruction or bleeding.

BRONCHOSCOPY

In the diagnosis of patients with pulmonary disease, bronchoscopy is the single most important examination for determining the cause of a roentgenographic abnormality. In addition, the recent development of flexible instruments has revolutionized bronchoscopy by rendering the procedure less strenuous for patients and by allowing wider visualization of the tracheobronchial tree. The rigid bronchoscope is preferred for therapeutic intervention, however, such as foreign-body removal or topical treatment of intraluminal lesions. Bronchoscopic examination of patients with persistent symptoms, such as hemoptysis, or patients with roentgenographic abnormalities permits inspection of intraluminal masses, ulcerations, mucosal changes, and injuries, as well as anatomic localization of bleeding. In addition, histologic examination of biopsy specimens and cytologic assessment of brushings and aspirates confirm visual and roentgenographic observations.

Indications

The diagnostic indications for bronchoscopy include abnormal chest roentgenograms, unresolved pneumonia, bronchial rupture, pulmonary infections, gastric aspiration, foreign body aspiration, hemoptysis, wheeze, obstruction, suspicious cytologic findings, smoke inhalation, and change in cough.

Some patients may have a combination of several indications. Patients with suspected bronchogenic carcinoma frequently have a change in cough, hemoptysis, and an abnormal chest roentgenogram. The most common indications for bronchoscopy are related to the diagnosis of a suspected malignant tumor.

Technique

Bronchoscopy is usually done using topical anesthesia. In preparation, the patient should have nothing to eat or drink for 6 to 8 hours and will benefit from mild sedation. The instrument is advanced under direct vision, through the vocal cords and into the trachea. The flexible bronchoscope may be passed through the endotracheal tube in an intubated patient with a two-way adapter. In addition to the examination of the area of interest, all airways should be inspected. It is advisable to examine the entire bronchial tree prior to manipulation with biopsy forceps, to avoid stimulating uncontrollable coughing or problematic bleeding. The passage of brushes and biopsy forceps into pathologic areas of lung not visible endoscopically is enhanced by fluoroscopic guidance. The accuracy of diagnosis is increased by collecting multiple specimens.[2] In addition, washings may be collected for cytologic examination; postbronchoscopy sputum specimens may be valuable diagnostically. The more centrally the pathologic lesion is located, the greater is the likelihood of visualization of that lesion during bronchoscopy. For nonvisualized peripheral lung masses and infiltrates, the size and anatomic proximity to bronchial distribution influence the probability of recovering diagnostically specific material. Because the examination is safe and direct, however, and because laboratory interpretation of the results is accurate, bronchoscopy should be done.

Although the sensitivity of the bronchoscopic examination depends on the nature of the primary problem, a negative examination should be considered as an indication for additional diagnostic procedure. Bronchoscopy may be done as an ambulatory procedure, but the majority of patients require extensive evaluation on an inpatient basis. The procedure is technically complex and requires special training and experience. To pass the instrument into the trachea and to examine the tracheobronchial airways adequately, the bronchoscopist must thoroughly understand the anatomic features of the area. Therefore, the procedure should be limited to specialists in pulmonary medicine, thoracic surgery, or head and neck surgery, with few exceptions. Complications are infrequent and include hemorrhage, perforation, pneumothorax, and infection.[3]

BRONCHOGRAPHY

Bronchography is almost a lost art. Requests for this procedure are unusual because endoscopic examination is more direct and because the incidence of bronchiectasis for which surgical treatment may be indicated has decreased. Bronchography may be helpful in patients with hemoptysis and in whom an anatomic or pathologic explanation cannot be established by other means. Obscure focal bronchial ectasia or other endobronchial lesions may be defined by contrast media as the cause of bleeding. The procedure is not difficult; it requires only topical anesthesia and the co-operation of the patient for successful instillation of radiocontrast media and bronchial filling. Occasionally, bronchography is the only diagnostic examination that provides positive information. The procedure should be done by a radiologist and is usually performed in hospitalized patients undergoing multiple diagnostic procedures.

NEEDLE ASPIRATION

Percutaneous needle biopsy of the lung to recover pathologic tissue for diagnosis has been used sparingly for many years. Because the insertion of a cutting needle into the lung to secure a core of tissue is frequently associated with pneumothorax or pulmonary hemorrhage, the procedure has not had widespread application.[4] Enthusiasm for percutaneous fine-needle aspiration of pulmonary masses, nodules, and infiltrates has been coincident with the development of cytopathologic techniques and improved instrumentation.[5] The diagnostic accuracy of this procedure is enhanced by the availability of roentgenographic guidance for needle placement. The procedure is helpful in determining a preoperative diagnosis in patients with elusive disorders and in precluding the need for an otherwise unbeneficial thoracotomy for diagnostic lung biopsy.

Indications

The primary indication for percutaneous fine-needle aspiration of pulmonary lesions is diagnosis of pulmonary diseases not established by sputum examination or bronchoscopy. The suitability of the procedure for diagnosis of pulmonary nodules is controversial if thoracotomy is otherwise indicated.

Technique

Prior to the insertion of the needle, the lesion should be localized roentgenographically, to determine the most direct access. The patient's skin is prepared, it is infiltrated with a local anesthetic agent, and the needle is inserted. Under fluoroscopic guidance, the needle tip is advanced into the area of abnormality. Suction is applied continuously while the aspirating needle is withdrawn from the chest, and the contents of the needle are submitted on glass slides for cytologic examination. The presence of unmanageable bleeding diathesis is the only contraindication to the procedure. Pneumothorax, which occurs in 20 to 25% of patients, transient minor hemoptysis, and asymptomatic, mild pleural effusion may complicate the procedure. Percutaneous fine-needle aspiration of lung lesions should be within the capability of any physician with access to and knowledge of the radiographic equipment necessary to localize and to monitor needle insertion.

In a large series of patients with malignant disease, a single aspiration recovered malignant cells in 87%; the positive yield was increased to 96% in patients who underwent the procedure twice.[5] The procedure was diagnostically sensitive (99%) for malignant disease; however, the specificity was less satisfactory (87%), and a finding of no malignant cells was not dependable. The presence of specific infective organisms, shown either microscopically or by culture, excludes a diagnosis of malignant disease. The procedure is well accepted by patients confronted with thoracotomy as an alternative. In view of the nature of the clinical problem, the complexity of diagnosis and management, and the care required after the procedure, patients who undergo percutaneous fine-needle aspiration biopsy of lung lesions should be hospitalized.

PLEURAL BIOPSY

The appearance of pleural effusion may indicate underlying, serious, treatable disease, dissemination of malignant tumor, or some self-limiting, temporary inflammation of the pleura. The examination of pleural fluid for cell content and character, as well as for chemical constituents, and the search for exogenous infecting agents is not often fruitful. Therefore, it is frequently necessary to proceed beyond aspiration of pleural fluid.

Closed-needle biopsy of the pleura is considered appropriate and safe if fluid is present in the pleural space. The procedure is hazardous if the pleural space is void of fluid. In anticipation of a need for tissue, thoracentesis should be done in conjunction with provisions for needle biopsy. The probability of success is enhanced by taking three to five specimens.[6] Although the diagnostic yield of this procedure is low, the avoidance of thoracotomy makes it worthwhile in patients for whom the diagnosis can be thereby established. Complications are rare, and injury to an intercostal blood vessel is avoidable.

THORACENTESIS

Thoracentesis should be considered for all patients with pleural fluid, including blood, for both diagnostic and therapeutic reasons. Exceptions to the foregoing general rule are rare. In addition to diagnostic examination of the pleural fluid, it is equally important to remove as much of the fluid as possible, to prevent subsequent fibrothorax or trapped lung. The most appropriate site for thoracentesis can be readily identified by co-ordinating the roentgenographic findings with surface landmarks on the chest. Rib interspaces are easily palpated over the anterior chest and are projected laterally or posteriorly to areas of fluid collection noted on the chest roentgenogram. The aspirating needle may be directed by ultrasonic findings, but this procedure is not usually necessary. When the patient's skin has been prepared and aseptically draped, one should infiltrate the skin and intercostal tissues with a local anesthetic agent. The aspirating needle, usually attached to a three-way stopcock, should be inserted into the pleural space. If pleural biopsy specimens are to be obtained, a special needle should be inserted and positioned, and a specimen should be secured on withdrawal of the needle. Our preference is to aspirate all available pleural fluid before terminating the procedure. Complications are rare; the most serious is vasovagal reflex fainting and hypotension.

Results of thoracentesis and pleural biopsy may be considered diagnostic only when positive information is obtained, such as the identification of an infective organism by microscopic examination or culture, the cytologic identification of malignant cells, the finding of specific pathologic change in pleural tissue, or the identification of chyle in the aspirate. The diagnostic yield overall of this procedure is low, except in patients with diffuse malignant disease. Nonetheless, the procedure can be performed at the patient's bedside by most physicians and is rarely associated with morbidity. Although the procedure could be done on an outpatient basis, the need for further studies and the diagnostic implications dictate that most patients be in the hospital.

MEDIASTINOSCOPY

Lymph nodes in the lung's lymph-drainage pathway are readily available for sampling and histologic examination. Lymph nodes in the supraclavicular area are exposed through a cervical incision. Paratracheal, subcarinal, or peribronchial lymph nodes may be approached by either mediastinoscopy or parasternal mediastinotomy. In the absence of physically palpable supraclavicular masses, mediastinal lymph nodes are more likely to provide representative diagnostic tissue in patients with lung diseases. Mediastinoscopy was developed specifically for this application, although some physicians prefer mediastinotomy.[7,8]

Technique

Mediastinoscopy is best conducted under general anesthesia with endotracheal intubation. Exploration to the level of the tracheal bifurcation is essential in most patients and is unsatisfactory without adequate anesthesia and airway control. Through a small, suprasternal skin-crease incision, the pretracheal fascia is opened, and a passage for the mediastinoscope is developed by finger dissection. The mediastinoscope is insinuated between the trachea and the great vessels; one must keep tracheal rings in the field of vision, to prevent injury to surrounding structures. The instrument is moved into position, for identification of the tracheal bifurcation and the subcarinal area. When anatomic structures have been identified, one dissects the lymph nodes in the areas of interest using the aspirating instrument. By careful dissection and with patience, mediastinal lymph nodes are identified and are prepared for biopsy. Each structure or tissue exposed for biopsy must be tested first by fine-needle aspiration, to minimize the possibility of injury to blood vessels in the mediastinum. Frozen-section examination of tissue recovered may be used advantageously to ensure removal of diagnostically representative material. In addition, decisions regarding immediate thoracotomy in patients with lung cancer may be guided by findings during mediastinoscopy.

Complications

Complications of mediastinoscopy are infrequent. The most feared technical error is hemorrhage and the threat of exsanguination. Although this error has been reported by others, we have not encountered bleeding that could not be controlled by pressure, minimal cauterization, and patience. We have observed pneumothorax and chylothorax requiring closed pleural-space drainage.

Indications

Mediastinoscopy has been used in the diagnosis of midmediastinal masses, diffuse lung disease, and lung cancer, as well as the staging of lung cancer. Positive histopathologic findings in mediastinal lymph nodes are usually accepted as diagnostically definitive. The finding of lymph nodes with hyperplastic changes or no pathologic features must be considered in view of the potential for sampling error. Tissue should be recovered for examination from all patients undergoing mediastinoscopy; otherwise, the procedure is inadequate. As with other diagnostic procedures, negative findings should lead to additional examinations.

Mediastinoscopy should be attempted only by surgeons who are familiar with the anatomic limitations and risks of the procedure and who are capable of the surgical management of complicating hemorrhage. The diagnostic sensitivity of the study depends on the particular disease and on the indication for mediastinoscopy. Representative tissue can be recovered from 99% of patients with sarcoidosis. The diagnostic yield in patients with bronchogenic carcinoma is low if all patients are so examined; however, when the test is limited to patients with roentgenographic evidence of hilar, subcarinal, or paratracheal masses, results are usually diagnostically rewarding. The role of computed tomography of the mediastinum in the preliminary determination of mediastinoscopically approachable lymph nodes or masses is currently under clinical evaluation.

Mediastinoscopy should be performed in a well-equipped operating room, and patients should be hospitalized for postoperative observation, to enable one to detect bleeding, pneumothorax, or other complications necessitating intervention. In the absence of complications, patients may be discharged the following day.

THORACOSCOPY

Thoracoscopy was frequently used in the past to establish therapeutic pneumothorax for patients with pulmonary tuberculosis. Under direct vision, through the thoracoscope, the physician produced lysis of adhesions between the visceral and the parietal pleura. Thoracoscopy was discarded when effective antituberculous chemotherapy became available.

Indications

The procedure has been recently reintroduced as a means of acquiring needed diagnostic tissue from the lung or pleura without performing a thoracotomy. Examination of tissue specimens may be critical to the accurate diagnosis of obscure but treatable intrathoracic diseases. Thoracoscopy, or pleuroscopy, has been used with increasing frequency in immune-compromised patients with pulmonary infiltrates and in patients with undiagnosed persistent or recurrent pleural effusion.[9,10]

Technique

Although the procedure may be performed using either local or general anesthesia, the examination is more satisfactory when general anesthesia and endotracheal intubation are administered. The sheath of the instrument is introduced through a small, intercostal incision, and a pneumothorax is created. The procedure may be technically impossible if the pleural space has been obliterated by adhesions between the lung and the chest wall. At times, one may consider an alternate site of entry. Pathologic areas suitable for biopsy are usually recognizable on visual examination. Several biopsy specimens may be removed, depending on the amount of tissue required for the studies contemplated. On completion of the procedure, a chest tube may be placed through the trocar insertion site, for drainage of the pleural space.

Thoracoscopy is a suitable alternative to limited thoracotomy for the diagnosis of diffuse, nonsurgical diseases of the lung and pleura. Successful outcome includes not only the probability that a specific positive diagnosis has been established, but also the exclusion by the pathologic findings of certain clinically suspected diseases. For example, the exclusion of *Pneumocystis carinii* infection or a finding of nonspecific pleuritis instead of malignant disease may be significant in the subsequent management of the patient.

Thoracoscopy should be performed by an experienced thoracic surgeon who is familiar with intrathoracic anatomic structures and who is comfortable working with instruments that limit one's vision. The procedure should be done in a well-equipped operating room and is limited to patients in the hospital. Closed pleural-space drainage may be required for several days after thoracoscopy. Complications are unusual. The most important complication, uncontrolled persistent bleeding, has not been a problem in our experience.

Thoracoscopy with lung or pleural biopsy allows one to make a diagnosis in more than 95% of patients. The diagnostic accuracy is high if the exclusion of specific, clinically suspected, treatable diseases is judged to be a positive finding. A limited comparison between specimens secured through the thoracoscope and those removed from the same lung by limited thoracotomy has shown no diagnostic discrepancy. Therefore, thoracotomy may be avoided in almost all patients with diffuse lung or pleural disease. Technical failures are limited to patients with lung adherence to the chest wall and obliteration of the pleural space.

DIAGNOSIS OF FOCAL LUNG LESIONS

A tentative diagnosis of lung cancer made on the basis of roentgenographic findings alone requires definitive etiologic and histopathologic confirmation. All too often, sputum specimens are nonspecific.

Therefore, one should select a minimally invasive procedure with a high probability of recovering diagnostic material.

The application of fine-needle aspiration is controversial. Enthusiasts cite the high diagnostic yield, the minimal associated morbidity, and the directness of the procedure; however, the procedure depends on the availability of an experienced cytopathologist for accurate interpretation of the aspirate. Bronchoscopy should be done prior to thoracotomy, to ensure the probability of a disease-free tracheobronchial tree after lung resection. Physicians who do not readily advocate percutaneous fine-needle aspiration prefer bronchoscopy with fluoroscopically guided transbronchial lung biopsy as the initial invasive diagnostic procedure; in their view, fine-needle aspiration should be reserved for patients in whom endoscopic attempts at diagnosis have failed and who are not candidates for thoracotomy and resection. In some patients with an established diagnosis of lung cancer, mediastinoscopy is useful in staging the extent of disease. The procedure is also beneficial in patients with relative contraindications to major lung resection, to establish objective evidence of the extension of disease to the mediastinal lymph nodes. Finally, in a few patients, thoracotomy may be the appropriate diagnostic procedure. Therefore, bronchoscopy or fine-needle aspiration, followed by mediastinoscopy in selected patients and subsequent thoracotomy, is the generally accepted sequence of diagnostic testing for lung masses and focal infiltrates.

DIAGNOSIS OF DIFFUSE PULMONARY DISEASE

Diagnostic material may be recovered from the lungs of patients with diffuse pulmonary disease by bronchoscopy, transthoracic needle aspiration, thoracoscopy, or surgical lung biopsy. In addition, the nature of the lung disease may be reflected pathologically in the mediastinal lymph nodes. The selection of diagnostic procedures and the sequence of application must be modified by clinical urgency. The immune-compromised patient may experience rapid progression of disease and often needs urgent or emergency diagnosis.

The diagnostic approach to immune-competent patients may proceed as outlined schematically in Figure 11–1. With each diagnostic step, a time lapse of 24 to 48 hours is usually required, to allow the laboratory or pathologists to report results. Therefore, in the immune-compromised patient, several steps must be eliminated to enable one to establish an early diagnosis. If the smears of sputum or transtracheal washing fail to show bacteria, an immediate bronchoscopic examination should be done. If a diagnosis is not evident within 24 hours, direct lung biopsy is indicated. In our experience, the use of thoracoscopy is ideal under these circumstances. Whether the patient's immune system is competent or compromised, sufficient material must be collected to distribute to all appropriate sections of the laboratory, including histopathology, bacteriology, virology, and parasitology.

DIAGNOSIS OF PLEURAL EFFUSIONS

Pleural effusions can be characterized as self-limited, persistent, or recurrent. A self-limited effusion may respond after thoracentesis and may require no further diagnostic investigation. Self-limited pleural effusion may herald the onset of serious disease, such as active pulmonary tuberculosis, however, and it should not be dismissed lightly. Certainly, persistent and recurrent pleural effusions demand diagnostic as well as therapeutic attention. Definitive, etiologic diagnosis is based on the identification of infective organisms, the cytologic identification of certain cells, or the histopathologic examination of tissue specimens. Histologic examination of the pleura is usually indicated at the time of initial thoracentesis. Closed, percutaneous needle biopsy of the parietal pleura is most safely accomplished in the presence of pleural fluid. Further, three to five specimens should be obtained, to maximize the probability of an accurate diagnosis. Failure to establish the diagnosis may require pleural biopsy under visual control, to increase sampling accuracy. This situation is a primary indication for thoracoscopy for those familiar with the procedure. Alternatively, one should consider pleural biopsy through a thoracotomy.

DIAGNOSIS OF MEDIASTINAL AND HILAR MASSES

Diagnostic possibilities are numerous and are wide ranging when evaluating patients with roentgenographic abnormalities of the mediastinum and lung hilar areas. Anatomic structures can be clearly defined on high-quality chest roentgenograms supplemented with special examination when needed. Vascular problems should be readily recognized. Masses in the anterior and posterior mediastinum should be approached definitively for both diagnostic and therapeutic management. Therefore, the real difficulties in diagnosis are limited to the midmediastinum, paratracheal, subcarinal, and lung hilar areas. These areas have major lymph node concentration, and the diseases commonly observed in these locations are not amenable to surgical treatment. Representative tissue obtained during mediastinoscopy may provide sufficient information to enable one to distinguish granuloma from lymphoma. Fine-needle aspiration, endoscopically di-

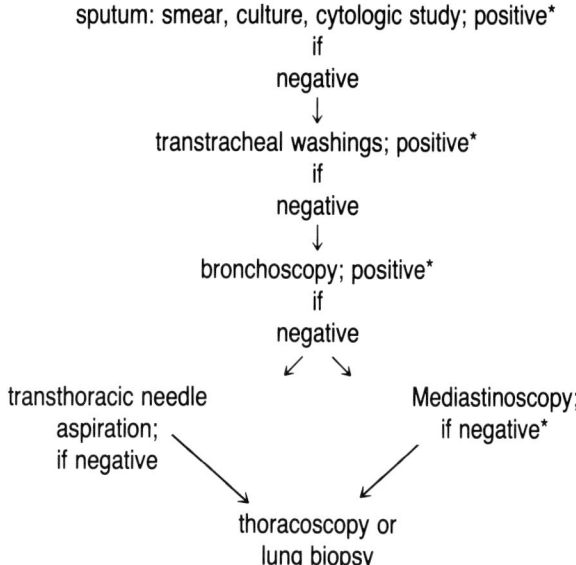

FIG. 11-1. Diagnostic approach to immune-competent patients with diffuse pulmonary disease.

rected through the trachea, is an alternative that may gain increasing popularity. The disadvantage of either approach is the minimal amount of tissue recovered in patients with mediastinal lymphoma; pathologists prefer to have a larger specimen.

REFERENCES

1. Thomas, P.A., Donnelly, J.C., Jr., and Haupt, G.J.: Rationale for selection and sequence of diagnostic surgical procedures in pulmonary disease. Surg. Clin. North Am., 53:617, 1973.
2. Kvale, P.A., Bode, F.R., and Kini, S.: Diagnostic accuracy in lung cancer: comparison of techniques used in association with flexible fiberoptic bronchoscopy. Chest, 69:752, 1976.
3. Credle, W., Smiddy, J., and Elliott, R.: Complications of fiberoptic bronchoscopy. Am. Rev. Respir. Dis., 109:67, 1974.
4. Forrest, J.V., and Sagel, S.S.: Cutting needle biopsies. Chest, 69:245, 1976.
5. Sagel, S.S., et al.: Percutaneous transthoracic aspiration needle biopsy. Ann. Thorac. Surg., 26:399, 1978.
6. Levine, J., and Cugell, D.W.: Blunt-end needle biopsy of pleura and rib. Arch. Intern. Med., 109:516, 1962.
7. Carlens, E.: Mediastinoscopy. Dis. Chest, 36:343, 1959.
8. McNeill, T.M., and Chamberlain, J.M.: Diagnostic anterior mediastinotomy. Ann. Thorac. Surg., 2:532, 1966.
9. Dijkman, J.H., et al.: Transpleural lung biopsy by the thoracoscopic route in patients with diffuse interstitial pulmonary disease. Chest, 82:76, 1982.
10. Canto, A., et al.: Thoracoscopy in the diagnosis of pleural effusion. Thorax, 32:550, 1977.

12

Upper Gastrointestinal Endoscopy

C. Thomas Bombeck

HISTORY

Upper gastrointestinal endoscopy is by no means a new diagnostic technique. The principle of the lighted endoscope was first applied in 1837 by Bergdorf. The true pioneer in modern endoscopy was Mickulicz who, in 1867, described the first angled endoscope. The next significant advance in endoscopy occurred at the turn of the century with the invention of the miniaturized light bulb. Using that light source, Jackson developed the modern rigid endoscope. The rigid instrument enabled the physician adequately to visualize the entirety of the esophagus, but only a small portion of the fundus of the stomach, and that only with great difficulty.

In 1922, Schindler made the next great advance when he developed the flexible-lens gastroscope, based on the principle that a linear series of small but convex lenses could transmit an image even though they were not exactly in line, but rather were curved. This advance led to the development of the first semiflexible gastroscope, which consisted of a rigid telescope with the flexible lens series located in the distal 25 cm of the tip. The optical quality of the transmitted image available with that endoscope has not been surpassed today. On the other hand, the endoscope was limited by its inflexibility, by the necessity for keeping the patient in an uncomfortable position with the neck hyperextended for long periods of time, and by the availability of only a right-angle side view from the tip of the endoscope with which to visualize most of the stomach. This last feature made Schindler's gastroscope useless for examination of the esophagus and added an element of danger to the examination of any structure because of the need to introduce the instrument blindly. Moreover, limitations in flexibility did not permit complete visualization of the entire stomach, but rather an intermittent view of the periesophageal fundus and the lesser curvature of the antrum. Finally, length limitations on the optical system did not permit examination of the duodenum.

In 1952, Hirschowitz, in conjunction with the ACMI Company of the United States, developed the first truly fiberoptic esophagogastroscope. At about the same time, several Japanese companies, most notably Olympus Optical, developed similar instruments. Since then, advances in endoscopic technology have been rapid. Instruments now available enable one to examine the entirety of the esophagus, the stomach, and the first, second, and third portions of the duodenum. These advances are by no means complete, and instruments are now under development for visualization of most of the small intestine as well.

Side by side with the development of the fiberoptic gastroscope came the gastrocamera. Initially, the gastrocamera of a miniaturized 4.0-mm camera mounted on the end of a control shaft that was fully flexible. The camera could be passed into the patient's stomach, and multiple photographs could be taken blindly. When these photographs were developed, an excellent view of the gastric mucosa could be obtained, but the view was always randomly oriented, and localization of any lesion depended on the chance inclusion of a gastroscopic landmark in the photograph.

The next step in this technology was inclusion of a fiberoptic image-transmitting bundle in the control shaft to allow manipulation of the camera under direct visual control. The image transmitted by those initial fiberoptic bundles was poor in resolution, but when supplemented by photographs taken with the endoscopic camera, it provided valuable diagnostic information. The best photographs currently available in atlases of and monographs on endoscopy are those taken with the gastrocamera.

The greatest advance in gastrocamera technology has recently been introduced by the Welch Allyn Company of the United States, who have developed a miniaturized television camera. This instrument has been incorporated into endoscopic apparatus for examination of the entire gastrointestinal tract. The camera, mounted in the tip of the instrument, provides a "real-time" image of the entire esophagus, stomach, and duodenum, with resolution much better than with any but the finest and most expensive fiberoptic viewing bundles. In addition, because the image is transmitted to a large color monitor rather than to a single eyepiece, it may be simultaneously viewed by many examiners and may be recorded for both archival and teaching purposes. At the present time, the durability of that instrument remains to be assessed. Because real-time imaging is obtained with the television camera, no fiberoptic viewing bundle is necessary.

Although the fiberoptic upper gastrointestinal endoscopes and the television endoscopes all provide excellent diagnostic information, they are limited in therapeutic application. Because of the necessity for fiberoptic light-carrying bundles as well as the fiberoptic viewing bundle or television-control apparatus in the endoscope, little space is available for channels to allow passage of large surgical instruments. Nonetheless, a whole family of miniaturized biopsy, grasping, snaring, washing, and brushing instruments has been developed. These instruments have not only enhanced the diagnostic quality of endoscopic devices, but they have also made possible endoscopic surgical procedures on the pancreas, biliary tract, and stomach. Discussion of the therapeutic application of these instruments is beyond the scope of this volume.

INSTRUMENTS

A number of different instruments are available for upper gastrointestinal endoscopy.

Rigid Esophagoscope

A brief mention of the rigid esophagoscope is warranted. Although many of the diagnostic functions of the rigid endoscope have been transferred to the fiberoptic instruments, the rigid instrument still has certain applications. Because its large lumen allows passage of much larger biopsy and grasping instruments than that of the fiberoptic endoscope, manipulation of foreign bodies in the esophagus is much more easily managed with the rigid endoscope. In addition, when insufflation of air into the esophagus or stomach may be dangerous, such as in patients with perforations, the rigid endoscope may be used because it depends for its view of the esophageal mucosa on obturation of the esophagus by the tip of the endoscope, rather than on distention of the organ. Thus, as the endoscope is advanced, a lesion may be visualized without the necessity of distending the esophagus with air.

Two types of these endoscopes are generally available, Jackson and Hollinger endoscopes. They are manufactured in a variety of sizes, to accommodate both adult and pediatric practice. These devices vary in the configuration of their tips, but most consist of a rigid metal tube with a light source at the tip in the form of a light bulb or a fiberoptic light-transmission bundle that may be passed down on a separate channel in the wall of the endoscope. The use of these instruments requires extreme cooperation on the part of the patient because they must be passed with the patient's head in the hyperextended position. Complete local anesthesia of the pharynx and of the hypopharynx is necessary. In some centers, all rigid-endoscopic examinations of the esophagus are carried out with the patient under general anesthesia. The incidence of esophageal perforation with these instruments during routine diagnostic examination approximates 5%.

Esophagogastroduodenoscope

The esophagogastroduodenoscope in current use may be called a true "pan endoscope." It is an end- or forward-viewing instrument that allows visualization of the lumen of the gastrointestinal tract as the instrument is introduced. Because of this feature, and because of the flexibility of the instrument as a result of fiberoptic construction, the incidence of perforation has been reduced to nearly the point of negligibility (.07%). The instrument is available in three different sizes. These are standard, slim, and pediatric.

STANDARD. The standard endoscope is 11 to 12 mm in diameter, is capable of biplanar flexion at the tip, is constructed with the forward-viewing lens in the tip of the instrument coupled to a fiberoptic bundle that terminates in an eyepiece system of lenses for the operator, and is further equipped with 2 fiberoptic light-transmission bundles and capabilities for biopsy, suction, washing, and air insufflation. Instruments vary in length from manufacturer to manufacturer, but they average about 145 cm. Because the standard instrument is stiff at the tip and is large, it is difficult to introduce into the patient's esophagus and is not easy for the patient to swallow. On the other hand, its size and relative rigidity allow it to be used to forcibly dilate strictures in various parts of the upper gastrointestinal tract. Furthermore, its large size allows incorporation of an extra channel through which another biopsy instrument may be passed simultaneously or of a large biopsy channel for the passage of larger-than-normal manipulative instruments. Finally, its size allows larger and more durable fiberoptic bundles to be used, as well as thicker and more adequate protection for the body of the instrument. When one considers that these instruments are expensive, features that lend to durability become important.

SLIM. Because of improvements in the optical quality of available fiberoptic bundles, owing primarily to diminution in the size of individual fibers in those bundles as well as to improvements in the methods of bonding fibers together to form a geometrically uniform bundle, slimmer and more flexible endoscopes have been developed. Each instrument manufacturer now produces these "slim" instruments, which have become the most widely used in diagnostic upper gastrointestinal endoscopy. They have all the features of the standard endoscope, but in improved versions. The tips of these instruments are fully flexible, to allow complete visualization of the entire stomach, a goal not always possible with the standard endoscope. At the present time, the biplanar tip deflection of the endoscope usually has 180 or 190° of retrograde flexion in one direction, 150° of flexion in the opposite direction, and at least 90° of flexion in the bisecting planar direction. These instruments are limited by a small biopsy channel. Several variations of these instruments, including oblique-viewing lenses at the tip or tiltable prisms in the tip for either forward or side viewing, have been introduced, but these devices have been associated with an unacceptable incidence of complications.

PEDIATRIC. Most manufacturers of endoscopes also produce a forward-viewing instrument with a slim fiberoptic viewing and light-transmission bundle system originally intended for pediatric use. In fact, the standard slim endoscope may be used in pediatric patients, even in infants, with nearly the same ease as pediatric endoscopes. Nonetheless, pediatric endoscopes have other applications because of their small, 7-mm diameter, which allows them to be introduced through strictures that do not admit passage of either a standard or a slim endoscope. These pediatric devices may also be used as carriers of other types of instrumentation mounted on the outside of the endoscope. One company has recently introduced a fabric and rubber balloon, for pneumatic dilatation, that is to be mounted on the outside of a pediatric endoscope. These endoscopes are limited by the small bundles available for light transmission that make complete illumination of a dilated stomach nearly impossible because of the narrow field of view of the small lens at the endoscope's tip. The biopsy channels of these pediatric instruments are even smaller than those of the slim endoscopes, so it is difficult to obtain adequate biopsy specimens with the instruments that can be passed through the channels. Nonetheless, because of their small size, pediatric instruments are much better tolerated by patients than standard endoscopes and are widely used in the evaluation of existing, known lesions. Most endoscopic facilities have a pediatric endoscope as a backup instrument.

Side-Viewing Versus End-Viewing Endoscopes

Although all early gastroscopes, such as the Schindler instrument, were side-viewing endoscopes, most recently trained endoscopists prefer to use end-viewing flexible fiberoptic endoscopes. Nonetheless, many individuals who have become skillful with the side-viewing endoscope prefer it to the end-viewing endoscope because of the ease with which it may be manipulated in examining the stomach. The primary application of the side-viewing flexible endoscope is manipulation and instrumentation of the ampulla of Vater. It is nearly impossible to intubate the ampulla with an end-viewing instrument because of the small diameter of the duodenum, whereas direct intubation with a side-viewing instrument in the hands of an experienced endoscopist is a matter of only 10 or 15 min because of the "en face" view provided. The side-viewing endoscope is unsurpassed for complete viewing of the entire stomach. With end-viewing endoscopes, it may be difficult to visualize the lesser curvature of the antrum and the area immediately around the gastroesophageal junction. Special maneuvers, such as the inversion maneuver, have been devised to lessen these difficulties, but the problems remain because of limitation in light sources and wide variations in stomach size from patient to patient. Use of the side-viewing endoscope does not impose these limitations. On the other hand, the side-viewing endoscope is essentially useless for diagnostic maneuvers in the esophagus. Further, in areas where blind passage of an instrument may lead to difficulty, the side-viewing endoscope simply "cannot see where it is going."

Various attempts have been made to combine the best features of end-viewing and side-viewing endoscopes. These developments include tiltable prisms in the tip of the endoscope, to convert the device from a side-viewing to an end-viewing instrument and incorporation of a mirror system in the tip of the endoscope, to allow one to view structures in an oblique direction rather than in the side- or end-viewing mode. These attempts have not succeeded, primarily because of the complexity of the mechanical systems. In the case of the oblique-viewing instrument, the endoscope has none of the advantages of the full end view or of the whole side view. Certain examinations can only be carried out with the side-viewing endoscope. The duodenum is simply not large enough to allow routine visualization of the ampulla of Vater, except in profile, with an end-viewing endoscope. A side-viewing endoscope enables one to obtain a direct "en face" view and allows direct manipulation of the ampulla. Maneuvers such as endoscopic cholangiopancreatography can only be performed with a side-viewing endoscope.

In conjunction with the side-viewing endoscope, several specialized devices have been produced for particular functions. These devices include directable cannulas for intubation of the ampulla of Vater, to allow contrast radiography of the pancreatic and biliary ductal systems, and snares, loops, and other devices for operative manipulation of the ampulla. A separate, small endoscope may even be passed through the biopsy channel of a larger side-viewing endoscope and into the ampulla of Vater, for direct visualization of the interior of the biliary tract. The miniature size of this instrument has made it expensive, and consequently, it has not become popular.

New Developments

Progress in the development of new endoscopes is continual. The last 5 years have seen significant improvement in the optical quality of the image transmitted by the fiberoptic bundle, as well as in the durability of the bundle itself. The primary limitation of all endoscopes has been the finite number of flexions through which a fiberoptic bundle may be stressed. Repeated flexions of the bundle lead to fatigue in the glass fibers of the bundle and in the bonding agents that maintain their orientation. Because of this characteristic, repeated use of any endoscope eventually leads to disorientation of the image or fracture of individual fibers in the bundle and causes blind spots in the image. The use of smaller and smaller fibers has lessened this difficulty, and improvement in the bonding agents has led to the production of more durable bundles. These improvements, in turn, increase the longevity of an endoscope and therefore decrease the relative cost of an endoscopic examination. The foregoing advances have also made possible the development of longer and longer endoscopes. At present, an enteroscope has been introduced and is under investigation in specialized centers for examination of most of the small bowel.

ENDOSCOPIC SPECIALIZATION

The practice of gastrointestinal endoscopy deserves mention. Because of the complexity of the instrumentation, as well as the complex and varied nature of the many diseases that may be encountered and diagnosed, the temptation has been strong for some physicians to devote their entire careers to gastrointestinal endoscopy. This practice has been widely regarded by both surgeons and gastroenterologists as a serious error. Gastrointestinal endoscopy should be used by both medical and surgical physicians specializing in the treatment of gastrointestinal disease. Endoscopy is an adjunct to the practice of gastrointestinal medicine and not an end in itself.

GASTROINTESTINAL ENDOSCOPIC LABORATORY

Because of the specialized nature of gastrointestinal endoscopic instruments, and because of their fragility, it has become necessary to develop a specialized locale for their use. In the past, it was customary to perform gastrointestinal endoscopic studies in radiology suites or in operating rooms, but neither setting is ideal for this purpose. Any institution that anticipates more than a token number of gastrointestinal endoscopic examinations should have a specialized laboratory for that purpose. Specialized tables designed for endoscopic studies allow easy mechanical manipulation of the patient, for ideal positioning for any examination.

Gastrointestinal assistants, who are usually nurses with extra training, have achieved identity as a paramedical group. Many of these individuals have become so experienced that, in some countries, they are the primary performer of the examination. Routine gastrocamera surveys are carried out in Japan by technicians without the intervention of a physician, except in the final analysis of the photographs. This situation is analgous to that in hospital radiology departments, in which radiographs are taken by technicians, but are read by radiologists.

The instruments themselves are delicate and require careful maintenance with a detailed knowledge of their structure and functions. The dedicated gastrointestinal assistant performs this function superbly, whereas the standard general nurse, even the operating-room-instrument nurse, has little knowledge of the principles of fiberoptics and less appreciation of the necessity for meticulous and painstaking cleaning of the instruments. Failure to follow these principles leads to the inevitable and early deterioration of an instrument and thereby makes it either useless or unavailable for further examinations.

Finally, although in the actual performance of any endoscopic examination, only one operator, the endoscopist, is required, the extra pair of hands provided by the assistant is valuable when specialized maneuvers, such as biopsy, are performed. The endoscopist obtains the biopsy specimen, and the assistant places it in fixative, labels the bottles, cleans the instruments, helps to pass the instruments, and helps to position the endoscope for the next biopsy. An endoscopic examination performed by an endoscopist alone may become cumbersome, time-consuming, and uncomfortable for the patient.

INDICATIONS

Several attempts have been made to define rigid indications for and contraindications to the performance of upper gastrointestinal endoscopy. The whole field is in such a state of flux with rapid advancements in instrument technology and increasing numbers of new findings regarding gastrointestinal disorders that such rules have proved unworkable. It is therefore possible only to say that gastrointestinal endoscopy is indicated whenever it may be helpful for the treating physician to view a disorder directly. The direct view of a lesion in the upper gastrointestinal tract is so superior to that provided by radiographic examination that, in many centers, endoscopy is replacing routine radiographic contrast studies of the upper gastrointestinal tract. Although it is not possible categorically to state conditions for which upper gastrointestinal endoscopy is not required, one may now name several conditions for which it is absolutely required. These conditions are discussed under the categories of the various organs of the gastrointestinal tract.

Esophagus

Any patient with dysphagia requires an upper gastrointestinal endoscopic examination as an integral and early part of the diagnostic evaluation. Symptoms relative to the esophagus are generally not specific and indicate only a problem with the organ, but not necessarily the nature of that problem. Patients with carcinoma of the esophagus may have nothing other than heartburn, and patients with esophagitis may primarily have dysphagia. Any patient with symptoms at all suggestive of esophageal involvement may therefore need to be evaluated endoscopically some time in the course of the examination. Patients with classic symptoms of heartburn and gastroesophageal reflux may have an endoscopic examination deferred while initial treatment is undertaken, but the presence of any aberrant symptoms immediately calls for endoscopy. If the symptoms of regurgitation persist despite adequate nonoperative therapy, then endoscopy must be performed.

Any patient for whom an operation is contemplated must be endoscopically evaluated prior to that operation, to determine the nature of the anatomic defect. Obviously, the differentiation between an obstructing carcinoma of the esophagus and an esophageal stricture requires endoscopic study and biopsy done under the most meticulous conditions. Even then, it may not be possible to distinguish between the two on early examination, and repeated studies may be required.

The specialized instance of the desmoplastic tumor of the esophagus, which produces an intense fibrous reaction and closely mimics stricture, requires further evaluation. In such a case, when the lesion is viewed from above and is seen to represent only a tight stricture, dilation of that stricture is necessary. These kinds of evaluations may be augmented by specialized techniques of brushing and washing the length of the esophagus, including the underside of the stricture, to permit cytologic examinations.

In the past, the presence of esophageal diverticula was a relative contraindication to the performance of upper gastrointestinal endoscopy. This consideration was valid when the instruments available were primarily side-viewing endoscopes and when the view provided by the instrument was such that the operator was required to pass the endoscope blindly through the esophagus before any meaningful view could be obtained. It was obviously possible to pass the instrument into the orifice of a diverticulum and to perforate it before the operator was aware of the location of the tip of the instrument. The newer end-viewing endoscope has largely resolved this difficulty; the orifice of the diverticulum may be visualized and may safely be bypassed during the insertion of the endoscope. In addition, diverticula have often been reported in association with neoplastic lesions, possibly because of the stagnant inflammation of the diverticulum from retained foodstuffs. Exclusion of such a diagnosis by examination is therefore a relative indication for endoscopic study.

The one possible contraindication is the high-lying pharyngoesophageal or Zenker's diverticulum. This particular lesion is located in the cricopharyngeus, which remains the one blind spot for passage of any endoscope. It is therefore possible to pass the instrument into the lumen of a Zenker's diverticulum without being aware of this deviation. Nonetheless, if adequate reason exists to suspect the presence of a concomitant lesion in the esophagus, even the patient with a Zenker's diverticulum should undergo endoscopy, but with great caution, to avoid perforation of that diverticulum.

The inflammatory diseases of the esophagus may only be differentiated by upper gastrointestinal endoscopy. Indeed, because of the wide use of this diagnostic technique, the number of diseases of the esophageal mucosa that can be detected has increased. Such lesions as cytomegalic inclusion disease of the esophagus or extensive herpes of the esophagus have only recently been described, although they have been present for many years. Esophageal bleeding, a special indication for gastrointestinal endoscopic examination, is discussed separately.

Stomach

The general rule is that any mass lesion in the stomach should be endoscopically examined. Although radiologists have obtained a reasonable degree of accuracy, 85% or better, in identifying mass lesions in the stomach, the remaining 15% and the high percentage of errors of identification lead to the recommendation that all mass lesions must be viewed directly. Coupled with biopsy and brush cytologic study, endoscopic examination has raised the accuracy of diagnoses of these lesions to nearly 100%. Detection of diseases such as early gastric cancer, as described in Japan, is a true child of the endoscopic age. The existence of such diseases was really not even suspected until routine endoscopy, usually for other reasons, showed a mucosal defect that could seldom be radiologically defined. When such a mucosal defect underwent biopsy, it showed either dysplastic changes of the gastric mucosal epithelium or true metaplasia, leading to diagnosis of carcinoma "in situ." Because of early detection of these lesions from routine endoscopic survey, the Japanese have raised the cure rate for all gastric carcinomas several fold and the cure rate for these particular lesions to 95%.

Gastric ulcer as an indication is still disputed. Although, at least in the United States, 97% of gastric ulcers discovered in the symptomatic patient are benign, and endoscopic differentiation of a carcinoma from these ulcers by the time they reach the ulcerated stage adds nothing to the survival rate, most endoscopists routinely examine patients with gastric ulcers. No real reason exists for this examination, except alleviation or confirmation of the fears of the patient and the physician. Depending upon the view of the individual physician, that indication may be sufficient. If a gastric ulcer heals with adequate therapy within the usually prescribed 4 to 6 weeks, then it is unlikely to be a carcinoma. This healing may be followed and confirmed radiologically; endoscopic examination is not necessary. Upper gastrointestinal examination may be justifiable in patients with symptoms that indicate a problem in the stomach, duodenum, or esophagus, although all other diagnostic techniques have failed to show a lesion. Several entities may only be detected endoscopically, including early gastric cancers and inflammatory lesion of the gastric mucosa that are too superficial to produce anatomic deformities of the stomach. Such disorders as acute gastritis, acute infectious gastritis, or drug-induced gastritis may only be seen endoscopically in the early stages.

Duodenum

In contrast to gastric ulcers, duodenal ulcers seldom require endoscopic examination. Carcinoma of the duodenum and, especially, ulcerated carcinoma of the duodenum are so rare that routine upper gastrointestinal endoscopic examination of a duodenal ulcer is not justified. The expense of the thousands of examinations that would be required to detect one carcinoma is not supportable. For this reason, when a patient has symptoms of a duodenal ulcer and is found to have such an ulcer on x-ray examination, upper gastrointestinal endoscopy is not indicated. Only when an operation is contemplated for the duodenal ulcer should endoscopy be used. The only reason for this recommendation is the advent of newer operations such as selective vagotomy. In this instance, endoscopy not only allows the detection of concomitant lesions that might require treatment at the time of operation, but also demonstrates the adequacy of the pyloric canal, which may be obstructed by the ulcer itself. If a standard endoscope may be passed through the pylorus, then the pyloric channel may be considered adequate, and operative procedures to improve gastric drainage will not be necessary. As in the stomach, the presence of any duodenal mass lesion is an indication for prompt endoscopy.

Pancreas

Upper gastrointestinal endoscopy, coupled with the specialized examination of endoscopic retrograde cholangiopancreatography, is absolutely indicated prior to the operative treatment of such diseases as chronic pancreatitis or carcinoma of the pancreas. Those specialized examinations allow anatomic definition of the pancreatic ductal system and, especially, assessment of the extent of involvement of that system by the primary disease. Such examinations dictate the type of operation to be performed. In the past, it was customary to carry out this radiographic examination on the operating table, with a cannula inserted directly into the ampulla of Vater through a duodenotomy. This maneuver requires a great deal of time, with attendant increases in anesthetic time and in the incidence of complications. Prior endoscopic examination makes this operative manipulation unnecessary. In centers equipped to perform the examination, cytologic investigation of the pancreatic fluid is also indicated when a diagnosis of carcinoma of the pancreas is likely.

Biliary Tract

Patients with obstructive jaundice that does not resolve promptly or that cannot be shown to be due to an obstructing stone require early endoscopic study. Only this examination shows such lesions as carcinoma of the ampulla of Vater in their curable stages.

Upper Gastrointestinal Bleeding

Upper gastrointestinal bleeding is discussed separately because it is usually impossible to determine the exact site of such bleeding. Opinions vary widely regarding the timing of endoscopic examinations in these patients. Some investigators, our own group among them, believe that upper gastrointestinal bleeding is an urgent indication for upper gastrointestinal endoscopic examination. The reason is that one patient may have multiple upper gastrointestinal lesions that are capable of bleeding. If the patient does not undergo an endoscopic examination during the active bleeding episode, it will not be possible to determine which lesion has bled. It is common in a large, city-hospital practice, in which many patients with alcoholism are seen, to encounter a patient with esophageal varices, acute alcoholic gastritis, and duodenal ulcer. If the patient does not undergo endoscopy during the active bleeding episode, then all three lesions will be described, but no one will know which one has bled. Because the treatment of each of these three lesions is different, one will not be able to determine the proper course of management.

On the other hand, investigators primarily engaged in large private-hospital practice have not had the foregoing experience. In that instance, a single lesion is usually encountered, and it makes no difference when the patient undergoes endoscopy because bleeding can usually be stopped with supportive measures. One may then proceed with an unhurried, detailed examination of the upper gastrointestinal tract, rather than the emergency examination in the middle of the night. The emergency examination obviously is fraught with more complications than the elective examination, and one cannot be as thorough. Investigations from these centers have indicated that emergency endoscopic examination has not changed the course of treatment in patients with upper gastrointestinal bleeding; these findings suggest that performing the examination as an emergency really has no marked benefit. On the other hand, the patient who requires an operation because of continued bleeding certainly benefits from an accurate preoperative diagnosis. Because it is not possible initially to predict which patients will continue to bleed, endoscopic examination should be done urgently, if not as an absolute emergency.

As a general rule, the type of bleeding dictates the type of examination. In patients with massive upper gastrointestinal hemorrhage sufficient to produce changes in vital signs and significant return of blood through a nasogastric tube, endoscopic examination cannot be satisfactorily performed. The large volume of blood trapped in the stomach makes visualization of the gastrointestinal mucosa nearly impossible. The suction ports of all standard endoscopic instruments are too small to allow adequate clearing of bleeding of this magnitude. The most useful examination in such a situation is frequently angiography, if one has time. If not, then the only appropriate examination is direct study of the interior of the gastrointestinal tract by exploratory laparotomy.

If the bleeding can be cleared by upper gastrointestinal lavage with iced saline solutions, then urgent endoscopic examination should be undertaken. In this instance, as soon as it is determined that the patient is bleeding from the upper gastrointestinal tract, a nasogastric tube should be inserted, and lavage should be begun. When the lavage fluid is pink and not red, then the lavage tube should be removed, and the endoscope should be inserted. This procedure allows at least gross determination of the general location of the bleeding site and thereby gives an indication of the nature of the bleeding lesion. Obviously, if the blood is returning from the duodenum through the pylorus, even though a duodenal ulcer may not be seen, the chances are almost overwhelming that the cause of the bleeding is a duodenal ulcer. Esophageal varices may be directly visualized under the same circumstances, and bleeding acute gastritis may also be readily seen and treated.

Finally, acute blood loss from the upper or lower gastrointestinal tract is frequently an indication for extensive endoscopic examination. When all other examinations have failed to enable one to make a diagnosis, even when a patient has no upper gastrointestinal symptoms, one must perform an endoscopic examination of the esophagus, stomach, and duodenum. The incidence of silent lesions of the esophagus, stomach, and duodenum is such that approximately 50% of the causes of acute gastrointestinal bleeding may be detected by this combination of endoscopic examinations.

CONTRAINDICATIONS

Contraindications to upper gastrointestinal endoscopy include situations in which the examination may add nothing to treatment and in which the examination itself may be harmful. In the first instance, we have already discussed duodenal ulcers, for which endoscopic examination is simply not required. The second type of contraindication, cases in which the examination might be harmful, has been steadily diminished by modifications in endoscopic techniques and by the introduction of newer and safer instruments. Other contraindications are systemic illness and specific lesions that may be aggravated by endoscopic examination.

The category of systemic illness includes recent myocardial infarction and severe obstructive pulmonary disease. Obviously, the introduction of an endoscope is a traumatic event for most patients, and such stress may be poorly tolerated by patients with severe cardiovascular disease. The introduction of an upper gastrointestinal endoscope is accompanied by electrocardiographic abnormalities in approximately 25% of patients over the age of 60 years. Whether these electrocardiographic abnormalities are artifacts produced by the presence of the endoscope immediately posterior to the heart or whether they are actual dysrhythmias produced by the trauma of the examination is questioned. Patients with severe obstructive pulmonary disease are at special risk during endoscopic procedures. The endoscope itself partially obstructs the airway by its size and by directly pressing against the larynx in passing through the piriform sinus. Laryngospasm may be caused by the endoscope, and accidental passage of the endoscope into the trachea may also produce severe respiratory complications. The potential for these complications dictates that all endoscopic laboratories be equipped with emergency facilities for cardiopulmonary arrest. For the same reason, intravenous access should be established prior to the performance of any endoscopic examination.

Lesions that may themselves be aggravated by an endoscopic examination include perforations of the gastrointestinal tract and other types of trauma. Perforations, whether in the esophagus, stomach, or duodenum, frequently seal spontaneously. Mucosal lesions are rarely detected for any kind of perforating ulcer because such ulcers are often acute and small. Further, they are surrounded by edema to a degree that obscures their internal presentation and their visualization by an endoscope. If the perforated organ is sufficiently distended to reduce this obstruction to endoscopic view, then the seal may be disrupted and the ulcer may thereby be reperforated. Suspected perforations are best examined by upper gastrointestinal radiography, with a combination of water-soluble contrast media and thin barium suspensions.

Chemical trauma to the upper gastrointestinal tract is considered a relative contraindication to endoscopy. In patients with severe lye burns of the esophagus and stomach, the local trauma to the organ may be converted to a perforation by the performance of an upper gastrointestinal endoscopic study. The endoscopic examination requires the insufflation of sufficient air to allow the manipulation of the instrument into the lumen of the organ. Unlike rigid endoscopy, which depends on obturation of the organ for visualization of the mucosa by the tip of the endoscope, fiberoptic endoscopy requires that the mucosa be moved away from the tip of the endoscope to become visible, that is, to be within the focal length of the viewing lens. Air is used for this purpose, and if one attempts to inflate an organ already severely burned by a chemical agent, that organ may simply "blow out." If, despite these risks, an upper gastrointestinal endoscopic study is still considered valuable, every precaution must be taken, including preparations for an emergency operation. Such examination should only be performed in a hospital.

Most foreign bodies cannot be removed with a fiberoptic endoscope. Although such things as bezoars may be broken up by using the endoscope as a battering ram, most foreign bodies large enough to produce symptoms cannot be removed with the instrumentation available. This limitation is imposed because of the size of the channel through which grasping instruments can be passed. Small foreign bodies, such as safety pins, may be snared and withdrawn with a fiberoptic endoscope. Other, larger foreign bodies simply cannot be grasped in this fashion and should be removed either by rigid endoscopy or laparotomy.

PREPARATION OF THE PATIENT

Preparation of the patient for upper gastrointestinal endoscopy is simple. For the usual diagnostic examination, the only preparation required is that the patient take no solid food for 12 hours before the examination. A patient may have clear liquids up until half an hour before the examination because these fluids empty rapidly from the stomach. When gastric emptying may be impaired, longer periods of abstention from all but clear liquids may be required, and in extreme situations, such as the patient with achalasia, clear liquids may be recommended for as long as 3 days. Even after such a prolonged clear-liquid diet, lavage of the upper gastrointestinal tract may be indicated before the examination. The endoscopic laboratory and, especially, the endoscopic laboratory technician should be prepared to carry out this manipulation.

Preoperative medication may or may not be given, depending on the attitude of the patient and the willingness of the examiner to spend time with the patient to allay anxieties regarding the examination. Generally, a 10- to 15-min explanation of the procedure to the patient of average intelligence precludes the necessity for pre-endoscopic sedation. When such a discussion is not possible, then sedation may be given in the form of intravenous meperidine or small doses of diazepam. Meperidine is preferred because it has a higher margin of safety than diazepam and its effects are easily reversible with naloxone. The usual intravenous dose for an adult is 25 mg, given over approximately 1 min.

Local anesthesia is usually administered in the form of an aerosol spray of either tetracaine or benzocaine. These local anesthetic agents are safer than previously used solutions of cocaine. One must use caution because too much local anesthesia may be induced if an excessive amount of the agent is given, and introduction of the endoscope may thereby be made difficult. The patient should be anesthetized with one or two sprays of the anesthetic agent, and then, as soon as the agent starts to become effective, the endoscope should be introduced. If much more time is allowed to elapse after spraying the hypopharynx, then the patient may be unable to swallow easily or to relax the pharyngeal constrictor muscles, and they will need to be obturated with the tip of the endoscope.

Intravenous access is generally established by insertion of a small-bore needle-tubing set, such as used in pediatric intravenous therapy. A standard intravenous infusion is not usually used; a simple heparin lock suffices. In the event of complications, this apparatus can be converted rapidly to a direct intravenous infusion. This apparatus also allows for a port of introduction for sedatives and other drugs.

All the foregoing preparations and manipulations are sufficiently simple and safe that the examinations may be performed in a multitude of locations, including the physician's office. Obviously, the standard emergency facilities for cardiopulmonary arrest must be available. Adequate suction devices to drive the endoscope and to allow clearing of the hypopharynx, in case the patient vomits, are required. In most centers, 75% of these examinations are done on an outpatient basis.

EXAMINATION TECHNIQUE

Although a full description of the technique of manipulation of upper gastrointestinal endoscopes is beyond the scope of this volume, a brief description of the procedure is relevant. The patient is usually placed on his left side on the endoscopy table, with his head supported by a pillow. The patient's pharynx, hypopharynx, and esophagus must be maintained on the same plane, to allow passage of the endoscope in a sharp curve through the mouth and into the upper esophagus.

The endoscope is introduced into the patient's hypopharynx, and the patient is requested to swallow it. Usually, one swallow is sufficient to pass the endoscope into the upper esophagus with little pressure. Once the endoscope is in the esophagus, the remainder of the examination involves manipulation of the instrument by the operator. The endoscope is simply advanced through the esophagus under direct visualization of the lumen. Anatomic deformities or mucosal lesions are noted as encountered. Any obstructing lesions or diverticula are avoided or are bypassed. The gastroesophageal junction is inspected, and the integrity of the squamocolumnar junction is determined. The endoscope is then introduced into the stomach, and the ease of passage through the lower esophageal sphincter is noted. When the endoscope reaches the patient's stomach, the operator uses endoscopic landmarks to determine the exact location of the endoscope. The primary landmark is the angulus or incisura angularis on the lesser curvature. In systematic fashion, the operator inspects the greater curvature and the posterior and anterior walls of the corpus of the stomach and then advances the endoscope into the pyloric antrum. Similarly, the greater curvature and the anterior and posterior walls of the antrum are inspected, and several maneuvers, including torsion of the endoscope, are used to examine the lesser curvature of the antrum. This area may be a blind spot that may not be adequately visualized with an end-viewing endoscope.

The pylorus is next inspected, and the endoscope is introduced through it. The ease of passage of the pyloric channel is noted. The first portion of the duodenum is carefully viewed, and the endoscope is then introduced into the second and third portions. This last maneuver may be carried out blindly; the endoscope is slipped across the duodenal mucosa until the lumen of the duodenum is visualized. The duodenum is frequently best visualized during withdrawal of the endoscope. The ampulla of Vater is noted, and its anatomic configuration is described. The endoscope is then withdrawn, and the duodenal bulb is reinspected as the endoscope passes through it. It is often helpful to position the endoscope proximal to the pylorus and to look at the duodenal bulb through the open pylorus.

The tip of the endoscope is next inverted, and the fundus and upper corpus of the stomach are inspected. With the endoscope in the fully flexed position, the instrument is rotated to allow a full view of the entire circumference of the gastroesophageal junction. The endoscope is then straightened, and stomach is aspirated of any air that may have been introduced during the examination. The endoscope is withdrawn into the esophagus, and the previous examinations are repeated on withdrawal of the instrument. Endoscopic findings should be reported with reference to a standardized method of examination of the entire upper gastrointestinal tract, to ensure that no portion escapes examination or description.

The single most important error in upper gastrointestinal endoscopy is failure to find an existing lesion. The most feared complication, perforation of the upper gastrointestinal tract, rarely occurs with the newer instruments. If the endoscopist does not follow a systematic procedure for inspecting the entire stomach, some portion of the mucosa will be missed during the examination, and if this portion harbors the lesion for which the endoscopic study has been performed, then the examination will be worthless and the patient will be harmed.

COMPLICATIONS

Complications include perforation, bleeding, and inadequate inspection of the gastric mucosa. Perforation is a rare complication of which the examiner must always be aware. The incidence of such perforation is inversely proportional to the experience of the examiner and to the ability of the patient to co-operate. The usual symptoms of gastrointestinal tract perforations follow perforation by the endoscope. After an endoscopic examination, the examiner must become aware of any atypical chest or neck pain in a patient or any unexplained signs of inflammation such as fever. When such signs occur, the examiner should proceed immediately to localize the perforation.

Patients with perforations anywhere in the esophagus may only have pain in the neck, and it is a serious error to assume that the perforation is therefore in the neck. It may be anywhere in the course of the esophagus. For this reason, when a perforation is suspected, that perforation should be localized radiographically. The patient should swallow water-soluble contrast material initially, to outline large perforations; thin barium is used to outline small perforations. If the perforation is large, the water-soluble contrast medium will enable one to see it, and the extravasation of medium will not be a problem because the water-soluble agent will be absorbed by the patient and excreted. Only when such large perforations are ruled out should thin barium be administered. Thin barium provides much better contrast and allows visualization of small perforations that are not shown by a water-soluble contrast agent. Moreover, if the perforation is small, leakage of the contrast material will also be minimal, and cleansing of the area at operation will be easier.

If the perforation is in the stomach or duodenum, then the usual signs of such perforation will be present. The special instance of perforation in the achlorhydric patient, especially of the upper stomach, should be noted. In such a patient, only an unexplained tachycardia may signal perforation, and the index of suspicion must then be high. The same measures are used as for the esophagus. When the perforation is lower in the stomach or in the duodenum in a patient who does secrete hydrochloric acid, then the signs of chemical peritonitis are unmistakable. In that instance, as indeed when all perforations are confirmed, prompt operation is required for adequate drainage of the area and for closure of the perforation when possible.

Serious bleeding is a rare complication of upper gastrointestinal endoscopy. Obviously, maneuvers such as biopsy of esophageal and gastric varices or vascular malformations of the stomach should be avoided, but such lesions are usually identifiable by gross inspection alone. Although the removal of biopsy specimens of most other lesions encountered during these examinations causes bleeding, the bleeding is usually minor. One should obtain a careful medical history, to rule out bleeding disorders in patients, before carrying out these examinations. Laboratory determinations of the clotting mechanism are not generally indicated, however. Great care should be exercised in biopsy of ulcers that have bled in the past, especially duodenal ulcers, of which biopsy is rarely indicated. Gastric ulcer, on the other hand, does require a biopsy for adequate differentiation from carcinoma, and the examiner should be prepared to control bleeding from the ulcer either by local application of styptic agents, such as norepinephrine, or by electrocoagulation of the bleeding point.

Finally, the third and most prevalent complication, failure to detect a lesion and thereby causing both patient and examiner to have a false sense of security, is avoided by rigid adherence to a systematic schedule of examination from point to point, to ensure visualization of every square centimeter of the gastric mucosa. Unlike other types of endoscopic studies, examination of the stomach is difficult because of the organ's size. The endoscope represents only one small point within a dilated "balloon," which may have a volume of 2 L. It is important to use every method of ensuring that the entire balloon is seen. No substitute exists for experience. For this reason, most endoscopy societies recommend a minimum number of supervised endoscopic examinations before an individual may be considered adequately trained in these techniques. The usual number is 100 upper gastrointestinal examinations, performed under supervision.

ENDOSCOPIC FINDINGS

Lesions commonly encountered in upper gastrointestinal endoscopy include esophageal varices, esophagitis with ulcerations, gastric ulcer, gastric carcinoma, gastritis, and duodenal ulcer. Obviously, many more lesions may be seen, and every endoscopist should be familiar with all of them before undertaking an endoscopic examination.

SUGGESTED READING

The scope of this chapter is far too broad to allow individual literature citations. The resultant bibliography would be as large as the chapter itself. Instead, the reader is referred to several of the more recent or more comprehensive monographs on the subject of fiberoptic endoscopy.

Ashizawa, S., and Kidokoro, T.: Endoscopic Color Atlas of Gastric Diseases. Bunkodo, Tokyo, 1970.
Berci, G.: Endoscopy. New York, Appleton-Century-Crofts, 1975.
Berry, L.H.: Gastrointestinal Pan-Endoscopy. Springfield, IL, Charles C Thomas, 1973.
Blackstone, M.O.: Endoscopic Interpretation. New York, Raven Press, 1984.
Cotton, P.B., and Williams, C.B.: Practical Gastrointestinal Endoscopy. Oxford, Blackwell Scientific Publications, 1982.
Demling, L., Ottenjann, R., and Elster, K.: Endoscopy and

Biopsy of the Esophagus and Stomach: A Color Atlas. Translated by K.H. Soergel. Philadelphia, W.B. Saunders, 1972.

Kasugai, T.: Endoscopic Diagnosis in Gastroenterology. Tokyo, Igaku-Shoin, 1982.

Papp, J.P.: Endoscopic Control of Gastrointestinal Hemorrhage. Boca Raton, CRC Press, 1981.

Tsuneoka, K., Takemoto, T., and Fukuchi, S.: Fiberscopy of Gastric Diseases. Baltimore, University Park Press, 1973.

13

Lower Intestinal Endoscopy

Herand Abcarian

The development of flexible fiberoptic colonoscopy in 1969 revolutionized the diagnosis, treatment, and surveillance of diseases of the colon. Whereas up to the late 1960s, the only way to assess the colon was with the barium enema, the colonoscope enabled the physician and surgeon to evaluate colonic diseases as accurately as rectal diseases could be assessed with the rigid proctosigmoidoscope.

Two techniques have been developed for examination of the colon with fiberoptic instruments: colonoscopy and flexible fiberoptic sigmoidoscopy. Because of the differences in the indications for and uses of the flexible fiberoptic colonoscopes and the shorter sigmoidoscopes, these two techniques are discussed separately.

COLONOSCOPY

The goal of colonoscopy is the examination of the entire colon from anus or an end stoma to the cecum or an ileocolic anastomosis. Additional procedures such as biopsy or polypectomy complement this examination. In the hands of an experienced endoscopist and with proper bowel preparation, this goal can be achieved in under 45 to 60 min in most patients. The procedure's safety has been well documented; the perforation rate is less than 0.5%, and the bleeding rate is less than 2% during polypectomy. The definite but slight risk of death from colonoscopy (0.06%) is worth mentioning, and the risk-to-benefit ratio must always be considered before submitting high-risk patients to colonoscopy and polypectomy.

It is estimated that colonoscopic polypectomy, when compared with polypectomy by colotomy, has reduced morbidity rates threefold and has decreased the associated mortality rate twentyfold.[1] The undeniable importance of these figures has established colonoscopy as an important diagnostic and therapeutic technique in patients with colorectal disease.

Total colonoscopy is considered in terms of a description of technique and a summary of indications, including applications for each indication.

Technique

The patient must be prepared for colonoscopy by a thorough cleansing of the colon. I generally prescribe either a 2-day preparation, consisting of magnesium citrate by mouth and cleansing enemas, or a 1-day preparation, consisting of 3 to 4 L of polyethylene glycol-electrolyte solution by mouth.

The examination is ideally performed in an endoscopy laboratory where trained assistance and resuscitative equipment are available, but it may be performed at the patient's bedside. The patient is usually sedated with meperidine or diazepam. The patient is placed on the examining table, usually in the left lateral position, although the patient may also be supine, and the position may be changed during the examination. Total colonoscopy is performed with an instrument 170 to 180 cm in length. By a combination of air insufflation and manipulation, the endoscope is passed to the cecum.

Indications for flexible colonoscopy can be classified by the three principal uses: diagnosis, therapy, and surveillance (Table 13–1).

Diagnostic Indications

NEOPLASTIC DISEASE. Colonoscopy is a key step in the diagnosis and treatment of neoplastic disease.[2] When a polyp is seen during a proctoscopic examination or is suspected on the basis of a barium enema study, colonoscopy is essential to exclude the presence of additional polyps, as occurs in 30% of patients. In symptomatic patients with barium enema findings that suggest a polyp, colonoscopy is the only diagnostic test that can ascertain or exclude the presence of colonic neoplasms.[3] If the polyp is amenable to snaring, endoscopic polypectomy will be the obvious therapeutic alternative. The incidence of invasive cancer in colonoscopic polypectomy series is about 5%.[4,5] In patients with large or sessile polyps, multiple biopsies, snare biopsy or piecemeal removal, or surface brushing and cystologic examination may be of great benefit.[2]

When cancer of the colon is suspected or proved, colonoscopy is of the utmost importance in the ex-

Table 13–1. Indications for Fiberoptic Colonoscopy

Indication	Condition	Purpose
Diagnosis	Neoplastic disease, benign or malignant	Confirmation of lesion by biopsy or polypectomy Exclusion of synchronous lesions
	Inflammatory bowel disease	Evaluation of extent of disease Evaluation of activity of disease Distinction between chronic ulcerative colitis and Crohn's disease Exclusion of "precancerous" dysplasia
	Diverticular disease	Evaluation of extent and severity of disease Distinction between diverticular disease and cancer
	Ischemic colitis	Confirmation of diagnosis, especially in the presence of stricture Evaluation of extent of disease
	Radiation-induced colitis	Evaluation of extent and severity of disease Exclusion of cancer in the presence of stricture
	Colonic stricture	Exclusion of cancer
	Vascular anomalies	Identification of abnormality
	Unexplained rectal bleeding or positive fecal occult blood test	Identification of origin, in patients with negative flexible fiberoptic sigmoidoscopy and double-contrast barium enema results
	Unexplained abnormality on barium enema study	Identification of abnormality
	Intraoperative conditions	Identification of problem during surgical procedures
	Disorders in children	Identification of condition
	Miscellaneous disorders	Diagnosis of conditions causing chronic abdominal pain or diarrhea
Therapy	Presence of polyp	Removal of polyp
	Bleeding	Control of bleeding from fulguration of polyp stalk or angiodysplasia, for example
	Presence of foreign body	Removal of foreign body
	Cecal volvulus	Reduction of volvulus
	Ogilvie's syndrome	Decompression of colon
Surveillance	Neoplastic disease	Observation of patients with metachronous polyps or cancer and cancer family syndrome
	Inflammatory bowel disease	Evaluation of mucosa, by biopsy, to exclude "precancer"
	Strictures	Follow-up of strictures caused by inflammatory bowel disease, diverticulitis, radiation-induced colitis, ischemic colitis, or anastomosis

clusion of synchronous polyps or cancers. In patients with malignant tumors of the right side, preoperative colonoscopy is mandatory to exclude a diagnosis of cancer in the left half of the colon that might otherwise remain after right hemicolectomy. When the presence of scirrhous carcinoma precludes total colonoscopy, a high-quality, air-contrast barium enema may be an acceptable substitute for preoperative colonoscopy. When no other lesion is palpable at the time of operation, total colonoscopy is indicated 6 months postoperatively, to exclude any synchronous polyps or cancerous tumors missed at the time of the original surgical procedure. Either way, once the colon has been "cleared" of any neoplastic lesions, colonoscopy for surveillance is needed only every second or third year. The incidence of metachronous cancer ranges from 5 to 10%.[6]

INFLAMMATORY BOWEL DISEASE. The colonoscope is the perfect instrument for assessing the extent of disease, severity of involvement, and response to treatment in patients with inflammatory bowel diseases.[7] Multiple biopsies obtained during the procedure may help one to differentiate chronic ulcerative colitis from Crohn's disease and other colitides.[8] In patients with longstanding inflammatory bowel disease, strictures can be examined to exclude the presence of malignant tumors, and target areas may undergo biopsy for detection of dysplastic or precancerous changes.[9,10] Although most such strictures have a benign cause, malignant disease should be suspected if the stricture is endoscopically rigid.[11]

DIVERTICULAR DISEASE. Colonoscopy can be helpful in the differentiation of symptomatic diverticular disease from irritable bowel syndrome. In patients with sigmoid strictures, the colonoscope is an important tool in excluding a diagnosis of co-existent cancer.[12] The major limitation is the inability to pass the instrument through the narrowed segment of colon in about 50% of these patients.[13] If an obstruction is treated with proximal colostomy, the addition of the antegrade route, through the stoma, to the conventional retrograde examination may be helpful. Colonoscopy plays a lesser role in the diagnosis of massive colonic bleeding secondary to diverticulosis. In such patients, radionuclide imaging and angiography are more accurate.

ISCHEMIC COLITIS. Endoscopic examination during an attack of ischemic colitis may clearly demonstrate a demarcation between normal and ischemic segments of the colon.[14] Biopsy specimens may have mucosal ulceration with dilated capillaries. In patients with postischemic strictures, endoscopic biopsy specimens showing hemosiderin-laden macrophages are diagnostic.[15]

RADIATION-INDUCED COLITIS. Radiation-induced injury to the colon may cause rectal bleeding, although symptoms may occur 20 to 30 years after radiation therapy.[15] Colonoscopy aids in assessing the extent and severity of injury. In patients with a prior history of pelvic radiation, colonoscopic examination helps one to exclude the possibility or recurrence or of a second primary cancer.

COLONIC STRICTURES. Although strictures may be the result of inflammatory bowel disease, diverticulitis, radiation-induced or ischemic colitis, or previous anastomosis, the primary purpose of colonoscopy in patients with such strictures is to exclude cancer in the narrow segment of the colon. The use of a small-caliber colonoscope may be necessary, to traverse tight strictures.

VASCULAR ANOMALIES. Vascular ectasias of the cecum have been implicated in bleeding of the lower gastrointestinal tract.[16] Angiodysplasias have also been associated with aortic valvular stenosis.[17] Colonoscopy not only complements angiography in documentation of the diagnosis, but also offers therapeutic benefits because smaller lesions may be successfully fulgurated by diathermy or argon laser photocoagulation.[18,19]

UNEXPLAINED RECTAL BLEEDING OR POSITIVE FECAL OCCULT BLOOD TESTING. If the results of flexible sigmoidoscopy and double-contrast barium enema studies are unclear, flexible colonoscopy may show the cause of bleeding in over 40% of these patients.[20] In addition, chronic blood loss and anemia in the elderly are commonly caused by angiodysplasia, which can be diagnosed and sometimes treated endoscopically.[18] Because an unexplained abnormality seen on a barium enema study may often be identified by colonoscopic examination, the need for repeated barium enemas at frequent intervals is obviated.

INTRAOPERATIVE COLONOSCOPY. Intraoperative colonoscopy is valuable in many situations.[21,22] Although the need for intraoperative colonoscopic examination decreases with the expertise of the endoscopist, the procedure may be of value in obviating the need for colotomy or resection, in limiting the scope of a planned operation, or in suggesting indications for a previously unplanned operation. A previous polypectomy site or the site of recurrent bleeding can be delineated.

PEDIATRIC COLONOSCOPY. Colonoscopy in pediatric patients is much less common than in adults. On some occasions, however, the technique is most useful. The major indications for colonoscopy in infants and children are unexplained rectal bleeding, therapeutic removal of colonic polyps, an unexplained abnormality seen on a barium enema study in a patient with diarrhea, bleeding or passage of mucus, and inflammatory bowel disease. Most colonoscopic studies can be performed with adult instruments, and the patient should receive suitable general anesthesia. Total colonoscopy is desirable in all cases because, in 20% of patients with left-sided polyps, more than one lesion can be found during the procedure.[23]

MISCELLANEOUS INDICATIONS. Colonoscopy may assist one in the diagnosis of a variety of problems, including unexplained abdominal pain, diarrhea, and the presence of extraluminal compression on the barium enema study. The procedure may also facilitate the endoscopic examination of the small bowel after total proctocolectomy (ileoscopy) and the examination of Koch pouch or ileoanal pouch anastomosis for inflammatory disease ("pouchitis").

Therapeutic Indications

POLYPECTOMY. Endoscopic polypectomy has revolutionized the treatment of polypoid disease of the colon and rectum. An experienced endoscopist, using the newest equipment and blended current and taking appropriate precautions, such as proper cleansing of the patient's colon, can perform multiple polypectomies safely. Colonoscopic polypectomy does not cause patients to lose much time from work. The endoscopic procedure has obviated the need for costly colotomy-polypectomy operations, with the inherent complications of general anesthesia and laparotomy. The major risks of colonoscopic polypectomy are bleeding (2%), and perforation (0.3%).[24] The incidence of these complications decreases dramatically with the experience and skill of the endoscopist.[1] The mortality rate associated with colonoscopic polypectomy is 0.06%.[24]

CONTROL OF BLEEDING. Snare strangulation of a polyp stalk that is bleeding actively after colonoscopic polypectomy is the ideal way to control the bleeding. The use of pressure for 5 to 10 min, without application of electric current, controls the bleeding without the additional risk of bowel perforation.[24] Should this method fail, diathermy or laser coagulation may be used.[18]

REMOVAL OF FOREIGN BODIES. The foreign bodies commonly encountered as a result of autoeroticism are usually too large to be removed with a colonoscope. Indeed, the use of the colonoscope to remove foreign bodies is unusual. Various plastic or rubber objects, such as enema tips, irrigation catheters, or dental prostheses, have been snared and removed during colonoscopy, however.

REDUCTION OF CECAL VOLVULUS. Using the same principles of and precautions for reduction of a sigmoid volvulus with a rigid or flexible sigmoidoscope, one may attempt to reduce a cecal volvulus with a flexible colonoscope. Frequently, however, the barium enema administered to confirm or to establish the diagnosis of cecal volvulus precludes the use of endoscopy for therapeutic purposes.

DECOMPRESSION OF COLON IN OGILVIE'S SYNDROME. Idiopathic colonic ileus or pseudo-obstruction (Ogilvie's syndrome) has been successfully decompressed by the use of the flexible colonoscope.[25] The generally poor health of these patients, the emergency necessitating colonic decompression, and the high risk of laparatomy and cecostomy make colonoscopic decompression an attractive alternative. Recurrent ileus and colonic distention can be prevented by the use of a sump tube decompressing stent left in the colon after colonoscopic decompression.[26]

Indications for Surveillance

NEOPLASTIC DISEASE. Although the appropriate frequency of postpolypectomy or postcolectomy endoscopic surveillance of the colon can be debated, the need for the surveillance itself is unquestioned. If the patient's colon is satisfactorily clear of all neoplastic disease on 2 consecutive annual or semiannual examinations, follow-up colonoscopy will not be needed for another 2 to 3 years.[24] On the other hand, endoscopic surveillance must be more frequent, and the age at which such examinations begin must be lower, in high-risk individuals, such as those with hereditary, site-specific colon cancers, or cancer family syndromes.

INFLAMMATORY BOWEL DISEASE. The need for surveillance of the entire colonic mucosa and for target biopsies to exclude early cancer or "precancer" is discussed in the previous paragraph. Criteria for frequency of surveillance and algorithmic approaches to the issue are well established in the literature.[27,28] Unfortunately, misinterpretation of these data has led to the abuse and overuse of colonoscopy by some endoscopists, who perform these examinations as often as every 3 months.

STRICTURES. All patients with strictures encountered by rigid sigmoidoscopy or by double-contrast barium enema studies must be followed with periodic regular endoscopic examinations, to exclude the presence or subsequent development of cancer, irrespective of the underlying disorder, that is, inflammatory bowel disease, diverticulitis, radiation-induced injury, ischemia, or postanastomotic conditions. If an adequate examination cannot be performed to rule out cancer conclusively, resection of the strictured segment will be indicated in patients who are unlikely to develop complications. The benefits of such an operation must be weighed against the possible complications in high-risk patients.

Contraindications and Limitations

Contraindications to therapeutic colonoscopy include the following: (1) lack of bowel preparation; (2) myocardial infarction within the past 6 months; (3) acute colitides, whether from inflammatory bowel disease, bacterial infection, or radiation; (4) acute sigmoid diverticulitis with localized abscess formation; and (5) possible hepatitis or acquired immune deficiency syndrome.

Time-consuming factors in colonoscopy include the following: (1) inexperience of the endoscopist; (2) poor bowel preparation; (3) prior pelvic or abdominal operations or radiation causing fixation of the colon; (4) extreme redundancy of the sigmoid or transverse colon; and (5) lack of co-operation on the part of the patient.

FLEXIBLE FIBEROPTIC SIGMOIDOSCOPY

Although flexible fiberoptic sigmoidoscopy was briefly used in the late 1960s,[29] the rapid development of colonoscopes overshadowed the flexible sigmoidoscope. In later years, when the flexible sigmoidoscope was reintroduced, many workers believed that this instrument had been supplanted by the modern colonoscopes.

In 1977, Bohlman and his associates, in a trial of 120 patients examined with both rigid and flexible sigmoidoscopes, showed that the depth of insertion of the flexible instruments was 2.5 times greater than that of the rigid devices, and rate of detection of significant pathologic features was 3 times as high.[30] Following this study, many other authors focused on the advantage of flexible sigmoidoscopy over rigid instrumentation in the office setting. Flexible sigmoidoscopy has gained enormous popularity in that context.[31]

Technique

Preparation for flexible sigmoidoscopy is less intense than for colonoscopy. I usually prefer bowel preparation with 2 commercially prepared enemas administered over 5 to 10 min. at 2 hours and 1 hour prior to the examination. The examination is usually performed with a flexible sigmoidoscope 65 cm in length and with the patient in the left lateral position. The indications for this technique are discussed in terms of diagnosis, therapy, and surveillance (Table 13–2).

Diagnostic Indications

NEOPLASTIC DISEASES. Because of the scattered distribution of colonic polyps, the only suitable instrument with which to examine and survey the entire colon is the colonoscope.[32] In many studies, however, diagnostic flexible fiberoptic sigmoidoscopy is adequate because it is three times more accurate than rigid sigmoidoscopy in the diagnosis of neoplastic disease. Given that the most difficult area of surveillance by barium enema is the redundant sigmoid colon, the flexible sigmoidoscope can be used in the physician's office to evaluate this structure.[33]

INFLAMMATORY BOWEL DISEASE. The short, 65-cm length of flexible sigmoidoscopes render them unsuitable for total colonic examination in patients with inflammatory bowel disease. In patients with ulcerative proctosigmoiditis, however, the progression or improvement of the disease can be easily assessed with this technique.

DIVERTICULOSIS OR DIVERTICULITIS. Many patients with sigmoid diverticulosis or even mild diverticulitis have symptoms that appear to be attributable to irritable bowel syndrome. In view of the increased incidence of diverticulosis and diverticulitis in persons under age 45, patients with frequent changes in bowel habits or left lower abdominal pain should undergo endoscopic examination, to rule out diverticular disease. This study is easily done in the physician's office, with minimal preparation.

ISCHEMIC COLITIS. Ischemic colitis following aortoiliac reconstruction is common. Patients with bloody diarrhea after aortoiliac operations may have an ischemic rectosigmoid colon. When these symptoms are neglected, frank gangrene of the sigmoid colon in a patient with a recently implanted arterial prosthesis is often fatal. On the other hand, an unnecessary sigmoid resection in a sick, postoperative patient can be equally hazardous. Ischemic colitis may improve spontaneously. Consequently, a gentle, bedside, low-pressure flexible sigmoidoscopy repeated at frequent intervals, if necessary, can be helpful in assessing the extent and degree of the ischemia. If the disease progresses despite conservative therapy, a well-timed, judicious operation may be lifesaving.

RADIATION-INDUCED PROCTOSIGMOIDITIS. Radiation therapy is increasingly used as a primary or adjuvant therapeutic technique for cancers of the prostate, cervix, uterus, or ovaries. The upper rectum and the sigmoid colon are often included in the field of radiation. Subsequent gastrointestinal symptoms, such as bloody diarrhea and tenesmus, can be evaluated with a flexible sigmoidoscope, to as-

Table 13–2. Indications for Flexible Fiberoptic Sigmoidoscopy (65 cm)

Indication	Condition	Purpose
Diagnosis	Neoplastic disease	Evaluation of "difficult" sigmoid colon
	Inflammatory bowel disease	Evaluation of ulcerative proctosigmoiditis
	Diverticulosis and diverticulitis	Distinction from irritable bowel syndrome
	Ischemic colitis	Evaluation following aortoiliac reconstruction
	Radiation-induced proctosigmoiditis	Evaluation of extent of disease
	Sigmoid stricture	Determination of cause
	Risk factors for examination	Office examination of high-risk patients
Therapy	Sigmoid volvulus	Reduction of volvulus
Surveillance	Inflammatory bowel disease	Evaluation of ulcerative proctosigmoiditis Determination of status after subtotal colectomy
	Neoplastic disease	Determination of status after subtotal colectomy
	Risk factors for colon disease	Follow-up of high-risk patients

sess the patient's response to the medical treatment of this complication.

SIGMOID STRICTURES. Sigmoid strictures caused by cancer, diverticulitis, inflammatory bowel disease, especially Crohn's disease, radiation, and ischemic colitis are easily diagnosed and evaluated with flexible fiberoptic sigmoidoscopy. Therapeutic plans, whether medical or surgical, may depend on the endoscopic findings as well as on clinical symptoms.

OFFICE PROCTOSIGMOIDOSCOPY. Office screening procedures should be performed in individuals at increased risk for colorectal cancer. This group includes: (1) men and women over 40 years of age; (2) those with a family history of colonic polyps or cancer; (3) patients with a previous history of polyps or cancer of the colon; (4) women with breast or genital cancer; (5) patients with longstanding inflammatory bowel disease; and (6) patients with inherited polyposis syndromes. Flexible sigmoidoscopy is preferable to rigid sigmoidoscopy because of the increase in the amount of colonic mucosa surveyed (2.5 times) and the higher diagnostic yield (3 times).

Therapeutic Indications

Endoscopic derotation of sigmoid volvulus is possible with the flexible sigmoidoscope, and it may be easier to guide the smaller-caliber tip of the instrument through the fulcrum of the twisted sigmoid, to facilitate reduction and decompression. Rigid sigmoidoscopes are often preferable, however, because one is thereby able to insert a long rectal or chest tube through the large lumen of the rigid sigmoidoscope, to splint the reduced volvulus.

Endoscopic polypectomy is not indicated with the flexible sigmoidoscope because of the need for total colonoscopy, to exclude the presence of additional neoplastic lesions, and because of the lack of proper bowel preparation and the possibility of explosion of combustible colonic gases.

Indications for Surveillance

Although long-term endoscopic surveillance of the rectum and sigmoid colon for metachronous neoplastic lesions is desirable, the use of the flexible sigmoidoscope is limited to patients with prior major colonic resections because of the short length of the instruments. Similarly, its use in surveillance of patients with inflammatory bowel disease is confined to patients with ulcerative proctosigmoiditis or those who have undergone previous subtotal colectomy. Follow-up flexible sigmoidoscopy, performed annually in the physician's office, in conjunction with fecal occult blood testing, is currently the standard of care in high-risk patients. After 2 negative examinations, the frequency of the procedure can be reduced to once every 2 or 3 years.

Contraindications and Limitations

Contraindications to flexible fiberoptic sigmoidoscopy are similar to those to flexible colonoscopy and include the following: (1) lack of or inadequate proper bowel preparation; (2) acute sigmoid diverticulitis; (3) acute radiation-induced colitis; and (4) recent myocardial infarction.

Factors limiting the procedure include the following: (1) inexperience of the endoscopist; (2) poor bowel preparation; (3) lack of co-operation of the patient; (4) prior pelvic operation or radiation; and (5) extreme redundancy of the sigmoid colon.

REFERENCES

1. Fruhemorgen, P., and Demling, L.: Complications of diagnostic and therapeutic colonoscopy in the Federal Republic of Germany. (Results of an inquiry.) Endoscopy, 11:146, 1979.
2. Winawer, S.J., et al.: Colonoscopic biopsy and cystology in the diagnosis of colon cancer. Cancer, 42:2849, 1978.
3. Winawer, S.J., et al.: Screening for colon cancer. Gastroenterology, 70:783, 1976.
4. Wolf, W.I., and Shinga, H.: Endoscopic polypectomy, therapeutic and clinicopathologic aspects. Cancer, 36:683, 1975.
5. Gillespie, P.E., et al.: Colonic adenomas—a colonoscopy survey. Gut, 20:240, 1979.
6. Morson, B.C.: Genesis of colorectal cancer. Clin. Gastroenterol., 5:3, 1976.
7. Dilawaei, J.B., et al.: Colonoscopy in the investigation of ulcerative colitis. Gut, 14:426, 1973.
8. Waye, J.D.: The role of colonoscopy in the differential diagnosis of inflammatory bowel disease. Gastrointest. Endosc., 23:150, 1977.
9. Morson, B.C., and Pang, L.S.C.: Rectal biopsy as an aid to cancer control in ulcerative colitis. Gut, 8:423, 1967.
10. Evans, D.J., and Pollack, D.J.: In situ and invasive carcinoma of the colon in patients with ulcerative colitis. Gut, 13:566, 1972.
11. Waye, J.D.: Colitis, cancer and colonoscopy. Med. Clin. North Am., 62:211, 1978.
12. Clerum, J., Agcnaut, D., and Tylgut, G.N.: Value of colonoscopy in the detection of sigmoid malignancy in patients with diverticular disease. Endoscopy, 9:228, 1977.
13. Dean, A.C.B., and Newell, J.P.: Colonoscopy in the differential diagnosis of carcinoma from diverticulitis of sigmoid colon. Br. J. Surg., 60:633, 1973.
14. Hunt, R.H., and Buchanan, J.D.: Transient ischemic colitis—colonoscopy and biopsy in diagnosis. J.R. Nav. Med. Serv., 65:15, 1979.
15. Morson, B.C., and Dawson, I.M.P.: Gastrointestinal Pathology. 2nd Ed. Oxford, Blackwell Scientific Publications, 1979.
16. Boley, S.J., et al.: Vascular ectasias of the colon. Surg. Gynecol. Obstet., 149:353, 1979.
17. Williams, R.C.: Aortic stenosis and unexplained gastrointestinal bleeding. Arch. Intern. Med., 108:859, 1961.
18. Hunt, R.H.: Angiodysplasia—an important cause of gastrointestinal bleeding in the elderly. Gut, 21:A460, 1980.
19. Fruhemorgen, P., et al.: Endoscopic laser coagulation of bleeding gastrointestinal lesions with report of the

first therapeutic application in man. Gastrointest. Endosc., 23:73, 1976.
20. Tedesco, F.J., et al.: Colonoscopic evaluation of rectal bleeding—a study of 304 patients. Ann. Intern. Med., 89:907, 1978.
21. Martin, P.G., and Forde, K.A.: Intraoperative colonoscopy: preliminary report. Dis. Colon Rectum, 22:234, 1979.
22. Bowden, T.A., Hooks, V.H., and Maasberger, A.R.: Intraoperative endoscopy. Am. Surg., 191:680, 1980.
23. Habr-Gama, A., et al.: Pediatric colonoscopy. Dis. Colon Rectum, 22:530, 1980.
24. Fruhemorgen, P.: Therapeutic colonoscopy. In Colonoscopy. Edited by R.H. Hunt and J.D. Waye. London, Chapman Hall, 1981, p. 199.
25. Bode, W.E., et al.: Colonoscopic decompression for acute pseudo-obstruction of the colon (Ogilvie's syndrome). Am. J. Surg., 147:243, 1984.
26. Nivatvongs, S., Vermeulen, F.D., and Fang, D.T.: Colonoscopic decompression of acute pseudo obstruction of the colon. Ann. Surg., 196:598, 1982.
27. Leonard-Jones, J.E., et al.: Prospective study of outpatients with extensive colitis. Lancet, 1:1065, 1974.
28. Leonard-Jones, J.E., et al.: Cancer in colitis: assessment of the individual risk by clinical and histological criteria. Gastroenterology, 73:1280, 1977.
29. Overholt, B.F.: Flexible fiberoptic sigmoidoscopy. Cancer, 19:80, 1969.
30. Bohlman, T.W., et al.: Fiberoptic pansigmoidoscopy: an evaluation and comparison with rigid sigmoidoscopy. Gastroenterology, 72:644, 1977.
31. Holt, R.W., and Wherry, D.C.: Flexible fiberoptic sigmoidoscopy in a surgeon's office. Am. J. Surg., 139:708, 1980.
32. Coller, J.A., Corman, M.L., and Veidenheimer, M.C.: Colonic polypoid disease: need for total colonoscopy. Am. J. Surg., 131:490, 1976.
33. Marks, G., et al.: Sigmoidoscopic examination with rigid and flexible fiberoptic sigmoidoscopes in the surgeon's office: a comparative prospective study of effectiveness in 1012 cases. Dis. Colon Rectum, 22:162, 1979.

14

Diagnostic Laparoscopy

George Berci

In abdominal surgery, it is important to visualize the problematic area, to palpate organs, and to remove tissue samples for histologic diagnosis. Formerly, diagnostic or exploratory laparotomy was the procedure of choice for exclusion or confirmation of the clinical suspicion of a pathologic entity.

Laparoscopy, which was introduced 70 years ago, has had enthusiastic support because it is not associated with the stress of surgical abdominal exploration.[1-4] Laparoscopy is performed through a stab incision, with a telescope as an extension of the surgeon's eye; local anesthesia is sufficient. Palpating fingers are replaced by a palpating probe advanced through a second stab incision into the abdominal cavity. Since the introduction of laparoscopy, its diagnostic accuracy in hepatology,[5-12] oncology,[13-20] and general surgery has been well established.[21-33]

Unfortunately, some surgeons are still reluctant to use laparoscopy to evaluate difficult abdominal problems. These surgeons generally rely on clinical findings, biochemical essays, simple or complex roentgenographic studies, radioactive scans, lavage, or diagnostic laparotomy.

Laparoscopy has been rediscovered in the field of gynecology. Apart from the tubal sterilization procedure, many laparoscopies are performed, to assess pelvic inflammatory disease and to detect malignant disease and other conditions. The development of a new image-relaying system (Hopkins rod lens*) has permitted the design of improved, smaller instruments for both adult and pediatric patients. This advance in technology should encourage one to re-evaluate this important examination for use in general surgery.

ALTERNATIVES TO LAPAROSCOPY

A number of alternatives to laparoscopy have been proposed for the nonoperative or semi-invasive examination of the peritoneal cavity.

Paracentesis

Puncture of the abdominal wall at one site or at four quadrants, to discover bleeding intra-abdominal vessels or organ perforations, is no longer performed.

Abdominal Lavage

Abdominal lavage is used for the rapid assessment of intra-abdominal hemorrhage in patients with blunt abdominal trauma. This examination has become an important adjunct in hospital emergency rooms. The major drawback is that not every hemoperitoneum needs exploration. Consequently, many (20%) unnecessary surgical explorations are performed in patients with multiorgan injuries who are elderly or who are at high risk.[34] Computed tomography enables one to detect hemoperitoneum accurately. In 19% of patients, however, surgical exploration shows no significant injury associated with the hemoperitoneum.[35] I elaborate further on this subject in the section of this chapter on emergency minilaparoscopy.

DIAGNOSTIC LAPAROSCOPY

Nothing is more valuable to a surgeon than to recognize a lesion and to perform a tissue biopsy. Laparoscopy should be considered, however, before resorting to diagnostic surgical exploration by formal laparotomy. The advantages and limitations of diagnostic laparoscopy constitute the basis for the indications and contraindications for the procedure.

Indications

1. Distinction between cirrhosis and chronic active or persistent hepatitis.
2. Verification of a suspicion of hepatocellular carcinoma in a patient with pre-existing liver disease.
3. Diagnosis of metastases or hepatomegaly of unexplained origin.
4. Evaluation of a palpable abdominal mass when a routine diagnostic workup does not suggest the cause.

---

*Distributed by Karl Storz Endoscopy America, Inc., Los Angeles, California

5. Staging of malignant tumors before surgical exploration; findings can alter planned treatment.
6. Provision of "second looks" in patients with malignant tumors; assessment of the potential effect of treatment.
7. Evaluation of ascites of unknown origin.
8. Determination of the presence of vascular insufficiencies in high-risk patients.
9. Evaluation of lymphogranulomatous disease.
10. Assessment of obscure abdominal diagnostic dilemmas, such as possible appendicitis in the elderly patients or in infants.

Contraindications

1. Acute abdominal distress with generalized peritonitis.
2. Mechanical or paralytic ileus.
3. Blood dyscrasias or nonresponding coagulopathies.
4. Large hiatal hernia.
5. Extreme obesity.

Conditions Requiring Special Precautions

Cardiovascular or respiratory insufficiencies alone are not contraindications to laparoscopy; however, the creation of a pneumoperitoneum must be performed with care. Existing dyspnea, cyanosis, or cardiac failure requires careful evaluation and the presence of an anesthesiologist to monitor the vital signs and hemodynamic status of these patients. Even in these critically ill patients, the procedure is much better tolerated than diagnostic surgical exploration.

Although previous surgical intervention is not a contraindication, the operator must be experienced and must know where to insert the pneumoperitoneum needle and the trocar.

Instrumentation

Laparoscopes require either a single- or a dual-puncture technique.

SINGLE-PUNCTURE APPROACH. An instrument for single-puncture laparoscopy incorporates a telescope with a biopsy or instrument channel. Therefore, the larger and wider trocar (11- to 12-mm) that must be used is more difficult to insert through the abdominal wall. Another drawback of single-puncture laparoscopy is the 0° or straightforward optic, which does not allow a proper view of corners and structures along the side of the end-scope, such as the dome of the liver. Furthermore, operation of the instrument channel does not permit independent maneuvers or movements. As soon as the manipulating instrument grasps or moves an organ, the view moves with it. This feature is a great disadvantage.

DUAL-PUNCTURE APPROACH. Because of the disadvantages of the single-puncture approach, I prefer the dual-trocar technique. This approach permits the introduction of a smaller (7-mm) and safer examining trocar that has a telescope with a forward oblique (30°) view. In difficult situations, when the working space is small or narrow, this instrument allows more extended observation, such as in the interspace between the rib cage and parietal peritoneum and the anterior surface of the liver. With rotation, corners or suspicious side areas can be scanned. The second, 4-mm trocar is introduced under visual control. Through this trocar, instruments for palpation, suction, coagulation, biopsy, or grasping can be introduced. The view obtained while working with this instrument is constant and is not affected by movements performed by palpating or other instruments introduced through the second, accessory trocar.[36] (Figs. 14–1 and 14–2).

Information to Patients

The patient or relatives should be informed in detail about the procedure, including risks, and alternatives. It should be made clear that, on rare occasions, a viscus is perforated, and surgical exploration is necessary. Fortunately, however, this complication is rare (0.2 to 0.3%). To put things into perspective for the patient, the surgeon should mention that diagnostic surgical exploration has a much higher complication rate than laparoscopy. The biopsy procedure should be explained. The patient should understand that pathologic intra-abdominal processes can be seen and can undergo biopsy, but retroperitoneal lesions cannot be discovered unless they protrude into the abdominal cavity. In such situations, one may attempt to perform a biopsy in an avascular area. Large lymph nodes in the mesenterium can be seen, and tissue samples can be obtained. In case of liver involvement, tissue from this organ can also enable one to determine the progress of the disease.

For medicolegal reasons, the patient's consent should be properly formalized, and the patient's knowledge of the process should be accurately recorded.

Preparation of Patient

The patient is kept in a fasting state from the previous night. In patients with cardiac or respiratory insufficiency, the surgeon should consult with appropriate colleagues. In particular, the anesthesiologist should be consulted for premedication and monitoring. The bladder of female patients undergoing examination for gynecologic disorders should always be evacuated because the second trocar is

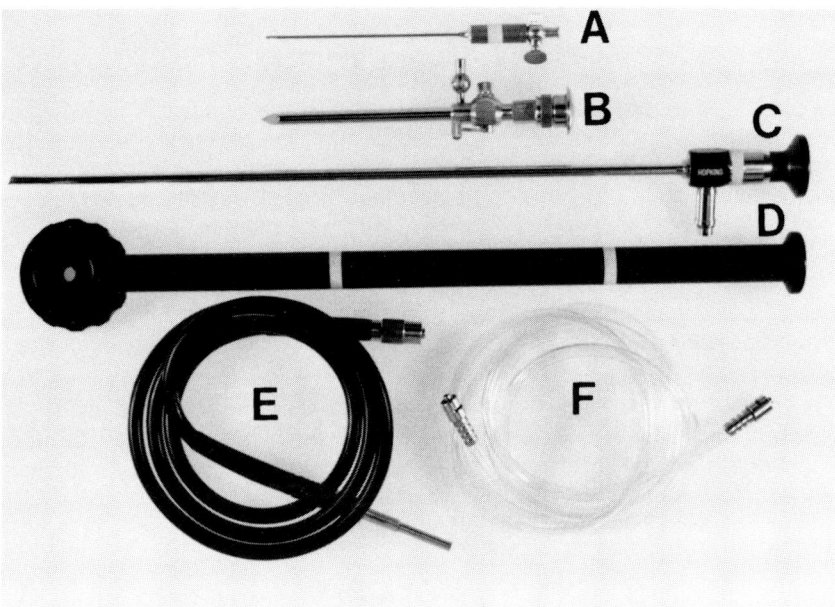

FIG. 14-1. Basic set of instruments for laparoscopy. A, Pneumoperitoneum needle with spring-loaded stylette; B, 7-mm examining trocar with stylette; C, 30° telescope with Hopkins rod-lens (distributed by Karl Storz Endoscopy America, Inc., Los Angeles); D, teaching attachment; E, fiberoptic (light) cable; and F, tube-connector to insufflator apparatus.

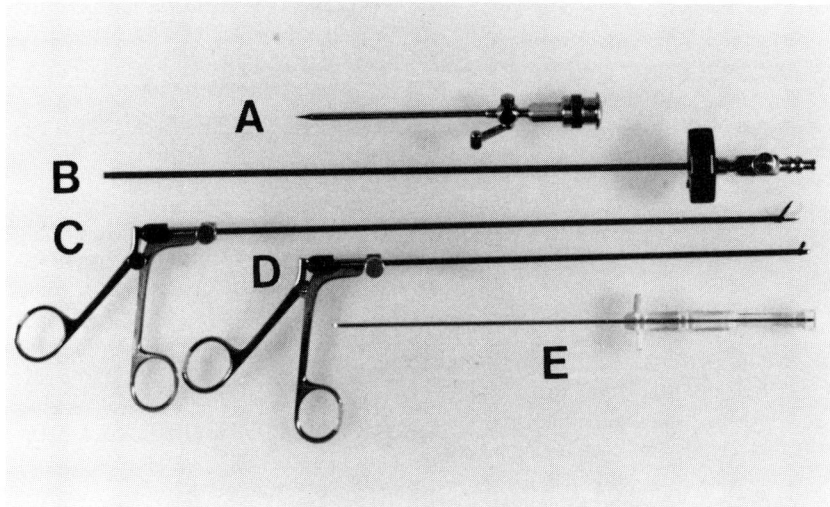

FIG. 14-2. Biopsy (second accessory instrument) set. A, 4-mm trocar with stylette; B, suction-coagulation-palpation probe; C, biopsy forceps with pointed jaws; D, biopsy forceps with sharp cutting (punchout) jaws; and E, Tru-Cut needle.

introduced superior to the symphysis pubica, and the perforation of a full bladder must be avoided.

Anesthesia

An attractive feature of laparoscopy is the use of local anesthesia with minimal intravenous premedication, in the form of diazepam or meperidine. Often, patients are severely ill or cachectic. It is a great advantage to be able to mobilize these patients on the following day or to discharge them from hospital 24 hours later. I prefer that intravenous medication be administered by the anesthesiologist when the patient is on the operating table. The depth of somnolence can thereby be better titrated. The patient should remain responsive. In addition to intravenous medication, local anesthetics are injected, and the needle to produce pneumoperitoneum or the trocar is passed without causing the patient pain. Laparoscopy is well tolerated by patients, and if proper intravenous medication is administered, the patient will hardly recall the procedure. Vital signs should be continuously monitored. A resuscitation cart should be available. In selected patients with severe respiratory or cardiac insufficiency, general anesthesia with controlled ventilation may be the best choice.

Facilities and Preparation of Instruments

I perform laparoscopy in a hospital operating room, but the procedure may be done in a clean endoscopy area, as long as resuscitation equipment is available and the patient's vital signs are continuously monitored.

The instruments should be checked beforehand by the operating room nurse and the surgeon. Nothing is more frustrating than discovering, when the patient has already been medicated, that important accessories are missing or that the telescope was damaged during the cleaning or sterilization process.

The patient's abdomen is surgically prepared and is draped, and the procedure is performed under sterile conditions.

Technique

Dual-puncture laparoscopy is performed in the following steps: (1) gas insufflation to produce a pneumoperitoneum; (2) insertion of an examining trocar; (3) preliminary inspection; (4) insertion of a second trocar; (5) examination and operative maneuvers; and (6) termination of procedure.

PNEUMOPERITONEUM. This maneuver is one of the most important steps during the procedure. If it is properly performed, the safety and efficiency of the examination will be ensured. I do not recommend the use of room air or oxygen because modern laparoscopic technique involves coagulation. If air, by chance, is injected into blood vessels, it may cause air emboli.[37,38] Gas, carbon dioxide or nitrous oxide, is therefore preferred. The gas is insufflated through the pneumoperitoneum needle with an insufflator apparatus. The site of insertion of the needle is important and depends on whether the patient has had a previous abdominal surgical procedure.

Careful examination of the abdomen prior to laparoscopy is important for detecting the borders of palpable masses, such as liver or spleen, and the presence of ascites. These data determine the site of approach. In patients with an intact abdomen, the linea alba, just inferior to the umbilicus, is the puncture site of choice. A small stab incision is made with the tip of a No. 11 blade, and the spring-loaded needle is introduced. It is necessary to attach a syringe filled with saline solution and to aspirate to make sure that the needle has not entered a blood vessel or the lumen of the intestine.[39] Gas is then introduced.

During the insufflation period, continuous monitoring of the patient's vital signs is obligatory. If a proper protective cushion of gas has been created, then trocar insertion will be safe. Every attempt should be made to ensure that this first phase of the examination is performed well. If the patient develops arrythmias, insufflation should be stopped; if these persist, the peritoneal cavity should be desufflated. Insufflation can be repeated when the patient's heart rhythm returns to normal.

INSERTION OF THE EXAMINING TROCAR. Once the pneumoperitoneum has been completed, the needle is withdrawn, and the small stab incision is slightly enlarged, to provide a tight fit around the examining trocar. The trocar is introduced with a drilling-pressing motion. A hissing noise through the hollow stylet indicates that the higher pressure zone has been entered. The stylet is removed, and a prewarmed telescope is advanced.

PRELIMINARY INSPECTION. Once the trocar has been inserted, the prewarmed telescope is carefully advanced. Observation should begin before the telescope protrudes through the trocar sleeve. The first landmark is the falciform ligament; its position in the midline or any displacement should be noted. Is fluid present or absent? When adipose tissue is observed at the tip of the trocar sleeve during insertion of the telescope, the trocar is probably in the preperitoneal fatty tissue, a possibility in obese patients. Before the procedure is continued, one should ensure that the trocar is in the proper area, as seen through the endoscope.

INSERTION OF THE SECOND TROCAR. When local anesthesia has been administered inferior to the right costal margin just lateral to the ledge of the rectus muscle, the second accessory (4-mm) trocar is introduced under visual control. This trocar's most useful tool is the palpation probe (Fig. 14–2), which also acts as a suction-coagulation cannula. Fluid samples are obtained for analysis. If much ascitic fluid is present, some may be evacuated by attaching a suction device to this hollow probe. As soon as the fluid is removed, it should be replaced by gas, to maintain the pneumoperitoneum.

EXAMINATION AND OPERATIVE MANEUVERS. During inspection of the liver, one should note the size of the lobes and the appearance of the liver's surface in terms of color, whether dark, greenish, or patchy, and texture, whether smooth, shiny, or irregular. Is the liver nodular? If so, what is the size and distribution of the nodules? Are they diffuse and symmetric, involving both lobes? On palpation with the probe, the consistency of the liver parenchyma, whether mushy or hard, is determined. The parietal peritoneum superior to the liver should be examined.

Normal peritoneum is shiny, with small-caliber vessels. Dilated veins on the parietal peritoneum, diaphragm, or falciform ligament indicate portal hypertension.

Under normal conditions, the spleen is covered with omentum and is not visible. At times, the omentum may be carefully moved from the splenic area, and a normal spleen may be seen. When the patient is in a reverse Trendelenburg position and is rotated to the right, one may see a large, protruding spleen in the left posterior gutter. It is not advisable to take tissue samples from this organ.

The undersurface of the liver is not visible under normal conditions. If seen, such a liver will be hypertrophied or displaced by a retroperitoneal process that will also narrow the space between the parietal peritoneum and the anterior surface of the liver. In some cirrhotic patients, the undersurface of the liver is visible and is firm on palpation. Obtaining biopsy specimens in the narrow working space is expedited by the use of a smaller biopsy set (Fig. 14–2).

The gallbladder is normally seen. Its size and appearance should be observed, and its resistance to compression should be noted. The finding of a whitish, dull organ or one covered with adhered omentum indicates previous or present cholecystitis. With the palpation probe, one may gently lift the right lobe of the liver beside the gallbladder, and one may partially inspect the undersurface. The same probe, from the same position and under visual control, can be advanced under the falciform ligament to the left side of the abdomen, and the entire left lobe can be lifted and the undersurface clearly observed up to the diaphragm.

If any lesion is discovered on the surface of the liver, the telescope should be advanced, to observe this area more closely. The likely site for biopsy should be palpated first to determine its consistency. If the lesion is cystic and bluish in appearance, a hemangioma or a cavernous malformation may be present, and biopsy should be avoided. Both lobes of cirrhotic livers should be systematically inspected to discover whether the diffuse micro- and macronodularity contains small, whitish lesions. Such a finding suggests malignant change, and a biopsy specimen should be obtained.

Inspection of the parietal peritoneum is easy and should be performed systematically. One should first examine the upper abdomen superior to both liver lobes and then the lower quadrants. The presence of small, whitish nodules, 1 to 3 mm in size, should cause one to suspect metastatic cancer, tuberculosis, or mesothelioma, and biopsy should be performed.

By turning the telescope 180° under visual control, the pelvic area can be observed. Use of a palpation probe is helpful in lifting individual loops of intestine; one may thereby discover a short, ischemic bowel segment resulting from vascular insufficiency in patients with a small amount of hemorrhagic fluid in the gutter.

In patients with gynecologic disorders, it is advisable to introduce, prior to laparoscopy, a suction cannula onto the cervix or cervical canal, to raise the uterus, to enable one to see the fallopian tubes. The fallopian tubes may then be grasped, and the ovaries may be easily visualized. The bulge of a Foley catheter in the bladder may act as a landmark.

TERMINATION OF PROCEDURE. Before the patient's abdomen is desufflated, one should reinspect the areas of manipulation and the biopsy specimens before the endoscope is withdrawn into the sheath. The operating table is lowered, and the area under the trocar and the area of insertion of the pneumoperitoneum needle are carefully scanned, to determine whether any injury has resulted from the insertion of these sharp instruments. The patient's abdomen is then desufflated, and the stab incisions are closed with metal clips. In patients with ascitic fluid, skin sutures are recommended (see the next section of this chapter.) The procedure can be completed within 20 to 30 min.

Clear liquids may be administered a few hours after the procedure, and the patient's diet may be slowly returned to normal. Bed rest is recommended on the day of the procedure. The patient's vital signs should be monitored every half-hour for 4 to 6 hours after laparoscopy.

Special Management of Ascites

The assumption that a trocar can be introduced safely in patients with ascitic fluid and a distended abdomen without pneumoperitoneum is a misconception. Air-containing intestine floats on top of the fluid level. Therefore, it is advisable to insufflate this type of abdomen to create a protective gas cushion. One must not immerse the pneumoperitoneum needle into the fluid because gas bubbles thereby created cannot be dispersed. The needle should be kept parallel to the patient's abdominal wall after penetration during insufflation, to prevent this complication. As soon as the telescope is advanced and vision is clear, one should introduce the second trocar and aspirate fluid under visual control. In patients with ascites, the umbilicus is more inferiorly placed than normally, and the abdominal wall is thin. The site of the pneumoperitoneum and trocar insertions should take this factor into account.

One must keep the stab incision tight, to avoid air leakage during the procedure. Once laparoscopy has been completed and the patient's abdomen has been desufflated, the incision is closed in two layers, subcutaneous tissue and skin.

Laparoscopy is a useful procedure in patients with

ascites of unknown origin or ascites resulting from liver disease because tissue samples can be obtained with much more accuracy than with a blind percutaneous technique.

Biopsy

The accessory trocar is introduced under visual control in relation to the lesion.[39] A suction, coagulation, and palpation probe is advanced, and the area to undergo biopsy is first palpated, to ensure that the lesion is not cystic. If bleeding on the liver's surface is observed after obtaining the biopsy specimens, the suction coagulation probe should be reintroduced, the bleeding site should be located, and the bleeding should be stopped. For patients with small metastatic nodules on the parietal peritoneum, diaphragm, or serosa of the bowel, one should use the punch forceps (Fig. 14–2). These areas do not bleed if one is careful and if tearing action by the punch forceps is avoided.

For intraparenchymal liver lesions, a cutting biopsy needle, as shown in Figure 14–2(E), is introduced beside the second trocar, and tissue cores are obtained. Again, bleeding vessels or oozing spots on the liver's surface may be compressed or coagulated under visual control. This method is much safer than blind percutaneous techniques. Avascular areas for biopsy can be selected on large masses, and dilated veins can be avoided.

Comparison with Other Techniques

In addition to these data, other advantages of laparoscopy are evident when compared to laparotomy or blind biopsy of peritoneal structures.

The dome of the liver is difficult, if not impossible, to see during abdominal surgical exploration, but it may be clearly observed through the telescope. During laparotomy, the surgeon's fingers slide over the liver's surface to palpate irregularities. Suspicious areas located more proximally are difficult to bring into view through an abdominal incision. The parietal peritoneum located over the liver as well as the diaphragm can be observed with ease through the endoscope.

The percentage of false-negative or uninformative liver biopsy results in patients with cirrhosis and tumors is higher with blind biopsy technique than with laparoscopic biopsy. Bleeding after biopsy can be observed and arrested by compression or coagulation under visual control. This safeguard is valuable in preventing such bleeding.

Although laparoscopy requires special skill and training, it may be acquired within the framework of a teaching program. If laparoscopy is peformed properly, with sound indications, it may enable one to establish a diagnosis with histologic proof and thereby to avoid surgical exploration, which has higher morbidity and mortality rates and requires extended hospitalization. Further, the surgeon may gain an impression of the feasibility of a surgical intervention.

Liver scans, ultrasound, and computed tomographic scans do not show metastases smaller than 1 cm. Ninety percent of metastatic leions involving the liver are visible. Peritoneal dissemination, metastases on the surface of the intestine, or implants on the diaphragm that are not visualized by imaging techniques are clearly seen through the laparoscope. Laparoscopy is also better for detecting a small accumulation of fluid (ascites), changes in color and architecture of the liver, circumscribed lesions, and surface changes in the liver or intra-abdominal organs. All this information can be obtained without undertaking surgical exploration.

Complications

In our experience with 608 laparoscopies, complications occurred in 10 patients, a morbidity rate of 1.6%. No one died. Two patients required emergency surgical exploration; one patient had tuberculous peritonitis, and the other had dense adhesions. Perforation of the bowel with the pneumoperitoneum needle resulted in massive bleeding in one patient, whereas in another patient, a branch of a mesenterial artery was injured. Both patients required surgical exploration and survived. In 2 patients, the pneumoperitoneum needle entered the intestinal lumen, as shown by aspiration of bowel contents; when the needle was relocated, the procedure was completed. A nasogastric suction tube was inserted, and each patient was observed closely and received intravenous fluids for a few days. No further sequelae developed. The remaining six complications were minor (Table 14–1). In a review of the literature, the reported mortality rate was 0 to 0.3%, with an incidence of morbidity of 1.3 to 2.0%.[40]

Table 14–1. Complications of Diagnostic Laparoscopy

Complication	No. of Patients (n = 608)
Bowel perforation*	1
Bleeding artery*	1
Perforation of small bowel with needle	2
Transient arrhythmia	4
Transient ileus	1
Metastatic implantation at trocar site	1
Death	0
	10 (1.6%)

*Both patients required surgical exploration

Table 14–2. Diagnostic Results of Laparoscopy

Result	No. of Patients (%) (n = 608)
Diagnosis established	555 (91.3%)
No disorder found	43 (7%)
Examination uninformative	10 (1.7%)
	608 (100%)

DIAGNOSTIC RESULTS

In 555 patients (91.3%) my colleagues and I were able to establish a diagnosis. In 43 patients (7.0%), no intra-abdominal disorder was found, and in 10 patients (1.7%), the examination was technically impossible because of adhesions or was not informative because of a variety of conditions (Table 14–2). In addition to these data, other advantages of laparoscopy are evident when the procedure is compared to laparotomy or blind biopsy of peritoneal structures.

MINILAPAROSCOPY IN BLUNT ABDOMINAL TRAUMA

Minilaparoscopy is preferred to peritoneal lavage.[41] The examination is performed in the hospital emergency room or intensive care unit, either while the patient is on a stretcher or at the patient's bedside. The aim is to reduce the incidence of unnecessary surgical exploration for abdominal trauma involving hemoperitoneum (20%). In a few patients with acute deterioration of neurologic signs or neurosurgical emergencies, the procedure may be done simultaneously with craniotomy in the operating room, with the patient under general anesthesia.

Anesthesia for this procedure, consisting of local anesthesia with premedication, and technique are the same as for diagnostic laparoscopy, except the instruments are miniaturized, as shown in Figure 14–3. The reason for a smaller trocar is ease and speed of introduction. Despite a smaller telescope, resolution provided by the optics enables one to see, for example, blood, fluid in the posterior gutter, or organ injuries that require surgical exploration.

INDICATIONS

Minilaparoscopy should be considered under the following circumstances in patients with abdominal trauma:

1. Mental obtundation for any reason, such as from head trauma, alcoholism, drug ingestion, or disease.
2. History or evidence of blunt abdominal trauma or abdominal stab wounds.
3. Unexplained hypotension.
4. Equivocal abdominal signs on physical examination.

Severely injured patients with multiple organ injuries require rapid and accurate diagnostic assessment of injuries and the setting of priorities for treatment. These factors influence the eventual outcome.

Abdominal lavage was initially performed by the percutaneous approach.[42] Because of incidental injuries to underlying organs, however, an open technique is now used.[43] In my opinion, lavage is an overly sensitive examination. The cell count level at which tests should be considered positive is still controversial.[44] A fine line exists between positive and negative results. The major drawback of abdominal lavage is that not every hemoperitoneum requires surgical exploration. Up to 20% of patients with positive results of lavage who undergo surgical exploration have no visceral injury or significant

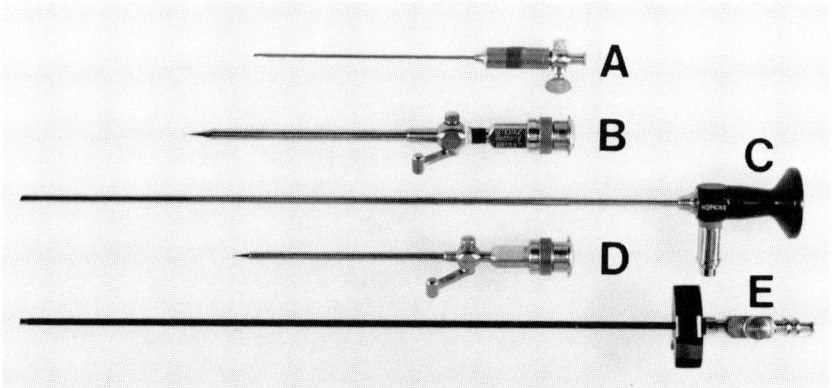

FIG. 14–3. Basic set of instruments for emergency laparoscopy. A, Pneumoperitoneum needle; B, 5-mm examining trocar with stylette; C, 30° telescope (4-mm) with Hopkins rod-lens (distributed by Karl Storz Endoscopy America, Inc., Los Angeles); D, second (4-mm) trocar with stylette; and E, suction-coagulation-palpation probe.

bleeding site. Therefore, no further intervention is necessary.[45,46] Even the introduction of computed tomography has not eliminated unnecessary laparotomy.[35]

Diagnostic Findings

Minilaparoscopy enables one to detect a variety of conditions, including hemoperitoneum, organ perforation, and splenic, liver, and penetrating injuries.

HEMOPERITONEUM. The mode of distribution of blood can provide clues to the location of the bleeding site. A good example is the pelvic area. The quantitive assessment of hemoperitoneum is difficult, but an impression can be gained based on the following findings:

Minimal Hemoperitoneum. A small amount of blood is seen in the lateral peritoneal gutters, or streaks of blood are discovered between intestinal loops. If the volume of blood remains unchanged and the search for a bleeding site is unsuccessful, this patient should be observed. If the bleeding site is found, it may be oozing, or the bleeding may have stopped. In the series of patients examined by my colleagues and myself, only half the bleeding sites were discovered in patients whose bleeding was minimal. Minute volumes of blood in the peritoneal cavity may suffice to provide a positive result from abdominal lavage.

Moderate Hemoperitoneum. A 5- to 10-mm blood level is found in the lateral gutters. The second accessory trocar should be immediately introduced under visual control after infiltration of local anesthetic, and the suction cannula should be advanced. Hemoperitoneum should be evacuated, and one should search systematically for the injury. The suction cannula is also used as a palpation probe. If an organ is bleeding, such as in a patient with a liver laceration, one should observe the injury through the laparoscope. If the bleeding is brisk, surgical intervention will be indicated. When a bleeding site is not discovered within 5 to 10 min of diligent searching, but the gutters refill with blood to the previous level, the bleeding vessel is probably not within the range of visualization and surgical intervention should be considered. Small lacerations that bleed slightly or are covered with a blood clot without bleeding can be managed by observation alone. The suction-coagulation probe may be used to assess oozing lesions, and coagulation may be applied in selected patients.

Severe Hemoperitoneum. If the initial pneumoperitoneum needle aspiration shows whole blood in the syringe during two or three attempts on various sites, or if laparoscopic observation discloses intestinal loops floating in or surrounded by a pool of blood, immediate operation will be indicated. In such patients, the level of blood in the lateral gutters reaches two or more fingerbreadths.

ORGAN PERFORATION. Yellowish fluid seen in the lateral gutters may be aspirated and analyzed for amylase and bile content, pH, and culture. In general, such fluid represents an indication for immediate operation. If several hours have elapsed between trauma and admission to hospital, and if injury to underlying organs cannot be seen, indirect signs should be sought, such as thickening, adherence, or inflammation of the omentum in a particular area or of intestinal loops. The palpation probe may help one to move such loops or omentum. Perforation of the retroperitoneal segment of the duodenum or pancreatic injuries will escape detection, however.

SPLENIC INJURIES. Splenic injuries are characterized by an accumulation of blood in the left gutter. The omentum covering the spleen is elevated by a pool of blood or by a blood clot that is bluish in appearance. Conservation of the spleen is desirable when possible.[47] Laparoscopy may show only minimal hemoperitoneum without significant bulging or bluish tint of the omentum. If the patient's vital signs are stable, and if a spleen scan denotes splenic injury, the patient may be managed nonoperatively under careful observation.

LIVER INJURIES. Deceleration injuries are frequently characterized by lacerations on the anterior surface of the liver, the dome of the liver, or the falciform ligament. The undersurface of the liver can be inspected with the palpation probe, which gently lifts the right and left lobes. If lacerations are discovered, the telescope should be advanced for close inspection under magnification for a few minutes. In patients with a small, oozing laceration, compression or coagulation may be used. If bleeding persists after a prolonged period of observation, laparotomy must be considered.

PENETRATING INJURIES. Laparoscopy is not performed in patients with gunshot wounds. Small or questionable penetrating stab wounds may be examined laparoscopically. In a recent review of patients with a stab wound of the abdomen, one-third underwent unnecessary surgical exploration.[48]

My approach is as follows: The skin edges of the wound are temporarily closed, to provide a seal for the pneumoperitoneum. The diagnosis of penetration through the parietal peritoneum may be either excluded or confirmed. The underlying area is inspected using the palpation probe; one should lift loops of the bowel and look for bleeding vessels, serosal injuries, leakage, or other signs of perforation or hemorrhage. In my limited experience with nine patients with stab wounds, I was able to avoid surgical exploration in six patients.

Diagnostic Results

My experience has been with 108 patients with blunt abdominal trauma. The results are summarized as follows:

NEGATIVE LAPAROSCOPY WITH NO EXPLORATION. In 54%, hemoperitoneum or abnormal yellow fluid was not observed. None of these patients subsequently required an exploratory laparotomy.

POSITIVE LAPAROSCOPY WITH NO EXPLORATION. In 25%, a minimal-to-moderate hemoperitoneum was discovered; no or minimal lesions were seen. These patients were observed in the hospital's intensive care unit. None of the patients required subsequent laparotomy.

POSITIVE LAPAROSCOPY WITH EXPLORATION. In 21%, severe hemoperitoneum was discovered. All underwent operation, and visual findings were confirmed during the surgical procedure. In all but one patient, the source of bleeding or the site of organ perforation was located by laparoscopy. One patient had 750 ml blood evacuated at operation, but the source of bleeding was not found.

Complications

One patient had a minimal amount of hemoperitoneum that was considered to be due to an injury to the omentum during trocar insertion. Fresh coagulum was seen around this area. Observation only was required.

In one comatose patient with a skull fracture, a minimal hemoperitoneum was found in the left lower quadrant. Later, a semisealed perforation of the rectosigmoid junction was discovered, and an operation was performed.

REFERENCES

1. Jacobaeus, V.H.C.: Kurze Uebersicht uber meine Erfahrungen mit der Laparo-Thorakoskopie. Munch. Med. Wochenschr., 38:2017, 1911.
2. Kelling, G.: Zur Coelioskopie und Gastroskopie. Arch. Klin. Chir., 126:226, 1923.
3. Kalk, H.: Erfahrungen mit der Laparoskopie. Z. Klin. Med., 111:303, 1929.
4. Ruddock, J.C.: Peritoneoscopy. Surg. Gynecol. Obstet., 65:623, 1937.
5. Zoeckler, S.J.: Peritoneoscopy—a revaluation. Gastroenterology, 34:969, 1958.
6. Herrera-Llerandi, R.: Peritoneoscopy: endoscopic refinement par excellence. Br. Med. J., 2:661, 1961.
7. Wildhirt, E.: Laparoskopie und Leberbiopsie. Wien. Med. Wochenschr., 5:66, 1970.
8. Rivera, R.A., and Boyce, H.W.: Peritoneoscopy: analysis of 150 cases. Am. J. Gastroenterol., 58:594, 1972.
9. Fritsch, W.P., et al.: Die Wertigkeit von Laparoskopie und Leberpunktion fur die Diagnostik chronischer Hepatopathien. Dtsch. Med. Wochenschr., 97:1635, 1972.
10. Balfour, T.W.: Laparoscopy in liver disease. Lancet, 1:612, 1976.
11. Dobrilla, G.: Laparoscopy in liver disease. Lancet, 1:1022, 1976.
12. Trujillo, N.P.: Peritoneoscopy and guided biopsy in the diagnosis of intraabdominal disease. Gastroenterology, 71:1083, 1976.
13. Coleman, M., et al.: Peritoneoscopy in Hodgkin disease: confirmation of results by laparotomy. JAMA, 236:2634, 1976.
14. Smith, W.G., Day, T.G., Jr., and Smith, J.P.: The use of laparoscopy to determine the results of chemotherapy for ovarian cancer. J. Reprod. Med., 18:257, 1977.
15. Cuschieri, A., Hall, A.W., and Clark, J.: Value of laparoscopy in the diagnosis and management of pancreatic carcinoma. Gut, 19:672, 1978.
16. Lightdale, C.J., and Hajdu, S.I.: Brush cytology of the liver and peritoneum at laparoscopy. Gastrointest. Endosc., 24:169, 1978.
17. Berek, J.S., Griffiths, C.T., and Leventhal, J.M.: Laparoscopy for second-look evaluation in ovarian cancer. Obstet. Gynecol., 58:192, 1981.
18. Ozols, R.F., et al.: Peritoneoscopy in the management of ovarian cancer. Am. J. Obstet. Gynecol., 140:611, 1981.
19. Bleiberg, H., LaMeir, E., and Lejeune, F.: Laparoscopy in the diagnosis of liver metastases in 80 cases of malignant melanoma. Endoscopy, 12:215, 1980.
20. McCallum, R.W., et al.: Laparoscopic diagnosis of peritoneal mesothelioma. Am. J. Dig. Dis., 24:170, 1979.
21. Berci, G.: Peritoneoscopy. Br. Med. J. 1:562, 1962.
22. Berci, G., et al.: A direct approach to the differential diagnosis of jaundice. Am. J. Surg., 126:372, 1973.
23. Gaisford, W.D.: Peritoneoscopy: a valuable technic for surgeons. Am. J. Surg., 130:671, 1975.
24. Cuschieri, A.: Value of laparoscopy in hepatobiliary disease. Ann. R. Coll. Surg. Engl., 57:33, 1975.
25. Berci, G.: Laparoscopy in general surgery. In Endoscopy. Edited by G. Berci. New York, Appleton-Century-Crofts, 1976.
26. Herbsman, H., Gardner, B., and Alfonso, A.: The value of laparoscopy in general surgery. J. Reprod. Med., 18:235, 1977.
27. Irving, A.D., and Cuschieri, A.: Laparoscopic assessment of the jaundiced patient: a review of 53 patients. Br. J. Surg., 65:678, 1978.
28. Friedman, I.H., and Wolff, W.I.: Laparoscopy: a valuable adjunct to the abdominal surgeon's armamentarium. Am. J. Surg., 135:160, 1978.
29. Wolfe, J.H.N., Behn, A.R., and Jackson, B.T.: Tuberculous peritonitis and role of diagnostic laparoscopy. Lancet, 1:852, 1979.
30. Hall, T.J., Donaldson, D.R., and Brennan, T.G.: The value of laparoscopy under local anaesthesia in 250 medical and surgical patients. Br. J. Surg., 67:751, 1980.
31. Lewis, A., and Archer, T.J.: Laparoscopy in general surgery. Br. J. Surg., 68:778, 1981.
32. Berci, G., and Jensen, D.: Laparoscopy for the hepatologist and surgeon. Acta Endosc., 12:3, 1982.
33. Deutsch, A.A., Zelikovsky, A., and Reiss, R.: Laparoscopy in the prevention of unnecessary appendicectomies: a prospective study. Br. J. Surg., 69:336, 1982.
34. Berci, G., et al.: Emergency mini-laparoscopy in abdominal trauma: an update. Am. J. Surg., 146(2):261, 1983.
35. Federle, M.P., et al.: Computed tomography in blunt abdominal trauma. Arch. Surg., 117:645, 1982.
36. Berci, G., et al.: The evaluation of a new peritoneo-

scope as a diagnostic aid to the surgeon. Ann. Surg., 178:37, 1973.
37. Jernstrom, P.: Air embolism during peritoneoscopy. Am. J. Clin. Pathol., 21:573, 1951.
38. Root, B., et al.: Gas embolism death after laparoscopy delayed by "trapping" in portal circulation. Anesth. Analg., 57:232, 1978.
39. Jensen, D., and Berci, G.: A new biopsy and documentation technique for laparoscopy. Gastrointest. Endosc., 17:150, 1981.
40. Vilardell, F., Seres, I., and Marti-Vicente, A.: Complications of peritoneoscopy: a survey of 1,455 examinations. Gastrointest. Endosc., 14:178, 1968.
41. Sherwood, R., et al.: Minilaparoscopy for blunt abdominal trauma. Arch. Surg., 115:672, 1980.
42. Root, H.D., et al.: Diagnostic peritoneal lavage. Surgery, 57:633, 1965.
43. Pachter, H.L., and Hofstetter, S.R.: Open and percutaneous paracentesis and lavage for abdominal trauma. Arch. Surg., 116:318, 1981.
44. Krausz, M.M., et al.: Peritoneal lavage in blunt abdominal trauma. Surg. Gynecol. Obstet., 152:327, 1981.
45. Soderstrom, C.A., DuPriest, R., and Cowley, R.A.: Pitfalls of peritoneal lavage in blunt abdominal trauma. Surg. Gynecol. Obstet., 151:513, 1980.
46. Peterson, S.R., and Sheldon, G.F.: Morbidity of a negative finding at laparotomy in abdominal trauma. Surg. Gynecol. Obstet., 148:23, 1979.
47. Morgenstern, L., and Shapiro, S.J.: Techniques of splenic conservation. Arch. Surg., 114:449, 1979.
48. Donaldson, L.A., Findlay, I.G., and Smith, A.: A retrospective review of 89 stab wounds to the abdomen. Br. J. Surg., 68:793, 1981.

15

Abdominal Paracentesis and Lavage for Trauma

John A. Barrett ■ Gary J. Merlotti

In the approach to the patient with abdominal trauma, the important question that confronts the surgeon is whether an indication exists for surgical exploration of the abdomen. This decision may be difficult, especially in patients with multiple injuries in whom the associated injuries make the diagnosis of intra-abdominal disorders difficult. The importance of detecting an intra-abdominal injury is obvious. In patients with head injuries, significant morbidity and mortality rates result from the failure to detect intra-abdominal injuries, a surprisingly frequent occurrence.[1] Abdominal paracentesis and lavage are valuable diagnostic aids in these situations. The purpose of this chapter is to review the indications, techniques, contraindications, and results of abdominal paracentesis and lavage in patients subjected to both blunt and penetrating trauma.

The decision to perform surgical exploration of a patient's abdomen following trauma is not necessarily based on the diagnosis of a specific intra-abdominal injury, but rather is based on the existence of an acute intra-abdominal problem that requires surgical intervention.[2] Not every patient with abdominal trauma needs to undergo diagnostic abdominal paracentesis and lavage. A patient who is in shock following penetrating abdominal trauma and who cannot be resuscitated, or who lapses into shock after the initial resuscitation, should immediately undergo surgical exploration of the abdomen, without paracentesis or lavage. Similarly, patients with gross peritonitis, or free air visible on abdominal films following blunt trauma, require urgent surgical intervention because such findings indicate the need for surgical exploration. Patients such as these, however, with clear indications for abdominal exploration, are the exception, rather than the rule. In the majority of patients with blunt abdominal trauma, no clear indication for surgical exploration is initially evident.

INDICATIONS IN BLUNT ABDOMINAL TRAUMA

Four major indications exist for abdominal paracentesis and lavage following blunt abdominal trauma.

Patients with Equivocal Abdominal Findings

The patient with obvious peritonitis does not require abdominal lavage. More common, however, is the patient who has some abdominal tenderness, but not overt peritonitis. It is frequently impossible to decide whether this tenderness is due to an associated intra-abdominal injury that requires exploration or whether it is merely caused by local abdominal wall tenderness that may be safely observed. Techniques such as tensing the abdominal muscles, in an attempt to differentiate deep from superficial abdominal tenderness, have been advocated,[3] but in our experience, these methods are unreliable. Such patients should therefore undergo diagnostic abdominal paracentesis and lavage.

Patients with Altered Levels of Consciousness

Patients with altered states of consciousness do not respond appropriately to abdominal examination. The determination of the existence of a significant intra-abdominal injury therefore depends on other reliable methods, such as paracentesis and lavage.[4-6] This group of patients includes not only those with head injuries who have decreased levels of consciousness, but also patients who are inebriated or whose responsiveness is altered by other drugs. Similarly, in the patient with spinal cord transection, an abdominal examination is diagnostically unreliable. A history of loss of consciousness is not itself an indication for abdominal lavage, however, provided the patient is alert and orientated at the time of the examination. The patient who remains obtunded requires the procedure.

Patients Unavailable for Continued Abdominal Observation

The most common reason for a surgeon's inability to observe patients at length is that these patients require surgical intervention for other, extra-abdominal injuries. These injuries are usually orthopedic in nature. Such patients may spend a long time under anesthesia. Deterioration of the patient's condition during the procedure may be attributed to the surgical operation in progress, rather than to a missed abdominal injury. The consequences may be disastrous.

Patients with Injuries Frequently Associated with Intra-abdominal Injuries

Patients with fractures of the lower ribs, the pelvis, or the spine, including fractures of the transverse processes of the lumbar vertebrae, frequently have associated abdominal injuries. Most of these patients have some degree of abdominal tenderness and require abdominal paracentesis or lavage on that basis alone.

TECHNIQUE FOR ABDOMINAL PARACENTESIS

Prior to abdominal lavage, one should perform abdominal paracentesis. Our technique is as follows: A No. 18 (1.5-inch) needle is mounted on a syringe and is introduced, after appropriate skin preparation, through the linea semilunaris at the lateral border of the rectus abdominis muscle, at the level of the anterior superior iliac spines. The needle is introduced at right angles to the skin and is slowly advanced until the peritoneal cavity is entered. This entry can be ascertained by the patient's complaint of pain, because the peritoneal lining is sensitive, and by a slight popping sensation.

Once the needle has entered the abdominal cavity, it should be released, and the needle's tip should be repositioned cephalad and caudad; the aspiration should then be repeated. It is not necessary to advance the needle's tip further into the abdominal cavity. Any blood present in the abdominal cavity is generally found immediately under the parietal peritoneal surface because of capillary attraction. Advancing the needle further into the abdominal cavity only increases the likelihood of intra-abdominal organ injury.

If the results of paracentesis are negative, the procedure should be repeated on the contralateral side. A positive result is characterized by the withdrawal of nonclotting blood from within the abdominal cavity. Although a positive abdominal result is a reliable indication for surgical exploration, a negative result in no way excludes the possibility of intra-abdominal injury. Almost 30% of patients with negative results of abdominal paracentesis have significant intra-abdominal injuries. The reason is that the most dependent portion of the abdominal cavity when the patient is supine is the pelvis. Blood gravitates toward the pelvis and may be missed by the needle. Therefore, the patient with a negative result of paracentesis should undergo peritoneal lavage.

TECHNIQUE FOR PERITONEAL LAVAGE

Prior to the performance of peritoneal lavage, one should pass a urinary catheter into the bladder, to decrease the likelihood of bladder injury. A nasogastric tube should be passed, and the patient's stomach should be decompressed. The skin of the lower abdomen should be shaved, prepared, and draped. An area 2 cm inferior to the umbilicus in the midline is anesthetized by infiltration of a local anesthetic agent containing 1% epinephrine, to decrease bleeding. Two methods of performing peritoneal lavage, the open method and the closed, percutaneous method, are in current use.

Open Method

The open method begins with a vertical incision through the skin and subcutaneous tissue to the linea alba. The linea alba is opened, and the peritoneum is grasped and divided. A peritoneal-dialysis catheter is passed under direct vision into the free abdominal cavity and is directed toward the pelvis. The catheter is aspirated, and if nonclotting blood is returned, the procedure is concluded, and the patient undergoes laparotomy. If no blood is returned, 1 L of lactated Ringer's solution is infused through the catheter (10 ml/kg in children). The patient's abdomen is gently agitated, or the patient is rolled slightly from side to side, unless this maneuver is contraindicated because of associated injuries. The container is then placed on the floor, and the lavage fluid is allowed to flow back into the container.

CLOSED METHOD

The closed method consists of passing a peritoneal catheter percutaneously into the abdominal cavity. Several techniques are available, but the most common involves the initial passage of a No. 18 needle into the abdominal cavity and directed toward the pelvis. A guidewire is passed through the needle, and the catheter is passed over the guidewire into the abdominal cavity. The catheter is aspirated, and if no nonclotting blood is returned, the abdomen is lavaged with lactated Ringer's solution, as in the open method.

CRITERIA FOR POSITIVE RESULTS OF LAVAGE

A number of criteria have been proposed to define a positive result of lavage. At one time, the criterion for surgical exploration was a lavage return so bloody that an observer could not read a newspaper through it. More sensitive and specific criteria have since been developed.[5,6] Results of peritoneal lavage are considered positive in patients with blunt abdominal trauma if any of the following criteria are met:

1. A red blood cell count greater than 100,000/mm^3 of unspun lavage return.
2. A white blood cell count greater than 500/mm^3 unspun of lavage return.
3. The presence of bile, bacteria, or feces (vegetable fibers) in the lavage return.

Should facilities for blood cell counts be unavailable, a red blood cell count of 100,000/mm^3 approximates a spun hematocrit of 2%. The advantage of peritoneal lavage over paracentesis is its high degree of accuracy when results are positive and its equally high reliability when results are negative. Many investigators have reported an accuracy rate of 97% or better.[4-6] These results pertain to patients with injuries that communicate with the free abdominal cavity, however. Peritoneal lavage cannot and should not be used to diagnose injuries limited to the retroperitoneum.

The reliability of percutaneous and open methods of peritoneal lavage has been compared.[7] Both methods are specific and sensitive, but the complication rate is greater with the percutaneous method. In the study by Patcher and Hofstetter, the complication rate with the open method was 2%, as compared to a 5% complication rate with the percutaneous (closed) method.[7] The advantage of the closed method is that it can be performed quickly, with a minimum of instrumentation, by an unassisted operator. The open method usually requires two people, with many instruments and lighting apparatus, and the procedure takes longer to perform.

CONTRAINDICATIONS TO PERITONEAL LAVAGE

The only absolute contraindication to peritoneal lavage is the presence of a clear indication for surgical exploration; such a patient should be moved to the operating suite as expeditiously as possible. Several relative contraindications to peritoneal lavage exist, however, as discussed in the following sections.

Pregnancy

Pregnancy can create two problems for peritoneal lavage. In patients who are in early pregnancy one may be concerned that the instillation of lavage fluid into the abdomen may induce a miscarriage. In fact, the fetus in early pregnancy is well protected, and the procedure does not appear to have any fetal effects. Thus, lavage is not contraindicated. A second problem is encountered in patients in late pregnancy who have undergone blunt abdominal trauma; the gravid uterus fills much of the abdominal cavity. Peritoneal lavage can still be performed between the fundus of the gravid uterus and the xiphoid process, however. An open technique is recommended in these patients.

Surgical Scars

The patient with abdominal incisions from prior operations presents problems to the surgeon considering a lavage procedure. Because of the presence of adhesions between the bowel and the abdominal scar, the risks of perforation of the intestine are increased. It is therefore advisable not to perform the lavage through the old scar. A patient who has a lower abdominal scar can undergo peritoneal lavage through the upper midline, and a patient with an upper abdominal scar may undergo lavage through the lower midline. The patient with a surgical scar from the xiphoid process to the symphysis pubica may undergo lavage through the lateral border of the rectus abdominis muscle. In all these patients, however, lavage should be performed by the open technique, to reduce the risk of perforation.

Another problem in patients with surgical scars is in interpretation of the results of lavage. A negative result in this situation cannot be trusted. The adhesions formed as a result of the prior operation may have divided the abdomen into several different compartments or loculations. The lavage fluid may remain trapped in one of these areas and may not mix with the traumatic bleeding that may be occurring in another isolated compartment. A negative result of lavage in these patients should therefore be viewed with caution. The criteria for positivity of peritoneal lavage are still reliable, however.

Pelvic Fracture

The decision to perform abdominal lavage in patients with pelvic fractures is often difficult. The problem lies not so much with the pelvic fracture itself, but rather with the associated pelvic hematoma. Pelvic fractures are frequently associated with pelvic hematomas, which may be large. The bleeding usually is venous in origin and begins posteriorly from the presacral plexus of veins.[8]

It is common for a pelvic hematoma that is retroperitoneal to extend anteriorly and to encircle the abdominal cavity completely. Blind percutaneous lavage in this situation may cause the lavage catheter to enter the hematoma instead of the free abdominal cavity. This error produces false-positive lavage results. If such a patient undergoes an exploratory laparotomy, the hematoma will be entered and decompressed. The loss of the tamponade effect produces massive venous bleeding, most of which comes from deep posterior presacral veins. Patients undergoing laparotomy have been exsanguinated because of this problem.

What, then, is to be done in the patient with a pelvic fracture? The integrity of the patient's intra-abdominal organs must be assessed. By physical examination of such patients, one may detect lower abdominal tenderness, but whether it is due to the pelvic fracture or to associated intra-abdominal injury may be difficult to decide. Moreover, these patients often have evidence of massive blood loss, and it may be impossible to distinguish between blood loss caused by the pelvic fracture, which should not be explored, and that caused by intra-abdominal bleeding, which should be explored.

Our answer is to perform a peritoneal lavage supraumbilically and by the open technique. The chances of placing the lavage catheter in the hematoma are thereby reduced. Even with these safeguards, a false-positive result is still possible, either because a small tear in the peritoneum overlying the pelvic hematoma allows free blood to enter the abdominal cavity, or diapedesis of red blood cells across the peritoneum is sufficient to give a positive result. Nonetheless, we advocate performance of the lavage; a negative result reliably rules out the diagnosis of significant intra-abdominal injury. If the result of lavage is positive, it cannot be trusted, and in such patients we obtain abdominal computed tomographic scans and, if necessary, angiograms, to assess the abdominal contents. The angiogram may also be of therapeutic use because if a bleeding artery in the pelvis is identified as the source of pelvic hematoma, arterial embolization of the vessel will be possible.

INDICATIONS IN PENETRATING ABDOMINAL TRAUMA

Although the role of peritoneal lavage in patients with blunt abdominal trauma is well accepted, its use in those who have undergone penetrating trauma is controversial. We therefore discuss the role of lavage in penetrating trauma of the abdomen under the headings of gunshot wounds and stab wounds.

Gunshot Wounds

Any patient with a gunshot wound that penetrates the abdominal cavity should undergo surgical exploration.[9] The chances of significant intra-abdominal injury are 98%.[9] Usually, penetration of the abdomen by the missile can be deduced from the path of the bullet, from the entry and exit wounds together, or from the entry wound and the retained missile. When victims are shot, they are unlikely to be in "normal anatomic position," so drawing a straight line from entry to exit may be dangerous. Patients with peritonitis, or free air visible on radiographs, however, have undergone intra-abdominal perforation. Surgical exploration without prior peritoneal lavage, is indicated in such patients.

In some patients, it is unclear whether the bullet penetrated the abdominal cavity. The management of these "tangential" gunshot injuries is controversial. Some trauma surgeons advocate local surgical exploration of the bullet tract by means of "tractotomy." Entry and exit wounds in these patients may be far apart and may not be easily connected. Moreover, a negative result of tractotomy does not rule out the possibility of associated "blast" injury to the intra-abdominal organs. Reports of intra-abdominal injury without penetration are rare,[10] but the fear of this blast effect has led some surgeons to advocate routine exploration of gunshot wounds that are in close proximity to the abdominal cavity. This method leads to a high rate of negative laparotomy, however, and laparotomy is not a benign procedure.[11]

Our approach to the problem is as follows. When the bullet has clearly penetrated the patient's abdominal cavity, we perform a laparotomy, with a 98% chance of finding significant intra-abdominal injury. When a gunshot wound appears tangential in nature, however, we perform peritoneal lavage.

Great care must be taken in the interpretation of lavage results in patients with penetrating trauma. Certainly, the presence of bile, bacteria, or vegetable matter produces a positive result and is an indication for surgical exploration. Similarly, a white blood cell count of greater than 500/mm^3 is an indication for exploration. The problem is in determining the number of red blood cells that signify a positive result of lavage in patients with penetrating trauma. In theory, even a single red blood cell in the lavage effluent should suggest abdominal penetration. Peritoneal lavage is much too sensitive for such a low threshold, however. The use of 100,000 cells, as in blunt trauma, appears to be too great. We use a figure of 10,000 red blood cells as an indication of penetration. In 235 consecutive patients, this technique has resulted in a 13% false-positive rate, but a 1% false-negative rate.[12] If the traditional figure of 100,000 cells had been used, the false-positive rate would have been 0%, but the false-negative rate would have been 10.4%. We are pleased with this degree of accuracy and prefer to perform unnecessary laparotomies in 13% of patients rather than to miss 10% of significant abdominal injuries.

Penetrating pelvic gunshot wounds are a special type of tangential abdominal wound. If one suspects abdominal penetration, lavage should be performed. Such injuries may damage the outlet tracts: the vagina, the bladder and urethra, and the rectum. Because injuries to the outlet tracts cannot always be recognized from within the abdominal cavity, all patients with penetrating pelvic gunshot wound should undergo careful vaginal examination by speculum, cystourethrography, and proctoscopic examination.

Stab Wounds

Patients with gunshot wounds of the abdominal cavity have a 98% chance of significant intra-abdominal injury.[9] The situation with stab wounds of the abdomen is different. Of all stab wounds of the abdomen, only approximately 50% enter the abdominal cavity; of these penetrating wounds, only approximately 50% cause significant intra-abdominal injury.[13] If we managed stab wounds as we do gunshot wounds and performed laparotomy on the basis of penetration alone, we would have a negative laparotomy rate of 50%. In some centers, this high rate is considered acceptable; the rationale is that a negative laparotomy for trauma is a benign procedure, and by using abdominal penetration as a criterion, no intra-abdominal injuries will be missed. Even when this policy is pursued, however, one is left with the problem of assessing penetration of the stab wound.

Some surgeons recommend local surgical exploration of the wound under these conditions and believe that penetration of the anterior fascia is significant.[14] Local wound exploration is not reliable, however. Victims of stabbing are not likely to have been wounded while in "normal anatomic position." Such persons usually crouch over to protect themselves. The entry wound in the skin may not therefore overlie the entry wound in the fascia, and local surgical exploration under the entry site in the skin may yield a false-negative result. In addition, even if an entry wound in the anterior fascia is discovered, it does not mean that the posterior fascia and peritoneum have been penetrated. Attempts to follow the tract of the stabbing implement through the body of the rectus abdominis muscle, while using local anesthesia and inadequate lighting, help, and instrumentation, are doomed to failure. The injection of contrast material into the tract of the stab wound, in an attempt to prove abdominal penetration, produces a high degree of false-negative results and is not reliable.[10] If abdominal penetration is used as the criterion for surgical exploration of stab wounds, we believe that peritoneal lavage is the most sensitive test, and use the same criteria as for gunshot wounds.

In our institution we do not surgically explore stab wounds of the abdomen on the basis of penetration alone because of the high incidence of negative laparotomies. We do not believe that negative laparotomy for trauma is a benign procedure. In a review of 178 negative laparotomies from the Trauma Unit at Cook County Hospital in Chicago, the mortality rate was 1.6%, and the complication rate was 19%. The incidence of intestinal obstruction within 6 months of a negative laparotomy for trauma was 4%.[11] Therefore, if the stab wound is to the anterior abdomen, that is, inferior to the costal margins, superior to the inguinal ligaments, and anterior to the midaxillary line, we perform laparotomy only when the patient has evidence of visceral injury, such as the following:

1. Shock.
2. Peritonitis.
3. Free air visible on abdominal radiographs.
4. Blood in the nasogastric tube or the rectum.
5. Evisceration of abdominal contents.
6. Abnormal intravenous pyelograms or cystograms.
7. Abnormal arteriograms or scans.
8. Retained stabbing implement.

Two types of stab wounds require special attention. The first is the stab wound to the lower chest. A wound inferior to the nipples but superior to the costal margin may have penetrated the abdomen. Unlike anterior abdominal stab wounds, thoracoabdominal wounds have penetrated the diaphragm to enter the abdomen. Because of the danger of diaphragmatic herniation through these wounds, injuries to the diaphragm should be repaired. Therefore, in patients with thoracoabdominal stab wounds, penetration of the abdominal cavity is an indication for surgical exploration because of the possibility of diaphragmatic injuries. All patients with such wounds should undergo abdominal lavage; if results are positive according to the criteria for abdominal penetration, one should perform an exploratory laparotomy. Other signs of diaphragmatic injury in these situations are the egress of lavage fluid from the chest tube and, if a chest tube has not been placed, the presence of an ipsilateral pleural effusion following abdominal lavage.

A similar situation pertains to posterior abdominal stab wounds. Stab wounds posterior to the midaxillary line inferior to the costal margins and superior to the iliac crests enter the abdomen through the retroperitoneum, if at all. Like the neck, this area contains important and vital structures within a limited space. Because of the danger of injury to major retroperitoneal vessels, colon, duodenum, or urinary tract, all stab wounds that penetrate the abdominal cavity through a posterior approach should be explored surgically. The usual criteria for a positive result of abdominal lavage for penetration pertain to these patients.

REFERENCES

1. Butterworth, J.F., et al.: Detection of occult abdominal trauma in patients with severe head injuries. Lancet, 2(8198):759, 1980.

2. Committee on Trauma, American College of Surgeons: Advanced Trauma Life Support. Chicago, American College of Surgeons, 1981, p. 75.
3. Committee on Trauma, American College of Surgeons: Advanced Trauma Life Support. Chicago, American College of Surgeons, 1981, p. 76.
4. Root, H.D., Hauser, C.W., and McKinley, C.R.: Diagnostic peritoneal lavage. Surgery, 57:633, 1965.
5. Fisher, R.P., Beveruin, B.C., and Engrav, L.H.: Diagnostic peritoneal lavage. Am. J. Surg., 136:701, 1978.
6. Powell, D.C., Bivins, B.A., and Bell, R.M.: Diagnostic peritoneal lavage. Surg. Gynecol. Obstet., 155:257, 1982.
7. Pachter, H.L., and Hofstetter, S.R.: Open and percutaneous paracentesis and lavage for abdominal trauma. Arch. Surg., 116:318, 1981.
8. Flint, L.: Definitive control of bleeding from severe pelvic fractures. Ann. Surg., 189:709, 1979.
9. Lowe, R.J., Saletta, J.D., and Read, D.R.: Should laparotomy be mandatory or selective in gunshot wounds of the abdomen? J. Trauma, 17:903, 1977.
10. Bowerman, J.W., and Smithwick, W.: Contrast examination of abdominal stab wounds. Radiology, 97:619, 1970.
11. Lowe, R.J., et al.: The negative laparotomy for abdominal trauma. J. Trauma, 12:853, 1972.
12. Merlotti, G., et al.: Peritoneal lavage in evaluating abdominal penetration. J. Trauma, 25(3):228, 1985.
13. Nance, F.C., Wennar, M.H., and Johnson, L.W.: Surgical judgment in the management of penetrating wounds of the abdomen. Ann. Surg., 193:639, 1981.
14. Thompson, J.S., Moore, E.R., and Moore, J.B.: The evolution of abdominal stab wound management. J. Trauma, 20:478, 1980.

16

Diagnostic Pulmonary Function Tests

Gwendolyn Graybar ▪ Elena Adler

Whether one uses elaborate, computerized, room-sized machines or a simple, handheld spirometer, pulmonary function tests quantitate respiratory status. The severity of pulmonary disease may be determined, as well as the patient's response to therapy. Various forms of mechanical respiratory support are prescribed, based on measured pulmonary parameters. Patients at risk for developing postoperative pulmonary complications may be identified because the incidence of such complications increases with the severity of preoperative pulmonary dysfunction. Pulmonary complications are leading causes of surgical morbidity and mortality. Further, surgical procedures are the leading precipitators of acute respiratory failure in the Western world.

INDICATIONS

Diagnostic pulmonary function tests are indicated for surgical patients in three situations.

First is the preoperative evaluation of patients with chronic lung disease who are to undergo a nonpulmonary surgical procedure. Upper abdominal operations have the highest incidence of postoperative pulmonary complications because such procedures are accompanied by the greatest derangement of pulmonary function in the postoperative period. Screening pulmonary function tests are thus indicated for patients with mild lung diseases who are scheduled to undergo upper abdominal, rather than more peripheral surgical, procedures. Additional risk factors for these complications include obesity, advanced age, smoking, sepsis, and shock.[1]

The second indication for pulmonary function testing is in the preoperative evaluation of patients who are to undergo lung resection. The purpose of the testing is to assess operability.

Third is the evaluation of surgical patients with acute respiratory failure.

SPECIFIC TESTS

Included in this discussion are tests of lung volume and capacity, tests of ventilation, gas-exchange determinations, and tests for diseases of the small airways.

Tests of Lung Volumes and Capacities

DYNAMIC LUNG VOLUMES. Lung volumes, the oldest measure of pulmonary function, were described by Henry Davy around 1800. These measurements continue to be the basis of all pulmonary function tests and have been referred to as the gold standard for identification and follow-up of patients with lung disease.[2]

Tidal volume (V_T) is the volume of air that enters and leaves the lungs during normal breathing. It is normally 6 ml/kg or about 10% of the total lung capacity (TLC) (Figs. 16–1 and 16–2).

Inspiratory reserve volume (IRV) is the maximum volume of air that can be inhaled over and above tidal volume. Expiratory reserve volume (ERV) is the maximum volume of air that can be forcefully exhaled following tidal exhalation. Normally, IRV is about 50%, and ERV is approximately 20% of TLC.

STATIC LUNG VOLUMES. TLC, residual volume (RV), and functional residual capacity (FRC) are referred to as static lung volumes and are not measured by spirometry. TLC and RV are calculated from measurements of FRC, and the dynamic lung volumes are measured by spirometry. Direct measurements of TLC and RV are both more strenuous for the patient and are less accurate than measurements of FRC. FRC is the volume of the lungs at the end of normal tidal volume and may be measured by: (1) closed-circuit helium dilution; (2) open-circuit nitrogen washout; or (3) body plethysmography.

With closed-circuit helium dilution, the patient breathes into a closed system with a spirometer filled with 10% helium. Helium is neither absorbed nor excreted. Therefore, the amount of helium after equilibrium of the patient's breathing and the spirometer equals the initial amount and permits calculation of the lung volume at FRC.

In the nitrogen-washout method, patients inhale 100% oxygen and exhale into a large spirometer such as a Tissot. They breathe until all the nitrogen in their lungs has been washed out into the spiro-

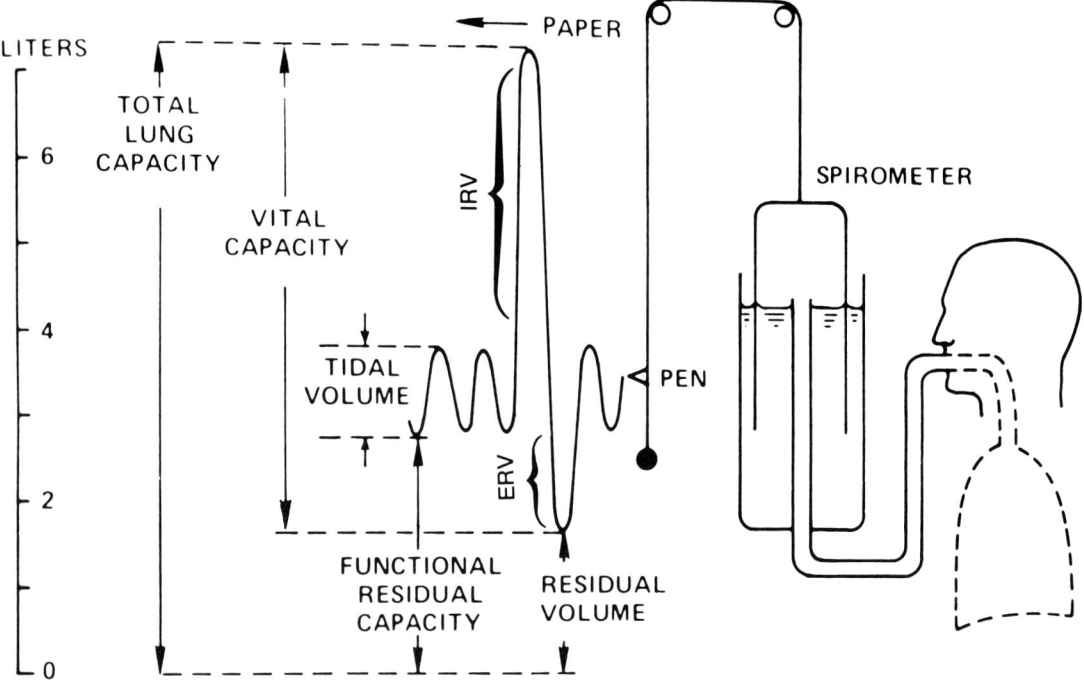

FIG. 16–1. Lung volumes as measured by spirometry. IRV and ERV, Inspiratory and expiratory reserve volume. (Adapted from West, J.B.: Respiratory Physiology—the Essentials. 2nd Ed. Baltimore, Williams & Wilkins, 1979.)

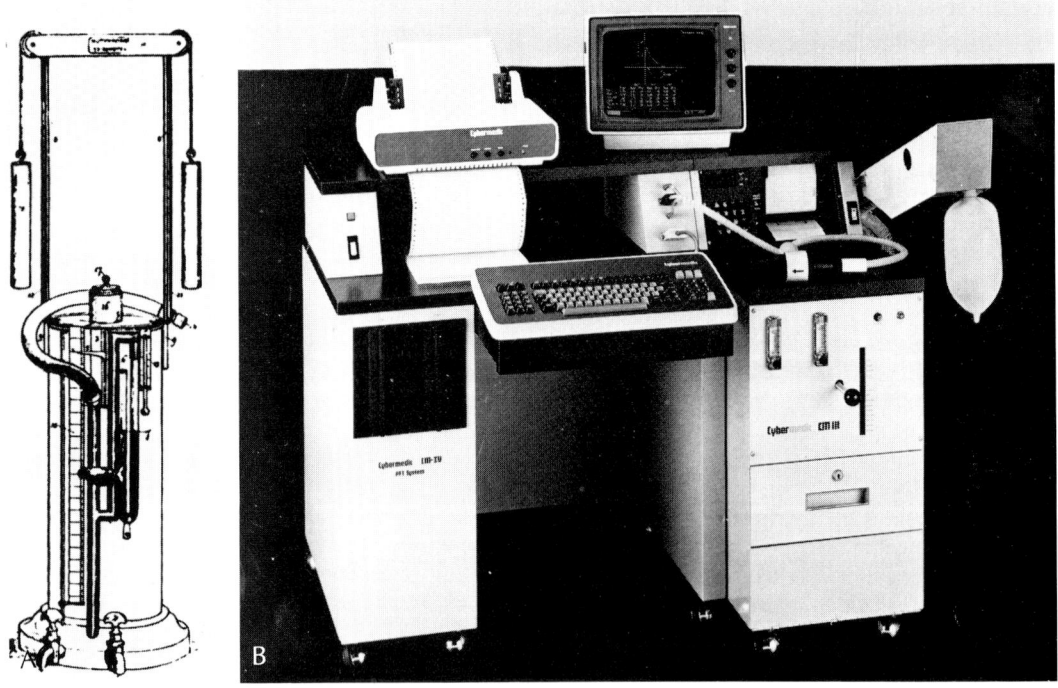

FIG. 16–2. Spirometers. *A*, Hutchinson's nineteenth-century device. *B*, A Cybermedic Unit in current use. (*A*, From Tisi, G.M.: Pulmonary Physiology in Clinical Medicine. Baltimore, Williams & Wilkins, 1980; *B*, From Cybermedic, Boulder, CO.)

meter. The beginning concentration of nitrogen in the lungs is known to be about 78%. The volume of exhaled gas and its nitrogen concentration are measured. FRC is then equal to the expired value times its percentage of nitrogen divided by 78%. The single-breath nitrogen-washout method uses a rapid nitrogen analyzer coupled with a pneumotachometer. FRC is calculated as previously discussed.

The nitrogen-washout technique shares with the helium-dilution method the disadvantage of measuring only ventilated lung volume. Therefore, patients with chronic obstructive pulmonary disease have falsely low FRC when measured by either of these methods. The nitrogen-washout technique has the following further disadvantages: (1) the concentration of nitrogen in the exhaled gases is low and may cause errors in calculated lung volumes; and (2) some of the expired nitrogen comes from body tissues.

Body plethysmography measures total thoracic gas volume, based on Boyle's law that for a gas at a constant temperature, the product of pressure and volume is constant. The plethysmograph measures gas volume in both ventilated and nonventilated lung areas. Therefore, the difference in FRC as measured by the plethysmograph and either the helium-dilution or nitrogen-washout method gives a measure of air trapping. A difference of more than 200 ml denotes significant air trapping. Because the body plethysmograph is not available in most hospitals, it is not considered part of routine, clinical pulmonary function testing.

Tests of Ventilation

FORCED EXPIRATORY SPIROGRAM. The forced vital capacity (FVC) maneuver differentiates among normal, obstructive, and restrictive patterns (Fig. 16–3). The patient rapidly and forcefully exhales from TLC to RV into a spirometer. The total amount exhaled (FVC) and that exhaled in the first three seconds (FEV_1, FEV_2, and FEV_3) are measured. FEV_1, which may be expressed as a percentage of FVC, is the most reproducible and thus the most valid flow rate in the FVC. The most effort-dependent portion of the curve is the first part. The first 200 ml are exhaled slowly because the inertia of both the lung-thorax system and the spirometer must be overcome. Forced expiratory flow, $FEF_{200-1,200}$, depends less on effort; FEF_{25-75} depends least on effort and is the most reproducible. Normal values for the FVC maneuver range from 80 to 120% of predicted for each value. Height is the closest anthropometric correlate. For adult males, height (cm) × 25 approximates predicted FVC, and for adult females, the equation is height (cm) × 20.

In patients with obstructive lung disease, expiratory flow rates are decreased, and hyperinflation results in increased RV, TLC, and RV/TLC. Mild airway obstruction may prolong only FEF_{25-75}, which is believed to reflect dysfunction of small airways. As the obstruction worsens, all flow rates fall below predicted. Pulmonary obstruction may be graded by the following decreases in FEF_{25-75}[3]: greater than 84%, no obstructive impairment; 80 to 84%, within the low range of normal limits; 65 to 79%, mild obstructive or no significant impairment; 50 to 64%, moderate obstructive impairment; 35 to 49%, severe obstructive impairment; and less than 35%, extreme obstructive impairment.

FEF_{25-75} deteriorates rapidly as obstructive lung disease worsens; in fact, this value may decrease exponentially.[4,5] Therefore, patients with severe obstructive lung disease do not show further large decreases in FEF_{25-75}. In such patients, measuring FEV_1/FVC as a percentage is useful, to monitor the decline in pulmonary function.[6]

In nonsmokers, FEV_1 declines gradually with age, and significant airway obstruction rarely develops. Smokers appear to fall into susceptible and nonsusceptible groups. FEV_1 in nonsusceptible smokers follows a pattern of decline similar to that in nonsmokers. Susceptible smokers have an exponential decline in FEV_1 and become disabled by obstructive lung disease. In persons who stop smoking before age 45, Fletcher and Peto found that the rate of decay in FEV_1 reverts to nonsusceptible-smokers' levels, and disability is unusual.[7] Thus, FEV_1 may be used to detect susceptible smokers in early middle age and, one hopes, to persuade them to stop.

Restrictive lung disease is characterized by a marked decrease in FVC and RV. Most restrictive lung diseases produce uniform reductions in all lung volumes and capacities. Conditions resulting in abdominal distention such as ascites, obesity, and pregnancy reduce ERV and FRC with normal inspiratory capacity; expiratory flow rates are normal or increased.

Grading of restrictive impairment is based on TLC, as follows[3]: greater than 120%, hyperinflation; 116 to 120%, high range of normal limits; 85 to 115%, within normal limits; 80 to 84%, within the low range of normal limits; 65 to 79%, mild restrictive impairment; 50 to 64%, moderate restrictive impairment; 35 to 49%, severe restrictive impairment; and less than 35%, extreme restrictive impairment.

FVC reflects the patient's ability to cough and to breathe deeply. It should be at least two to three times tidal volume. Next to the match test, FVC is the most readily accessible measure of ventilatory reserve.[8]

When persons in screening programs are found to have abnormal results of spirometry and are notified of this situation, they stop smoking at a rate approximating that achieved at smoking-cessation

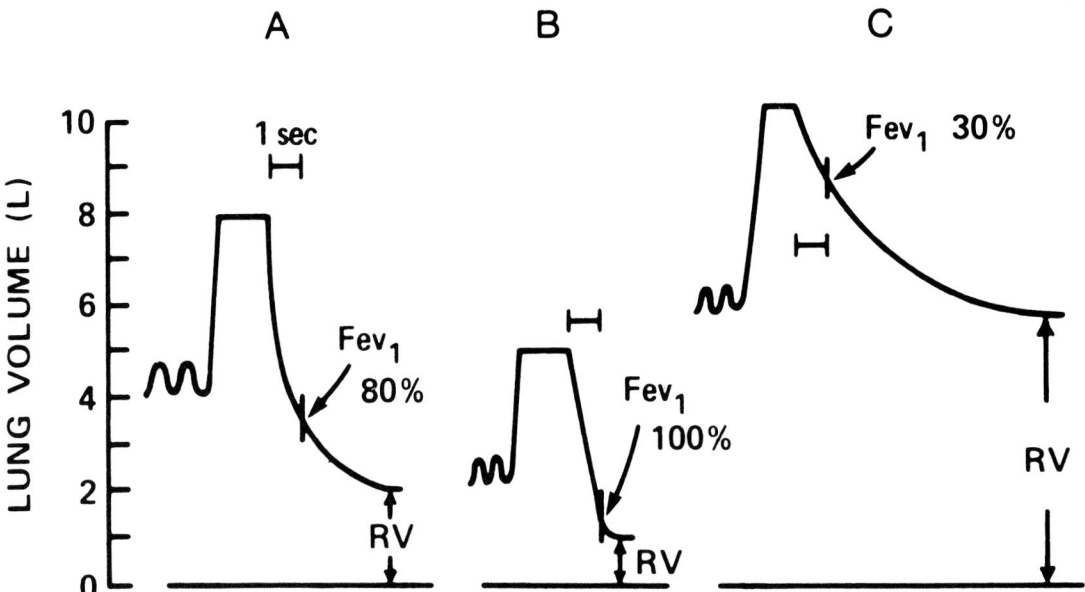

FIG. 16–3. Three clinical patterns based on forced vital capacity (FVC): Normal (A), restrictive (B), and obstructive with hyperinflation (C). RV, Residual volume; FEV_1, forced expiratory volume in 1 sec. (Adapted from Tisi, G.M.: Pulmonary Physiology in Clinical Medicine. Baltimore, Williams & Wilkins, 1980, p. 66.)

clinics.[9] Comprehensive pulmonary rehabilitation programs for patients with severe chronic obstructive pulmonary disease bring about statistically significant improvements in vital capacity, MVV, resting Pa_{O_2}, and exercise tolerance.[10] Surgeons whose middle-aged patients have abnormal results of preoperative screening spirometry may be in a unique position to influence their patients' longevity. By combining these abnormal results with the emotional drama of the perioperative period, surgeons may convince patients to quit smoking. Cessation of smoking a week or two preoperatively does little to decrease the incidence of postoperative pulmonary complications.[1] Nonetheless, attempts to inspire a patient to stop smoking are worthwhile; even overnight cessation improves a patient's oxygen-carrying capacity by eliminating carboxyhemoglobin.

MAXIMUM VOLUNTARY VENTILATION. Many believe that maximum voluntary ventilation (MVV) is the best predictor of postoperative pulmonary complications.[2,11–14] MVV is measured with a spirometer and is the maximum amount of air that can be breathed in 1 min. It is actually measured over a period of 10 to 15 sec and is then extrapolated to 1 min. The maneuver, which exaggerates air trapping, depends on the intangible variables of co-operation, motivation, and stamina of the patient and may therefore anticipate how closely the patient will adhere to a respiratory-care regimen. The normal value is 150 L/min; MVV less than 45 L/min is of grave prognostic significance in a postoperative patient. MVV should be about 40 times FEV_1; if MVV is much lower than that, it indicates a lack of effort on the part of the patient. MVV is the most strenuous spirometric test and may be uncomfortable for the patient with significant air trapping. Because many argue that the measurement is not a true "pulmonary" function test, MVV is not included in routine spirometry as frequently as it was in the past.

TECHNICAL ASPECTS OF SPIROMETRY. Dynamic lung volumes, FVC, and MVV are measured with a spirometer, a simple gas-volume recorder. As seen in Figure 16–1, the common, water-filled spirometer has a bell floating in water. It closely resembles the instrument used by John Hutchinson in the 1840s,[15] as seen in Figure 16–2. As air enters the spirometer, the bell rises, lowering the pen by the pulley.

In addition, dry spirometers are available, such as the wedge-bellows apparatus and the piston-rolling-seal spirometers. In general, the water-filled spirometers are less expensive but require more of the technician's time for measurement and calculation. Electronic, dry spirometers are available with microprocessors that perform all calculations and offer possible interpretations. Complete pulmonary function testing previously took 3 hours, but now it may be done in several minutes. The least-accurate spirometers generally are the least-expensive electronic spirometers.

Lung volumes may also be measured by pneumotachometers, or flow-sensing devices. One of the simplest and smallest is the Wright respirometer. It is handheld and nonelectric and hence has become popular for bedside monitoring, particularly in the hospital recovery room and intensive care units. This instrument enables one to measure volume between flow rates of 3 and 300 L/min. Therefore, lung volumes in patients with low flow rates are underestimated. Another disadvantage is that the device is easily broken when forcefully blown into by individuals with healthy lungs.[16]

Many factors influence predicted "normal values." Advancing age decreases predicted vital capacity, whereas increased height increases this value. Non-Caucasians have vital capacity values about 15% lower than Caucasians.[17,18] The Cotton Dust Standards of the United States Occupational Safety and Health Administration, which are for industrial surveillance, specify that the predicted FEV_1 and FVC for blacks be multiplied by 0.85.[19] The United States Department of Labor's recommendations regarding disability state that identical tables should be applied to whites and blacks, however.[20] Clausen has summarized arguments for and against standardization of pulmonary function tests.[21] The foregoing example suggests the need for such standardization, as well as some of the problems when government agencies attempt to formulate standards.

These racial differences have been attributed to variations in thoracic configuration and diaphragmatic position. Similar variations may also explain the normal lower values for women.

The type of spirometer used also influences results. All results should be corrected to body temperature and pressure for saturated gas (BTPS). The BTPS correction usually increases volumes 8 to 10% and may be crucial when determining disability, as well as operability for cancer.

Each laboratory should carefully choose its predicted normal regression equations from studies based on similar testing equipment, methods, and patients. Minimum recommended performance standards for spirometry have been developed by the American Thoracic Society and the American College of Chest Physicians.[3,22,23] Criteria for technically satisfactory studies may be found in these recommendations.

Despite modern equipment, precision remains elusive. Variability among patients results from diurnal rhythm as well as from random, unexplained causes. Pulmonary function is worst in the morning; FEV_1 and airway resistance improve later in the day.[24] The surgeon may delay the start of a surgical procedure in patients with chronic obstructive pulmonary disease, to wait for an optimal time of day and to allow respiratory therapy to be performed several times.

Pulmonary function tests may be affected by irritants and bronchodilators. Clinicians must emphasize to patients the importance of not smoking, drinking coffee, using bronchodilators, or inhaling irritants such as cold air or traffic pollution in the several hours preceding pulmonary function tests, lest the results be misleading.

Nearly all pulmonary function tests require the active participation and compliance of the patient. The abilities of the technician who instructs the patient and performs the tests may have more impact on the results than the equipment, methods, or reference values. The technician should combine the qualities of a personal confidant, a biomedical engineer, and a football coach. The technician must assess and must report the patient's effort in performing pulmonary function tests.

The cost of spirometry varies widely. The major determining factors are the spirometer itself, which may cost between $500 and $50,000, the technician, and the time for testing and calculation. Costs of the various pulmonary function tests are given in Table 16–1.

One must not assume that the most advanced piece of equipment guarantees the highest standard of care. Instrumentation improves the level of care only when it is appropriate to the situation and when it is selected, maintained, and used by personnel who understand and respect the equipment and who know how to respond in the event of the unexpected. The patient's well-being depends on these factors.[25] In fact, equipment for pulmonary function testing should be chosen for its simplicity.

FLOW VOLUME LOOPS. The patient exhales forcibly and then inhales to TLC. The results are displayed by plotting flow rate on the vertical axis and volume on the horizontal axis, as seen in Figure 16–4. The flow at 50% vital capacity (VC) (V_{max} 50%) approximates that of FEF_{25-75}. In normal persons, inspiratory and expiratory flow rates at 50% are equal; that is, the mid-VC ratio is nearly 1 (Fig. 16–4,A). This shape, from 75% VC to RV, is nearly independent of the patient's effort; flow is determined by the elastic recoil of the lungs and by the flow-resistive properties of the small airways. Patients with chronic obstructive pulmonary disease have slower flow rates and lower peak flow rates than other persons (Fig. 16–4,B). Further, they do not have a plateau. Restrictive lung disease decreases lung volumes, but flow rates remain normal (Fig. 16–4,C).

Three types of upper airway obstruction may be identified from flow volume loops. First is fixed obstruction, such as by tracheal stenosis or goiter (Fig. 16–4,D). Second is variable extrathoracic obstruction, such as from vocal cord paralysis or polyps, tracheal masses, or foreign bodies (Fig. 16–4,E).

Table 16-1. Summary of Pulmonary Function Tests

Tests	Indication	Complexity	Airway	Effort	Normal Values*	Cost**
Lung volumes and capacities VC VT IRV ERV	To assess obstructive or restrictive disorders and risk of postoperative pulmonary complications (PPC)	Simple bedside units available for immobile patients	Large	Dependent	5 L 6 ml/kg or 10% of TLC 50% of TLC or 3 L 20% of TLC or 1.2 L	$60; $90 if pre- and postbronchodilation
FRC nitrogen washout	To measure the functional residual capacity	Complex; subject to errors; amount of N_2 is miniscule to measure; endogenous N_2 produced FRC may be falsely low	Only ventilated airways	Dependent	FRC, 2.4 L RV, 1.2 L FRC/TLC, 20%	$38.50
helium dilution	To calculate RV + TLC		Ventilated and non-ventilated airways	Dependent	RV/TLC, 20%	$44.00
body plethysmography		Complex; box must be airtight				
Tests of Ventilation Expiratory Flow Rates FEV_{1-2-3}	To assess obstructive lung disease and reversibility with bronchodilators	Simple, with a spirometer	Large	Dependent	80 to 120% of FVC	Included with lung volumes
FEV_{25-75}	To assess obstruction of small airways, such as in smokers		Small	Independent	84% of FVC	
MVV	To predict PPC To assess restrictive and obstructive disease	Simple, with a spirometer, but with patient's co-operation; uncomfortable for patient	Large	Dependent	>150 L/min	$60
flow volume loops	To assess fixed and variable airway obstruction, chronic obstruction and restrictive disease	Simple	Large	Dependent	See Fig. 16-3	
Tests for Gas Exchange						
Arterial blood gases	To evaluate alveolar exchange; as a base line To predict PPC	Simple	Alveolar-capillary	Independent	pH 7.35 to 7.45 P_{CO_2} 35 to 45 P_{O_2} 80–100	Included in cardio-pulmonary profile; $1.50
Qs/Qt	To measure shunt To determine level of PEEP	Requires Swan Ganz Catheter	Alveolar-capillary	Independent	<5% <15% for optimal PEEP	$55
Single-breath CO diffusing capacity	To evaluate alveolar and capillary damage in patients with hypoxia	Simple, although breath holding may be difficult in patient with SOB	Alveolar-capillary	Dependent		
Split lung function tests Xenon ventilation and perfusion studies	To assess operability of patients for lung resection	Complex; requires expensive radiologic equipment and radiation exposure	All air-filled spaces; large, small alveoli	Independent	Equal ventilation and perfusion throughout both lungs	$225
Macroaggegate perfusion scans ^{131}iodine-tagged albumin and-technecium-tagged ferric chloride	To assess contribution of diseased lungs to test results	Perfusion scans less complicated than ventilation	Airways not examined	Independent		$175
unilateral pulmonary artery occlusion	To predict postoperative pulmonary function and thus to determine whether patient can tolerate lung resection	Invasive, uncomfortable for patient; requires cardiac catheterization laboratory	Perfusion study, not airway examination	Independent	If pulmonary artery pressure of >35 mm Hg or Pa_{O_2} <45 mm/Hg develops during arterial occlusion, then patient is not a candidate for lung resection	$175

* Based on 70 kg
** Based on 1983 Tulane Medical Center prices

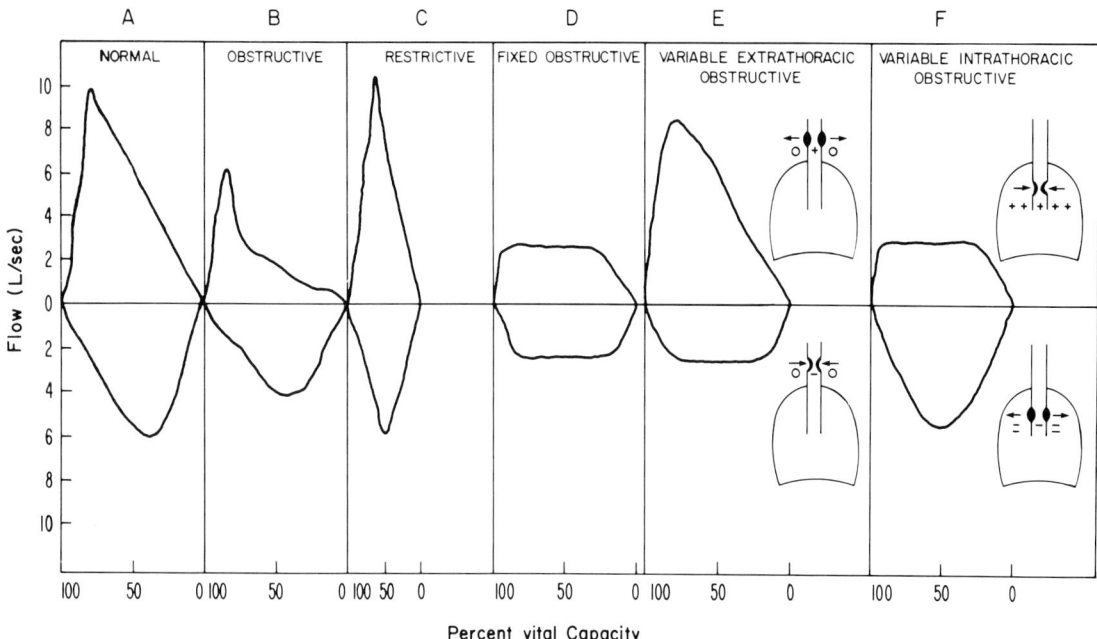

FIG. 16-4. Normal and abnormal flow volume loops. A, Normal; B, obstructive; C, restrictive; D, fixed obstructive; E, variable extrathoracic obstructive; and F, variable intrathoracic obstructive.

Third is variable intrathoracic obstruction, such as that caused by tumors (Fig. 16-4,F).

In patients with fixed obstruction, both inspiratory and expiratory flow rates are decreased. Expiratory flow rate plateaus near TLC and appears as a square wave. Inspiratory flow rate plateaus near 50% VC. The mid-VC ratio is nearly 1 because both inspiration and expiration are equally affected.

In patients with variable extrathoracic obstruction, forced exhalation causes tracheal pressure to become positive and thereby decreases the obstruction and dilates the airway. During forced inspiration, tracheal pressure is lower than around the airway; it increases the obstruction and narrows the trachea while lowering inspiratory flow rates. The mid-VC ratio is greater than 1.

In patients with variable intrathoracic obstruction, the opposite occurs; during exhalation, pleural pressure exceeds intratracheal pressure. The result is a decrease in the expiratory flow rate and thus in the mid-VC ratio.

Upper airway obstruction clinically may mimic asthma. Nearly every pulmonary physician can recall a patient who was treated without success for "asthma" when th diagnosis was upper airway obstruction. Flow volume loops help one to distinguish among various forms of obstruction and may indicate the need for surgical intervention.

Tests for Gas Exchange

BLOOD GASES. Oxygen, carbon dioxide, and hydrogen ion measurements are referred to as "blood gases." These measurements are nonspecific, but they indicate the severity of the patient's pulmonary dysfunction. In the absence of metabolic alkalosis, Pa_{CO_2} greater than 50 mm Hg is believed to be the most reliable predictor of postoperative pulmonary complications,[26,27] as well as indicating minimal reserve.[28] Metabolic alkalosis is the most common blood-gas abnormality in hospitalized patients, however, and 80% of these patients retain carbon dioxide in compensation.

The patient's acid-base status may be determined by measuring Pa_{CO_2} and pH and by plotting the patient's blood-gas values on various nomograms. That of Grogono and colleagues is one of the easiest to use and to understand (Fig. 16-5).[29] This nomogram eliminates curved lines, nonlinear axes, and confusing in vitro terminology.

Blood-gas analysis is available in nearly all hospitals. The test itself is simple to perform; however, the technician's time and skill are needed in obtaining the arterial and mixed venous specimens.

Computers may be used to interpret the results of blood-gas measurement. Although the majority of physicians are confident in their ability to interpret blood gases, in a simple exercise at a large, university-affiliated hospital, fewer than 40% consistently gave the correct answers.[30] The computer offers not only an aid to diagnosis but also suggestions for appropriate therapeutic intervention. In smaller hospitals, such a computer offers a degree of accuracy that may not otherwise be possible. In larger

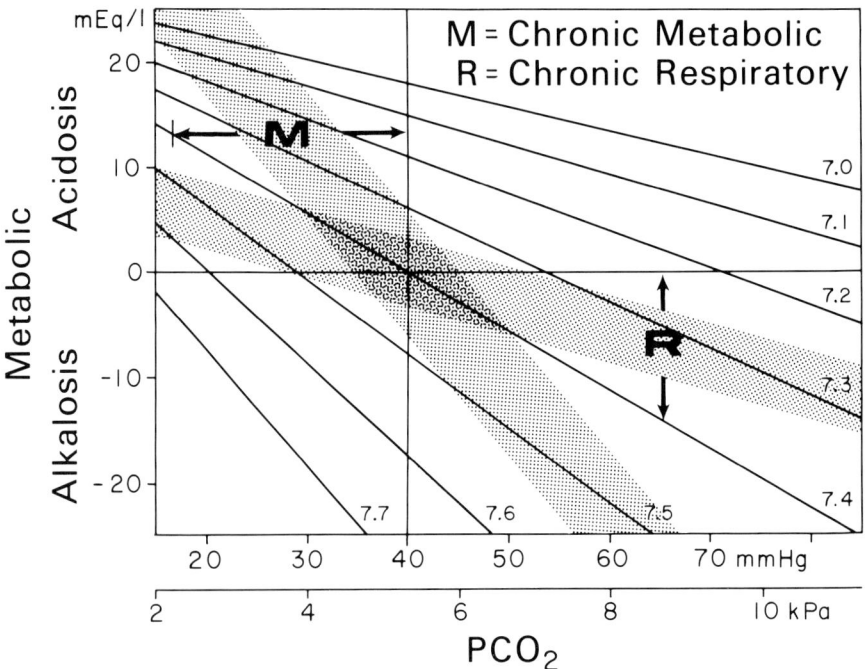

FIG. 16–5. Acid-base nomogram. M, Chronic metabolic; R, chronic respiratory. (From Grogono, A.W., et al.: An in vivo representation of acid base balance. Lancet, 2:499, 1976.)

hospitals, it frees pulmonary specialists from a tedious, time-consuming task.

One of the most important reasons to obtain blood gases in the preoperative patient is to establish a base line for later reference. Because anesthesia and surgical procedures impair pulmonary function, it is useful to have a postoperative goal in surgical patients. This concept is particularly important in view of the recent advances in the treatment of adult respiratory distress syndrome (ARDS); aggressive ventilatory techniques with positive end-expiratory pressure (PEEP) are used to maintain near-normal pulmonary function, such as a shunt (Qs/Qt) of less than 15%.[31] This goal may be impossible in patients with pre-existing pulmonary dysfunction.

DIFFUSION CAPACITY. Diffusion capacity ($D_{L_{CO}}$) measures the lung's ability to conduct a gas from the alveoli to the capillaries. The presence of severe hypoxia may indicate measurement of $D_{L_{CO}}$. Carbon monoxide has diffusion characteristics similar to those of oxygen. Diffusion capacity is measured by the single-breath carbon monoxide test. The patient takes a deep inspiration of a low concentration of carbon monoxide. This maneuver is followed by a 10-sec period of breath holding, followed by measurements of inspired and expired carbon monoxide. The volume of gas in the lung is determined, as well as the uptake of carbon monoxide from the lung. The $D_{L_{CO}}$ determination may be performed simultaneously with the single-breath nitrogen washout test for FRC. No blood samples are required, but the results must be corrected for hemoglobin values. $D_{L_{CO}}$ is reduced in the presence of destruction of the alveolar-capillary network, such as in patients with pulmonary consolidation, fibrosis, or edema.

Tests for Diseases of the Small Airways

Chronic obstructive lung disease begins in the smallest peripheral airways. Asymptomatic young smokers develop progressive pathologic changes, including terminal bronchiolitis and bronchiectasis, goblet-cell hyperplasia with subsequent mucus plugging, and obstruction of the peripheral airways.[32,33]

Conventional spirometry assesses large-airway function. The patient must have widespread pulmonary damage before results of spirometry will be abnormal. Therefore, various tests have been developed to aid in the determination of early disease of the small airways. These tests include closing volume, frequency-dependent dynamic compliance, FEF_{25-75}, and volume of isoflow with flow-volume loops.[34]

With the exception of the FEF_{25-75}, these tests appear to have little value in the diagnosis of surgical patients. Thus, tests for dysfunction of the small airways are currently most useful as epidemiologic or behavior-modification tools. A history of smoking is as reliable a predictor of postoperative pulmonary complications.[2] Acute viral upper respiratory infections also cause dysfunction of the small airways, as measured by these tests.[35] Because patients who are to undergo lung resection must have far-advanced lung dysfunction to be denied operation, the foregoing tests are not indicated in the preoperative evaluation.

EVALUATION OF PATIENTS FOR LUNG RESECTION

Provided the remaining lung is normal, pneumonectomy should not be associated with cardiorespiratory failure. Carcinoma of the lung is now the leading indication for lung resection. Boushy and coworkers reported that 70% of patients with lung cancer had symptoms of chronic obstructive lung disease, and 20% had abnormal results of pulmonary function tests.[36]

Resectability is defined as the technical ability to remove the tumor. Contraindications to resectibility are the presence of distant metastases and contiguous spread to areas that cannot be resected, such as the diaphragm and the superior vena cava.

Operability is the patient's ability to tolerate lung resection without cardiorespiratory failure. Screening spirometry and blood-gas measurements help one to identify patients at high risk for cardiorespiratory failure. The risk criteria include the following: FVC less than 50% predicted; FEV_1 less than 50% FVC or less than 2 L; MVV less than 50% predicted; RV/TLC greater than 50%; $D_{L_{CO}}$ less than 50%; and arterial P_{CO_2} greater than 45 mm Hg. In addition, patients over 60 years of age have increased rates of postoperative morbidity and mortality. Poor predictors of the postoperative course include resistance, compliance, work of breathing, elastic recoil, and duration of anesthesia.[36]

The foregoing function tests can predict neither lung function after pneumonectomy nor the patient's postoperative course. Patients should not be denied a possibly curative operation based on these parameters alone. Given the dismal outlook for patients with lung cancer who do not undergo operation, high-risk patients should have split function tests to determine operability. If the lung to be removed contributes little to the patient's overall pulmonary function, then an operation will be less risky.

Results of radioisotopic lung scanning correlate well with those of bronchospirometry. Radiospirometry requires less of the physician's time, placement of an endobronchial tube is unnecessary, and discomfort to the patient is minimal. Estimation of regional lung function with bronchospirometry uses the Fick equation, with its technical and physiologic uncertainties. For these reasons, radiospirometry has replaced bronchospirometry in predicting postpneumonectomy lung function.

Pulmonary perfusion scans are the simplest, most readily available tests for determining differential lung perfusion. Either ^{131}iodine (^{131}I)-macroaggregated albumin or ^{99m}technetium (^{99m}Tc)-ferric hydroxide macroaggregates are injected intravenously. They lodge in the pulmonary capillaries and give a measure of pulmonary perfusion as the lungs are scanned. Postpneumonectomy FEV_1 and other functions may then be calculated using the formula of Neuhaus and Cherniack (postpneumonectomy FEV_1 = prepneumonectomy FEV_1 × fraction of contralateral lung, as measured by ^{99m}Tc perfusion).[37,38]

^{133}Xenon radiospirometry measures perfusion, ventilation, and lung volume. Both quantitative and qualitative information on regional ventilation and perfusion are obtained. Xenon, an insoluble gas, is injected intravenously and is inhaled. These tests require sophisticated machinery and expertise, as well as special handling of the radioactive xenon gas, but they allow accurate prediction of postoperative lung function.[39] One problem with xenon radiospirometry is that it is performed at rest, and a nonresting FEV_1 is predicted. Precision might be increased if the measurements of ventilation distribution and lung volume were made during forced breathing, such as during an exercise test.[40]

Results of the lateral-position test correlate well with results obtained from macroaggregate scanning.[41] This test may be useful in hospitals lacking radionuclide scanning capabilities. Problems with the lateral-position test include some patients' inability to be supine or to be placed in a lateral decubitus position. Further, unilateral chest wall or pleural abnormalities result in disparate compliances and decreasing the test's reliability.

Potential pulmonary vascular conditions may be estimated preoperatively by temporary balloon occlusion of the pulmonary artery during cardiac catheterization while the patient is at rest and during exercise. On occlusion of the artery, if the mean pulmonary artery pressure exceeds 35 to 40 mm Hg or the systemic arterial P_{O_2} is less than 45 mm Hg, then patients will not be able to tolerate pneumonectomy. Although this procedure most realistically predicts postpneumonectomy function, it is the most invasive diagnostic test of pulmonary function, and Tisi believes it should only be done in patients with pulmonary hypertension secondary to primary pulmonary vascular disease or in patients with chronic obstructive pulmonary disease whose pulmonary hypertension is not explained by the underlying disease.[2]

Olsen and associates prospectively studied 56 patients for lung resection who were identified as being at high risk by screening spirometry and blood-measurement gas.[42] These researchers used the following arbitrary criteria for operability: (1) a predicted postpneumonectomy FEV_1 of 800 ml, (2) a mean pulmonary artery pressure on balloon occlusion and exercise of less than 35 mm Hg, (3) or a systemic Pa_{O_2} greater than 45 mm Hg. Thus, patients with marked pulmonary dysfunction underwent surgical procedures. The risk seemed worthwhile, however, given that these patients would almost certainly die without operation.[43] Seventeen of Olsen's patients subsequently underwent pneumonectomy, with a 17.6% mortality rate, and 13 patients underwent lobectomy, with a 7.7% mortality rate. An additional 12 patients who underwent operation had lesions that were not resectable. Of the patients who underwent lung resection, 59% were still living 1 to 3 years postoperatively.

The mortality rates in Olsen's study were better than those previously described for patients with similar pulmonary dysfunction.[36] Pulmonary artery balloon occlusion would thus seem justified when the predicted postpneumonectomy FEV_1 is less than 800 ml.

Lockwood found that the incidence of postoperative bronchopleural fistulas was closely correlated with the preoperative RV and RV/TLC ratio.[44] This association was attributed in part to the abnormal intrapleural pressures in patients with advanced chronic lung disease and in part to emphysematous changes in the large airways.

ASSESSMENT OF VENTILATORY RESERVE

An assessment of the patient's ventilatory reserve is crucial to the determination of anesthetic and operative risk.

In normal patients at rest, the work of breathing comprises about 5% of total body oxygen consumption ($\dot{V}_{O_2}$). The percentage increases disproportionately with increased minute ventilation (Fig. 16-6). Patients with chronic obstructive pulmonary disease expend a greater percentage of their $\dot{V}_{O_2}$ on the work of breathing. The closer a patient's tidal volume is to vital capacity, the greater is the percentage of total oxygen consumption used for the work of breathing, and the less reserve is available in situations of stress.

Tidal volume, minute volume, and vital capacity may be readily measured at the patient's bedside, for assessment of ventilatory reserve even in the most critically ill patients. A tidal volume of 3 ml/kg and a vital capacity twice that are generally considered adequate for weaning a patient from mechanical support and for extubation. Patients with a V_E greater than 12 L/min usually require continued mechanical ventilatory support.

Patients with chronic obstructive pulmonary disease should undergo intensive preoperative pulmonary preparation, as described by Gracey.[11] FEV_1/FVC should increase within several days. The

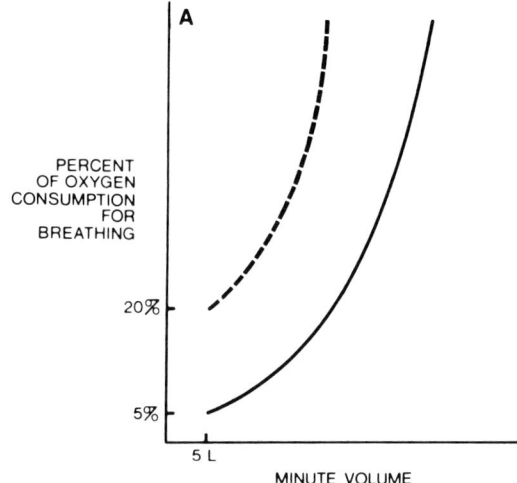

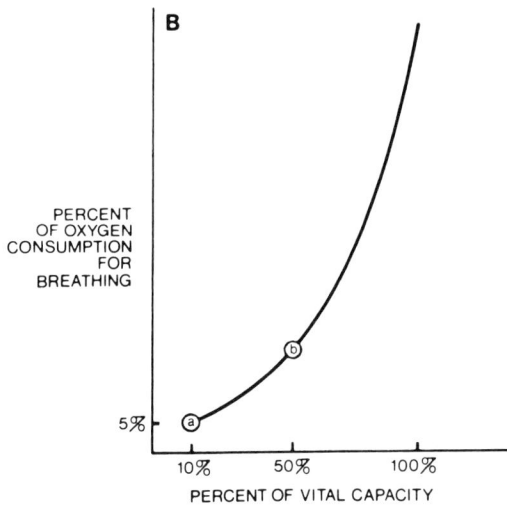

FIG. 16-6. The work of breathing in relation to minute volume (V_T) and vital capacity (VC). A, The solid line represents a normal person and the dotted line a patient with chronic obstructive pulmonary disease. B, Point a represents a V_T of 500 ml with a VC of 5 L; point b shows a V_T of 500 ml with a VC of 1 L. (Reproduced with permission from Shapiro, B.A., Harrison, R.A., and Walton, J.R.: Clinical Application of Blood Gases. 3rd edition. Copyright © 1982 by Yearbook Medical Publishers Inc., Chicago.)

incidence of postoperative pulmonary complications decreases, and the hospital stay and cost are reduced. Gracey's patients who did not show an improvement in spirometric values did poorly postoperatively, and many of these patients required prolonged mechanical ventilation.

ACKNOWLEDGMENTS

We extend special thanks to Harry S. Kaufman III, R.R.T., for his technical assistance and to H. William Barkman, M.D., for reviewing the manuscript.

REFERENCES

1. Schmidt, G.: Prophylaxis of pulmonary complications following abdominal surgery, including atelectasis,

1. ARDS and pulmonary embolism. Surg. Annu., 9:29, 1977.
2. Tisi, G.M.: Pulmonary Physiology in Clinical Medicine. Baltimore, Williams & Wilkins, 1980.
3. American College of Chest Physicians Committee on Pulmonary Physiology: Grading of pulmonary function impairment by means of pulmonary function tests. Dis. Chest, 52:270, 1967.
4. Sobol, B.J., Park, S.S., and Emirgil, C.: Relative value of various sprirometric tests in the early detection of chronic obstructive pulmonary disease. Am. Rev. Respir. Dis., 107:753, 1973.
5. Emirgil, C., and Sobol, B.J.: Long term course of chronic obstructive pulmonary disease: a new view of the mode of functional deterioration. Am. J. Med., 51:504, 1971.
6. Sobol, B.J., and Emirgil, C.: The first second-timed vital capacity and the course of obstructive lung disease. Chest, 72:81, 1977.
7. Fletcher, C., and Peto, R.: The natural history of chronic airflow obstruction. Br. Med. J., 1:1645, 1977.
8. Dines, D.E., and Fowler, W.S.: Comparison of the match test and Vitalor with standard pulmonary function tests. Minn. Med., 51:33, 1968.
9. Hepper, N.G.G., et al.: Chronic obstructive pulmonary disease: a community oriented program including professional education and screening by a voluntary health agency. Am. Rev. Respir. Dis., 121:97, 1980.
10. Petty, T.L., et al.: Objective functional improvement in chronic airway obstruction. Chest, 57:216, 1980.
11. Gracey, D.R., Divertie, M.B., and Didier, E.P.: Preoperative pulmonary preparation of patients with chronic obstructive pulmonary disease. Chest, 76:123, 1979.
12. Gaensler, E.A., et al.: The role of pulmonary insufficiency in mortality and embolism following surgery for pulmonary tuberculosis. J. Thorac. Surg., 29:163, 1955.
13. Stein, M., and Cassara, E.L.: Preoperative pulmonary evaluation and therapy for surgery patients. JAMA, 211:787, 1970.
14. Mittman, C.: Assessment of operative risk in thoracic surgery. Am. Rev. Respir. Dis., 84:197, 1961.
15. Hutchinson, J.: On the capacity of the lungs and on the respiratory functions, with a view of establishing a precise and easy method of detecting disease by the spirometer. Trans. Med. Chir. Soc. Lond., 29:137, 1846.
16. Ruppel, G.: Manual of Pulmonary Function Testing. 3rd Ed. St. Louis, C.V. Mosby, 1982.
17. Horvath, E.P.: Manual of Spirometry in Occupational Medicine. Cincinnati, NIOSH. 1981.
18. Lapp, N.L., et al.: Lung volumes and flow rates in black and white subjects. Thorax, 29:185, 1974.
19. Cotton Dust Standard. Federal Register, Vol. 43, No. 122, June 23, 1978.
20. Coal Workers Disability Standard. Federal Register, Vol. 45, No. 42, February 29, 1980.
21. Clausen, J.L. (Ed.): Pulmonary Function Testing: Guidelines and Controversies. Equipment, Methods, and Normal Values. New York, Academic Press, 1982.
22. Gardner, R.M.: American Thoracic Society statement—Snowbird workshop on standardization of spirometry. Am. Rev. Respir. Dis., 119:831, 1979.
23. American College of Chest Physicians Committees on Environmental Health and Respiratory Physiology. The assessment of ventilatory capacity. Chest, 67:959, 1975.
24. Butler, J.: The pulmonary function test—cautious overinterpretation. Chest, 79:438, 1981.
25. Bauman, R.: How to Choose the Best Equipment for the Operating Room and Critical Care Unit. Medical Products Reference Anesthesiology and Critical Care. Boston, Warren, Gorham & Lamont, 1982, p. 25.
26. Milledge, J.S., and Nunn, J.F.: Criteria of fitness for anesthesia in patients with chronic obstructive lung disease. Br. Med. J., 3:670, 1975.
27. Cain, H.D., Stevens, P.M., and Adoniya, R.: Preoperative pulmonary function and complications after cardiovascular surgery. Chest, 76:130, 1979.
28. Segall, J.J., and Butterworth, B.A.: Ventilatory capacity in chronic obstruction related to carbon dioxide tention. Scand. J. Respir. Dis., 47:215, 1966.
29. Grogono, A.W., Byles, P.H., and Hawke, W.: An in vivo representation of acid base balance. Lancet, 2:449, 1976.
30. Hingston, D.M., et al.: A computerized interpretation of arterial pH and blood gas data: do physicians need it? Respir. Care, 27:809, 1982.
31. Civetta, J.M., and Kirby, R.R.: Criteria for optimal PEEP. Respir. Care, 22:1171, 1977.
32. Niewoehner, D.E., Kleinerman, J., and Rice, D.B.: Pathologic changes in the peripheral airways of young smokers. N. Engl. J. Med., 291:755, 1974.
33. Cosio, M.G., Hale, R.A., and Niewoehner, D.E.: Morphologic and morphometric effects of prolonged cigarette smoking in the small airways. Am. Rev. Respir. Dis., 122:265, 1980.
34. McFadden, E.R., et al.: Small airway disease: an assessment of the tests of peripheral airway function. Am. J. Med., 57:171, 1974.
35. Hall, W.J., et al.: Pulmonary mechanics after uncomplicated influenza A infection. Am. Rev. Respir. Dis., 113:141, 1976.
36. Boushy, S.F., et al.: Clinical course related to preoperative and postoperative pulmonary function in patients with bronchiogenic carcinoma. Chest, 59:383, 1971.
37. Neuhaus, H., and Cherniack, N.S.: A bronchospirometric method of estimating the effect of pneumonectomy on the maximum breathing capacity. J. Thorac. Cardiovasc. Surg., 55:144, 1968.
38. Olsen, G.N., Block, A.J., and Tobias, J.A.: Prediction of post pneumonectomy pulmonary function using quantitative lung scanning. Chest, 66:13, 1974.
39. Kristersson, S., Lindell, S.E., and Svanberg, L.: Prediction of pulmonary function loss due to pneumonectomy using ^{133}Xe-radiospirometry. Chest, 62:694, 1972.
40. Benumof, J.L., and Alfery, D.D.: Pulmonary function testing. In Anesthesia. Vol. 1. Edited by R.D. Miller. New York, Churchill Livingstone, 1981, p. 1363.
41. Walkup, R.H., et al.: Prediction of postoperative pulmonary function with the lateral position test: a prospective study. Chest, 77:24, 1980.
42. Olsen, G.N., et al.: Pulmonary function evaluation of the lung resection candidate: a prospective study. Am. Rev. Respir. Dis., 111:379, 1975.
43. Hyde, L., et al.: Natural course of inoperable lung cancer. Chest, 64:309, 1973.
44. Lockwood, P.: The relationship between preoperative lung function test results and postoperative complications in carcinoma of the bronchus. Respiration, 30:105, 1973.

17

Cardiac Function Studies

William S. Frankl

In one short chapter, it is virtually impossible to do justice to such disparate cardiovascular procedures as electrocardiography, cardiac catheterization, and bedside hemodynamic monitoring. In fact, entire books have been written about each of these techniques. Thus, what follows is, by necessity, the barest of outlines, and more complete works on these subjects must be consulted for an in-depth appreciation of the complexities of these studies. Nonetheless, this chapter serves as an introduction to these procedures and affords the reader an overview.

For the sake of convenience, the chapter is divided into three sections, each with its own set of references. Hemodynamic monitoring is the last section, following naturally from its beginnings in cardiac catheterization. Electrocardiography is the first section because it is the oldest modern clinical function study of the cardiologist.

SECTION 1
ELECTROCARDIOGRAPHY

Potential Variables in Interpretation

The electrocardiogram is one of the oldest diagnostic tests in cardiology (Fig. 17–1). It was first applied to humans by Einthoven in 1906 and was initially considered to be a precise method for diagnosing a host of cardiac diseases and arrhythmias. With the development of newer and more sophisticated techniques, however, it has become clear that the electrocardiogram is not an accurate tool in cardiac diagnosis. Although electrocardiography has its place in cardiac diagnosis, one must be aware of its many limitations.

The interpretation of the electrocardiogram is influenced by a number of variables that are rarely applied in the interpretation. These variables are described in the following paragraphs.

Age

Age is perhaps the most important variable because the R-wave and S-wave amplitudes diminish with age, and the QRS axis shifts to the left with age. In addition, the PR interval increases, whereas the QRS duration is essentially unchanged. Many of these changes parallel the increased incidence of cardiac disease with age. In addition, aging is frequently associated with pulmonary emphysema, abnormalities of chest configuration, greater motion of the heart in the thorax, and alterations in conductivity through the chest wall and mediastinal structures.[1–3]

Sex

Up until about age 60, women have lower amplitudes of R, S, and T waves than men, especially in

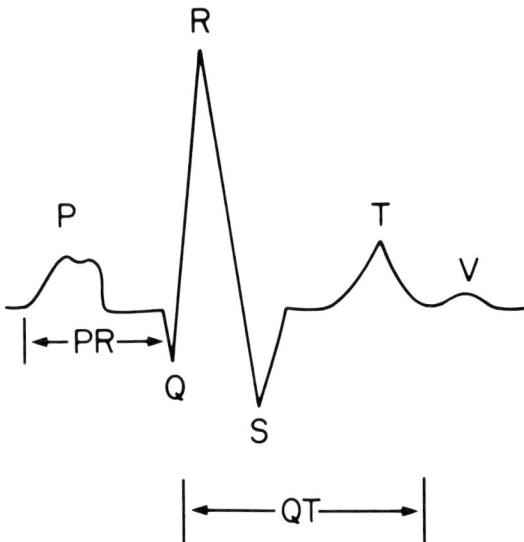

FIG. 17–1. The normal electrocardiogram showing the P, QRS, T, and V waves and the usual measurements, namely, PR interval, QRS duration, and QT interval.

the precordial leads. A reduced or absent set of initial anterior QRS forces is also more common in women. The PR interval, the QRS duration, and the QT intervals are usually shorter in women. The J point and ST segments are often more superiorly and posteriorly directed than in men. These differences between men and women are thought to be due to differences in chest-wall configuration, smaller heart size, increased total-body-fat content, the presence of ample breast tissue, and reduced metabolic rates and hemoglobin levels. Older women are more likely to have osteoporosis, and with the collapse of vertebrae, the heart may come closer to the chest wall; the subsequent increase in R wave amplitude may suggest a false diagnosis of hypertrophy.[1,4-6]

Weight

Increasing body weight is associated with a shift of the QRS axis leftward in the frontal plane, along with a reduction in R-wave and T-wave amplitude. A reduction in body weight, and especially body weight under normal, is associated with a more vertical QRS axis. Many mechanisms have been postulated for the effect of body weight on the electrocardiogram, including total-body-fat content, chest configuration, posture, and altered tissue conductivity.[1]

Height

The anatomic and resulting electrical position of the heart determines the QRS and T-wave amplitudes in the frontal and horizontal planes and the transitional zone of the precordial leads. Although age, body weight, and chest configuration may be the main contributors to the orientation of the electrical position, the QRS axis in the frontal plane is determined primarily by the anatomic position of the heart.[7]

Race

Normal values for the electrocardiogram vary among different races. Blacks have a shorter QRS duration, an increased QRS amplitude, and a more posteriorly directed T-wave vector than whites.[5]

Physiologic variables

Hemoglobin and hematocrit, body temperature, exercise conditioning, emotional state, hyperventilation, food intake, especially the ingestion of a meal that is high in carbohydrates, smoking, high altitude, blood pressure, intracardiac pressures, and heart size all affect the electrocardiogram.[1,8]

Technical variations

The fidelity of the electrocardiographic instrument, the conducting medium used under the electrodes and the variation in the positioning of the precordial electrodes, and the width of the patient's sternum may all influence the electrocardiogram. In addition are differences of opinion among observers, errors in measurement of intervals, and variations in the baseline of the electrocardiogram. These technical problems may produce an enormous variability in given tracings.

The relationship of the traditionally placed precordial leads with the actual anatomic position of the heart varies from person to person. Electrocardiographic machines differ in their ability to respond to small deflections or to rapid rates of deflection. Q waves that may appear to be significant on one machine may be slurred into the R wave on another machine. ST-segment depressions in the precordial leads may not represent ischemia, but rather an altered frequency response of the machine. If the electrodes are corroded and are not kept scrupulously clean, artifactual changes may be produced on the electrocardiogram. When alcohol, rather than a conducting material, is used, the result may be improper contact of the electrode with the skin and artifactual changes in voltage. Similarly, interobserver variation may be profound; these discrepancies may average up to 30%. The same observer may interpret the same electrocardiogram differently on different days. Observers may disagree on the measurement of intervals and amplitudes. The error of measurement further complicates the human interpretation of the electrocardiogram.

Computer programs have been designed to overcome these difficulties in interpretation.

The computer appears to be better than a well-trained cardiologist in measuring intervals, amplitudes, and axis, and it appears to be more consistent in application of criteria. The ability of a computer to make interpretations, to compare tracings, to read technically poor tracings, and to apply clinical findings to the electrocardiographic diagnosis is much poorer than that of a cardiologist, however. The use of computer interpretation should be combined with careful review by skilled cardiologists, to improve the overall interpretation of electrocardiograms.[1,9-12]

Diurnal Variations

The QRS and T-wave amplitude and the QRS axis vary from day to day. This change is most profound in small deflections such as the amplitudes of Q and R waves. Durations of QRS complex and T wave are less affected. This phenomenon may explain the possible variations in criteria for left ventricular hypertrophy or inferior wall myocardial infarction from day to day.[13]

Because of the many variables that affect the electrocardiogram, interpretations of abnormalities must be guarded. Correlation of the electrocardiogram with more sophisticated techniques, such as cardiac catheterization and angiography, electrophysiologic studies, echocardiography, radioisotopic scans, statistical methods, and improved pathologic techniques, may improve the diagnostic capabilities of the electrocardiogram in the future.

ATRIAL AND VENTRICULAR ABNORMALITIES

The normal P wave is composed of 2 forces, namely, an initial inferoanterior and leftward force caused by right atrial depolarization and a later inferior, leftward, and posterior deflection due to the left atrium (Fig. 17–2A). Right atrial activation time ranges from 20 to 45 msec, and left atrial depolarization ranges from 30 to 90 msec. The resultant normal P-wave vector averages about +60° in the frontal plane and is seen best in standard lead II. The normal P wave is anterior in the horizontal plane and produces a biphasic configuration in precordial lead V$_1$ (Fig. 17–2B). The normal P-wave duration should be 0.20 sec or less, and the P wave has a normal height of 2.5 mm or less.[14–17] The exact cause of atrial abnormalities is unknown, but the most recent studies suggest that P-wave changes are due to interatrial electrical conduction defects, and previous attempts at correlation with changes in wall structure, pressure, or volume, all of which could alter interatrial electrical conduction, make this theory attractive.[18]

Right Atrial Abnormality

The diagnosis of right atrial abnormality is made when tall, peaked P waves greater than 2.5 mm in height and less than 0.11 sec in duration are seen in lead II or V$_1$ (Fig. 17–3). This pattern has previously been dubbed "P pulmonale." Although this abnormal P-wave pattern is seen in patients with chronic lung disease and diseases predominantly of the right heart, it may also be seen in patients with various disorders that usually affect the left atrium and not the right atrium. Thus, the pattern of right atrial abnormality is not specific in favoring the right atrium over the left, and therefore the term "P pulmonale" is rarely used.[19,20]

Left Atrial Abnormality

Patients with left atrial abnormality have a posteriorly directed P-wave vector in the horizontal plane and an increase in the duration of the P wave (Fig. 17–4). The P wave in lead II is generally greater than 2.5 mm in amplitude and is longer than 0.12 sec in duration. Notching of the P wave may be seen in any lead, with a 0.04-sec or more separation of the peaks. Two other criteria are the Macruz index (P-wave duration divided by PR segment greater than 1.6) and the Morris index (product of the depth in mm and duration in sec of the terminal negative deflection of the P wave in lead V$_1$ greater than minus 0.4 mm/sec). The Morris index is probably the most sensitive and specific measurement used to detect left atrial abnormality. A P-wave duration greater than 0.12 sec is probably the second most accurate measurement. Notching of the P wave is not a reliable criterion because it is frequently present normally and is affected by the technical quality of the electrocardiogram. The Macruz index is less sensitive and less specific than the other criteria and cannot be applied when patients

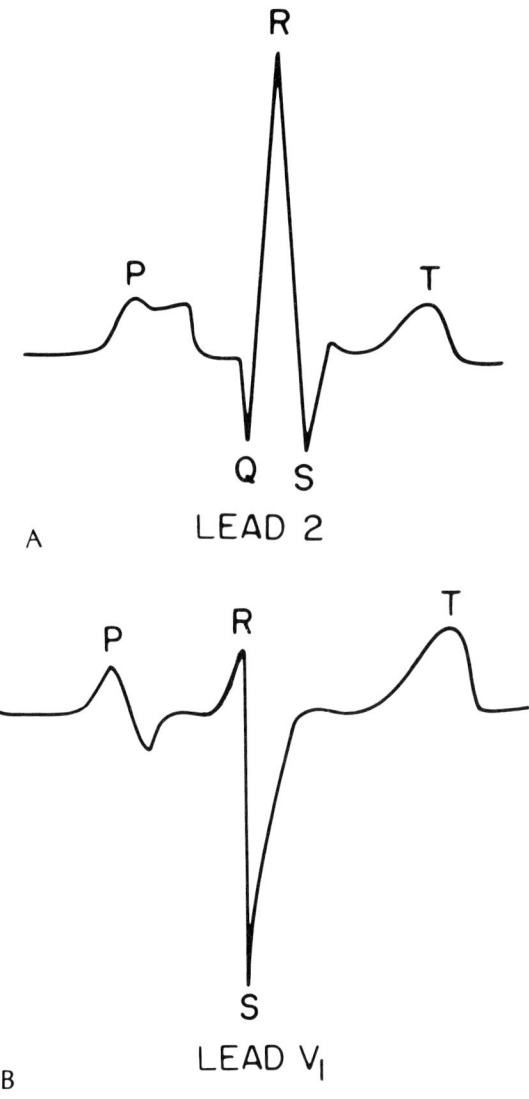

FIG. 17–2. A, The usual configuration of the P wave in standard lead 2, illustrating its two major components. The initial component is due to right atrial depolarization, and the second component is due to left atrial depolarization. B, The usual configuration of the P wave in precordial lead V$_1$, illustrating its two major components. The initial upward-directed deflection is due to right atrial depolarization, and the second downward-directed deflection is due to left atrial depolarization.

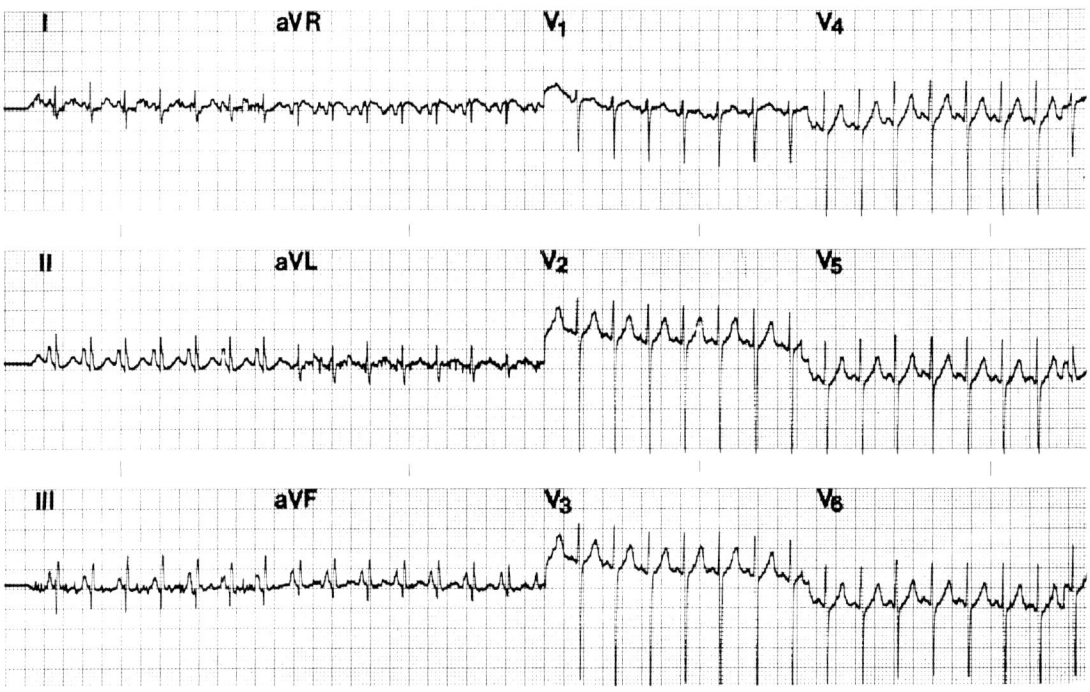

FIG. 17-3. Right atrial abnormality. The P wave is tall and peaked in standard leads 2, 3, and aVF in a patient with acute pulmonary embolism and right atrial overload. The P-wave vector in the frontal plane is directed rightward.

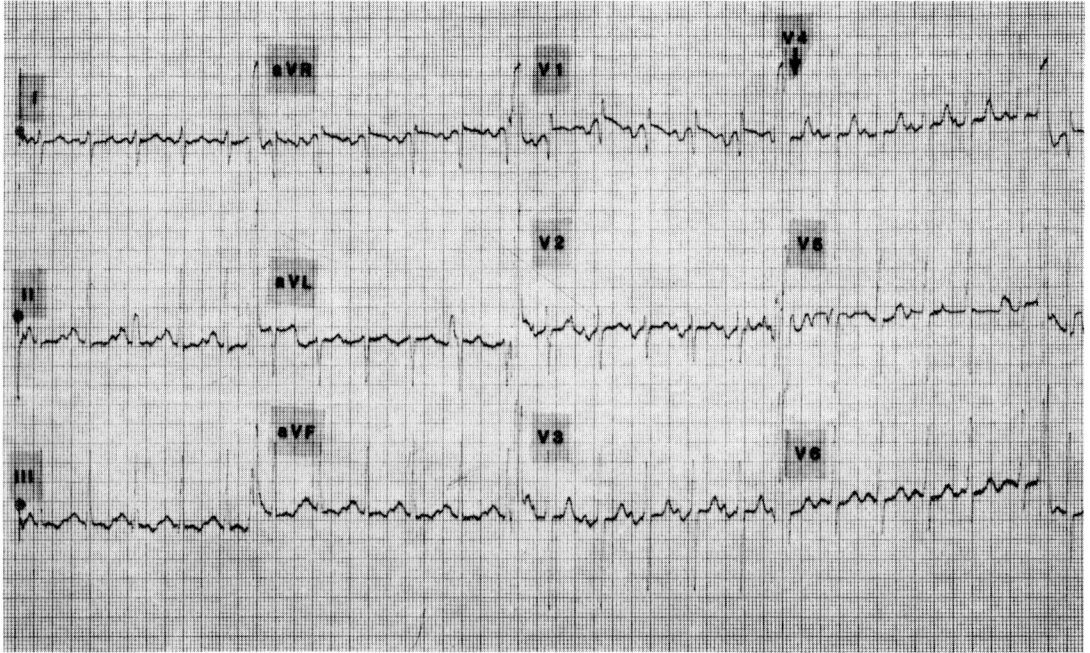

FIG. 17-4. Left atrial abnormality. The P wave is wide and notched; the second component of the P wave is much larger than the first in standard leads 2, 3, and aVF, with a deeply inverted terminal deflection of the P wave in V_1. This tracing, from a patient with severe mitral stenosis, also shows right axial deviation in the frontal plane and right ventricular hypertrophy.

are receiving digitalis therapy. All these criteria often lead to false-negative and false-positive results.[15,21-23]

Left Ventricular Hypertrophy

The electrocardiographic findings in patients with left ventricular hypertrophy include the following: (1) left atrial abnormality; (2) increased voltage, especially in leads aVL and V_5 and V_6; (3) a shift in the QRS vector to the left, posteriorly and superiorly; (4) a prolongation of left ventricular activation time (intrinsicoid deflection); and (5) secondary ST-segment and T-wave changes with a vector in an opposite direction to the mean QRS vector (Fig. 17-5).

These multiple effects of left ventricular hypertrophy on the electrocardiogram have led to the development of a number of point scores for making the diagnosis. Most common are the criteria of Romhilt and Estes. Space does not permit a review of these criteria, but the interested reader should consult the many articles on this subject.[14-17,24,25]

With the foregoing criteria, an autopsy-proved diagnosis of left ventricular hypertrophy is made electrocardiographically in fewer than 60% of patients. The limb leads are less sensitive but more specific than precordial leads, and although the point-score system of Romhilt and Estes is the most satisfactory approach to the diagnosis, incidence of false-negative results is still 46%. The correlation between the cardiac anatomic structures and the electrocardiogram is poor for numerous reasons, such as the multiple variations of normal and the differences in age, sex, body build, race, and weight, all of which influence the amplitude of the QRS complex. Changes in the QRS voltage can be produced by numerous physiologic alterations. For example, patients with longstanding left ventricular hypertrophy and associated congestive heart failure may develop right ventricular hypertrophy, which subtracts from the alterations in voltage and vector direction produced by left ventricular hypertrophy and causes a false-negative electrocardiogram for left ventricular hypertrophy. Changes in intracavity size in patients with congestive heart failure, myocardial infarction, left bundle branch block, and left anterior hemiblock and changes in metabolic and electrolyte status may all make the diagnosis of left ventricular hypertrophy impossible. Therefore, cardiologists are relying more on the echocardiogram, and occasionally the vectorcardiogram, to aid them in making the diagnosis.[1,24-44]

Right Ventricular Hypertrophy

The electrocardiographic diagnosis of right ventricular hypertrophy is even more difficult than that of left ventricular hypertrophy (Fig. 17-6). Criteria include the following: (1) right atrial abnormality; (2) a QRS vector displaced to the right, anteriorly, and

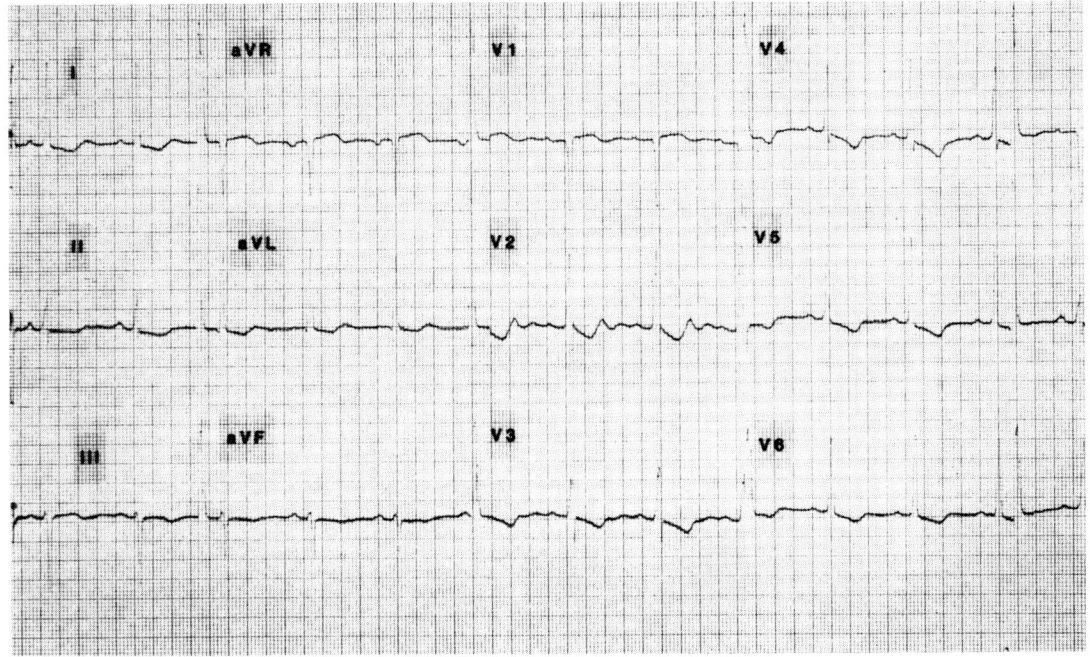

FIG. 17-5. Left ventricular hypertrophy (LVH) in a patient with severe systemic hypertension. One sees left axial deviation in the frontal plane, a 20-mm R wave in aVL, voltage criteria for LVH in the precordial leads (SV_1 and RV_6), and secondary ST-T wave changes.

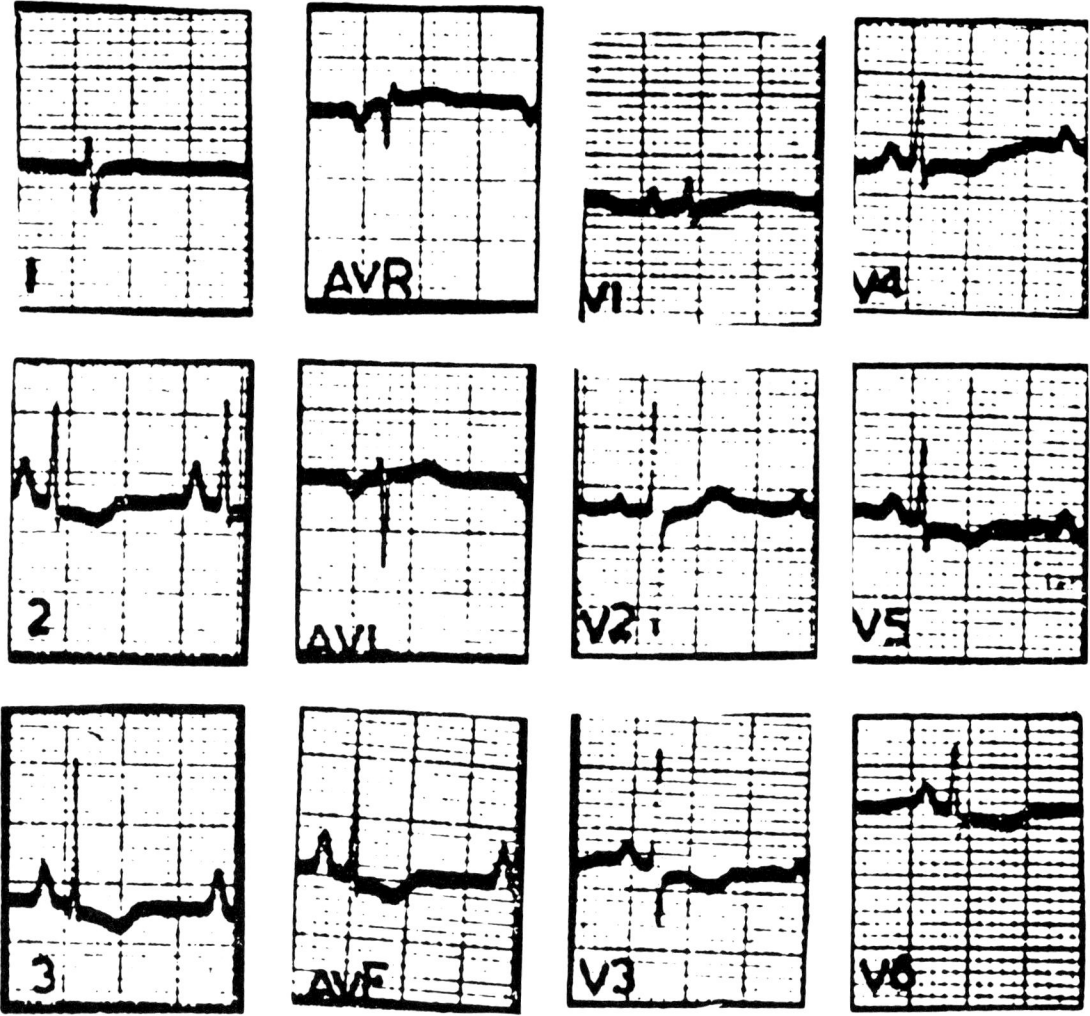

FIG. 17-6. Right ventricular hypertrophy (RVH) in a patient with longstanding atrial septal defect. One sees right axial deviation in the frontal plane of both the P-wave vector and the QRS vector. The P wave shows classic right atrial abnormality (tall and peaked in leads 2, 3, aVF and deeply inverted in aVL. In V_1, one sees an Rs wave, which also indicates RVH.

either superiorly or inferiorly, although occasionally it may be displaced to the right, posteriorly, and either inferiorly or superiorly; when clockwise rotation of the transverse loop on the vectorcardiogram occurs, right ventricular hypertrophy is severe; (3) increase in right ventricular forces especially in the right precordial leads; (4) prolonged right ventricular activation time (intrinsicoid deflection V_1); and (5) displacement of the ST segment and T-wave vector to the left, posteriorly, and either superiorly or inferiorly. These changes are not as pronounced as in left ventricular hypertrophy because the ST segment and T-wave vector may be small and may only be present when a patient has advanced right ventricular hypertrophy.

Scott and his colleagues have developed a number of criteria based on the foregoing findings. Again, space does not permit an in-depth discussion of this material. Although these criteria are specific in adults, they have a low degree of sensitivity. The most useful criteria are right-axis deviation in the frontal plane greater than $+110°$, an R/S ratio in V_1 greater than 1, and an R/S amplitude ratio in V_6 less than 1. Using these three criteria, right ventricular hypertrophy can be accurately diagnosed, but false-positive findings are frequent.[14-17,32,45-51]

It is difficult to make a diagnosis of right ventricular hypertrophy in the adult because of the marked predominance of left ventricular forces. Although the thickness of the right ventricle may double in size, left ventricular forces still predominate. Thus, the diagnosis of right ventricular hypertrophy is complicated in its earliest stages. It is easier to make a diagnosis of right ventricular hypertrophy with the electrocardiogram in patients with congenital heart disease, however.

A false-negative electrocardiogram may occur because of left ventricular hypertrophy, right or left bundle branch block, or anteroseptal myocardial infarction. A false-positive diagnosis of right ventricular hypertrophy can be made in the presence of right bundle branch block, posterior myocardial infarction, chronic lung disease, left posterior hemiblock, type-A Wolff-Parkinson-White syndrome, dextrocardia, or acquired abnormalities in placement of the heart in the thorax.[32,48,52,53]

Many of the changes that occur in true right ventricular hypertrophy are found in patients with chronic obstructive pulmonary disease (see Fig. 17–3). The electrocardiographic criteria usually associated with chronic obstructive pulmonary disease are as follows: (1) an enlarged P wave that is vertically oriented, usually between +75 and +90° in the frontal plane; (2) increased voltage of the S waves in the lateral leads; (3) a QRS vector shifted rightward in the frontal plane; and (4) normal or minimally abnormal ST-segment and T-wave changes.

Additional findings include a small R wave in right precordial leads and a shift in the transition zone, with the result that the R wave will be no larger than the S wave until V_5 or V_6; it is possible that the R wave may not exceed the S wave in those leads. One may also see an S_1, S_2, S_3 pattern with a large S wave in the left precordial leads. All the criteria for right ventricular hypertrophy may also appear in lead VI, especially if the patient has severe chronic obstructive pulmonary disease.[14–17,44–58]

A correlation exists between the electrocardiographic criteria and the severity of the pulmonary disease. Almost all patients with significant symptomatic pulmonary disease have electrocardiographic changes that fit one or more of the criteria already discussed. P-wave changes seem to be the earliest diagnostic abnormality.[59]

The most significant problem in differentiating between changes resulting from pulmonary disease and those due to pure right ventricular hypertrophy is that ventricular hypertrophy is a late finding in pulmonary disease and is not frequently diagnosed. Thus, right ventricular hypertrophy can be diagnosed only when the patient has right axis deviation beyond 110°, right bundle branch block, and the classic criteria.[54,55,60]

Another problem is the differentiation of the right ventricular hypertrophy of chronic lung disease from pulmonary embolism. As already noted, the electrocardiographic pattern is determined primarily by left ventricular forces. Usually, only overwhelming events on the right side of the heart have a demonstrable effect on the electrocardiogram.[61,62] A massive pulmonary embolism, however, can alter the electrocardiogram in the following ways: (1) production of atrial or ventricular arrhythmias; (2) shift of the P-wave vector to the right and increase; (3) shift of the mean QRS vector either to the right or to the left, more often to the right; (4) shift of the initial portion of the QRS complex superiorly, posteriorly, and to the left; (5) shift of the terminal portion of the QRS complex superiorly, posteriorly, and to the right; and (6) production of ST segment and T-wave changes. Similarly, some nonspecific changes may be seen, including the S_1, Q_3, T_3 pattern, the $S_{1,2,3}$ pattern, either complete or incomplete, right bundle branch block, a shift of the transition zone to the left, ST-segment elevation or depression in the right precordial leads, T-wave inversions in the right precordial leads, and Q waves in the inferior and anteroseptal areas, with or without ST-segment and T-wave changes, which may be confused with infarction. These alterations have been thought to be due to acute dilatation of the right heart and to secondary changes induced by alterations in coronary blood flow and hypoxia (Fig. 17–7).

In patients with acute pulmonary embolism, ST-segment depression or T-wave inversions are the most common electrocardiographic abnormalities. "Classic" changes of acute pulmonary embolism are seen only in up to 20% of patients with documented cases. In fact, the electrocardiogram is normal in more than 20% of patients with documented acute pulmonary embolism.[63]

SPECIFIC CARDIAC ABNORMALITIES
Mitral and Aortic Valve Disease

The P wave is often helpful when one is assessing the severity of valvular heart disease. Left atrial abnormality correlates well with intra-atrial conduction defects, which appear with increased atrial volume and pressure. In patients with rheumatic heart disease, however, left atrial abnormality may also be due to the rheumatic myocarditis rather than to pressure and volume abnormalities. In patients with mitral stenosis, left atrial abnormality correlates with left atrial pressure, left atrial size, the gradient across the mitral valve, and the mitral valve area (see Fig. 17–4). In patients with mitral regurgitation, on the other hand, left atrial abnormality does not correlate with mean left atrial pressure or with the degree of regurgitation, but is associated only with severe, longstanding mitral regurgitation.[64–68] Atrial fibrillation is frequently seen in patients with mitral valve disease, both stenosis and regurgitation; the reversibility of this arrhythmia may be related to the degree of structural change in the atria. Some correlation exists between the size of the fibrillatory

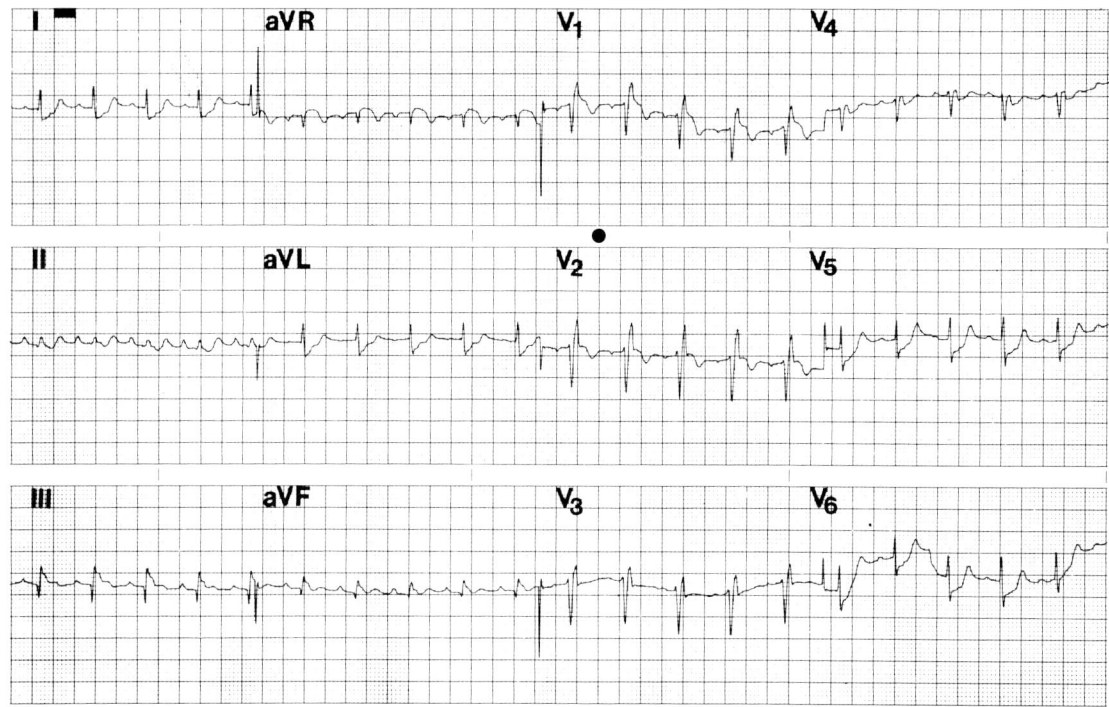

FIG. 17-7. Acute pulmonary embolus. Present are sinus tachycardia, S_1-Q_3, complete right bundle branch block, and ST segment elevation in V_1 to V_3, with T-wave inversions in V_1 and V_2.

waves and the presence of rheumatic valvular disease. If the fibrillatory waves are greater than 1 mm in amplitude, then rheumatic disease, rather than other forms of heart disease, may be present.[69] When a surgical procedure is performed in a patient whose mitral stenosis is not far advanced, the left atrial abnormality seen in the P wave may actually revert to normal.[70]

Left atrial abnormality occurs in a large percentage of patients with aortic valve disease, especially when they have predominant aortic stenosis. The presence of left atrial abnormality appears not to be related to left atrial hypertrophy or to left atrial pressure, but rather to aortic valve gradient and the degree of left ventricular hypertrophy. A large terminal negative deflection of the P wave in V_1 appears to correlate with left atrial pressure, whereas the duration of the P wave seems to correlate with left atrial size.[64,67,71,72]

The QRS complex correlates poorly with the presence of valvular disease. As mentioned previously, right ventricular forces are cancelled by left ventricular forces even when right ventricular hypertrophy is present. Fewer than 20% of patients with mild pulmonary hypertension have electrocardiographic criteria for right ventricular hypertrophy. Generally, however, more than half the patients whose right ventricular systolic pressure exceeds 70 mm Hg, have evidence of right ventricular hypertrophy on the electrocardiogram; if the systolic pressure exceeds 110 mm Hg, almost all patients will have electrocardiographic signs of right ventricular hypertrophy. Thus, pulmonary hypertension must be advanced in the presence of mitral stenosis to cause electrocardiographic changes indicating right ventricular hypertrophy.[73] On the other hand, a rightward shift of the QRS axis beyond 60° in the frontal plane is correlated with a mitral valve area of 1.3 cm² or less.[74]

Aortic stenosis must be moderate to severe before the electrocardiogram becomes abnormal. In fact, in patients with congenital aortic stenosis, the obstruction may be severe without causing electrocardiographic changes. A pattern of left ventricular hypertrophy is present in over 90% of patients with severe aortic stenosis, although occasionally, false-negative electrocardiograms may occur (Fig. 17-8). The age of the patient is important because voltage criteria for left ventricular hypertrophy become more specific during advancing years, especially over the age of 60 years.[66,75,76] When severe aortic regurgitation is present, left ventricular hypertrophy is frequently seen on the electrocardiogram, with marked secondary ST-segment and T-wave changes (Fig. 17-9).

In patients with mitral regurgitation, the QRS and T-wave abnormalities have a poor correlation with the degree of regurgitation. The more chronic the

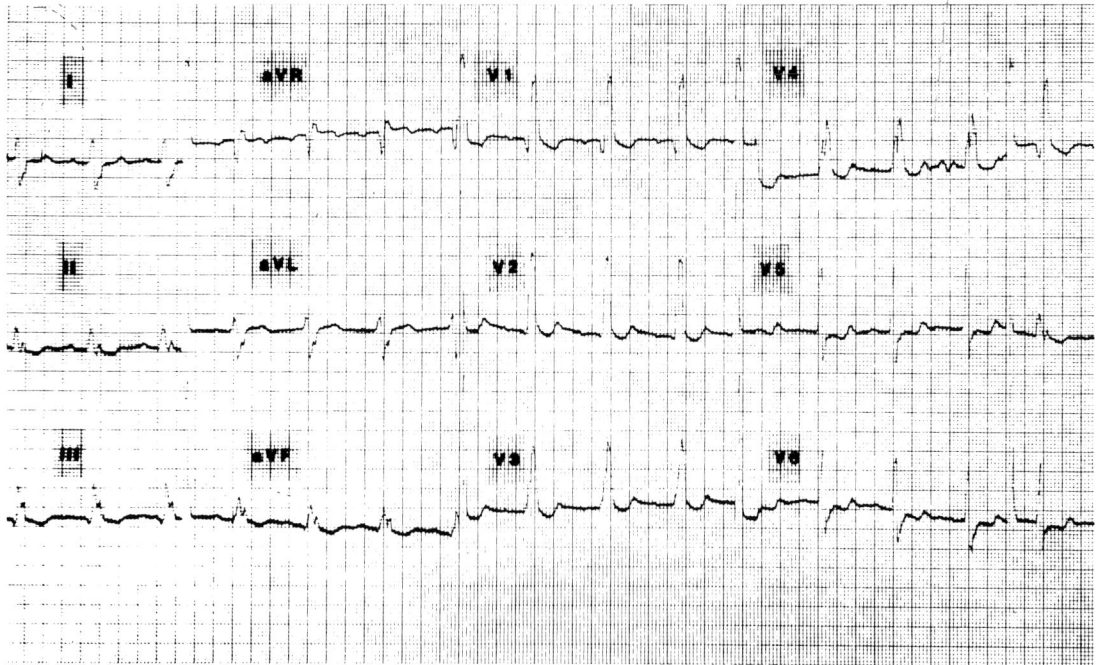

FIG. 17–8. Aortic stenosis. Although most patients have left ventricular hypertrophy, occasional patients with severe aortic stenosis develop intraventricular conduction abnormalities that cloud the diagnosis. This tracing was taken from a patient with severe isolated aortic stenosis and a 110-mm Hg gradient across the aortic valve. The tracing shows bifascicular block (right bundle branch block and left posterior hemiblock, that is, right bundle branch block and right axis deviation in the frontal plane).

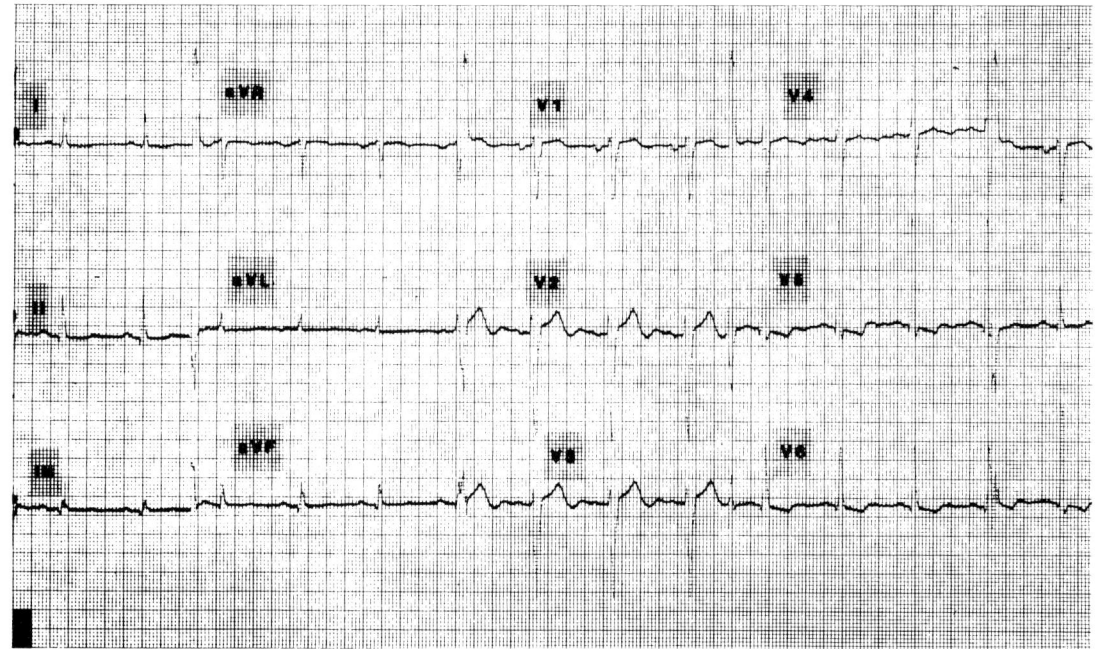

FIG. 17–9. Aortic regurgitation. Tracing from a patient with 4+ aortic regurgitation. Left ventricular hypertrophy (LVH) with voltage criteria is seen in the precordial leads. Left atrial abnormality is present in leads 2 and V_1. Secondary ST and T wave changes are due to LVH.

disease, the more likely it is that signs of ventricular hypertrophy will appear on the electrocardiogram. Despite the presence of chronic left ventricular volume overload, left ventricular hypertrophy is said to occur in only 30 to 70% of patients. The left ventricular hypertrophy seen in mitral regurgitation is more likely to be associated with a normal QRS axis or a somewhat rightward axis in the frontal plane than with left-axis deviation. Of course, patients with severe, acute mitral regurgitation do not have electrocardiographic changes of left ventricular hypertrophy.[66,68] In patients with papillary muscle dysfunction, the electrocardiographic findings are variable and are usually associated with only nonspecific ST-segment and T-wave abnormalities, although evidence for infarction, especially inferior or posterior infarction, may be seen.[77-80]

Electrocardiographic abnormalities are frequent in patients with mitral valve prolapse. Inversion of the T waves is most common in leads II, III, and aVF and is less common in leads V_4 through V_6. The ST segment may be depressed in the inferior leads, and QT prolongation may occur as well. Both atrial and ventricular arrhythmias may be seen, including premature atrial and premature ventricular beats, sinus arrest, atrial fibrillation, and ventricular tachycardia.[81-84]

Cardiomyopathies

ASYMMETRIC SEPTAL HYPERTROPHY. This disorder is also known as hypertrophic obstructive cardiomyopathy. At least 70% of asymptomatic patients with asymmetric septal hypertrophy and 90% of symptomatic patients have abnormal electrocardiograms. The abnormalities include left atrial abnormality, biatrial abnormality, left ventricular hypertrophy, secondary ST-segment and T-wave changes, and large Q waves in leads II, III, and aVF, producing a pattern of pseudoinferior-wall myocardial infarction, or large Q waves in the anterior precordial leads resulting in a pattern of pseudoanterior-wall myocardial infarction. These large Q waves are thought to be due to septal hypertrophy. A pre-excitation pattern of the Wolff-Parkinson-White syndrome is present in some patients with asymmetric septal hypertrophy (see the section on pre-excitation later in this chapter). Similar electrocardiographic findings are seen in patients with the nonobstructive and provokable types of asymmetric septal hypertrophy.[85-92]

CONGESTIVE CARDIOMYOPATHY. Unlike the hypertrophic variety, the congestive forms of cardiomyopathy have nonspecific electrocardiographic manifestations. These features include left atrial abnormality in just over 50% of patients, prolonged PR interval, complete heart block, left-axis deviation, complete left bundle branch block, complete right bundle branch block, low voltage, or left ventricular hypertrophy. Abnormal Q waves may be seen in leads II, III, and aVF, suggesting inferior wall infarction, or in lead I and aVL, suggesting lateral wall infarction. Q waves may be absent in leads I, aVL, and V_5 and V_6, suggesting fibrosis in the septum or an incomplete left bundle branch block. ST-segment and T-wave abnormalities are present in almost all patients with congestive cardiomyopathy and are nonspecific. Such abnormalities are generally related to a pattern of left ventricular hypertrophy or bundle branch block. Atrial fibrillation and ectopic ventricular beats are frequent.[86,89,91,93-101]

Pericarditis

The electrocardiographic changes in patients with pericarditis vary during acute and chronic stages of the disease; these changes also depend on whether a pericardial effusion is present, its size, and the presence of constriction. In acute pericarditis (Fig. 17-10), findings include the following:[102-106] (1) ST-segment elevations in leads I, II, aVL, aVF, and V_2 through V_6; (2) evolutionary ST-segment and T-wave changes, which can last from a few days to a few weeks until the ST segment is once more isoelectric; (3) an elevated PR segment in aVR and a depressed PR segment in the midprecordial leads; (4) T-wave inversions, especially in the left precordial lead; and (5) atrial tachyarrhythmias. Pericardial effusion is associated with the following changes:[105-107] (1) P waves that are wide and notched; (2) atrial tachyarrhythmias, especially atrial fibrillation; (3) right-axis deviation; (4) left atrial abnormality; (5) posterolateral T-wave inversions; and (6) low voltage of the QRS complex and T waves, with flat or inverted T waves.

Low voltage is not a helpful finding in the diagnosis of pericardial effusion of constriction, but electrical alternans is almost diagnostic of a large pericardial effusion. This condition is caused by swinging of the heart in a pendular fashion in the effusion. Almost all patients with chronic constrictive pericarditis have an abnormal electrocardiogram, as indicated previously. When acute pericarditis is present, a differential consideration is the early repolarization pattern, most often seen in black persons. When ST-segment elevation is seen only in the mid-precordial leads and when the ST-segment vector is to the right of both the QRS and T vectors, early repolarization is likely.[108,109]

Ischemic Heart Disease

As electrocardiographic diagnosis of myocardial infarction can be based on one or more of the following criteria: (1) current of injury originating from the area of infarction and resulting in ST-segment elevation or depression, depending on the location

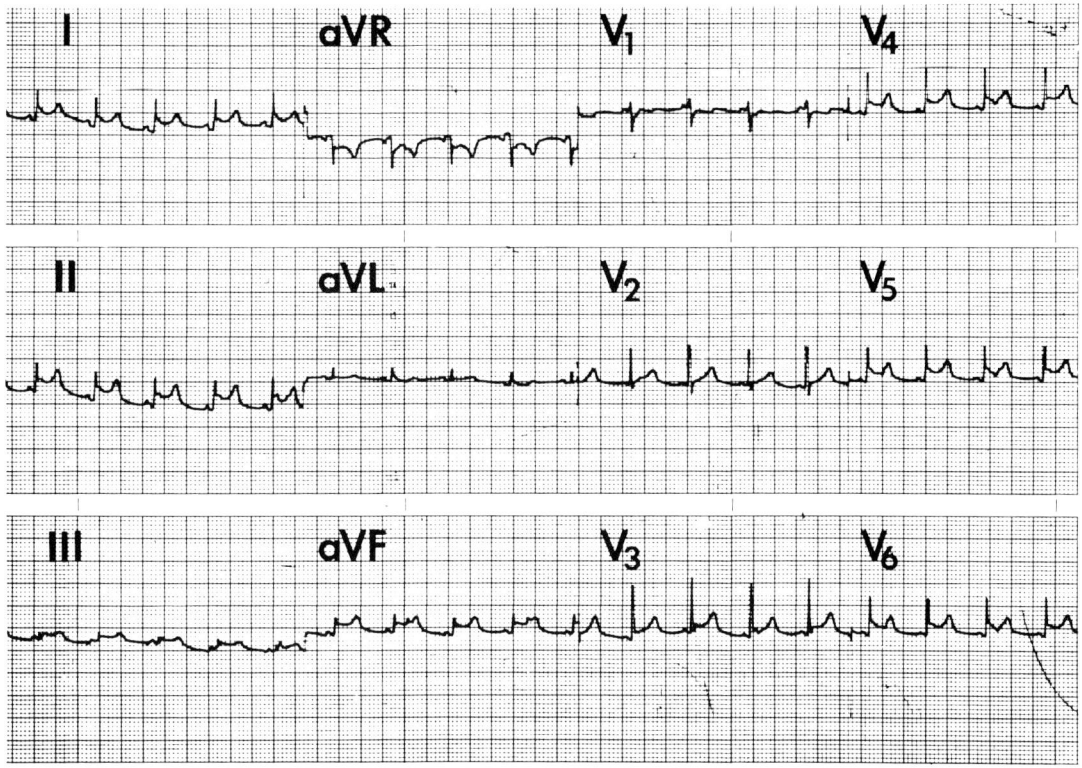

FIG. 17–10. Acute pericarditis. Tracing in a patient with acute viral perimyocarditis. Note the concave upward ST segment elevations in leads 1, 2, 3, aVF, and V_2 to V_6. ST segment depression is seen only in lead aVR.

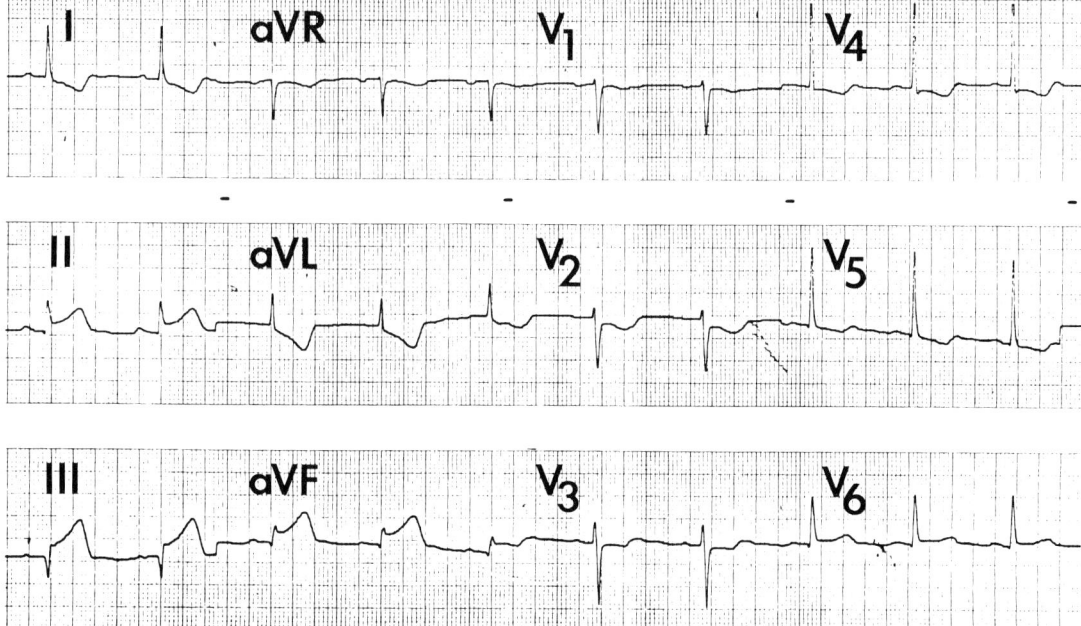

FIG. 17–11. Acute transmural myocardial infarction. ST segment elevations are seen in leads 2, 3, aVF, and V_6, with Q waves already present in leads 3 and aVF. One sees reciprocal ST segment depressions in leads 1, aVL, and V_2 to V_5. These changes occurred in a patient with an acute transmural inferolateral infarction.

and the leads subserving the infarcted area; (2) wide and deep Q waves in leads subserving the infarcted area; and (3) tall, hyperacute T waves directed toward the infarcted area, with later deep T-wave inversions, indicating that the T-wave vector has rotated away from the infarcted region (Fig. 17–11). The age of the infarction is predicated on the stage of evolution of the ST-segment and the T wave seen in the usual course of the infarction. The term "acute infarction" generally means those of 3 days' duration or less, "recent infarction" indicates those of 1 month's duration or less, and "old infarction" denotes one that has been present for 1 to 3 months. When one cannot ascertain the age of the infarction, the term "age undetermined" is used.[14,17,20–22]

The site of infarction is determined by the classic electrocardiographic findings in particular electrocardiographic leads. Changes in V_1 and V_2 indicate a septal infarction. Changes in V_3 and V_4 alone suggest an anterior infarction. Anterolateral infarction is suggested by changes in lead I, aVL, and in leads V_3 through V_6. An extensive anterior infarction is indicated by changes in lead I and in leads V_1 through V_6. An apical infarction is suggested by changes in leads II and III and in aVF, and V_3 and V_4. An inferior infarction produces changes in leads II and III and in aVF. An inferolateral infarction is indicated by changes in leads II and III, aVF, aVL, and leads V_5 and V_6. In patients with a posterior infarction, one sees a tall, wide R wave in leads V_1 and V_2. Patients with a posterolateral infarction have changes in leads I, aVL, V_1, and V_6.

Myocardial infarction can also be classified according to its location in the heart wall, whether transmural, subendocardial, or subepicardial. The ST-segment vector points away from an injured subendocardial area and toward an injured subepicardial area. Thus, ST-segment depression may be seen in patients with anterior or inferior subendocardial injury, and ST-segment elevation may be observed in patients with anterior or inferior subepicardial injury. A change in the initial portion of the QRS complex indicates a transmural infarction, whereas changes in the ST segment and the T wave without QRS complex changes suggest a nontransmural infarction. The electrocardiogram allows one to fairly reliably, but not quantitatively, localize the infarction. In fact, with the electrocardiogram, one may frequently miss the diagnosis of myocardial infarction and of coronary artery disease. For example, infarction of the atria and the right ventricle often do not appear on the electrocardiogram. Similarly, in attempting to correlate electrocardiographic with coronary angiographic results, one may find marked discrepancies. Severe double- or triple-vessel disease has been found in 65% of patients with a normal electrocardiogram. On the other hand, Q waves do not necessarily indicate that coronary artery disease is present. In one study, more than 50% of patients with patterns of anterior wall infarction and more than 25% of those with a pattern of inferior wall infarction had negative coronary angiograms.[110–113] The correlation of infarction patterns with ventricular asynergy or dyssynergy on the left ventriculogram has been variable.[114,115]

The physician encounters other problems when trying to diagnose myocardial infarction on the basis of the electrocardiogram. Classic changes of acute myocardial infarction may disappear, resulting in a normal electrocardiogram, or the pattern may become nonspecific. The reasons for such changes are not entirely clear, although shrinkage of the infarction, a new "opposing" infarction with the development of left ventricular hypertrophy, and a bundle branch block are possible explanations.[116–123]

ST-segment elevation during acute myocardial infarction resolves in about 95% of patients with inferior infarctions and in about 40% of those with anterior infarctions within 2 weeks. ST-segment elevations that persist beyond 2 weeks usually do not resolve and often indicate the presence of a ventricular aneurysm. Although continued ST-segment elevation is specific for ventricular aneurysm, it is not a sensitive measurement because many patients with ventricular aneurysms do not have ST-segment elevation.[115,124]

Although acute and evolving ST-segment and T-wave changes may run their "natural course," ST-segment changes may be transient, as indicated by ambulatory monitoring. In the presence of coronary artery spasm, ST-segment elevation may be due to intense myocardial ischemia. Such coronary artery spasm may occur in a normal coronary artery or may be superimposed on varying degrees of anatomic coronary artery obstruction. Changes in the ST segment and the T wave may be transient in patients with significant coronary artery disease during periods of both symptomatic and a symptomatic ischemia. Therefore, an electrocardiogram taken during an episode of chest pain may or may not show characteristic ST and T-wave changes, and characteristic ST and T-wave changes may be observed in the absence of symptoms. Thus, the electrocardiogram is not a sensitive indicator of myocardial ischemia.

The utility of the electrocardiogram in the diagnosis of coronary artery disease has been enhanced by the use of the exercise electrocardiogram in conjunction with thallium scanning. The reader is directed to an exhaustive review of exercise testing and its capabilities.[125]

Pre-Excitation Syndrome

Although it is outside the scope of this chapter to discuss the diagnosis of arrhythmias in detail, we

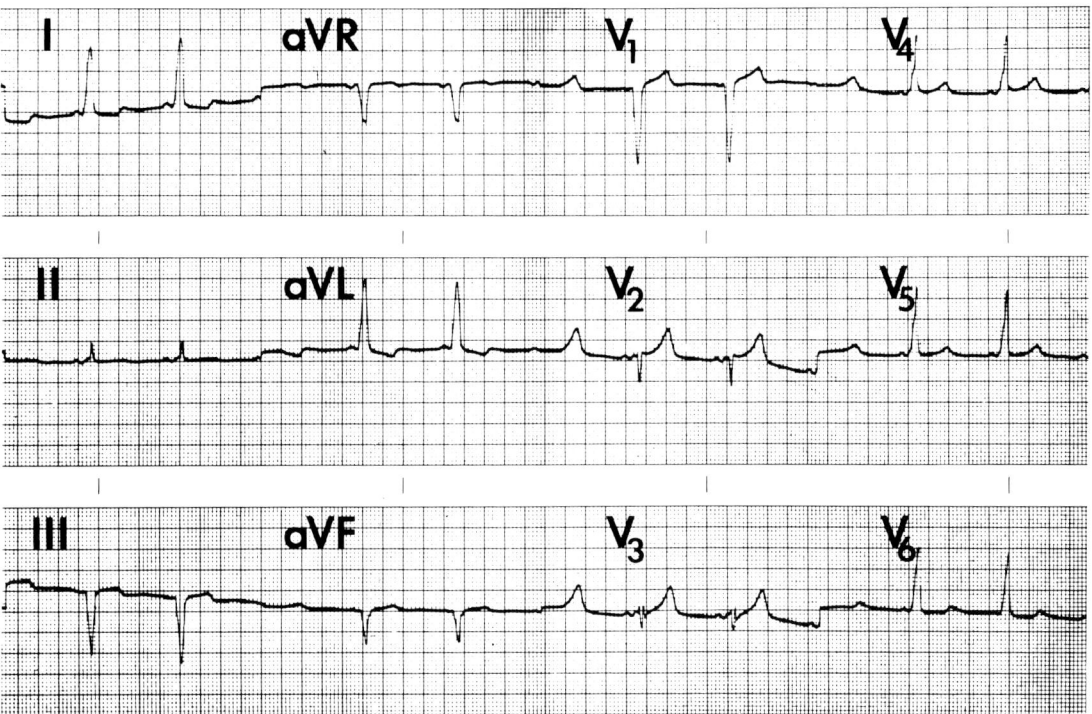

FIG. 17–12. Wolff-Parkinson-White (WPW) syndrome showing a short PR interval measuring 0.08 sec and a QRS duration of 0.12 sec. One clearly sees a delta wave in leads 1, 2, and V_4 to V_6. A pseudoinferior wall infarction pattern is noted. The patient had severe recurrent supraventricular tachyarrhythmias during which the WPW configuration of the QRS disappeared.

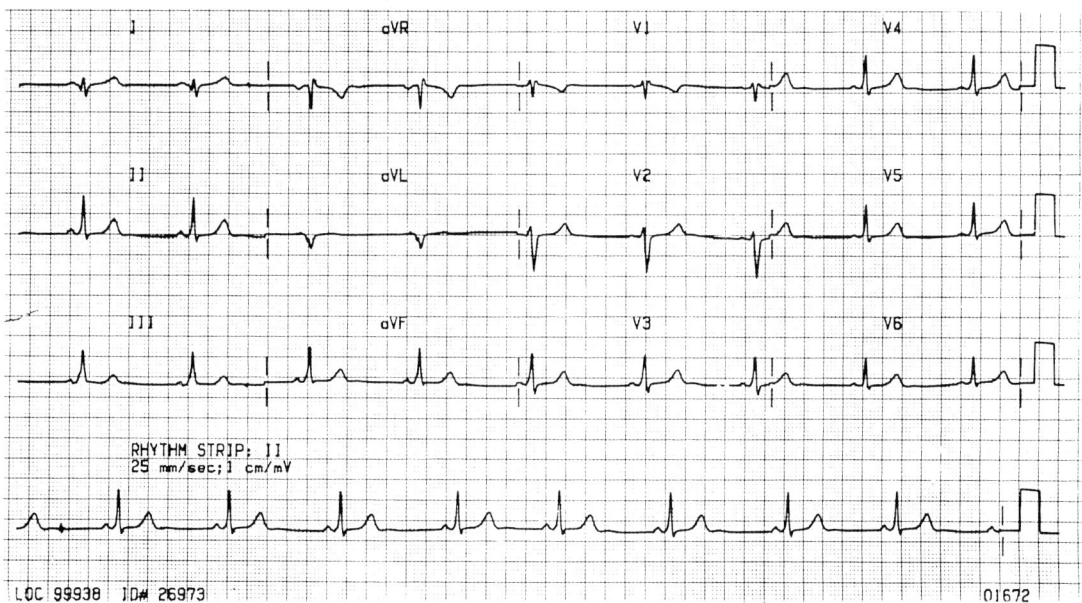

FIG. 17–13. Lown-Ganong-Levine (LGL) syndrome, with a short PR interval at 0.08 sec. The QRS duration is normal at 0.09 sec. The patient had occasional episodes of supraventricular tachycardia.

shall briefly outline the pre-excitation syndrome, which produces characteristic electrocardiographic changes and is frequently associated with arrhythmias. The pre-excitation syndrome exists when the normal atrioventricular nodal pathway is bypassed, to cause early activation of the ventricles. Three well-defined varieties of the pre-excitation syndrome are recognized, although with increasingly sophisticated electrophysiologic investigations, other forms are becoming evident. The most widely accepted varieties include the Wolff-Parkinson-White syndrome (Fig. 17–12), the Lown-Ganong-Levine syndrome (Fig. 17–13), and the pre-excitation syndrome associated with Mahaim fibers. In the Wolff-Parkinson-White syndrome, an accessory pathway is present outside the atrioventricular node. Patients with the Lown-Ganong-Levine syndrome have a specific intra-atrial tract that enters the inferior aspect of the atrioventricular node and allows early excitation of the His bundle. The Mahaim fibers are a discrete muscle bundle that connect the inferior atrioventricular node, the His bundle, or the bundle branches directly to the ventricular myocardium. These three types of pre-excitation have characteristic electrocardiographic findings. Patients with the Wolff-Parkinson-White syndrome have a short PR interval and a prolonged QRS complex, with slurring of the initial component of the QRS complex. This initial slurring is known as a delta wave. The QRS complex in Wolff-Parkinson-White syndrome results from a fusion beat caused by the combined conduction through the atrioventricular node and the accessory pathway. The Lown-Ganong-Levine syndrome is recognized by a short PR interval of under 110 msec in adults and 80 to 90 msec in children, with a normal QRS complex. Pre-excitation through the Mahaim fibers is recognized by a normal PR interval with a prolonged QRS and a delta wave.[126-130]

These patients may have an abnormal electrocardiogram with no clinical symptoms, or they may have multiple tachyarrhythmias. Similarly, latent pre-excitation with abnormalities may be seen on the electrocardiogram only occasionally, and the propensity for tachyarrhythmias may be proved only by electrophysiologic testing in such patients.

REFERENCES

1. Simonson, E.: Differentiation between Normal and Abnormal in Electrocardiography. St. Louis, C.V. Mosby, 1961.
2. Simonson, E.: The effect of age on the electrocardiogram. Am. J. Cardiol., 29:64, 1972.
3. Mihalick, M.J., and Fisch, C.: Electrocardiographic findings in the aged. Am. Heart J., 87:117, 1974.
4. Simonson, E., et al.: Sex differences in the electrocardiogram. Circulation, 22:598, 1960.
5. Nemati, M., et al.: The influence of constitutional variables on orthogonal electrocardiograms of normal women. Circulation, 56:989, 1977.
6. Nemati, M., et al.: The orthogonal electrocardiogram in normal women: implications of sex differences in diagnostic electrocardiography. Am. Heart J., 95:12, 1978.
7. Dougherty, J.D.: The relation of the frontal QRS axis to the anatomic position of the heart. J. Electrocardiol., 3:267, 1970.
8. Goldberg, E.: Mechanical factors and the electrocardiogram. Am. Heart J., 93:629, 1977.
9. Pipberger, H.V., et al.: Recommendations for standardization of leads and of specifications for instruments in electrocardiography and vectorcardiography. Circulation, 52:11, 1975.
10. Burchell, H.B., and Reed, J.: A test experience with a machine-processed electrocardiography diagnosis: the recognition of "normal" and some specific patterns. Am. Heart J., 92:773, 1976.
11. Caceres, C.A.: Limitations of the computer in electrocardiographic interpretation. Am. J. Cardiol., 38:362, 1976.
12. Caceres, C.A.: Present status of computer interpretation of the electrocardiogram: a 20 year overview. Am. J. Cardiol., 41:121, 1978.
13. Willems, J.L., Poblete, P.F., and Pipberger, H.V.: Day-to-day variation of the normal orthogonal electrocardiogram and vectorcardiogram. Circulation, 45:1057, 1972.
14. Grant, R.P.: Clinical Electrocardiography: The Spatial Vector Approach. New York, McGraw-Hill, 1957.
15. Massie, E., and Walsh, T.J.: Clinical Vectorcardiography and Electrocardiography. Chicago, Yearbook Medical Publishers, 1960.
16. Hurst, J.W., and Myerburg, R.J.: Introduction to Electrocardiography. New York, McGraw-Hill, 1973.
17. Chou, T., Helm, R.A., and Kaplan, S.: Clinical Vectorcardiography. 2nd Ed. New York, Grune & Stratton, 1974.
18. Josephson, M.E., Kastor, J.A., and Morganroth, J.: Electrocardiographic left atrial enlargement. Am. J. Cardiol., 39:967, 1977.
19. Chou, T., and Helm, R.A.: The pseudo P-pulmonale. Circulation, 32:96, 1965.
20. Surawicz, B., et al.: Taskforce. I: Standardization of terminology and interpretation. Am. J. Cardiol., 41:130, 1978.
21. Macruz, R., Perloff, J.K., and Case, R.B.: A method for the electrocardiographic recognition of atrial enlargement. Circulation, 17:882, 1958.
22. Morris, J.J., Estes, E.H., and Whalen, R.E.: P-wave analysis in valvular heart disease. Circulation, 29:242, 1964.
23. Termini, B.A., and Lee, Y.: Echocardiographic and electrocardiographic criteria for diagnosing left atrial enlargement. South. Med. J., 68:161, 1975.
24. Romhilt, D.W., and Estes, E.H.: A point-score system for the ECG diagnosis of left ventricular hypertrophy. Am. Heart J., 75:752, 1968.
25. Romhilt, D.W., Bove, K.E., and Norris, R.J.: A critical appraisal of the electrocardiographic criteria for the diagnosis of left ventricular hypertrophy. Circulation, 40:185, 1969.
26. Johnson, J.C., Horan, L.G., and Flowers, N.C.: Diagnostic accuracy of the electrocardiogram. Cardiovasc. Clin., 8:25, 1977.
27. Scott, R.C., et al.: Left ventricular hypertrophy. Circulation, 11:89, 1955.
28. Chou, T., et al.: Specificity of the current electrocar-

29. Carter, W.A., and Estes, E.H.: Electrocardiographic manifestations of ventricular hypertrophy: a computer study of ECG-anatomic correlations in 319 cases. Am. Heart J., 68:173, 1964.
30. Dower, G.E., Horn, H.E., and Ziegler, W.G.: On electrocardiographic-autopsy correlations in left ventricular hypertrophy: a simple post mortem index of hypertrophy proposed. Am. Heart J., 74:351, 1967.
31. Abbasi, A.S., et al.: Left ventricular hypertrophy diagnosed by echocardiography. N. Engl. J. Med., 289:118, 1973.
32. Scott, R.C.: Ventricular hypertrophy. Cardiovasc. Clin., 5:220, 1973.
33. Bennett, D.H., and Evans, D.W.: Correlation of left ventricular mass determined by echocardiography with vectorcardiographic and electrocardiographic voltage measurements. Br. Heart J., 36:981, 1974.
34. Morganroth, J., et al.: Electrocardiographic evidence of left ventricular hypertrophy in otherwise normal children. Am. J. Cardiol., 35:278, 1975.
35. Bahler, A.S., et al.: Correlations of electrocardiography and echocardiography in determination of left ventricular wall thickness: a study of apparently normal subjects. Am. J. Cardiol., 39:189, 1977.
36. Browne, P.J., et al.: The echocardiographic correlates of left ventricular hypertrophy diagnosed by electrocardiography. J. Electrocardiol., 10:105, 1977.
37. Dunn, F.G., et al.: Pathophysiologic assessment of hypertensive heart disease with echocardiography. Am. J. Cardiol., 39:789, 1977.
38. Dolgin, M., et al.: The electrocardiographic diagnosis of left ventricular hypertrophy: correlation with quantitative angiography. Am. J. Med. Sci., 273:301, 1977.
39. McFarland, T.M., et al.: Echocardiographic diagnosis of left ventricular hypertrophy. Circulation, 57:1140, 1978.
40. Kilty, S.W., and Lepeschkin, E.: Effect of body build on the QRS voltage of the electrocardiogram in normal man. Circulation, 31:77, 1965.
41. Walker, C.H., and Rose, R.L.: Importance of age, sex and body habitus in the diagnosis of left ventricular hypertrophy from the precordial electrocardiogram in children and adolescents. Pediatrics, 28:705, 1961.
42. Ishikawa, K., Berson, A.S., and Pipberger, H.V.: Electrocardiographic changes due to cardiac enlargement. Am. Heart J., 81:635, 1971.
43. Dunn, R.A., Zenner, R.J., and Pipberger, H.V.: Serial electrocardiograms in hypertensive cardiovascular disease. Circulation, 56:416, 1977.
44. Holt, J.H., Barnard, A.C., and Kramer, J.O.: A study of the human heart as a multiple dipole source. IV. Left ventricular hypertrophy in the presence of right bundle branch block. Circulation, 56:391, 1977.
45. Selzer, A.: Limitations of the electrocardiographic diagnosis of ventricular hypertrophy. JAMA, 195:1051, 1966.
46. Walker, I.C., Helm, R.A., and Scott, R.C.: Right ventricular hypertrophy. I. Correlation of isolated right ventricular hypertrophy at autopsy with the electrocardiographic findings. Circulation, 11:215, 1955.
47. Walker, I.C., Scott, R.C., and Helm, R.A.: Right ventricular hypertrophy. II. Correlation of electrocardiographic right ventricular hypertrophy with the anatomic findings. Circulation, 11:223, 1955.
48. Scott, R.C.: The electrocardiographic diagnosis of right ventricular hypertrophy: correlation with the anatomic findings. Am. Heart J., 60:659, 1960.
49. Scott, R.C.: The correlation between the electrocardiographic patterns of ventricular hypertrophy and the anatomic findings. Circulation, 21:256, 1960.
50. Roman, G.T., Walsh, T.J., and Massie, E.: Right ventricular hypertrophy. Am. J. Cardiol., 7:481, 1961.
51. Ray, C.T., Horan, L.G., and Flowers, N.C.: An early sign of right ventricular enlargement. J. Electrocardiol., 3:57, 1970.
52. Goodwin, J.F., and Abdin, Z.H.: The cardiogram of congenital and acquired right ventricular hypertrophy. Br. Heart J., 21:523, 1959.
53. Booth, R.W., Chou, T., and Scott, R.C.: Electrocardiographic diagnosis of ventricular hypertrophy in the presence of right bundle branch block. Circulation, 18:169, 1958.
54. Scott, R.C.: The electrocardiogram in pulmonary emphysema and chronic cor pulmonale. Am. Heart J., 61:843, 1961.
55. Phillips, J.H., and Burch, G.E.: Problems in the diagnosis of cor pulmonale. Am. Heart J., 66:818, 1963.
56. Fowler, N.O., et al.: The electrocardiogram in cor pulmonale with and without emphysema. Am. J. Cardiol., 16:500, 1965.
57. Oram, S., and Davies, P.: The electrocardiogram in cor pulmonale. Prog. Cardiovasc. Dis., 9:341, 1967.
58. Kamper, D., et al.: The reliability of electrocardiographic criteria of chronic obstructive lung disease. Am. Heart J., 80:445, 1970.
59. Littmann, D.: The electrocardiographic findings in pulmonary emphysema. Am. J. Cardiol., 5:339, 1960.
60. Scott, R.C., et al.: The electrocardiographic pattern of right ventricular hypertrophy in chronic cor pulmonale. Circulation, 11:927, 1955.
61. Spodick, D.H.: Electrocardiographic responses in pulmonary embolism. Am. J. Cardiol., 60:695, 1972.
62. Stein, P.D., et al.: The electrocardiogram in acute pulmonary embolism. Prog. Cardiovasc. Dis., 17:247, 1975.
63. Urokinase-Pulmonary Embolism Trial. Circulation, 47-48 (Suppl. II):II-1, 1973.
64. Sutnick, A.I., and Soloff, L.A.: P wave abnormalities as an electrocardiographic index of hemodynamically significant aortic stenosis. Circulation, 28:814, 1963.
65. Kasser, I., and Kennedy, J.W.: The relationship of increased left atrial volume and pressure to abnormal P waves on the electrocardiogram. Circulation, 39:339, 1969.
66. Rios, J.C., and Goo, W.: Electrocardiographic correlates of rheumatic valvular disease. Cardiovasc. Clin., 5:247, 1973.
67. Rios, J.C., and Leet, C.: Electrocardiographic assessment of valvular heart disease. Cardiovasc. Clin., 18:161, 1973.
68. Bentivoglio, L.G., et al.: An electrocardiographic analysis of 65 cases of mitral regurgitation. Circulation, 38:572, 1970.
69. Skoulos, A., and Horlick, L.: The atrial F wave in various types of heart disease and its response to treatment. Am. J. Cardiol., 14:174, 1964.
70. Calatagud, J.B., et al.: P wave changes after open heart mitral commissurotomy for isolated mitral stenosis. Angiology, 19:238, 1968.
71. Morris, J.J., et al.: P wave analysis in the electro-

cardiographic diagnosis of left ventricular hypertrophy. Circulation, 32 (Suppl. 2):154, 1965.
72. Gooch, A.S., et al.: Analysis of the P wave in severe aortic stenosis. Chest, 49:549, 1966.
73. Cueto, J., et al.: Vectorcardiographic studies in acquired valvular disease with reference to the diagnosis of right ventricular hypertrophy. Circulation, 33:588, 1966.
74. Hugenholtz, P.G., et al.: The spectrum of pure mitral stenosis—hemodynamic studies in relation in clinical disability. Am. J. Cardiol., 10:773, 1962.
75. Wood, P.: Aortic stenosis. Am. J. Cardiol., 1:553, 1958.
76. Shah, P.N.: Clinical-electrocardiographic correlations: aortic valve disease and hypertrophic subaortic stenosis. Cardiovasc. Clin., 8:151, 1977.
77. Bashour, F.A.: Mitral regurgitation following myocardial infarction. Chest, 48:113, 1965.
78. Heikkila, J.: Mitral incompetence as a complication of acute myocardial infarction. Acta Med. Scand. (Suppl. 475):182, 1967.
79. Burch, G.E., DePasquale, N.P., and Phillips, J.H.: The syndrome of papillary muscle dysfunction. Am. Heart J., 75:399, 1968.
80. Harrison, D.C., Isaeff, D.M., and DeBusk, R.F.: Papillary muscle syndrome. DM, 1:3, 1972.
81. Popock, W.A., and Barlow, J.B.: Postexercise arrhythmias in the billowing posterior mitral leaflet syndrome. Am. Heart J., 80:740, 1970.
82. Jeresaty, R.M.: Mitral valve prolapse-click murmur syndrome. Prog. Cardiovasc. Dis., 15:623, 1973.
83. Malcolm, A.D., et al.: Clinical features and investigative findings in the presence of mitral leaflet prolapse. Br. Heart J., 38:244, 1976.
84. Wei, J.Y., et al.: Mitral valve prolapse syndrome and recurrent ventricular tachyarrhythmias. Ann. Intern. Med., 89:6, 1978.
85. Estes, E.H., et al.: Electrocardiographic and vectorcardiographic findings in idiopathic hypertrophic subaortic stenosis. Circulation, 26:714, 1962.
86. Hollister, R.M., and Goodiver, J.F.: The electrocardiogram in cardiomyopathy. Br. Heart J., 25:357, 1963.
87. Frank, S., and Braunwald, E.: Idiopathic hypertrophic subaortic stenosis: clinical analysis of 126 patients with emphasis on the natural history. Circulation, 37:759, 1968.
88. Whiting, R.B., et al.: Idiopathic hypertrophic subaortic stenosis in the elderly. N. Engl. J. Med., 285:196, 1971.
89. Bahl, O.P., and Massie, E.: Electrocardiographic and vectorcardiographic patterns of cardiomyopathy. Cardiovasc. Clin., 4:95, 1972.
90. Maron, B.J., et al.: Asymmetric septal hypertrophy in childhood. Circulation, 53:9, 1976.
91. McMartin, D.E., and Flowers, N.C.: Clinical-electrocardiographic correlations in diseases of the myocardium. Cardiovasc. Clin., 8:191, 1977.
92. Savage, D.D., et al.: Electrocardiographic findings in patients with obstructive and non-obstructive hypertrophic cardiomyopathy. Circulation, 58:402, 1978.
93. Pinto Lima, F.X., Spiritus, O., and Tranchesi, J.: Arrhythmias and vector electrocardiographic analysis of complete bundle branch block in Chagas' disease: a study of 103 autopsied cases. Am. Heart J., 56:501, 1958.
94. Burch, G.E., and DePasquale, N.: A study at autopsy of the relation of absence of the Q wave in leads I, aVL, V_5 and V_6 to septal fibrosis. Am. Heart J., 60:336, 1960.
95. Brigden, W.: Cardiac amyloidosis. Prog. Cardiovasc. Dis., 7:142, 1964.
96. Rosenbaum, M.R.: Chagasic myocardiopathy. Prog. Cardiovasc. Dis., 7:199, 1964.
97. Marriott, H.J.L.: Electrocardiographic abnormalities, conduction disorders and arrhythmias in primary myocardial disease. Prog. Cardiovasc. Dis., 7:99, 1964.
98. Massumi, R.A., et al.: Primary myocardial disease. Circulation, 31:19, 1965.
99. Corne, R.A., et al.: Significance of marked left axis deviation. Am. J. Cardiol., 15:605, 1965.
100. Hamby, R.I., and Raia, F.: Electrocardiographic aspects of primary myocardial disease in 60 patients. Am. Heart J., 76:316, 1968.
101. McDonald, C.D., Burch, G.E., and Walsh, J.J.: Alcoholic cardiomyopathy managed with prolonged bed rest. Ann. Intern. Med., 74:681, 1971.
102. Surawicz, B., and Lasseter, K.C.: Electrocardiogram in pericarditis. Am. J. Cardiol., 26:471, 1970.
103. Spodick, D.H.: Diagnostic electrocardiographic sequences in acute pericarditis. Circulation, 48:575, 1973.
104. Spodick, D.H.: Electrocardiogram in acute pericarditis. Am. J. Cardiol., 33:470, 1974.
105. Fowler, N.O.: The electrocardiogram in pericarditis. Cardiovasc. Clin., 5:256, 1973.
106. Spodick, D.H.: Pathogenesis and clinical correlations of the electrocardiographic abnormalities of pericardial disease. In Clinical Electrocardiographic Correlations. Edited by J.C. Rios. Philadelphia, F.A.Davis, 1977.
107. McGregor, M., and Baskin, E.: Electrical alternans in pericardial effusion. Circulation, 11:837, 1955.
108. Kazemias, T.M., and Wasserburger, R.H.: Pericarditis revisited. J. Electrocardiol., 4:62, 1971.
109. Spodick, D.H.: Differential characteristics of the electrocardiogram in early repolarization and acute pericarditis. N. Engl. J. Med., 295:523, 1976.
110. Martinez-Rios, M.A., et al.: Normal electrocardiogram in the presence of severe coronary artery disease. Am. J. Cardiol., 25:320, 1970.
111. Horan, L.G., Flowers, N.C., and Johnson, J.C.: Significance of the diagnostic Q wave of myocardial infarction. Circulation, 43:428, 1971.
112. Hilsenrath, J., et al.: Pitfalls in prediction of coronary arterial obstruction from patterns of anterior infarction on the electrocardiogram and vectorcardiogram. Am. J. Cardiol., 29:164, 1972.
113. Redy, K., et al.: Severity and distribution of coronary artery disease in patients with normal resting electrocardiograms. J. Electrocardiol., 7:115, 1974.
114. Williams, R.A., et al.: Electrocardiographic, arteriographic and ventriculographic correlations in transmural myocardial infarction. Am. J. Cardiol., 31:595, 1973.
115. Bodenheimer, M.M., Banka, V.S., and Helfant, R.H.: Q waves and ventricular asynergy: predictive value and hemodynamic significance of anatomic localization. Am. J. Cardiol., 36:615, 1975.
116. Woods, J.D., Lawne, W., and Smith, W.G.: The reliability of the electrocardiogram in myocardial infarction. Lancet, 2:265, 1963.
117. Skjaeggestad, O., and Molne, K.: Electrocardiogram in patients with healed myocardial infarction disclosed at autopsy. Acta Med. Scand., 179:23, 1966.
118. Burns-Cox, C.J.: The occurrence of a normal elec-

trocardiogram after myocardial infarction. Am. Heart J., 75:572, 1968.
119. Willems, J., Draulans, J., and DeGeest, H.: An appraisal of the Minnesota code in "inferior" myocardial infarction. J. Electrocardiol., 3:147, 1970.
120. Canner, P.L., Berge, K.G., and Klimt, C.R.: The coronary drug project. Circulation, 47(Suppl. 1):1, 1973.
121. Toutouzas, P., et al.: The electrocardiogram and vectorcardiogram in the diagnosis of the old inferior myocardial infarction. J. Electrocardiol., 6:319, 1973.
122. Conde, C.A., et al.: Disappearance of abnormal Q waves after aortocoronary bypass surgery. Am. J. Cardiol., 36:889, 1975.
123. Madias, J.E., and Gorlin, R.: The myth of acute "mild" myocardial infarction. Ann. Intern. Med., 86:347, 1977.
124. Mills, R.M., et al.: Natural history of ST segment elevation after acute myocardial infarction. Am. J. Cardiol., 35:609, 1975.
125. Chung, E.K.: Exercise Electrocardiography: A Practical Approach. Baltimore, Williams & Wilkins, 1983.
126. Narula, O.S.: Wolff-Parkinson-White syndrome: a review. Circulation, 47:872, 1973.
127. Gallagher, J.J., et al.: Wolff-Parkinson-White syndrome: the problem, evaluation and surgical correlation. Circulation, 51:767, 1975.
128. Ferrer, M.I.: Pre-Excitation. Mt. Kisco, NY, Futura Publishing, 1976.
129. Sung, R.J., et al.: Clinical and electrophysiologic observations in patients with concealed accessory atrioventricular bypass tracts. Am. J. Cardiol., 40:839, 1977.
130. Chung, E.K.: Wolff-Parkinson-White syndrome: current views. Am. J. Med., 62:252, 1977.

SECTION 2
CARDIAC CATHETERIZATION

HISTORICAL REVIEW

Cardiac catheterization probably goes back to efforts made in the nineteenth century to catheterize animals. This technique was important in developing many of the principles of cardiac physiology, including pressure recordings and the application of the Fick method for the measurement of cardiac output. Forssman passed the first catheter into the heart of a human, namely, himself. He passed a ureteral catheter into the venous system and advanced it under fluoroscopic guidance into the right atrium. He then walked to the hospital radiology department, to document the position of the catheter with a chest roentgenogram.[1] Klein catheterized the right ventricle of 11 patients and measured cardiac output using the Fick principle in 1930.[2] It was Cournand, however, who brought cardiac catheterization into modern use, and many workers since have added to and have refined the technique. Because space does not allow a discussion of the contributions of these many workers, the reader is directed to these original works, which are monumental contributions to important cardiac procedures.[3-18]

INDICATIONS

Cardiac catheterization today is usually a combined procedure, including both hemodynamic and angiographic techniques, to define a clinically suspected cardiac abnormality. Catheterization is used to evaluate both the anatomic and physiologic state of the heart and the presence or absence of associated abnormalities. The risks of the procedure must be weighed against the benefits. The need to perform cardiac catheterization most often arises when a patient has reached a critical stage in the development of a disease. Cardiac catheterization is used to establish an accurate diagnosis and to determine the need, timing, and risks of surgical procedures. The risks of catheterization should be small, when compared to the information obtained, which is absolutely necessary if cardiac surgery is contemplated. An incorrect diagnosis may be fatal to the patient, or the presence of an unsuspected additional abnormality may prolong the procedure and may be associated with unexpected complications. The operating room is not a place for surprise findings. Therefore, cardiac catheterization must provide the surgical team with a precise and complete outline for the surgical approach and thus must enable one to perform a careful and maximally efficient operative procedure.

The following is a discussion of the indications for cardiac catheterization.

Patients in Whom Diagnosis is Reasonably Certain but Interventions are Required

In these patients, one needs to define the extent and severity of the disease and the requirements for a surgical procedure. The presence of associated conditions, for example, such as coronary artery disease in patients with valvular or congenital heart disease or, conversely, valvular disease in patients with coronary artery disease, must be known. One should also assess the determinants of prognosis, for example, left ventricular function. Other patients in this category are those who continue to have pain after an acute myocardial infarction, those who are undergoing acute thrombolysis for acute myocardial infarction, and those who are potential candidates for percutaneous transluminal coronary angioplasty.

Patients in Whom Diagnosis is Obscure or Uncertain

Certain categories of patients require catheterization to establish a diagnosis that cannot be made clinically or by less invasive testing.

UNEXPLAINED CHEST PAIN. This indication is for clear delineation of the presence or absence of obstructive coronary artery disease, of coronary artery spasm (ergonovine testing), of mitral valve prolapse as a cause of the pain, or of normal coronary arteries.

SHUNTING. In these patients, one must ascertain the magnitude and location of shunts.

CARDIOMYOPATHIES. Although some cardiologists are content with the clinical diagnosis of congestive cardiomyopathy, it is often necessary to perform cardiac catheterization to differentiate congestive cardiomyopathy of obscure origin from ischemic cardiomyopathy, which may be relieved by a bypass operation. Another form of cardiomyopathy is asymmetric septal hypertrophy, which may require cardiac catheterization. Although the diagnosis is generally made with the aid of echocardiography, it may be necessary to determine the degree of obstruction, the patient's short-term response to the administration of beta-adrenergic blocking agents, or the appropriateness of provocative interventions when obstruction is not obvious.

DIFFERENTIATION OF CONSTRICTIVE PERICARDITIS FROM RESTRICTIVE CARDIOMYOPATHY. At times, it is necessary to make such a distinction.

Assessment of Surgical Results

Since the advent of coronary artery bypass surgery, it has been occasionally necessary to recatheterize patients who have undergone the surgical procedure if they develop recurrent chest pain suggestive of angina pectoris. Under these circumstances, one should look for the patency of the grafts, as opposed to the development of new disease in the patient's native circulation. Similarly, after valve replacement, it may be necessary to recatheterize a patient, to assess the presence of prosthetic valvular dysfunction.

Follow-up of Myocardial Infarction

More and more patients undergo catheterization after myocardial infarction, even though they are asymptomatic or only mildly symptomatic. This procedure is undertaken to evaluate "other vessel disease" that may require a bypass operation. In addition, the evaluation of left ventricular function and the determination of "other vessel disease" may be valuable when one advises patients on further medical therapy and on their ability to resume normal activity.

Research

Cardiac catheterization is also a research tool. For example, one may wish to evaluate a patient's hemodynamic response to investigational agents that are used in the treatment of congestive heart failure. Such procedures must be well supervised and must be undertaken with a protocol that is carefully evaluated by an institutional review board and with a clear indication of the patient's "informed consent."

CONTRAINDICATIONS

The safety of cardiac catheterization has improved over the years. In fact, acute myocardial infarction, cardiogenic shock, recurrent ventricular tachycardia, and congestive heart failure are no longer absolute contraindications to the procedure.[19-22] The only really absolute contraindication is the refusal of the mentally competent individual to consent to the procedure. Numerous relative contraindications exist, however.

Recurrent Ventricular Arrhythmias

The presence of these arrhythmias makes the procedure more hazardous and the interpretation of ventricular function more difficult. Therefore, catheterization should be delayed, if possible, until these arrhythmias are suppressed, to allow safer and more precise intervention.

Severe Hypertension

Because cardiac catheterization predisposes patients with severe hypertension to ischemia, hypertension should be controlled as much as possible before the procedure is undertaken.

Left Ventricular Failure

In patients with elevated left ventricular end-diastolic pressure, acute pulmonary edema may result from the administration of the angiographic dye, which presents a large preload to the left ventricle. Therefore, if at all possible, left ventricular failure should be treated prior to the procedure.

Fever

In the febrile state, hemodynamic responses may be exaggerated, and infections may spread. It is therefore prudent to investigate the cause of the fever and to treat the patient appropriately before cardiac catheterization is undertaken.

Severe Anemia

Hemodynamic responses are accelerated in patients with anemia, and findings during cardiac catheterization may be inaccurate. In addition, bleeding may occur at the site of arterial puncture and may further aggravate the anemic state. Therefore, it is advisable to correct the patient's anemia before cardiac catheterization, if at all possible.

Digitalis Toxicity and Hypokalemia

Digitalis toxicity enhances the possibility of refractory arrhythmias and should be corrected before cardiac catheterization. The same is true for hypokalemia. Both disorders should be corrected prior to catheterization because of increased arrhythmogenic potential especially when these two conditions occur concomitantly.

Renal Failure

The presence of uremia is a strong relative contraindication to angiography. Although hemodynamic measurements may be made, the use of the angiographic dye, which is nephrotoxic, predisposes the patient to acute tubular necrosis. Therefore, except under extenuating circumstances, vigorous hydration and correction of the uremic state should be undertaken prior to cardiac catheterization.

Acute Myocardial Infarction

A patient should not undergo cardiac catheterization if acute myocardial infarction is present, unless some type of acute surgical intervention is contemplated. Cardiac catheterization, may therefore be indicated for any of the following reasons: (1) thrombolysis during acute myocardial infarction; (2) mitral valve replacement because of acute mitral regurgitation, as a result of acute papillary muscle rupture; (3) repair of an acute, acquired ventricular septal defect; or (4) bypass operation for continued pain.

Anticoagulation

If coagulation is abnormal, then cardiac catheterization should be postponed, especially if the percutaneous route is to be used. The effects of heparin, of course, can be reversed easily and safely during catheterization, but a prolonged prothrombin time due to the use of oral anticoagulants is entirely different. It is preferable to postpone the procedure rather than to administer vitamin K because the vitamin is slow to take effect, and later hypercoagulability may result. This possibility is especially dangerous if the patient already has a prosthetic valve(s) in place. If reversal of the effects of anticoagulant drugs is required on an emergency basis, fresh-frozen plasma should be used. In patients who are receiving oral anticoagulant agents on a long-term basis, the anticoagulant should be discontinued 48 to 72 hours prior to admission to the hospital, and heparin therapy should be instituted on admission to the hospital. Heparin is then discontinued 6 hours prior to the procedure. If patients who are taking oral anticoagulant agents on a long-term basis have not discontinued the medication prior to hospital admission, it is probably safe to proceed with cardiac catheterization if the patient's prothrombin time is less than 18 sec. Nevertheless, the entire question of cardiac catheterization in the face of anticoagulation is controversial, and the reader is referred to several contradictory articles on this subject.[23–27]

REQUIRED RADIOLOGIC EQUIPMENT

A modern cardiac catheterization laboratory consists of a number of important elements, including an x-ray generating system, an image intensifier, an image-recording system consisting of a video camera, a monitor, and a 35-mm cinefluorographic camera. Radiologic physics and technique are reviewed in Chapter 1. In the cardiac catheterization laboratory, the difference in the densities between the catheter and the surrounding tissue allows one to visualize the location of the catheter. The image intensifier converts x-ray photons into lower-energy photons in the visible light spectrum, and amplification of the image thereby occurs. A cesium-iodide phosphor screen is most often used in the catheterization laboratory and usually absorbs 50% or more of the radiation produced. These phosphor screens vary from 5 to 12 inches in diameter, and many intensifier systems have 2 or 3 interchangeable screens of differing size that can be selected by the operator, to adjust for different degrees of magnification, as required.[28–30]

CHOICE OF APPROACH

In modern cardiac catheterization laboratories in the United States, two main approaches to passage of the catheter are used. These are direct exposure of an artery and vein and a percutaneous approach, which includes the trans-septal procedure. By the use of either approach, or with a combination, the great vessels and all the cardiac chambers can be entered in almost all instances. Each method has advantages and disadvantages, and actually, the methods are not mutually exclusive. Rather, they are complementary, and the cardiologist who performs these procedures should be proficient in either approach.

In the direct approach, one cuts down on the brachial artery and the basilic vein at the elbow. The percutaneous approach involves entry into the femoral artery and vein in the groin. The direct brachial approach is distinctly advantageous in patients with coarctation of the aorta or with peripheral vascular disease involving the abdominal aorta or the iliac or femoral arteries, or those in whom thrombosis of the femoral vein or the inferior vena cava is suspected. The direct brachial approach may also have advantages in the obese patient, in whom the percutaneous femoral approach may be technically complex and in whom bleeding after the procedure may be difficult to control. Some workers prefer the brachial appproach in patients with aortic regurgitation or significant hypertension, as well as in those taking anticoagulants. These three groups of patients have an increased incidence of bleeding with the percutaneous approach. Moreover, the brachial approach may allow for better control of the catheter, greater potential selection of catheters, and easier exchange of a catheter when clotting occurs within its lumen.

On the other hand, the percutaneous femoral approach has certain advantages. An arteriotomy and arterial repair are not required, as with the brachial approach. It is possible to perform the procedure repeatedly at intervals, whereas the brachial approach should probably not be repeated more than once or twice in the same artery. Infection and thrombophlebitis at the catheterization site are much rarer with the percutaneous approach, and surgical repair of the skin is not necessary. This approach should be used in patients with absent or reduced radial and brachial pulsations and when the direct brachial approach is unsuccessful. It is also probably better in patients with severe aortic stenosis in whom retrograde catheterization is impossible. In these instances, the trans-septal approach may be the only way to obtain data.[14,15,23,24,31]

HEMODYNAMIC MEASUREMENTS

The contractile force of the myocardium is transmitted through blood as a pressure wave. An important objective of cardiac catheterization is the accurate measurement of the forces, and thus the pressure waves, produced by the various cardiac chambers. The pressure wave is a complete periodic fluctuation in force per unit area, with a cycle that consists of a time interval from the onset of one wave to the onset of the next.[32-35]

Technique

Fluid-filled catheters are used to measure these waveforms. With the use of these catheters, an external-pressure transducer is required to detect changes in pressure at the tip of the catheter and to transmit these changes to the transducer by the fluid-filled column in the catheter. A pressure transducer is a diaphragm that is deformed in a linear fashion by the application of pressure within a given physiologic range. When the diaphragm is deformed, electrical resistance changes within the transducer and with the use of a Wheatstone bridge circuit, this change in resistance within the transducer is converted into an electrical potential that is subsequently amplified and is recorded as an analog signal indicating the pressure applied to the transducer. The Wheatstone bridge is operated by an excitation voltage supplied by the pressure amplifier. Variable resistance control enables one to achieve a zero electrical potential when no pressure is applied and allows the transducer to be balanced. The system is calibrated by applying a known pressure to the transducer with a mercury manometer and by recording the analog voltage output. The sensitivity of the amplifiers can be adjusted, to allow a given pressure to correspond to a given deflection of the recorder. Because movement of the transducer diaphragm is required for a voltage output for any given pressure, a volume of fluid must move through the catheter connecting the system to the transducer to effect a pressure recording. Such flow produces a low-frequency resonance in the system that should exceed the significant frequencies contained in the intracardiac pressure recording. For clinical purposes, a system with a frequency response that is flat to 10 to 12 Hz and with a resonant frequency exceeding this level is satisfactory.

When one uses a fluid-filled catheter attached to a transducer, the transducer registers zero pressure when the catheter tip is at the same height as the transducer. If the catheter tip is elevated above the transducer, a positive pressure will be recorded, and this pressure will increase as the elevation is increased. A negative pressure of a similar magnitude will be produced if the catheter tip is progressively lowered below the height of the transducer. These effects are produced by gravitational forces acting on the fluid column in the catheter and the specific gravity of mercury. Thus, the transducer must be placed at approximately the level of the patient's heart, usually the midchest. If the transducer is located at a different height, attachment of a second fluid-filled catheter to the transducer and positioning of the tip of the catheter at the zero level will allow proper calibration of the transducer in relation to the catheter tip position within the heart.

The pressures measured within the heart are not necessarily the true transmural pressures, owing to the normal intrathoracic negative pressures, which range between 0 and −8 mm Hg with normal respiration. Despite all precautions for accurate placement, inaccuracies in the pressure waveform may occur, possibly because of motion of the catheter within the heart and great vessels that produces the artifact of catheter whip. Catheter whip is common within the pulmonary arteries and is difficult to eliminate. To minimize the effect of artifact, micromanometer-tipped catheters may be used and are of special importance in research work, in which precise measurements are required.

Normal and Abnormal Waveforms

Important information is obtained by examining the pressure curves and by recognizing normal and abnormal waveforms.

The right atrial pressure is made up of two major positive deflections, the A wave and the V wave (Fig. 17–14A). The A wave is produced by atrial systole and follows the P wave of the electrocardiogram. As pressure falls from the peak of the A wave, the X descent is recorded. The A wave is followed by a

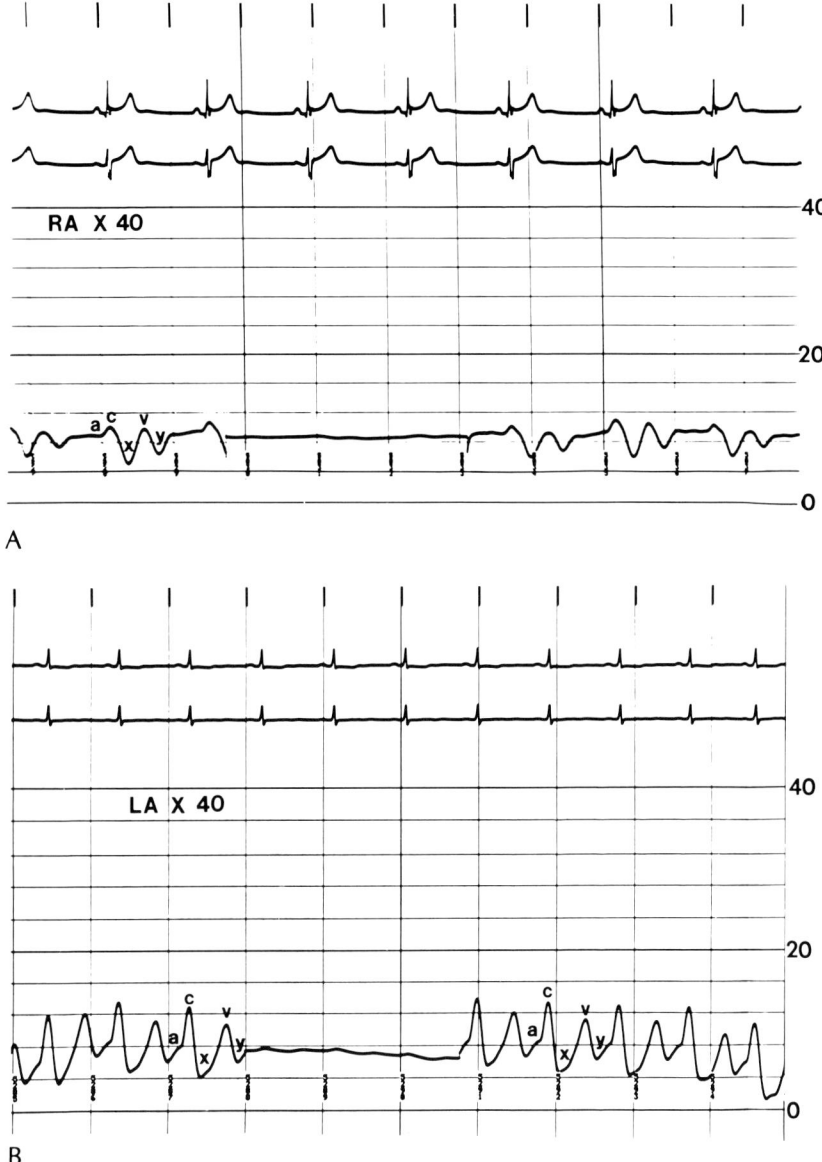

FIG. 17-14. A, Normal right atrial (RA) pressure tracing recorded during cardiac catheterization. For a detailed explanation, see the text. In all figures showing pressure waveforms, electrocardiographic tracings are shown at the top of the figure, and the pressure curves appear at the bottom. B, Normal left atrial (LA) pressure tracing recorded during cardiac catheterization. The various deflections are the same as found in the right atrium (see text), although the pressures are higher. This recording was made when the right heart catheter crossed a patent foramen ovale. Left atrial pressures are not usually recorded during routine cardiac catheterization.

small, positive deflection called the C wave, caused by tricuspid valve closure. After the C wave, right atrial pressure continues to decline because of atrial relaxation, even though the atrium is filling with blood; at this point, the tricuspid valve is closed. When atrial relaxation is finally complete, at the end of the X descent, pressure in the right atrium starts to rise as atrial filling continues because of peripheral venous return. The rise in right atrial pressure during right ventricular ejection is called the V wave and reaches a peak just prior to tricuspid valve opening. When the tricuspid valve opens, the contents of the right atrium empty into the right ventricle, and pressure in the atrium declines. This phenomenon is known as the Y descent. After the Y descent, pressure in the atrium is equilibrated with ventricular diastolic pressure and slowly increases as the ventricle fills. Left atrial pressure is similar to right atrial pressure, except it is normally higher (Fig. 17–14B).

The right ventricular pressure pulse is made up

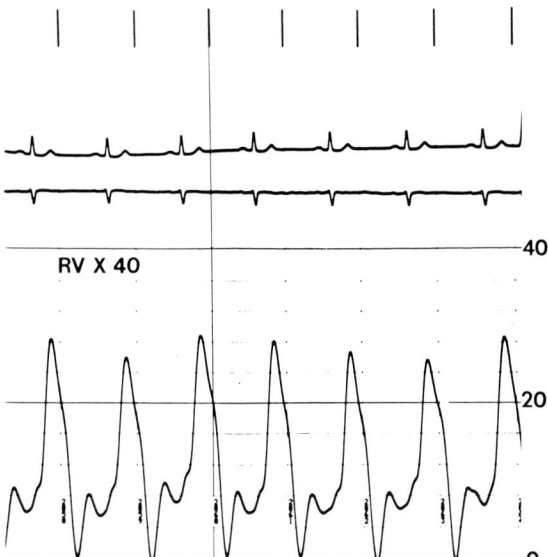

FIG. 17–15. Normal right ventricular (RV) pressure tracing during cardiac catheterization. For a detailed explanation, see the text.

of an early, rapid-filling wave during which about 60% of ventricular filling occurs. This wave is followed by a slow-filling period, which makes up about 25% of ventricular filling, and then by the atrial systolic wave, the A wave, which makes up about 15% of ventricular filling. During diastole, as mentioned previously, right atrial and right ventricular pressures are approximately equal, because of the low resistance to flow across the tricuspid valve. Two pressures are generally measured in the right ventricular pressure tracing, namely, the peak systolic pressure and the end-diastolic pressure immediately after the A wave (Fig. 17–15).

The pulmonary artery waveform consists of a systolic pressure resulting from the flow of blood into the pulmonary artery from the right ventricle (Fig. 17–16). As right ventricular ejection is completed, the pressure in the pulmonary artery falls, and the pulmonary valves close when the right ventricular pressure is less than the pulmonary artery pressure. This process results in the incisura on the pressure waveform. The pressure in the pulmonary artery then gradually drops as blood flows through the pulmonary arteries and veins into the left atrium and ventricle. The lowest point of this pressure in late diastole is called the end-diastolic pulmonary artery pressure. The three pressures recorded in the pulmonary artery trace are the peak-systolic pressure, the mean pulmonary artery pressure, and the end-diastolic pressure.

The pulmonary artery "wedge" pressure, or pulmonary capillary pressure, has a waveform similar to that of left atrial pressure, but it is damped and delayed because of transmission through the cap-

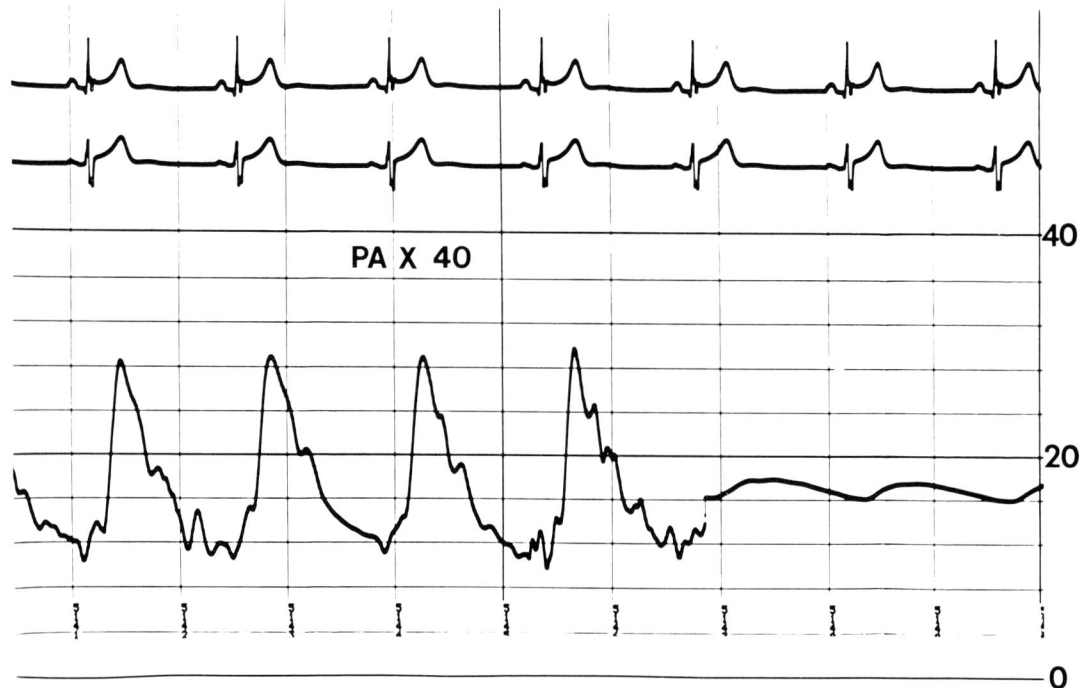

FIG. 17–16. Normal pulmonary artery (PA) pressure during cardiac catheterization. For a detailed explanation, see the text.

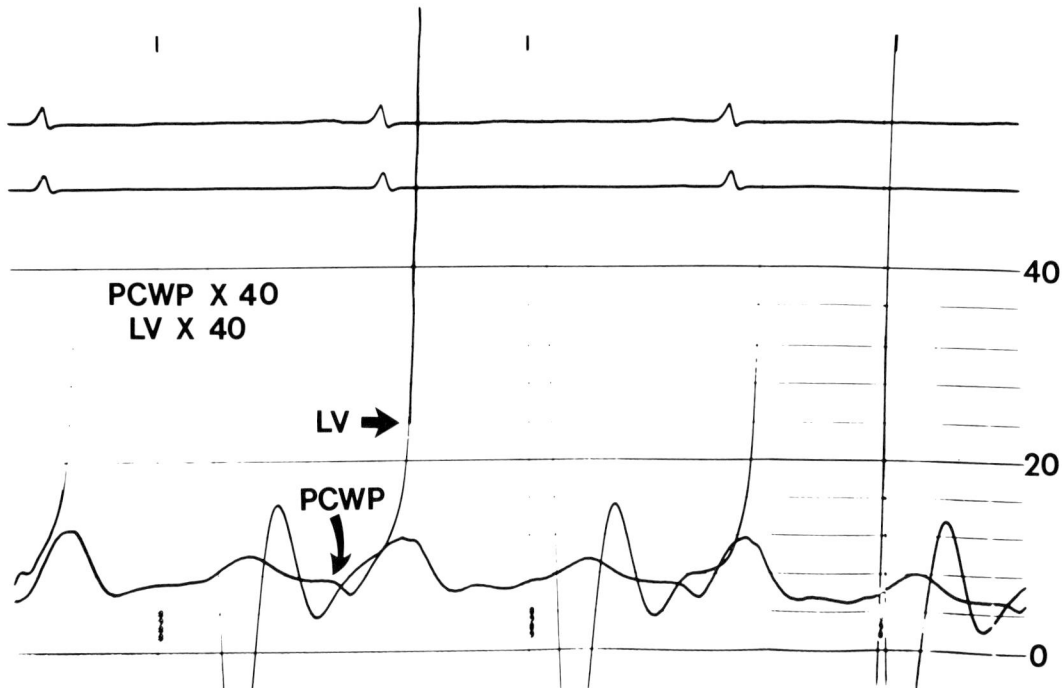

FIG. 17–17. Normal pulmonary capillary wedge pressure (PCWP) recorded simultaneously with left ventricular (LV) pressure during cardiac catheterization. No difference is observed between the PCWP and the LV end-diastolic pressures. For a detailed explanation, see the text.

illary vessels of the lung. A normal pulmonary capillary wedge pressure waveform should show A and V waves, which reflect left atrial systole and left atrial filling during left ventricle systole, respectively. C waves are often not seen on the wedge tracing. The peak A and V waves are generally measured, as well as the mean pressure. The end-diastolic pulmonary artery and mean pulmonary artery wedge pressures are approximately equal, but the mean pulmonary artery pressure is always higher than the mean wedge pressure. Unless trans-septal catheterization is performed, the pulmonary artery wedge pressure is generally used to approximate left atrial pressure. This calculation can be a source of error, however, if the catheter is not adequately "wedged." The wedged position should be confirmed by an arterial oxygen sample, which should be the same as fully oxygenated arterial blood (Fig. 17–17).

The left ventricular waveform is similar to that of the right ventricle, although pressures are normally higher because of the difference in wall thickness and compliance of the two ventricles (Fig. 17–18).

The central aortic pressure is made up of a systolic wave and an incisura that indicates closure of the aortic valve, and it is followed by a gradual fall in pressure as the blood flows from the aorta through the peripheral arterial capillary and venous vessels. Aortic pressure is generally measured at peak systole, at the end of diastole and as a mean pressure (Fig. 17–19).

The peripheral arterial pressure in the brachial or femoral artery has a waveform similar to that of the central aorta. Because of resonance within the arterial system, the peripheral arterial pressure has a wider pulse pressure and a higher peak-systolic pressure than the central aorta. The mean pressure, however, is usually about the same as the central aortic pressure.

Various cardiac diseases produce different abnormal pressure tracings. For example, in patients with valvular aortic stenosis, a pressure gradient is noted between the left ventricle and the aorta (Fig. 17–20). The aortic pressure wave is slow and delayed, when compared to the left ventricular pressure. Aortic regurgitation is marked by near equalization of aortic and left ventricular pressures at the end of diastole. One sees a widening of the aortic pressure and a slurring of the aortic incisura (Fig. 17–21). Mitral stenosis is characterized by a diastolic pressure gradient, as measured by the difference between the pulmonary arterial wedge pressure and the left ventricular end-diastolic pressure. This gradient may increase with exercise. In patients with mitral stenosis and sinus rhythm, a marked difference exists between the large, left atrial "A" wave and the small or absent A wave in the left ventricular pressure tracing (Fig. 17–22).

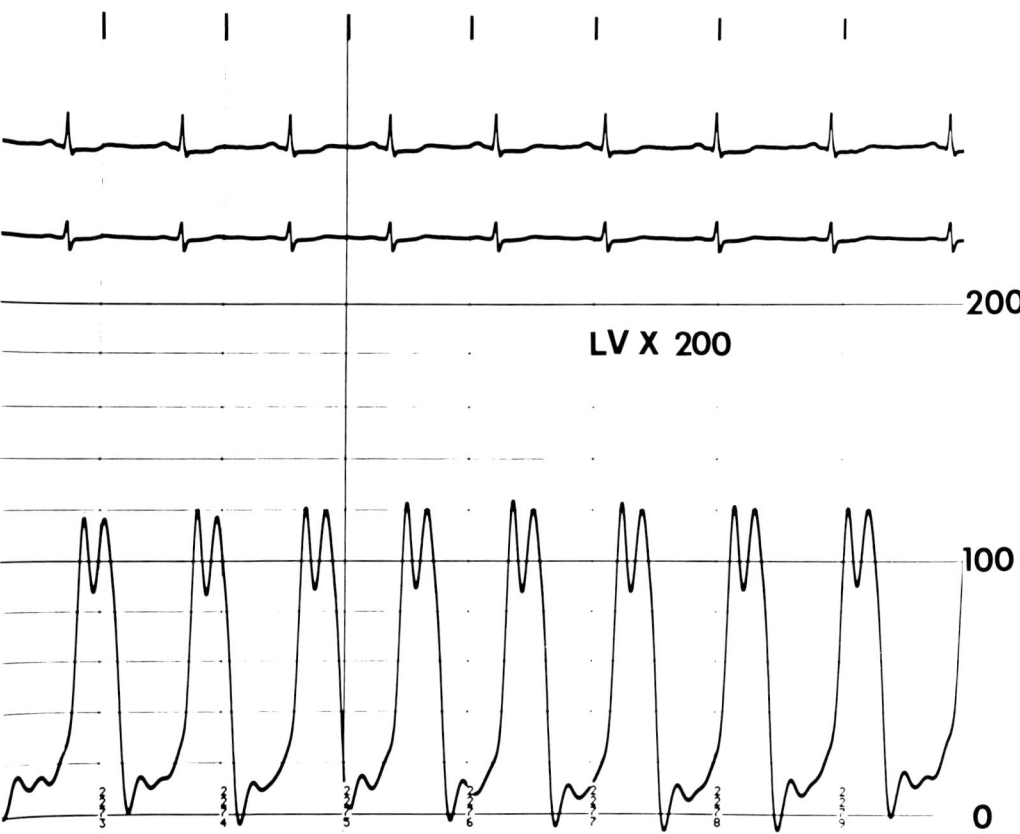

FIG. 17-18. Normal left ventricular (LV) pressure recorded during cardiac catheterization. For a detailed explanation, see the text.

Mitral regurgitation is characterized by a large V wave in the pulmonary artery wedge tracing. The size of the V wave is increased because the left atrium is in the process of filling during systole not only with blood entering from the pulmonary veins, but also with blood regurgitating across the mitral valve (Fig. 17-23). The accurate evaluation of mitral valve function by the measurement of simultaneous pulmonary artery wedge and left ventricular diastolic pressures assumes that the wedge pressure reflects both the phasic and the mean left atrial pressure.

In patients with asymmetric septal hypertrophy, one may also see a large systolic pressure gradient, but the timing and the upstroke of the left ventricular and aortic pressures are virtually identical. Prominent A waves are also seen in this condition, as well as in true valvular aortic stenosis. Pulmonary and tricuspid stenosis and pulmonary and tricuspid regurgitation are measured during right heart catheterization. This measurement is often achieved by rapid pullback of the catheters from the pulmonary artery, through the right ventricle and into the right atrium. Much more precise measurement of simultaneous pressures can be achieved by using double-lumen right heart catheters, however, which permit monitoring of pressures on opposite sides of the tricuspid valve or pulmonary outflow tract and the pulmonary valve.

The pressure gradient may rise with exercise because cardiac output is normally increased by an increase in heart rate, and especially in the presence of mitral stenosis, the left atrial-left ventricular pressure gradient may increase markedly with a concomitant marked rise in pulmonary arterial pressure. On occasion, this finding allows one to identify what appears to be only mild mitral stenosis and to delineate its severity, which may have been missed without exercise. Similarly, exercise exaggerates mitral and tricuspid regurgitation and enables one to recognize much more severe regurgitation than is suggested when the patient is at rest.

ANGIOCARDIOGRAPHY

To visualize the anatomic structures of the heart, a radiodense material must be injected into the blood to contrast it with the cardiac soft tissues. Serial films rapidly obtained record the flow of the opacified blood through the heart, to provide information regarding the anatomic features of the car-

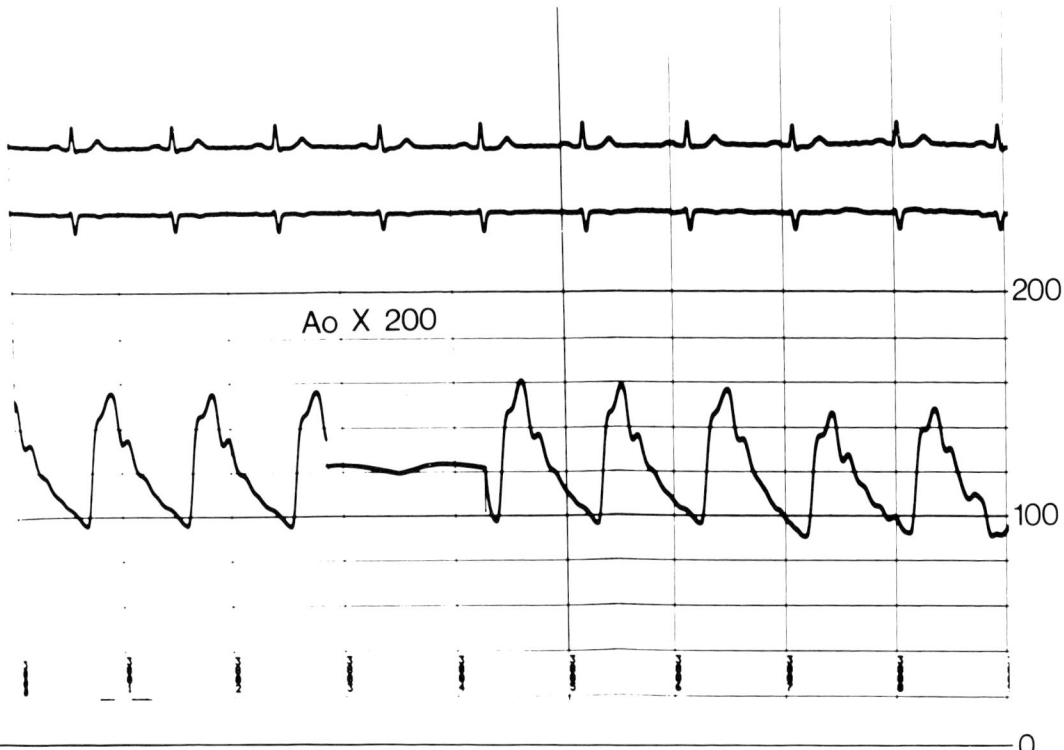

FIG. 17-19. Normal central aortic (Ao) pressure recorded during cardiac catheterization. For a detailed explanation, see the text.

diac chambers, their function, and the pattern of blood flow through the heart and great vessels.

Contrast material consists of a water-soluble organic iodine-containing compound. The degree of opacification depends on the concentration of contrast material and on the speed of injection. High iodine concentration increases the viscosity and makes injection more difficult. Therefore, moderately concentrated contrast material is preferable to a denser but thicker compound. The contrast material must be introduced rapidly and as close to the area to be studied as possible, to prevent dilution.

The radiologic equipment used for angiocardiography may include a roll-film or cut-film changer, which produces beautifully contrasted images; however, the necessity to slide the patient over the changer for each angiographic injection lengthens the procedure and moves the patient out of the fluoroscopic field. Image intensifiers have supplanted film changers, and the image on the output screen is photographic with a 35-mm cinefluorographic camera, usually at a rate of 30 to 60 frames/sec. Some workers use 100- to 105-mm film, at a rate of 6 to 12 frames/sec.

As the images are recorded on film, they can also be seen on a television monitor, to provide fluoroscopic control. Multiple views are usually required to obtain the most detailed outline of anatomic structures. Because the amount of contrast material that can be safely given is limited, it is often difficult to obtain an adequate study without biplane equipment. Consequently, it is optimal to have biplane equipment unless the cardiac catheterization laboratory is designed exclusively for coronary arteriography. No single set of views is best for all conditions. Angle views are obtained by turning the patient or by rotating the tube, depending on the available equipment. The number and types of views often depend on the skill and experience of the angiographer performing the study. An experienced angiographic team with up-to-date equipment is a necessity for a modern cardiac catheterization laboratory.[36-39]

MEASUREMENTS OF CARDIAC OUTPUT

Many methods are used to measure cardiac output, but the two most common are the Fick oxygen method and the dye-dilution technique.

Fick Oxygen Method

This method is based on the principle that the total uptake or release of any substance by an organ is determined by blood flow and by the arteriovenous

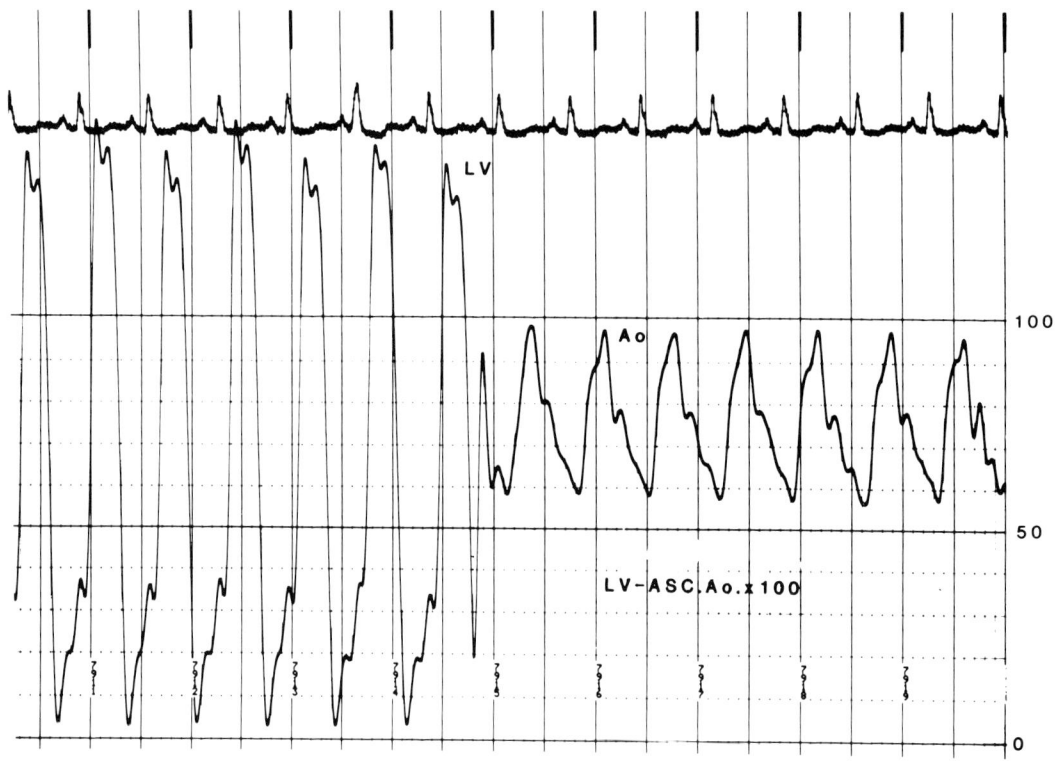

FIG. 17–20. Moderately severe aortic stenosis. Pullback across the aortic valve from left ventricle into the ascending aorta (ASC.Ao), showing a 50-mm Hg gradient across the aortic valve. LV, Left ventricular pressure, Ao, aortic pressure.

concentration difference of that substance. The substance released to the blood by the lungs is oxygen, and the blood flow to the lungs can be measured by the arteriovenous difference of oxygen across the lungs and by the consumption of oxygen per minute. When no intracardiac shunt exists and if the pulmonary blood flow equals the systemic blood flow, the Fick principle is a measure of systemic blood flow as well. Oxygen consumption is usually determined by measuring the oxygen extracted by the lungs during a given period of time. This determination assumes a steady state in which oxygen consumption and cardiac output are constant during the period of measurement. Usually, oxygen consumption is measured by the collection of all the air expired by a patient over a 3-min period. Milliliters of oxygen consumed per liter of expired air comprise the difference between the oxygen content of room air and the oxygen content of the collected expired air corrected for barometric pressure. Minute ventilation is estimated by dividing total volume of air expired by the number of minutes that the expired air was collected. Oxygen consumption can then be calculated as the product of the milliliters of oxygen consumed per liter of expired air and the liters of expired air per minute of collection. Oxygen consumption in milliliters per minute is generally divided by body surface area, to correct for differences in oxygen consumption rate that might be due to variations in body size. Normal basal oxygen consumption index is between 110 and 150 ml oxygen/min/m^2 body surface area. Oxygen consumption may be erroneously estimated if expired air collection is incomplete because of a poorly fitting mouthpiece or a perforated eardrum.

The arteriovenous oxygen difference across the lungs is calculated as the difference between the oxygen content of pulmonary artery blood and that of systemic arterial blood; pulmonary venous blood cannot be sampled easily. Pulmonary arterial blood is used for the determination of the mixed venous blood oxygen content, which is measured usually by oximetry. The oxygen content of blood is determined as the product of the oxygen saturation and the theoretic oxygen-carrying capacity of hemoglobin. The arteriovenous oxygen content difference is then calculated as the arterial minus the venous oxygen content. Cardiac output is determined by dividing oxygen consumption by the arteriovenous oxygen difference. The cardiac index is obtained by dividing oxygen consumption in milliliters per minute per square meter by the arteriovenous oxygen difference. The normal range for the cardiac index is 2.5 to 4.2 L/min/m^2. The total error in measurement of cardiac output by the Fick method is about 10%. The Fick method is most accurate in patients with

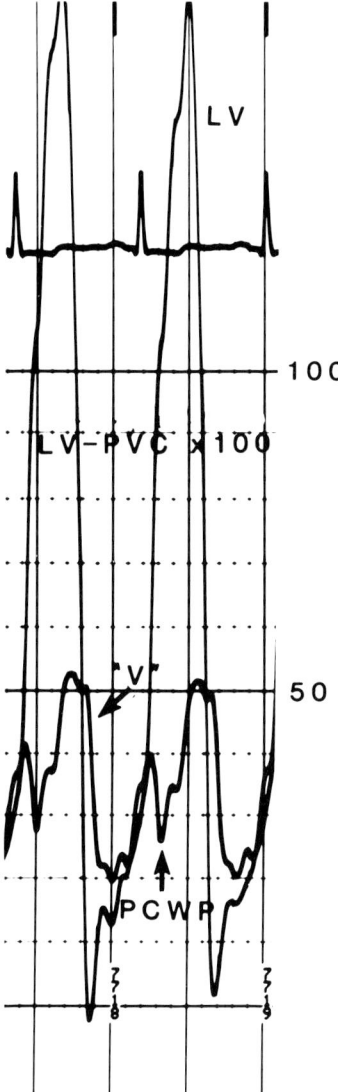

FIG. 17-21. Severe aortic regurgitation with a mean pulmonary capillary wedge pressure (PCWP) of 36 mm Hg and a left ventricular (LV) pressure of 160/35 mm Hg. A large "V" wave is seen in the PCWP tracing. The patient has severe pulmonary hypertension as well, with pulmonary artery pressure of 80/36 mm Hg, with a mean of 50 mm Hg.

a low cardiac output in whom the arteriovenous oxygen difference is great.[35,40–45]

Dye-dilution Method

Stewart first reported a dye-dilution method for the measurement of cardiac output.[46] Today, indocyanine green is the most widely used dye, but a thermodilution method using cold saline solution as the indicator is gaining popularity. When indocyanine green dye is injected rapidly into the pulmonary artery, its appearance and concentration in arterial blood are recorded from a brachial, radial, or femoral

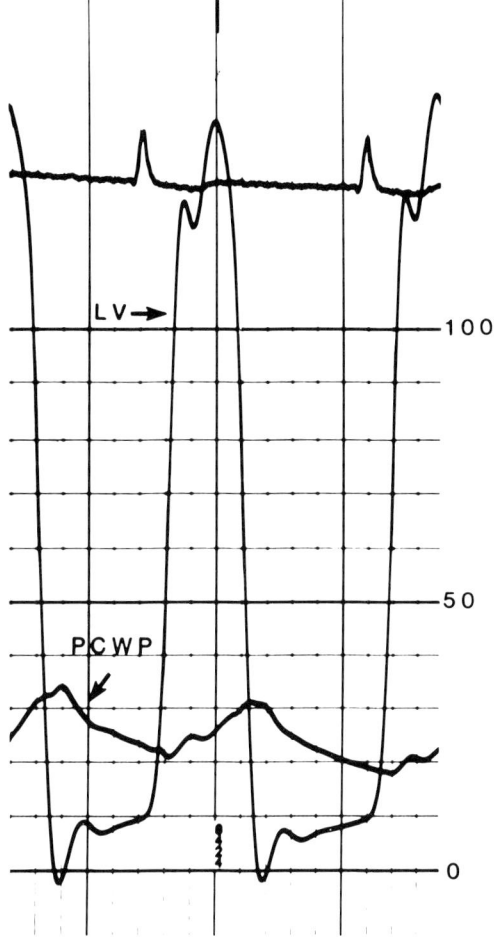

FIG. 17-22. Severe mitral stenosis. A 10-mm Hg end-diastolic gradient is seen across the mitral valve. The cardiac output is low, and the mitral valve area is calculated at 0.8 cm². PCWP, pulmonary capillary wedge pressure; LV, left ventricular pressure.

artery. This method results in a time-concentration curve that demonstrates a rapid rise to a peak, followed by a gradual decline in concentration, and later by a secondary rise due to dye recirculation (Fig. 17-24). The first-pass curve is displayed on semilogarithmic paper by extrapolating the early linear part of the descent plot, to ignore the recirculation. The cardiac output is the quantity of indicator injected, divided by the product of the average concentration of the indicator during the first pass and the total duration of the curve. Thus, C.O. = $\frac{I}{C \times T}$, where I = quantity of indicator injected, C = average concentration of indicator during the first pass, and T = the duration of the curve. Results of the dye-dilution method correspond to those of the Fick method. The dye-dilution method is least ac-

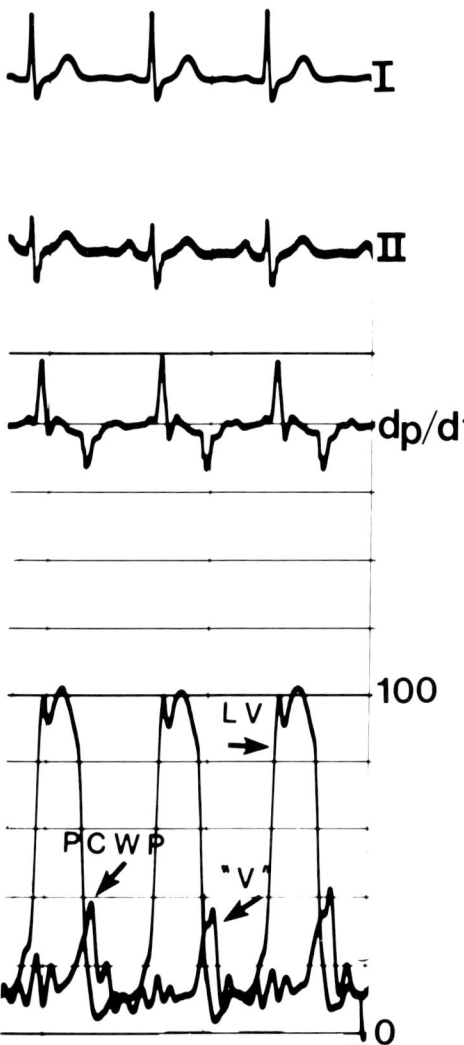

FIG. 17–23. Severe mitral regurgitation resulting from chronic papillary muscle dysfunction. Note the large "V" waves in the pulmonary capillary wedge tracing. PCWP, pulmonary capillary wedge pressure; LV, left ventricular pressure.

curate in patients with low cardiac output, severe valvular regurgitation or shunts, however. Thus, the two methods are complementary, and the decision to use one or the other is predicated on the cardiac disease to be studied. Because the thermodilution method can be used repeatedly without any buildup of dye or any recirculation problems, it is becoming more popular.[45–56]

Angiographic Cardiac Output

Left ventricular end-diastolic and end-systolic volumes can be estimated by quantitative left ventricular angiography, which allows for the determination of left ventricular stroke volume. Thus, cardiac output can be estimated as the product of stroke volume and the heart rate during the angiogram. This method is inaccurate in patients with atrial fibrillation and significant valvular regurgitation, however, and is definitely less accurate then the Fick or dye-dilution methods.

ASSESSMENT OF INTRACARDIAC SHUNTS

Intracardiac shunts can usually be detected, localized, and quantified precisely during cardiac catheterization. Although one usually suspects the presence of a shunt prior to cardiac catheterization,

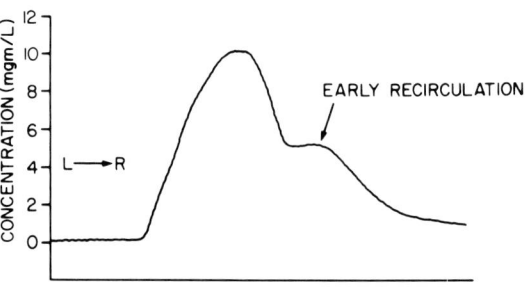

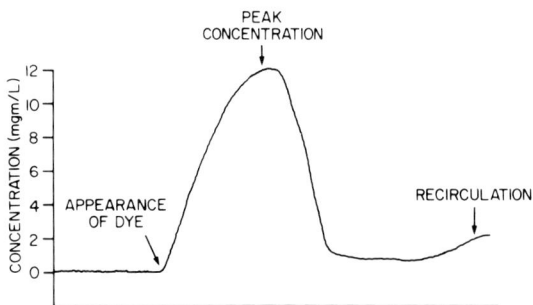

FIG. 17–24. Normal first-pass indocyanine dye curve for determination of cardiac output. For a detailed explanation, see the text.

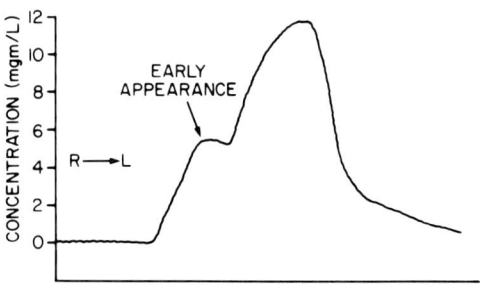

FIG. 17–25. First-pass indocyanine dye curve in a patient with left-to-right shunt (A) and right-to-left shunt (B). The left-to-right shunt produces early recirculation of dye. The right-to-left shunt is apparent because of the early appearance of dye. For a detailed explanation, see the text.

one must search for a shunt when arterial oxygen desaturation is found or when a patient's pulmonary oxygen saturation is inordinately high. In patients with a left-to-right shunt, as seen with atrial or ventricular septal defects and patent ductus arteriosus, pulmonary blood flow is generally increased over systemic blood flow, and the pulmonary artery oxygen saturation is greater than the true mixed venous blood saturation. The exact anatomic location of the shunt is determined by taking multiple oxygen samples as the catheter progresses from the superior vena cava to the pulmonary artery. The oxygen-saturation method is not sensitive to small shunts, however.

On the other hand, the hydrogen-sensitive platinum-tipped electrode catheter that measures DC voltage changes can be used to detect the early appearance of hydrogen in small left-to-right intracardiac shunts. Indocyanine green dye injected into the pulmonary artery with sampling from the femoral artery also may enable one to detect small left-to-right shunts. Indocyanine green dye produces early recirculation on the downslope of the dye curve in patients with left-to-right shunts and early appearance of dye on the upslope of the curve in those with right-to-left shunts (Fig. 17-25). In right-to-left shunts, the arterial blood is unsaturated, and the point of shunting can be detected by sampling from each of the left heart chambers and by noting which is the first to show the desaturation. Because it is difficult to enter the pulmonary vein and the left atrium, small right-to-left shunts can best be determined by injecting-indocyanine green dye into the vena cava and by noting the early appearance of the dye on the upslope of the dye curve.[35,57-61]

Shunts may be quantified during cardiac catheterization. Pulmonary blood flow (Q_p) is determined as oxygen consumption divided by the pulmonary venous oxygen content (PV_{O_2}) minus the pulmonary artery oxygen content (PA_{O_2}). If the pulmonary vein cannot be entered, systemic arterial oxygen content may be used.

$$Q_p = \frac{O_2 \text{ consumption (ml/min)}}{\underset{(ml/L)}{PV_{O_2}} - \underset{(ml/L)}{PA_{O_2}}}$$

Systemic blood flow (Q_s) is calculated as oxygen consumption divided by systemic arterial oxygen content (SA_{O_2}) minus mixed venous oxygen content.

$$Q_s = \frac{O_2 \text{ consumption (ml/min)}}{\underset{(ml/L)}{SA_{O_2}} - \underset{(ml/L)}{\text{mixed venous } O_2}}$$

The shunt flow itself is then calculated as Q_p minus Q_s. If the shunt is left to right, the value is positive, whereas it is negative if the shunt is purely right to left. When a bidirectional shunt is present, more complicated formulas must be used.[37]

CALCULATION OF VASCULAR RESISTANCE

Vascular resistance may be calculated for both the systemic and pulmonary vascular beds. The systemic vascular resistance (SVR) equals 80 times the difference of the mean aortic (Ao) and mean right atrial (RA) pressure divided by systemic blood flow (Q_s). Pulmonary vascular resistance (PVR) is 80 times the difference between the mean pulmonary artery (PA) and the mean left atrial or pulmonary capillary wedge pressure (PCWP) divided by pulmonary blood flow (Q_p).

$$SVR = \frac{80 \, (Ao - RA)}{Q_s}$$

$$PVR = \frac{80 \, (PA - PCWP)}{Q_p}$$

These values can be corrected for body size by multiplying them by body surface area, and they are usually expressed in metric terms as dyne/sec/cm^{-5}. The cardiac output as measured by the Fick or the dye-dilution method is used in calculating blood flow; however, in the presence of an intracardiac shunt in which the pulmonary and systemic blood flows are unequal, the blood flow through each circuit must be measured separately in the calculation of resistance. As noted previously, the pulmonary artery wedge pressure is used to approximate mean left atrial pressure. The normal value for systemic vascular resistance is 1130 ± 178 dyne/sec/cm^{-5}. The normal pulmonary vascular resistance is 67 ± 23 dyne/sec/cm^{-5}. Abnormal systemic and pulmonary vascular resistances are seen in several conditions, and are especially important in the evaluation of pulmonary hypertension. Marked fixed elevations in pulmonary vascular resistance in patients with severe mitral stenosis and pulmonary hypertension or in those with congenital heart disease and shunts may contraindicate surgical procedures. Thus, it is important to determine whether the increased resistance is fixed. Oxygen inhalation, infusions of acetylcholine, infusions of tolazoline-hydrochloride, and exercise have all been used to lower resistance.

It is often valuable, in patients with mitral stenosis, to consider both total pulmonary resistance and pulmonary vascular resistance. Total pulmonary resistance includes the pulmonary vascular resistance and the resistance to flow across the mitral valve. Normally, these values are almost equal. In mitral stenosis, however, the resistance to flow produced by the narrowed mitral orifice is significant, and although total pulmonary resistance may be elevated, pulmonary vascular resistance may only be mildly to moderately elevated. This finding suggests that the patient would benefit from relief of mitral stenosis, with a distinct possibility that pulmonary hypertension would be corrected.

EVALUATION OF VALVE AREAS

The evaluation of valvular stenosis not only depends on detecting pressure gradients, but also depends on determining valve areas. Equations for the aortic and mitral valve areas were developed by Gorlin and Gorlin and were later modified by Cohen and Gorlin.[62,63] At low flow rates, these formulas may be inaccurate, and in addition, in the presence of valvular regurgitation, a falsely low valve-area calculation may be derived because the actual valve flow per beat is more than the flow calculated from systemic cardiac output. Thus, valve areas that are calculated in patients with regurgitation across a stenotic valve should be considered as minimal; the valve area is usually larger than calculated. The pressure gradient across the valve is a more accurate measure than calculation of valve area in assessing valvular stenosis. Calculation of the valve area is a useful clinical tool and should be done when possible, however.

ELECTROPHYSIOLOGIC STUDIES

Space does not permit a detailed discussion of the current literature on electrophysiologic testing and pacing. Suffice it that these studies use catheters with multiple electrodes and have helped us to define conduction abnormalities, arrhythmias, bypass tracts, therapy of arrhythmias, and the need for temporary and permanent transvenous pacing. Catheters are passed through the right femoral vein and the right brachial vein into the right atrium and the right ventricle for multiple recordings pacing studies, to determine the origin and inducibility of arrhythmias. The left ventricle has also been used for recordings of conduction abnormalities and of inducibility of ventricular tachyarrhythmias.[64–73]

PREPARATION AND PREMEDICATION OF THE PATIENT

In preparing the patient for cardiac catheterization, one should first explain the proposed procedure fully, in terms that the patient will understand. The cardiologist must specifically outline the risks, including allergic reactions to the dye, thrombosis at the site of catheter entry, myocardial infarction, cerebrovascular accident, and death. At the same time, one should emphasize that in a well-equipped, modern, active cardiac catheterization laboratory, these complications occur in less than 1% of procedures. The discomforts that the patient may experience and the length of the procedure should be reviewed. The patient's coagulation status, blood count, electrocardiogram and chest roentgenogram should be carefully assessed preoperatively. Diazepam, diphenhydramine, or meperidine may be used for sedation. The patient should have had no food after midnight if the procedure is to be done in the morning. If the procedure is to be done in the afternoon, a liquid breakfast may be given. The patient should be evaluated by the catheterization team on the evening before the procedure, to select the method of approach most suitable for the information desired.

CATHETERIZATION PROTOCOL

Each catheterization laboratory should have well developed and clear protocols to be followed by the team of cardiologists, nurses, and technicians. After the patient's antecubital fossae and the right groin are scrubbed with appropriate antiseptic solutions, the patient should be covered with sterile drapes, and arterial and venous lines should be inserted. Hemodynamic measurements should precede angiographic studies, to obtain physiologic values as close to the basal state as possible because the injection of dye alters the physiologic status. Pressures and oxygen saturation should be measured and recorded, and several determinations of cardiac output should be obtained before angiography. Finally, angiographic examination should be performed, to delineate anatomic abnormalities.

COMPLICATIONS

Cardiac catheterization has many possible complications, including death, significant arrhythmias, severe hypotension, laceration and thrombosis of arteries and veins, perforation of the heart, knotting of catheters around anatomic structures, embolic phenomena, serious allergic reactions, bleeding, pneumothorax, and significant vagal reactions.[24,74–91] In a past multicenter study, the overall incidence of complications in adult and pediatric patients was 3.4%.[24] The complications were much more common in infants, occurring in 9%. The incidence of death was 0.44% (55 patients out of 12,367), and this complication was more common in infants than in older patients. Today, all forms of these complications are even less common.

Death may be due to a number of complications, including tamponade, which is much more common with the trans-septal approach, acute myocardial infarction, especially if coronary angiography is performed, perforation of the aorta, severe vagal reactions, severe hypotension due to acute blood loss, and ventricular fibrillation.

Perforation of the heart is much more likely to occur with right ventricular catheterization, especially in the right ventricular outflow tract and the apex. Problems with the catheters include knotting of the catheter around valves, both native and prosthetic, clotting, and pyrogenic reactions. Emboli may be due to either clot or air. Significant vagal reactions may occur at any time; patients usually respond to atropine and to the administration of fluids to restore volume.

The brachial arterial approach is much more likely to be associated with arterial thrombosis, which occurs in about 2 to 3% of patients. This incidence is directly related to the duration of the catheterization, the number of catheters used, the presence of underlying arterial disease, and the technique of repair of the artery. The transfemoral approach is associated with 3 to 4% of local complications, including thrombosis, distal embolization, the development of a false aneurysm, and hemorrhage.

Contrast material may be injected intramurally if the catheter tip is entrapped by trabeculae and is thereby prevented from recoiling during the injection. The full force of the contrast material from the catheter is deposited against the endocardium, and small intramural dissections may occur and are usually of no consequence. If an important portion of the conduction system is involved, however, arrhythmias may result. Large intramural deposits may cause myocardial infarction, although these intramural deposits are not usually important.

All contrast media have some degree of toxicity, especially nephrotoxicity and central nervous system toxicity. Some patients have mild allergic reactions, usually in the form of urticaria; anaphylactic reactions are rare. Sensitivity testing is of no value in predicting who will have an allergic reaction to the dye.[92] If the patient has a history of a previous allergic reaction to iodine-containing dyes, or if the patient has a history of asthma or other allergic reactions associated with dye, however, one should administer premedication with corticosteroids. Allergic reactions short of bronchospasm usually can be managed with antihistamines or short-term administration of corticosteroids. Occasionally, a patient may have an anaphylactic reaction that requires epinephrine, vasopressor agents, intubation, and assisted ventilation.

Central nervous system toxicity has been reported and may be manifested as seizures. Such seizures can be treated successfully with either diazepam or barbiturates.

As mentioned earlier, all iodine-containing contrast material has some nephrotoxicity. One must therefore be careful about the amount of contrast material given in the patient with borderline or clearly abnormal renal function. In addition, all such patients should be well hydrated before the angiographic study is performed.

REFERENCES

1. Forssman, W.: Die Sondierung des rechten Herzens. Klin. Wochenschr., 8:2085, 1929.
2. Klein, O.: Zur Bestimmung des zirkulatorischen Minutensvolumen nach den Fickschen Prinzip. Munch. Med. Wochenschr., 77:1311, 1930.
3. Cournand, A.F., and Ranges, H.S.: Catheterization of the right auricle in man. Proc. Soc. Exp. Biol. Med., 46:462, 1941.
4. Cournand, A.F., et al.: Measurement of cardiac output in man using the technique of catheterization of the right auricle or ventricle. J. Clin. Invest., 24:106, 1945.
5. Richards, D.W.: Cardiac output by the catheterization technique in various clinical conditions. Fed. Proc., 4:215, 1945.
6. Dexter, L., et al.: Studies of congenital heart disease. II. The pressure and oxygen content of blood in the right auricle, right ventricle, and pulmonary artery in control patients with observations on the oxygen saturation and source of pulmonary "capillary" blood. J. Clin. Invest., 26:554, 1947.
7. McMichael, J., and Sharpey-Schafer, E.P.: The action of intravenous digoxin in man. Q. J. Med., 13:1123, 1944.
8. Stead, E.A., Jr., and Warren, J.V.: Cardiac output in man: analysis of the mechanisms varying the cardiac output based on recent clinical studies. Arch. Intern. Med., 80:237, 1949.
9. Stead, E.A., Jr., Warren, J.V., and Brannon, E.S.: Cardiac output in congestive heart failure: an analysis of the reasons for lack of close correlation between the symptoms of heart failure and the resting cardiac output. Am. Heart J., 35:529, 1948.
10. Bing, R.J., et al.: Catheterization of the coronary sinus and the middle cardiac vein in man. Proc. Soc. Exp. Biol. Med., 66:239, 1947.
11. Wood, E.H., et al.: General and special techniques on cardiac catheterization. Proc. Staff Meetings Mayo Clin., 23:494, 1948.
12. Zimmerman, H.A., Scott, R.W., and Becker, N.D.: Catheterization of the left side of the heart in man. Circulation, 1:357, 1950.
13. Seldinger, S.I.: Catheter replacement of the needle in percutaneous arteriography: a new technique. Acta Radiol., 39:368, 1953.
14. Ross, J., Jr.: Transseptal left heart catheterization: a new method of left atrial puncture. Ann. Surg., 149:395, 1959.
15. Ross, J., Jr., Braunwald, E., and Morrow, A.G.: Transseptal left atrial puncture: a new technique for the measurement of left atrial pressure in man. Am. J. Cardiol., 3:653, 1959.
16. Sones, F.M., Jr., et al.: Cinecoronary arteriography. Circulation, 20:773, 1959.
17. Sones, F.M., Jr., and Shirey, E.K.: Cinecoronary arteriography. Mod. Concepts Cardiovasc. Dis., 31:735, 1962.
18. Swan, H.J.C., et al.: Catheterization of the heart in man with use of a flow-directed balloon-tipped catheter. N. Engl. J. Med., 283:447, 1970.
19. Diamond, G., Marcus, H., and McHugh, T.: Catheterization of the left ventricle in acutely ill patients. Br. Heart J., 33:489, 1971.
20. Rackley, C.E., and Russell, R.P.: Left ventricular function in acute myocardial infarction and its clinical significance. Circulation, 45:231, 1972.

21. Gold, H.K., Leinbach, R.C., and Sanders, C.A.: Intraaortic balloon pumping for ventricular septal defect or mitral regurgitation complicating acute myocardial infarction. Circulation, 47:1191, 1973.
22. Levine, F.H., Gold, H.K., and Leinbach, R.C.: Management of acute myocardial ischemia with intraaortic pumping and coronary bypass surgery. Circulation, 56 (Suppl. 3):61, 1977.
23. Mortensen, J.D.: Clinical sequelae from arterial needle puncture, cannulation and incision. Circulation, 35:1118, 1967.
24. Braunwald, E., and Swan, H.J.C.: Cooperative study on cardiac catheterization. Circulation, 37(Suppl. 3):1, 1968.
25. Mendel, D.: A Practice of Cardiac Catheterization. Oxford, Blackwell Scientific Publications, 1968, p. 119.
26. Kloster, F.E., Bristow, J.D., and Seaman, A.J.: Cardiac catheterization during anticoagulant therapy. Am. J. Cardiol., 28:675, 1971.
27. Walker, W.J., et al.: Systemic heparinization for femoral percutaneous coronary arteriography. N. Engl. J. Med., 288:826, 1973.
28. Selman, J.: The Fundamentals of X-Ray and Radium Physics. 6th Ed. Springfield, IL, Charles C Thomas, 1980.
29. Sprawls, P., Jr.: The Physical Principles of Diagnostic Radiology. Baltimore, University Park Press, 1977, p. 1.
30. Reuter, F.G.: Physician and patient exposure during cardiac catheterization. Circulation, 58:134, 1978.
31. Cope, C.: Technique for transseptal catheterization of the left atrium: preliminary report. J. Thorac. Surg., 37:482, 1959.
32. Wood, E.H., et al.: Measurement of pressures in man by cardiac catheters. Circ. Res., 2:294, 1954.
33. Fry, D.L.: Physiologic recording by modern instruments with particular reference to pressure recording. Physiol. Rev., 40:743, 1960.
34. Grossman, W., McLaurin, L.P., and Stefadourous, M.A.: Left ventricular stiffness associated with chronic pressure and volume overloads in man. Circ. Res., 35:793, 1974.
35. Grossman, W.: Cardiac Catheterization and Angiography. 2nd Ed. Philadelphia, Lea & Febiger, 1980.
36. Williamson, D.E.: Experimental determination of flow equation in catheters for cardiology. Am. J. Roentgenol. Radium Ther. Nucl. Med., 94:704, 1965.
37. Intersociety Commission for Heart Disease Resources: Optimal resources for examination of the chest and cardiovascular system: catheterization-angiographic laboratories. Circulation, 53:A-1, 1976.
38. Elliott, L.P., et al.: Axial cineangiography in congenital heart disease. II. Specific lesions. Circulation, 56:1084, 1977.
39. Bargeron, L.M., Jr., et al.: Axial cineangiography in congenital heart disease. I. Concept, technical and anatomic considerations. Circulation, 56:1075, 1977.
40. Visscher, N.B., and Johnson, J.A.: The Fick principle: analysis of potential errors in its conventional application. J. Appl. Physiol., 5:635, 1953.
41. Thomassen, B.: Cardiac output in normal subjects under standard basal conditions: the repeatability of measurements by the Fick method. Scand. J. Clin. Lab. Invest., 9:365, 1957.
42. Barratt-Boyes, B.G., and Wood, E.H.: The oxygen saturation of blood in the venae cavae, right heart chambers, and pulmonary vessels in healthy subjects. J. Lab. Clin. Med., 50:93, 1957.
43. Selzer, A., and Sundrann, R.B.: Reliability of the determinations of cardiac output in man by means of the Fick principle. Circ. Res., 6:485, 1958.
44. VanSlyke, D.D., and Neill, J.M.: The determination of gases in blood and other solutions by vacuum extraction and manometric measurements. J. Biol. Chem., 8:654, 1962.
45. Guyton, A.C., Jones, C.E., and Coleman, T.G.: Circulatory Physiology: Cardiac Output and its Regulation. 2nd Ed. Philadelphia, W.B. Saunders, 1973.
46. Stewart, G.N.: Researches on the circulation time and on the influences which affect it. IV. The output of the heart. J. Physiol., 22:159, 1897.
47. Kinsman, J.M., Moore, J.W., and Hamilton, W.F.: Studies on the circulation. I. Injection method; physical and mathematical considerations. Am. J. Physiol., 89:322, 1929.
48. Moore, J.W., et al.: Studies on the circulation. II. Cardiac output determinations; comparison of the injection method with the direct Fick procedure. Am. J. Physiol., 89:331, 1929.
49. Hamilton, W.F., et al.: Comparison of Fick and dye dilution methods of measuring the cardiac output in man. Am. J. Physiol., 153:309, 1948.
50. Doyle, J.T., et al.: An evaluation of the measurement of the cardiac output and of the so-called pulmonary blood volume by the dye-dilution method. J. Lab. Clin. Med., 41:29, 1953.
51. Eliasch, H., et al.: Comparison of the dye dilution and the direct Fick methods for the measurement of cardiac output in man. Scand. J. Clin. Lab. Invest., 7(Suppl. 20):73, 1955.
52. Rahimtoola, S.H., and Swan, H.J.S.: Calculation of cardiac output from indicator-dilution curves in the presence of mitral regurgitation. Circulation, 31:711, 1965.
53. Branthwaite, M.A., and Bradley, R.D.: Measurement of cardiac output by thermal dilution in man. J. Appl. Physiol., 24:434, 1968.
54. Ganz, W., et al.: A new technique for measurement of cardiac output by thermodilution in man. Am. J. Cardiol., 27:392, 1971.
55. Shepherd, R.L., Higgs, L.M., and Glancy, D.L.: Comparison of left ventricular and pulmonary arterial injection sites in determination of cardiac output by indicator dye dilution technique. Chest, 62:175, 1972.
56. Reddy, P.S., et al.: Determinants of variation between Fick and indicator dilution estimates of cardiac output during diagnostic catheterization: Fick vs. dye outputs. J. Lab. Clin. Med., 87:568, 1976.
57. Dexter, L., et al.: Studies of congenital heart disease. I. Technique of venous catheterization as a diagnostic procedure. J. Clin. Invest., 26:547, 1947.
58. Swan, H.J.C., and Wood, E.H.: Localization of cardiac defects by dye dilution curves recorded after injection of T-1824 at multiple sites in the heart and great vessels during cardiac catheterization. Proc. Staff Meetings Mayo Clin., 28:95, 1953.
59. Hyman, A.L., et al.: A comparison study of the detection of cardiovascular shunts by oxygen analysis and indicator dilution methods. Ann. Intern. Med., 56:535, 1962.
60. Castillo, C.A., et al.: Simulated shunt curves. Am. J. Cardiol., 17:691, 1966.
61. Dalen, J.E.: Shunt detection and measurement. In Cardiac Catheterization and Angiography. Edited by W. Grossman. Philadelphia, Lea & Febiger, 1974, p. 96.
62. Gorlin, R., and Gorlin, S.G.: Hydraulic formula for calculation of the area of the stenotic mitral valve, other

cardiac valves, and central circulatory shunts. Am. Heart J., 41:1, 1951.
63. Cohen, M.V., and Gorlin, R.: Modified orifice equation for the calculation of mitral valve area. Am. Heart J., 84:839, 1969.
64. Scherlag, B.J., et al.: Catheter technique for recording His bundle activity in man. Circulation, 39:13, 1969.
65. Damato, A.N., et al.: Recordings of specialized conducting fibers (AV nodal, His bundle, and right bundle branch) in man using an electrode catheter technique. Circulation, 39:435, 1969.
66. Rosen, K.M., et al.: Bundle branch and ventricular activity in man: a study using catheter recording of left and right bundle branch potential Circulation, 43:193, 1971.
67. Miller, R.N.S., et al.: Studies of intra-atrial conduction in bipolar atrial and His electrograms. Br. Heart J., 35:604, 1973.
68. Denes, P., et al.: The effects of cycle length on cardiac refractory periods in man. Circulation, 49:32, 1974.
69. Wittig, J.H., and Boineau, J.P.: Surgical treatment of ventricular arrhythmias using epicardial, transmural, and endocardial mapping. Ann. Thorac. Surg., 20:117, 1975.
70. El-sherif, N., Scherlag, J.B., and Lazzara, R.: Electrode catheter recordings during malignant ventricular arrhythmia following experimental acute myocardial ischemia. Circulation, 51:1003, 1975.
71. Josephson, M.E., Horwitz, L.N., and Farshidi, A.: Continuous local electrical activity: a mechanism of recurrent ventricular tachycardia. Circulation, 59:659, 1978.
72. Frankl, W.S., and Greenspon, A.: Electrophysiologic testing: clinical applications. Cardiovasc. Clin., 13(3):301, 1983.
73. Josephson, M.E.: Ventricular Tachycardia: Mechanisms and Management. Mount Kisco, NY, Futura Publishing, 1982.
74. Lang, E.K.: A survey of the complications of percutaneous retrograde arteriography: Seldinger technique. Radiology, 81:257, 1963.
75. Hey, B., Jr., Dyrda, I., and Joyner, C.R.: Entanglement of a cardiac catheter on a heart valve prosthesis. N. Engl. J. Med., 275:434, 1966.
76. Wilson, W.J., Lee, G.B., and Amplatz, K.: Biplane selective coronary arteriography via percutaneous transfemoral approach. Am. J. Roentgenol., 100:332, 1967.
77. O'Brien, K.P., Glancy, D.L., and Brandt, P.W.T.: Cardiac catheterization: indications, current techniques, and complications. Australes. Radiol., 14:378, 1970.
78. Bristow, J.D., et al.: Late heparin-induced bleeding after retrograde arterial catheterization. Circulation, 37:393, 1968.
79. Jeresaty, R.M., and Liss, J.P.: Effects of brachial artery catheterization on arterial pulse and blood pressure in 203 patients. Am. Heart J., 76:481, 1968.
80. Kloster, F.E., Bristow, J.D., and Griswold, H.E.: Femoral artery occlusion following percutaneous catheterization. Am. Heart J., 79:175, 1970.
81. Campion, B.C., et al.: Arterial complications of retrograde brachial arterial catheterization. Mayo Clin. Proc., 46:589, 1971.
82. Murphy, T.O., Piper, C.A., and Anderson, C.L.: Complications of left heart catheterization. Am. Surg., 37:472, 1971.
83. Takaro, T., Pifarre, R., and Wuerflein, R.D.: Acute coronary occlusion following coronary arteriography: mechanisms and surgical relief. Surgery, 72:1018, 1972.
84. Chahine, R.A., Herman, M.V., and Gorlin, R.: Complications of coronary arteriography: comparison of the brachial to the femoral approach. Ann. Intern. Med., 76:862, 1972.
85. Gupta, P.K., and Haft, J.I.: Complete heart block complicating cardiac catheterization. Chest, 61:185, 1972.
86. Machleder, H.I., Sweeney, J.P., and Barker, W.F.: Pulseless arm after brachial artery catheterization. Lancet, 1:407, 1972.
87. Eshaghy, B., et al.: Mediastinal and retropharyngeal hemorrhage: a complication of cardiac catheterization. JAMA, 226:427, 1973.
88. Stanger, P., et al.: Complications of cardiac catheterization of neonates, infants and children. Circulation, 50:595, 1974.
89. Goodman, D.J., et al.: Thromboembolic complications with the indwelling balloon-tipped pulmonary arterial catheter. N. Engl. J. Med., 291:777, 1974.
90. Nicholas, G.G., and DeMuth, W.E.: Long-term results of brachial thrombectomy following cardiac catheterization. Ann. Surg., 183:436, 1976.
91. Dawson, D.M., and Fisher, E.G.: Neurologic complications of cardiac catheterization. Neurology, 27:496, 1977.
92. Pendergrass, H.P., et al.: Reactions associated with intravenous urography: historical and statistical review. Radiology, 71:1, 1958.

SECTION 3
BEDSIDE HEMODYNAMIC MONITORING

FLOW-DIRECTED CATHETERS

Flow-directed catheters were originally constructed for clinical use without fluoroscopy.[1-5] These original catheters frequently failed, however, because of the length of time it took to pass them into the pulmonary artery. Withdrawal of blood samples was difficult, and clotting was a frequent problem. Ventricular arrhythmias were also common during the passage of the catheters. The development of balloon-tipped, flow-guided catheters by Swan, Ganz, and Forrester overcame most of these problems.[6]

The catheter, with a balloon inflated at its tip as a guide, is carried by the circulation from the great intrathoracic veins into the pulmonary artery or into other areas of the vascular bed. These Swan-Ganz, flow-directed catheters have revolutionized our ability to monitor acutely ill patients at the bedside.

The inflated balloon protrudes over the tip of the catheter itself (Fig. 17-26). This feature prevents the tip of the catheter from coming into repeated contact with the endocardium by manipulation or with the action of the beating right ventricle, thus avoiding damage to the endocardium or the induction of arrhythmias. The pulmonary artery pressure and pulmonary artery wedge pressure are obtained

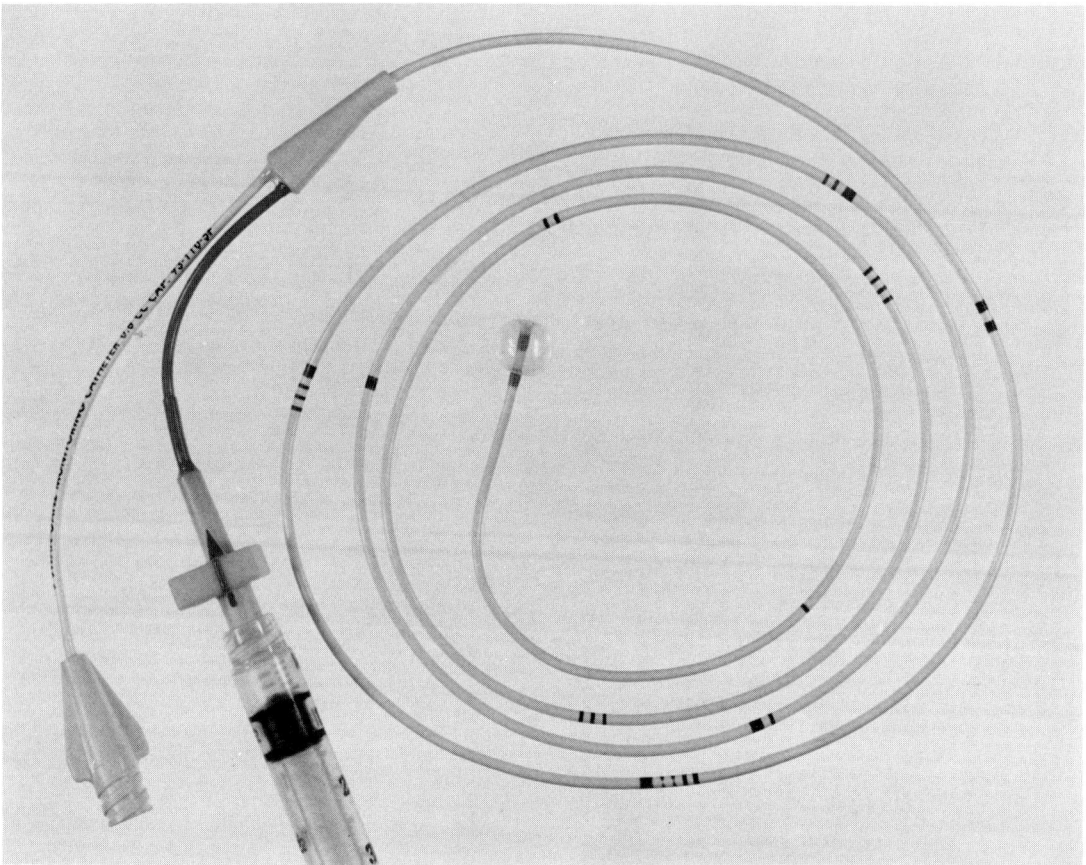

FIG. 17-26. Swan-Ganz catheter, showing an inflated balloon. For details, see the text.

from the same position without repeated manipulations merely by inflating and deflating the balloon. The catheter is made of polyvinyl chloride and has a soft, pliable shaft that softens further at body temperatures. The balloon opening is 1 to 2 mm from the tip. The usual catheter is 110 cm long and is either 5 or 7 French in external diameter. Each of these catheters has two lumens. One is small, for inflating the balloon, and the other is large, with an opening at the tip of the catheter for measuring pressures and withdrawing blood samples. The 7-French catheter has a preformed curvature at the balloon tip to enhance its ability to pass through the right ventricle. Shorter 60- to 70-mm catheters are manufactured in 4- to 5-French diameters for pediatric use. Also available are triple-lumen catheters that are 110-cm long and 7-French in external diameter; these catheters have both proximal and distal ports, which permit simultaneous measurement of right atrial and pulmonary artery or pulmonary wedge pressures. All these catheters have balloons constructed such that inflation with 0.8 ml gas produces a protrusion above and around the tip of the catheter. The catheter is radiopaque, thus fluoroscopic visualization is possible.

INDICATIONS FOR FLOW-GUIDED CATHETERIZATION

Adults

ROUTINE CARDIAC CATHETERIZATION. The Swan-Ganz catheter has achieved acceptance in cardiac catheterization laboratories because passage into the right ventricle and pulmonary artery can often be accomplished in the same time or in less time than with the use of semirigid, nonfloating catheters and with a lower incidence of serious arrhythmias.[6,7] Pressure tracings are taken as the catheter moves through the right atrium and the right ventricle and into the pulmonary artery, until a pulmonary capillary wedge pressure is obtained (Fig. 17-27).

CARDIAC CARE UNITS. The ability to catheterize the pulmonary artery at the patient's bedside without the need for fluoroscopy and with a low incidence of serious arrhythmias allows rapid and accurate assessment of cardiac performance in seriously ill patients. The most frequent use of the Swan-Ganz catheter is in the hospital's cardiac care unit. Recording pressures from the pulmonary artery and

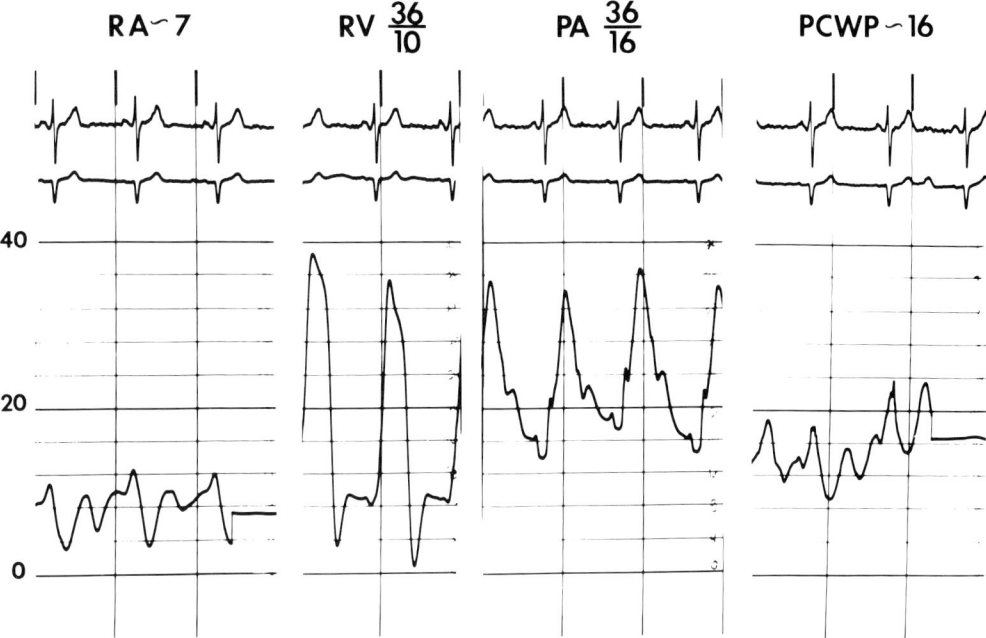

FIG. 17-27. Normal values found in the Swan-Ganz catheterization of a patient with uncomplicated acute myocardial infarction. RA, Right atrial pressure; RV, right ventricular pressure; PA, pulmonary artery pressure; PCWP, pulmonary capillary wedge pressure. For details, see the text.

from the pulmonary capillary wedge position and sampling blood from the right heart facilitate the diagnosis of acute mitral regurgitation due to papillary muscle dysfunction or rupture (Fig. 17-28), rupture of the interventricular septum (Fig. 17-29), right ventricular infarction (Fig. 17-30), and pulmonary embolism. The use of cardiac catheterization in the patient with myocardial infarction has improved our ability to treat these patients and has improved survival rates. These catheters are also used in the management of patients with unstable angina or severe congestive heart failure, in whom drugs may be administered more appropriately with the knowledge of their effect on hemodynamics. Flow-directed catheters with special electrodes may enable one to recognize arrhythmias and may also be used for emergency pacing.[6,8,9]

SURGICAL PATIENTS. The use of the flow-directed catheter permits hemodynamic monitoring for intraoperative and postoperative fluid management, evaluation of ventricular function, and the diagnosis of pulmonary embolism.[10-12]

Infants and Children

The small, flow-directed catheters are more flexible and may be used to measure cardiac output and pressures. These catheters have been used in children in whom the exact anatomic features of the cardiac chambers are not known because of complex congenital abnormalities, such as transposition of the great vessels. Other uses are for passage of the catheter into the left atrium, left ventricle, and aorta, to avoid retrograde arterial catheterization in patients with partial or total anomalous pulmonary venous return, and in patients with the Wolff-Parkinson-White syndrome or Ebstein's anomaly, in whom catheter manipulation may produce arrhythmias.[13-16] When a flow-directed catheter enters the aorta or any large artery, however, care must be taken to avoid occlusion of a major vessel such as the carotid artery or the descending aorta. This complication may be avoided by continuous pressure monitoring and by partial deflation of the balloon to maintain its position.

TECHNIQUE

Prior to insertion of the catheter, the balloon should be tested by inflating it up to 0.8 ml with saline solution, to ensure the balloon's integrity. The catheter may be inserted in a number of ways. The percutaneous route may be used if a large enough vein can be found; a cut-down technique is also possible. The antecubital, internal jugular, subclavian, and femoral veins may be used. The catheter may be advanced about 40 cm when the right antecubital vein is used and 50 cm when the left antecubital vein is used. The balloon is then inflated and is advanced under continuous pressure and electrocardiographic monitoring.

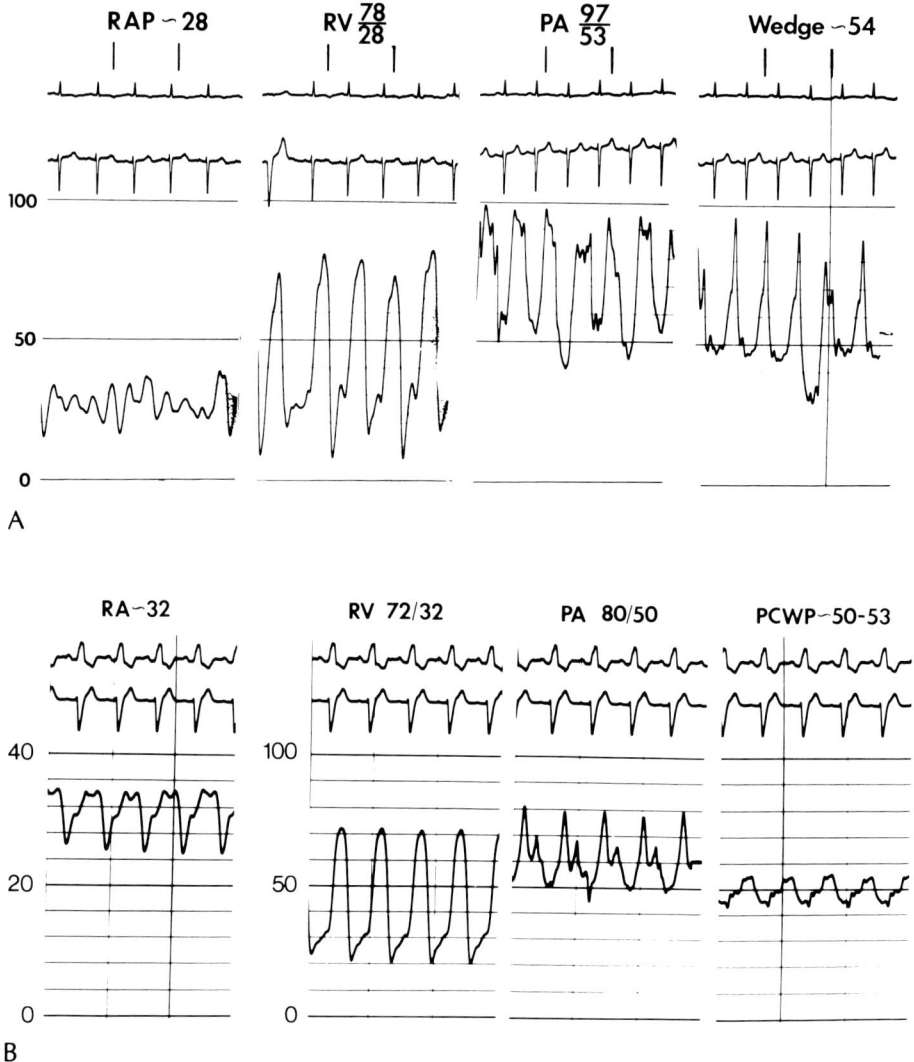

FIG. 17-28. *A,* Swan-Ganz catheterization recorded in a patient with acute mitral regurgitation due to severe papillary muscle dysfunction during acute inferior wall myocardial infarction. Note the elevated right heart pressures, with huge "V" waves seen in the "wedge" tracing as tall, sharp, spiking deflections. RAP, Right atrial pressure; RV, right ventricular pressure; PA, pulmonary artery pressure; Wedge, mean pulmonary capillary wedge pressure. *B,* Swan-Ganz catheterization recorded in a patient with acute mitral regurgitation due to papillary muscle dysfunction during acute inferior wall myocardial infarction. Note the high right heart pressures, but the absence of large "V" waves in the pulmonary capillary wedge (PCWP) tracing. RA, Right atrial pressure; RV, right ventricular pressure; PA, pulmonary artery pressure.

Air is generally used to inflate the balloon, but if any chance exists that the catheter may pass into the left side of the heart or into a systemic artery, carbon dioxide should be used. Carbon dioxide diffuses through Latex, however, and causes the balloon to deflate within several minutes, with protrusion of the tip of the catheter above the balloon. Thus, if the catheter has not been inserted successfully within 2 min after balloon inflation, the balloon should be reinflated with another 0.8 ml carbon dioxide. The inflation volume needed to obtain a pulmonary capillary wedge pressure may vary with time. The contractions of the right ventricle may advance the catheter tip into a smaller branch of the pulmonary artery and, therefore, the volume of air required to obtain a satisfactory wedge pressure may be much smaller. In such a case, inflation of the balloon to its full capacity may produce overdistention and potential damage to the pulmonary artery wall. It may also result in a false elevation of the wedge pressure or damping. Thus, it is necessary to inflate the balloon gradually while continuously monitoring the pulmonary artery pressure. Inflation of the balloon should be discontinued

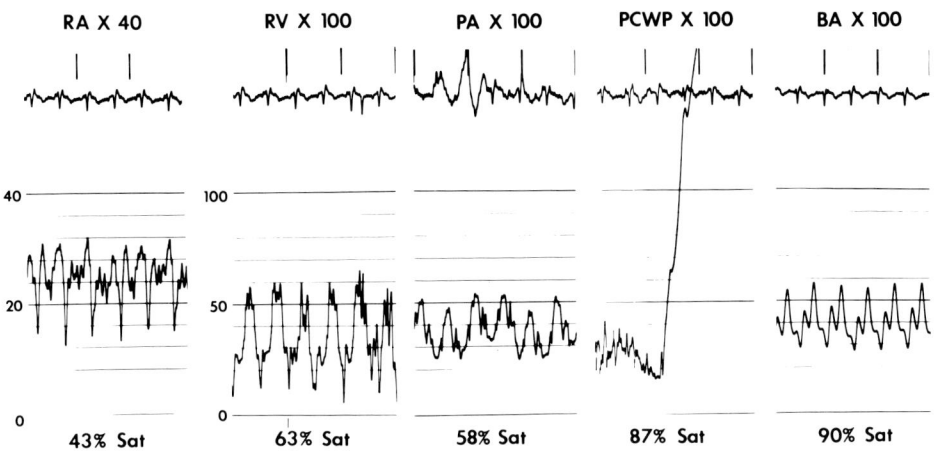

FIG. 17-29. Swan-Ganz catheterization in a patient with ventricular septal rupture during an acute inferior wall infarction. Diagnosis is made by the presence of elevated right heart pressures and an oxygen "step-up" at the ventricular level (43% in right atrium and 63% in right ventricle). Ventricular septal rupture and acute mitral regurgitation may mimic each other clinically and even hemodynamically. The differential is made with the Swan-Ganz catheter by the detection of the oxygen "step-up" in the right ventricle, which is present with the ventricular septal rupture but not with the acute mitral regurgitation. RA, Right atrium; RV, right ventricle; PA, pulmonary artery; PCWP, pulmonary capillary wedge pressure; BA, brachial artery.

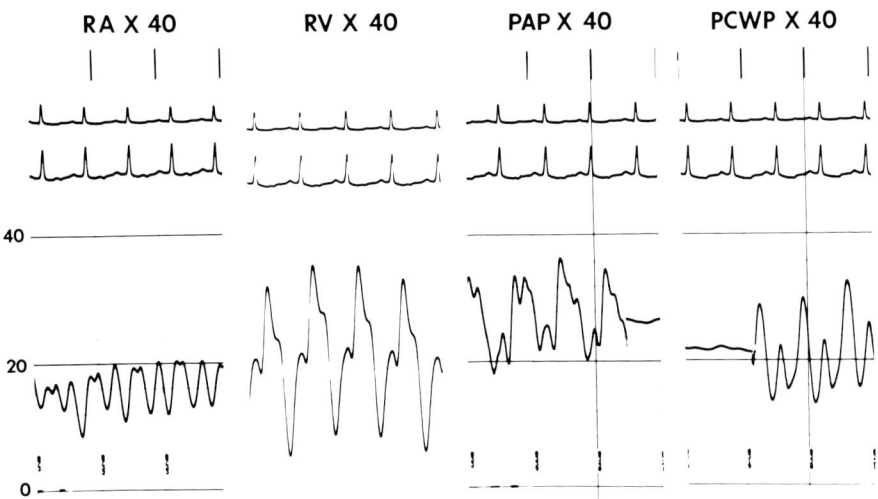

FIG. 17-30. Swan-Ganz catheterization in a patient with right ventricular infarction seen as part of the syndrome of acute inferoposterior myocardial infarction. The right atrial mean pressure, right ventricular end-diastolic pressure, pulmonary artery diastolic pressure, and mean pulmonary capillary wedge pressure are all equilibrated and are essentially equal. One sees a so-called "dip and plateau" in the right ventricular pressure tracing. This entire hemodynamic pattern closely resembles constrictive pericarditis, but the differentiation should be obvious in the setting of acute inferior wall myocardial infarction. RA, right atrium; RV, right ventricle; PAP, pulmonary artery pressure; PCWP, pulmonary capillary wedge pressure.

immediately as soon as one notes a change from pulmonary artery to pulmonary capillary wedge pressure.

It is necessary to confirm a pulmonary capillary wedge position by aspirating the blood from the catheter tip and by observing an oxygen saturation of 95% or greater. Technical difficulties may cause confusion, however. If the pulmonary capillary wedge pressure is obtained from a large pulmonary artery, it is often necessary to withdraw between 5 and 15 mm of blood before the fully oxygenated pulmonary capillary blood enters the syringe. The reason is that blood is present in the pulmonary artery between the catheter tip and the pulmonary capillary network and must be withdrawn before obtaining confirmation by oxygen saturation.

It may be difficult to maneuver the standard flow-directed catheter into the pulmonary artery in patients with a large right heart chamber. Various maneuvers may be undertaken to pass the catheter, including use of the Valsalva maneuver, deep inspiration, and stiffening of the catheter by flushing it with iced solutions.

USES AND INTERPRETATION

Pressures

Pressures obtained from the tip of flow-directed catheters after occlusion of the pulmonary artery by the inflated balloon are virtually identical to those recorded by conventional catheters in the pulmonary capillary wedge position. In the absence of mitral valve disease and pulmonary vascular hypertension, the pulmonary capillary wedge pressure is an accurate indicator of mean left atrial pressure and therefore of left ventricular end-diastolic pressure. Because pulmonary artery end-diastolic pressure is only about 1 to 3 mm higher than mean pulmonary capillary wedge pressure, pulmonary artery end-diastolic pressure is often used as an indicator of mean left atrial pressure in patients without mitral valve disease or pulmonary hypertension. On the other hand, if the pulmonary artery end-diastolic pressure exceeds the pulmonary capillary wedge pressure by 6 mm Hg or more, pulmonary arterial vascular disease should be suspected. Similarly, in patients with severe mitral regurgitation with large V waves, the mean pulmonary capillary wedge pressure is often greater than the pulmonary artery end-diastolic pressure.

Cardiac Output

Cardiac output is measured through flow-directed catheters by the use of the thermodilution technique. This method is similar to the dye-dilution technique and is based on the principle of the injection of a cold material at one point in the circulation and the measurement of the change in intravascular temperature beyond that point (Fig. 17–31). Saline solution or dextrose and water at room temperature, or ice-cold saline solution, is injected rapidly into the superior vena cava, the inferior vena cava, or the right atrium in quantities of 10 ml in adults and 5 ml or less in children. The Swan-Ganz, flow-directed, thermodilution catheter has a triple lumen: a large lumen that opens at the tip for measurement of the pulmonary artery and pulmonary capillary wedge pressures, a second large lumen that opens 30 cm from the tip for injection of the cold saline solution or dextrose and water, and a small lumen for inflation of the balloon. A small thermistor for the measurement of the blood temperature in the pulmonary arteries is located 4 cm from the tip. The thermodilution method is accurate and is particularly advantageous in the management of severely ill patients because it does not require withdrawal and reinfusion of blood or arterial puncture.[17,18] The indicator is inert and inexpensive, calibration is simple and accurate, recirculation is minimal, and the primary curve is suitable for computer analysis of cardiac output.

Placement of Temporary Ventricular Pacing Electrodes

Flow-directed catheters with two platinum electrodes mounted at the tip of the catheter are ideal for temporary pacing. As the catheter is inserted, the intracardiac electrogram is recorded from the tip of the electrode and indicates the location of the catheter. When a right ventricular electrogram is seen, the balloon is deflated, to prevent it from floating into the pulmonary artery. The catheter tip is then advanced to the apex of the right ventricle. Two models of this catheter are available. One model is designed for insertion from the femoral vein and has a J-shaped tip for greater stability when it is placed in the apex of the right ventricle (Fig. 17–32). The other type is designed for insertion through the superior vena cava and is a straight catheter. Bedside insertion of these flow-directed pacing catheters may be performed quickly and accurately with the use of the electrocardiogram from the electrode tip as the guide.

Intracavitary Electrocardiography

Some flow-directed catheters not only record pulmonary artery and pulmonary capillary wedge pressures, but also provide the ability to monitor the intracavitary electrocardiogram from the right atrium and the right ventricle. Platinum electrodes are mounted on the Swan-Ganz catheter at 26 and 28 cm for monitoring right atrial intracavitary electrocardiograms. With the use of appropriate filters, 50- to 300-Hz filters for the right atrium and 15- to 300-Hz filters for the right ventricle, one may record stable intercavitary electrocardiograms. This advance is important because it allows for a more rapid and precise diagnosis of arrhythmias. In the future, it may enable one to devise more accurate alarm systems based on heart rate and, ultimately, more accurate means of computer analysis of cardiac rhythms.

COMPLICATIONS

Rupture of the Balloon

Should the balloon rupture, the flotation properties of the catheter would be lost. The injection of air into the right heart chambers or into the pulmonary artery is probably of no consequence, except in children with congenital heart disease who may have right-to-left shunting.

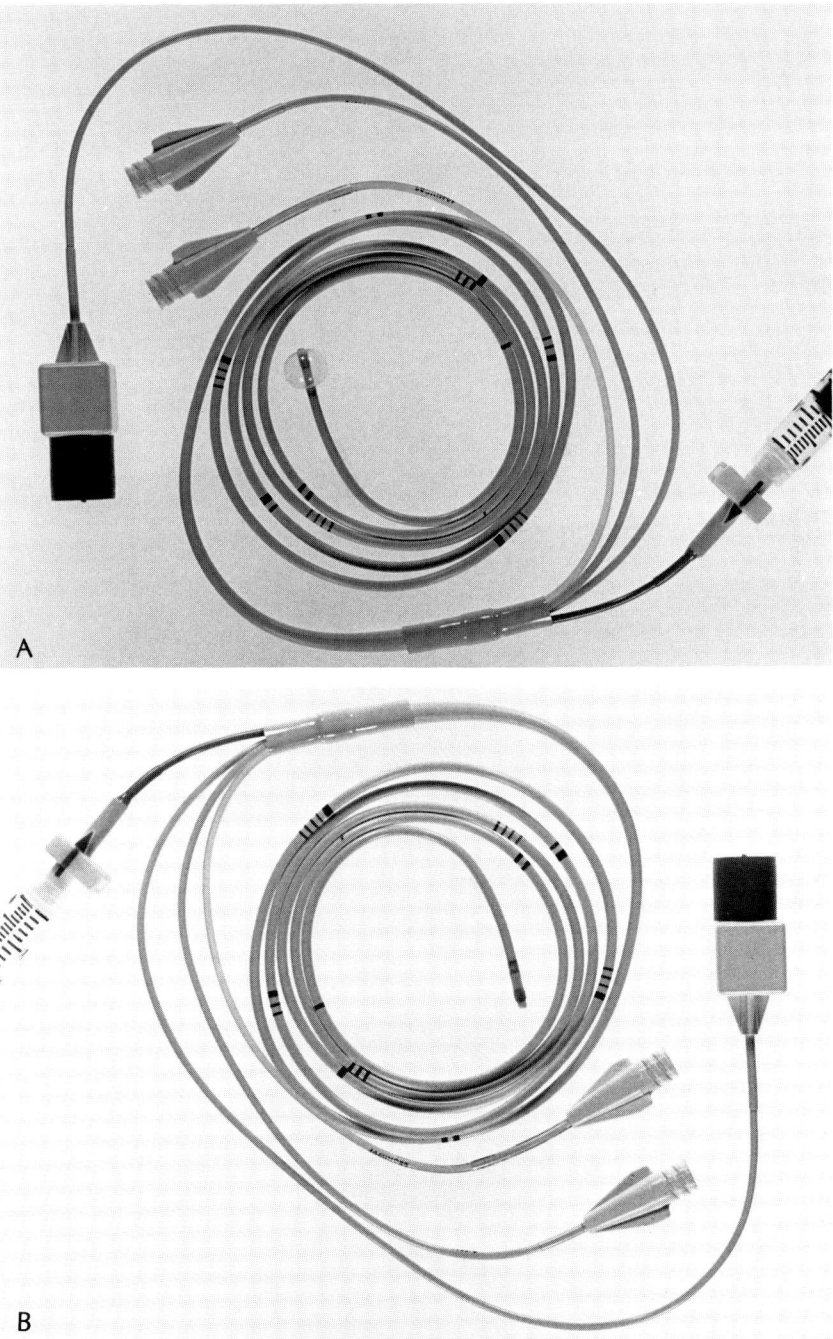

FIG. 17–31. Thermodilution Swan-Ganz catheter for cardiac output determinations with balloon inflated *(A)* and deflated *(B)*. For details, see the text.

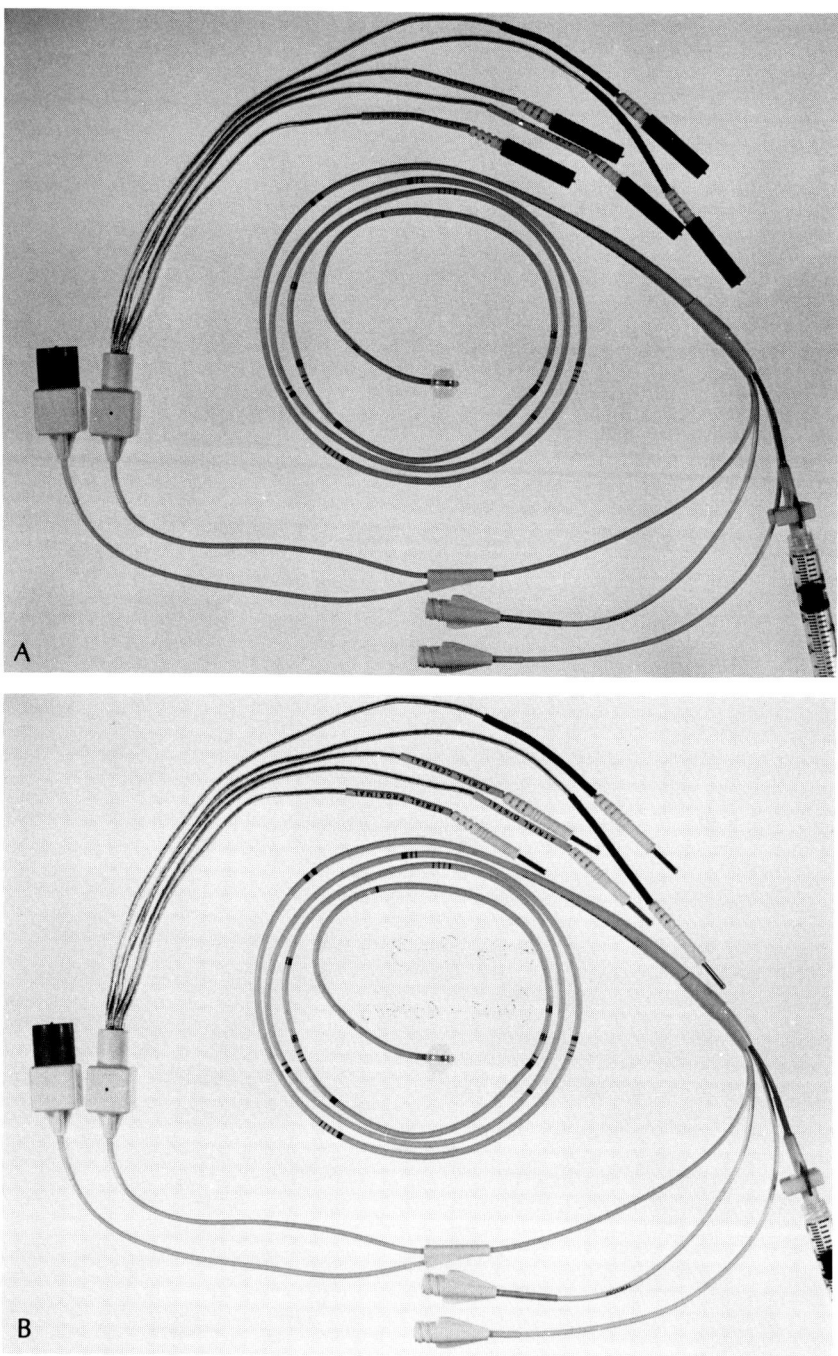

FIG. 17–32. Inflated Swan-Ganz catheter for pacing and thermodilution cardiac output determinations with (A) and without (B) covers for the electrodes. For details, see the text.

Pulmonary Artery Infarction

Ideally, the catheter tip should be placed in either the right or left main branches of the pulmonary artery. Even when the balloon is deflated, these flow-directed catheters usually advance into a distal branch because of right ventricular contraction. Pulmonary artery wedging may occur inadvertently and, if unrecognized, may result in segmental pulmonary infarction. Thus, the catheter tip pressure must be carefully monitored by frequent observation of the pressure curve, fluoroscopy, and chest roentgenograms. The best position for the catheter is one in which inflation of the balloon to full capacity will produce a change from pulmonary artery to pulmonary capillary wedge pressure. Medical personnel should understand the significance of an apparently damped pressure indicating pulmonary artery wedging, and one should determine the location of the catheter.

Pulmonary Artery Perforation

Pulmonary artery rupture and fatal pulmonary hemorrhage may be caused by flow-directed balloon tipped catheters.[19,20] To reduce risk, the balloon should be inflated gradually and under visual inspection of the pulmonary artery waveform. Inflation should be discontinued as soon as one notes a change from pulmonary artery to pulmonary capillary wedge pressure. The balloon should remain inflated for only brief periods of time, especially in patients who have pulmonary hypertension. A large amount of fluid may be accidently injected under high pressure into the balloon and may rupture the pulmonary artery. To prevent this complication, the syringe with air or carbon dioxide should remain attached to the lumen for balloon inflation.

Arrhythmias

Significant arrhythmias are not common during insertion of Swan-Ganz catheters. As previously mentioned, the reason probably is that the right ventricular endocardium is protected from the catheter tip by the inflated balloon. Nonetheless, a defibrillator should be by the patient's bedside when the Swan-Ganz catheter is inserted.

Knotting of the Catheter

Intercardiac knotting of Swan-Ganz catheters has been reported.[21,22] Knotting is likely due to a loop in the right ventricle. Because the catheter is soft, it may be withdrawn to the site of vein insertion, and a small incision may be made to remove the tightened knot from the vein. This method of removal is not always possible, however, and the catheter may have to remain in place permanently. The development of ventricular arrhythmias during right atrial pressure recording suggests the complication of knotting. If right ventricular or pulmonary artery pressure is not recorded when the catheter has been advanced 15 cm from the right atrium or the right ventricle, it is likely that a loop has formed in the right atrium or right ventricle, and the catheter should be withdrawn and the procedure repeated.

Miscellaneous Complications

All the usual complications of cardiac catheterization can occur with flow-directed catheters. These complications include infection, thrombophlebitis, and clotting within the catheter. To prevent these complications a continuous, slow perfusion of heparinized 5% dextrose and water should be maintained. Other complications reported with flow-directed catheters include pulmonary thromboembolism, pulmonary valve injury, and ruptured chordae tendineae of the tricuspid valve.[23-25]

ACCEPTANCE BY THE PATIENT

It is obvious that the use of flow-directed catheters is indicated primarily in patients who are seriously ill; such patients generally accept the necessity for this invasive procedure. The most common complaint is the stiffness that results from keeping the arm or leg in a stationary position. If complications arise, the level of the patient's acceptance is reduced.

COST

Because patients who require flow-directed catheterization are in a hospital intensive care unit, the overall cost of their care is high. The catheters themselves cost $26.50 for an ordinary Swan-Ganz catheter, $80.00 for the thermodilution Swan-Ganz catheter, and $220.00 for the pacing Swan-Ganz catheter. These costs are trivial in patients in whom monitoring of intracardiac pressures may be lifesaving.

REFERENCES

1. Dotter, C.T., and Straub, K.R.: Flow-guided cardiac catheterization. Am. J. Roentgenol., 88:27, 1962.
2. Bradley, R.D.: Diagnostic right-heart catheterization with miniature catheters in severely ill patients. Lancet, 2:941, 1964.
3. Carr, I., and Wells, B.: Coaxial flow-guided catheterization of the pulmonary artery in transposition of the great arteries. Lancet, 2:318, 1966.
4. Winkler, J.B., and Duprey, R.: Pulmonary angiography using a flow-guided catheter: construction and applications. Radiol. Technol., 39:23, 1967.
5. Scheinman, M.M., Abbott, J.A., and Rapaport, E.: Clinical uses of a flow-directed right heart catheter. Arch. Intern. Med., 124:19, 1969.
6. Swan, H.J.C., Ganz, W., and Forrester, J.: Catheterization of the heart in man with use of a flow-directed balloon-tipped catheter. N. Engl. J. Med., 283:447, 1970.

7. Steele, P., and Davies, H.: The Swan-Ganz catheter in the cardiac laboratory. Br. Heart J., 35:647, 1973.
8. Mond, H.G., Hunt, D., and Sloman, G.: Hemodynamic haemodynamic monitoring in the coronary care unit using the Swan-Ganz right heart catheter. Br. Heart J., 35:635, 1973.
9. Swan, H.J.C., and Ganz, W.: The use of balloon-tipped flow-directed catheters in monitoring patients with acute myocardial infarction. In Myocardial Infarction. Edited by E. Corday and H.J.C. Swan. Baltimore, Williams & Wilkins, 1973.
10. Cerra, F., Milch, R., and Lajos, T.Z.: Pulmonary catheterization in critically ill surgical patients. Ann. Surg., 177:37, 1973.
11. Rosenbaum, R.W., et al.: The importance of pulmonary artery pressure monitoring. Surg. Gynecol. Obstet., 136:261, 1973.
12. Civetta, J.M., and Gabel, J.C.: Flow-directed pulmonary artery catheterization in surgical patients: indications and modifications of technique. Ann. Surg., 176:753, 1972.
13. Kelly, D.T., Krovetz, L.J., and Rowe, R.D.: Double-lumen flotation catheter for use in complex congenital cardiac anomalies. Circulation, 44:910, 1971.
14. Stanger, P., et al.: Use of the Swan-Ganz catheter in cardiac catheterization of infants and children. Am. Heart J., 83:749, 1972.
15. Black, J.F.S.: Floating a catheter into the pulmonary artery in transposition of the great arteries. Am. Heart J., 84:761, 1972.
16. Jones, S.M., and Miller, G.A.H.: Catheterization of the pulmonary artery and transposition of the great arteries using a Swan-Ganz flow-directed catheter. Br. Heart J., 35:298, 1973.
17. Branthwaite, M.A., and Bradley, R.D.: Measurement of cardiac output by thermodilution in man. J. Appl. Physiol., 24:434, 1968.
18. Ganz, W., et al.: A new technique for measurement of cardiac output by thermodilution in man. Am. J. Cardiol., 27:392, 1971.
19. Lapin, E.S., and Murray, J.A.: Hemoptysis with flow-directed cardiac catheterization. JAMA, 220:1246, 1972.
20. Pape, L.A., Haffajee, M.B., and Markis, J.E.: Fatal pulmonary hemorrhage after use of the flow-directed balloon-tipped catheter. Ann. Intern. Med., 90:344, 1979.
21. Lipp, H., O'Donoghue, K., and Resnekov, L.: Intracardiac knotting of a flow-directed catheter. N. Engl. J. Med., 284:220, 1971.
22. Meister, S.G., et al.: Knotting of a flow-directed catheter about a cardiac structure. Cathet. Cardiovasc. Diagn. 3:171, 1977.
23. Goodman, D.J., et al.: Thromboembolic complications with the indwelling balloon-tipped pulmonary arterial catheter. N. Engl. J. Med., 291:777, 1974.
24. Smith, W.R., Glauser, F.L., and Jemison, P.: Ruptured chordae of the tricuspid valve: the consequence of flow-directed Swan-Ganz catheterization. Chest, 70:790, 1976.
25. O'Toole, J.D., et al.: Pulmonary-valve injury and insufficiency during pulmonary artery catheterization. N. Engl. J. Med., 301:1167, 1979.

18

Prolonged Esophageal pH Monitoring

Luigi Bonavina ▪ Tom R. DeMeester

Gastroesophageal reflux accounts for approximately 75% of esophageal disorders and is among the most challenging diagnostic and therapeutic problems in benign esophageal disease. Prolonged esophageal pH monitoring is a diagnostic test for this disorder that is designed to quantitate the actual time during which the esophageal mucosa is exposed to refluxed acid gastric juice over a 24-hour period. This method provides objective evaluation of gastroesophgeal reflux by combining an analysis for reflux, clearance, and relation of symptoms to changes in intraesophageal pH. The 24-hour esophageal pH monitoring test combines 3 tests: (1) a quantitative pH reflux test, by recording the degree and pattern of esophageal acid exposure; (2) an acid-clearance test, by recording the duration of each reflux episode and by evaluating the ability of the body of the esophagus to clear refluxed acid; and (3) an endogenous acid-perfusion test (Bernstein), by assessing the time relationship of a reflux episode with heartburn experienced by the patient. Atypical symptoms of the disorder can be evaluated as well, by correlating these symptoms to the drops in esophageal pH associated with reflux.

Extensive clinical experience has proved the reliability and diagnostic usefulness of 24-hour esophageal pH monitoring in evaluating symptoms suggestive of GER disease.[1] Because of recent developments in ambulatory instrumentation for continuous esophageal pH monitoring, this test may become the initial and only evaluation required for identification of abnormal esophageal acid exposure and may thus become basic to the diagnosis of esophageal disorders.

TECHNIQUE

A pH probe is passed through the patient's nose and is positioned 5 cm above the superior border of the distal esophageal sphincter, which has already been located by infusion manometry.[2] A reference electrode is placed on the patient's anterior chest wall. The pH probe and reference electrode are connected to a pH meter and a strip-chart recorder or an ambulatory solid state microprocessor-based recorder. The system is standardized at pH values of 4.0 and 7.0.

Written instructions are given to patients, and they are specifically asked to record symptoms such as heartburn, regurgitation, belching, coughing, wheezing, and chest pain on the strip chart with a pencil or by pushing buttons on the microprocessor (Table 18–1). They are asked to note when they start and finish eating and when they drink. It is necessary to indicate changes in body position. While upright, patients are allowed to sit in a chair, stand, or walk about within the length of the leads of the machine. With the ambulatory apparatus there is no limitation on the patient's activity. Coffee and tea drinking and cigarette smoking are forbidden during the test, nor may the patient have carbonated beverages. A normal diet is served, unique only in the absence of food and beverages with a pH value less than 5.0 or greater than 6.0. A typical menu is shown in Table 18–2.

On completion of the test, the esophageal pH probe is advanced, to sample the pH of the stomach. The probe is then removed, and the calibration of the system is verified with standard pH solutions.

A typical esophageal pH monitoring record is shown in Figure 18–1. Acid reflux is defined as occurring whenever the esophageal pH drops below 4. The tracing is read by counting the number of reflux episodes and by measuring the duration of each episode in minutes. From these data, 6 components of the 24-hour record are tabulated: (1 to 3) the percentage of the time that the esophagus was exposed to pH less than 4 for the total 24-hour period and for the time spent in the upright and supine positions; (4) the total number of reflux episodes; (5) the number of reflux episodes lasting longer than 5 min; and (6) the duration of the longest reflux episode.

Similar measurements are made for alkaline reflux, according to the number and duration of episodes during which the esophageal pH rose above 7. Normal values for these components have been obtained from healthy volunteers and are shown in

*Table 18–1. Twenty-four-hour Esophageal pH Monitoring:
Instructions to the Patient*

Dear Patient:

The test you are having is important to you because it helps your doctor to determine the effectiveness of the valve at the lower end of your esophagus in preventing the leakage of acid from your stomach back into your esophagus. The results will form a basis for your future treatment. It is essential that certain instructions be followed; otherwise, we run the risk of drawing wrong conclusions from the test.

It is necessary that you do not take any *antacids* or *laxatives* during this test. Any medications should be checked by your doctor before you take them. We would like you to take all your meals during the period of the test from the dietician's specially controlled "pH diet." *No substitutions are allowed.* This is to control the acidity/alkalinity of the food entering your stomach. Please *do not* take any extremely *HOT OR COLD DRINKS;* otherwise, the delicate and expensive test probe may be damaged. The only liquids you may have are room-temperature water or milk with meals and room-temperature water between meals. *Do not* take any carbonated beverages, tea, or coffee. *SMOKING IS NOT ALLOWED DURING THE STUDY.* The machine should not be disconnected or switched off for any reason. You may either use a bedside commode or walk the whole cart into the bathroom. Please record the following on the chart paper *when it occurs:*

1. Body position: We prefer that you remain upright for 12 continuous hours and lie flat (with one pillow only) for 12 continuous hours. While upright, you may sit in a chair, sit vertically in bed, stand, or walk about within the length of the leads of the machine. Should it be necessary for you to change your position from upright to supine, kindly try to spend at least 2 hours in that position before alternating. Be sure to record this change by drawing a line with the pen.
2. Start of a meal.
3. End of a meal.
4. Drink of water between meals.
5. Vomiting, regurgitation, or belching.
6. Symptoms during the test, especially "heartburn," cough, wheezing, or any type of pain. This is important.

If you have any questions, please contact the nurse.

Thank you for helping us. The test will be of benefit in the diagnosis and treatment of your esophageal disorder.

Table 18–2. 24-hour Esophageal pH Monitoring: Diet

BREAKFAST	LUNCH	DINNER
Sugar	Sugar	Sugar
Salt	Salt	Salt
Pepper	Pepper	Pepper
Margarine × 3	Margarine × 2	Margarine × 2
1 cup Cream of Wheat	Cream of chicken soup	Cream of mushroom soup
2 slices of toast	Roast beef with gravy	Chicken breast supreme
1 cup 2% milk	Baked potato	Whipped potatoes
	Buttered green beans	Buttered carrots
	1 slice white bread	1 slice white bread
	Vanilla ice cream	Vanilla ice cream
	1 cup 2% milk	1 cup 2% milk

NOTES:

1. No substitutions or additions.
2. Only room-temperature water to be taken with meals or between meals; no fruit juices, coffee, tea, or carbonated beverages.

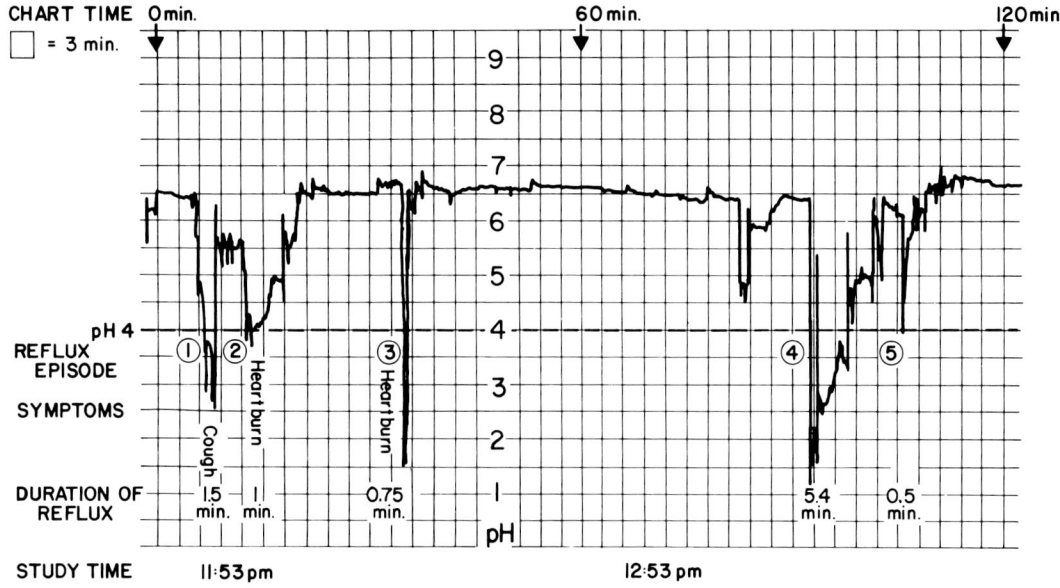

FIG. 18–1. Reproduction of a portion of a 24-hour pH record showing 5 (circled numbers) reflux episodes indicated by a drop in pH to below 4.0, the symptoms that occur concomitant with the reflux episode, and the duration of each reflux episode as measured by the chart speed.

Table 18–3. Normal Values for the 24-Hour Esophageal pH Monitoring Test

Total time pH < 4	< 4.2%
Upright time pH < 4	< 6.3%
Supine time pH < 4	< 1.22%
No. of reflux episodes	< 50
No. of reflux episodes longer than 5 min	3 or less
Duration of longest reflux episode	< 9.2 min
Overall acid score	< 17.92

Table 18–3. The upper limit of normal for the 6 components has been set at 2 standard deviations above the mean of that measured in control subjects.[3,4] An overall value for the 24-hour pH test is determined by calculating the 24-hour pH score. This score is obtained by referring to the scoring tables for the 6 major components of the 24-hour analysis and by recording the appropriate score for the measured value of each component. The scores are added, and a total score is obtained. A number exceeding the sum of scores for the normal upper limit of each component indicates an abnormal score. Recordings made with the microprocessor can be processed with a computer software program (see p. 363).

In reading the tracing, one must take care to note the relation of the recorded symptoms to the intraesophageal pH. This relationship often provides a valuable clue to the cause of atypical symptoms of esophageal disease.

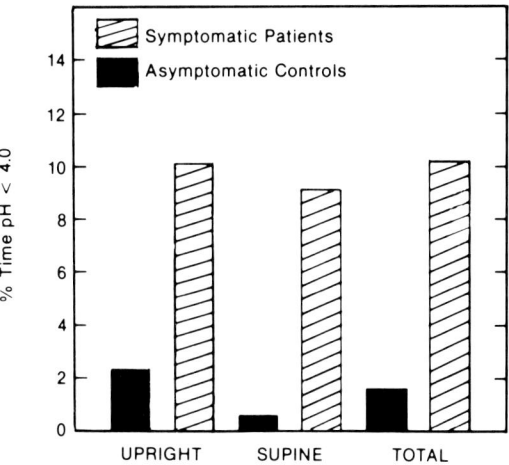

FIG. 18–2. Comparison of acid exposure time in asymptomatic control subjects and in symptomatic patients. Symptomatic subjects experience more acid exposure to esophageal mucosa than control subjects.

RATIONALE AND INDICATIONS

From observations made in normal control subjects, it is clear that everyone experiences gastroesophageal reflux at times, especially after meals. A distinct difference exists between this physiologic reflux and pathologic reflux, as shown in Figure 18–2. Supine nocturnal reflux is rare in normal people.

Patterns of Abnormal Reflux

By analyzing the results of prolonged esophageal pH monitoring in a variety of patients with symptomatic reflux and its complications, several patterns of abnormal reflux have been identified[5] (Fig. 18–3). Ten percent of patients with an abnormal acid score have abnormal reflux only in the upright position and are termed "upright refluxers." Twenty-six percent have reflux only in the supine position and are termed "supine refluxers." Sixty-four percent have reflux both in the upright and supine positions and are termed "combined" or "bipositional refluxers." Upright reflux is characterized by reflux episodes that are of short duration because of the aid of gravity and salivatory excretion on clearance of the refluxed gastric juice. Supine reflux is characterized by few reflux episodes, which are of long duration because of the loss of gravity and reduced swallowing and salivatory excretion during sleep.

The incidence of esophagitis progressively increases from 33% in upright refluxers to 46% in supine refluxers to 75% in combined refluxers. Similarly, the severity of esophagitis progressively rises with the type of reflux, and the natural history of the disease varies accordingly.[6] Only 4% of upright refluxers develop strictures, as compared to 20% of combined refluxers. Determining the pattern of reflux is of a great benefit in selecting therapy.

Patients with pure upright reflux are usually aerophagic and experience reflux caused by repetitive belching. A biphasic gastric-emptying pattern is common in these patients. An initial delay is followed by a rapid period of gastric emptying; this pattern suggests the presence of pyloric or duodenal disease and an overall disturbance of gastrointestinal motility. These patients often have symptoms suggestive of an irritable colon. Patients with pure upright reflux should be treated medically because a surgical antireflux procedure in these patients is associated with a high incidence of the gas-bloat syndrome.

Excessive acid exposure in patients who are symptomatic while supine is associated with reflux episodes of longer duration; this finding indicates impaired acid clearance from the esophagus when patients are recumbent. Patients with only supine reflux should be treated initially with medical therapy. Bethanechol, 25 mg taken prior to going to bed, and a 6-inch elevation of the head of the patient's bed, help to increase esophageal clearance of reflux acid during the night.[7] The addition of cimetidine reduces gastric acid secretion at night and helps to control symptoms.

Patients with combined reflux, have the most severe disease. One may attempt medical therapy, but patients with this pattern of reflux who have a severe mechanical defect of the cardia may develop a stricture while they are receiving intensive medical treatment[8] and should undergo a surgical antireflux procedure.

Relation of Symptoms to Reflux Episodes

One of the most important aspects of the 24-hour esophageal pH monitoring test is the relation of symptoms experienced during the monitoring period to the occurrence of a reflux episode. Symptoms may be unrelated to a reflux episode, they may immediately precede a reflux episode, or they may follow an episode. In approximately 30% of patients, the symptom to be evaluated does not occur during the monitored period, and remonitoring may be necessary.

Among 48 patients who underwent 24-hour esophageal pH monitoring for unexplained respiratory symptoms, 8 had positive test results for reflux, with documented episodes of aspiration, characterized by a drop in esophageal pH, followed by an acid taste in the mouth and the onset of cough or wheezing spell, during the monitored period (Fig. 18–4). Five of these patients noted complete relief of symptoms when a surgical antireflux procedure was performed. In the remaining 40 patients, the

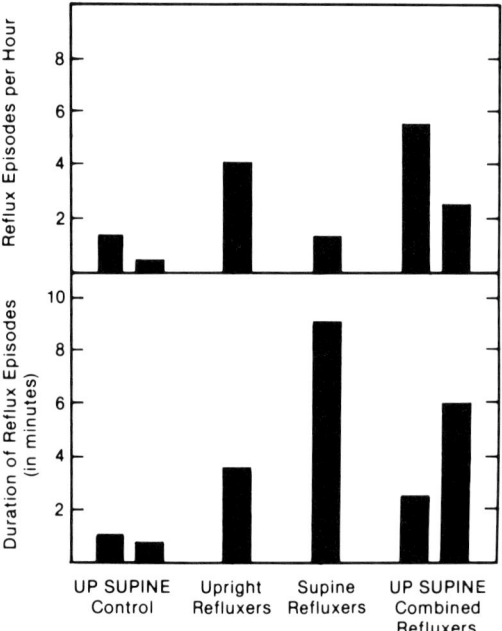

FIG. 18–3. Relationship of reflux pattern with number and duration of reflux episodes in symptomatic patients and asymptomatic persons. Symptomatic patients experience more reflux episodes of longer duration than healthy volunteers. Supine reflux episodes have the longest duration and may be the most detrimental.

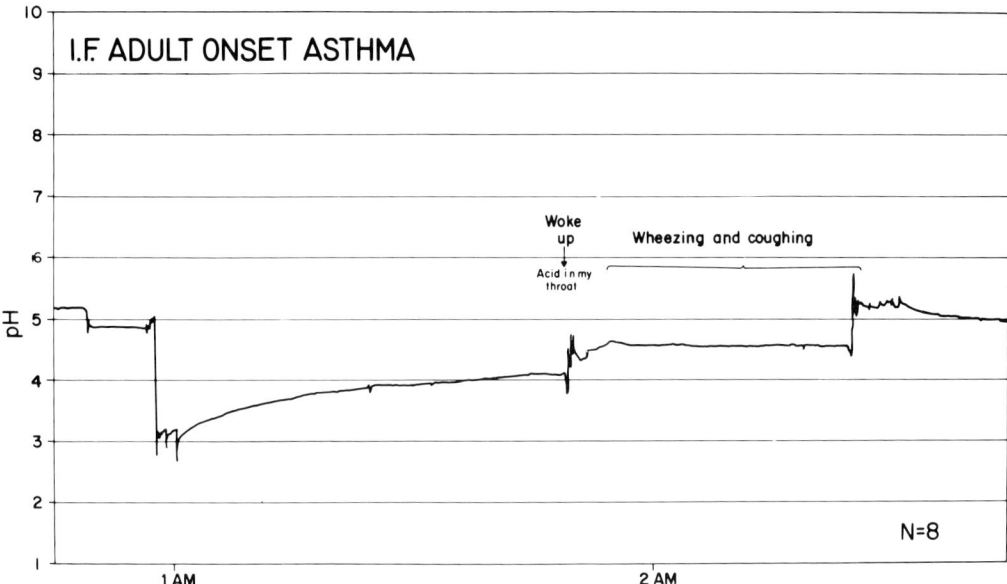

FIG. 18–4. A portion of a 24-hour pH record of a patient (I.F.) with asthma. One sees the relationship between a nocturnal reflux episode and the onset of respiratory symptoms.

respiratory symptoms induced the reflux episode, were unrelated to the reflux episodes, or failed to occur during the monitored period.[9]

Fifty patients who had had an episode of severe chest pain sufficient to require coronary angiography to rule out heart disease and who were subsequently shown to have normal coronary arteries underwent 24-hour esophageal pH monitoring. In 23 of these patients, or 46%, the 24-hour test results suggested a diagnosis of reflux. Seventy-three percent of these patients noted total abolition of chest pain by surgical or medical antireflux therapy. Patients whose chest pain coincided with a reflux episode documented on 24-hour pH monitoring had a 100% response to treatment.[10]

An additional 11 patients had previously undergone coronary artery bypass grafting without relief of their chest pain, even though the grafts were patent. Evidence of gastroesophageal reflux disease, as assessed by 24-hour esophageal pH monitoring, was present in 7 patients, and in 4 patients, the onset of chest pain was associated with a reflux episode (Fig. 18–5). All patients were completely free of chest pain after fundoplication.

Seventy-four percent of patients evaluated for symptoms following gastric operations had unrecognized gastroesophageal reflux, which caused postgastrectomy syndrome.[11] Similarly, in 62% of patients with recurrent symptoms after esophageal myotomy and in 63% of patients with symptoms after an antireflux procedure, symptoms were due to the failure to control reflux, as assessed by prolonged esophageal pH monitoring.[1] Endoscopic examination does not allow one to detect gastroesophageal reflux reliably in these patients, and the 24-hour esophageal pH monitoring test was invaluable in helping to solve these difficult clinical problems and thereby in helping to provide a rational basis for management.

Indications for Monitoring

Current indications for 24-hour esophageal pH monitoring are as follows:

1. The presence of typical symptoms of gastroesophageal reflux when the diagnosis is in question or when the pattern of reflux needs to be identified.
2. The presence of atypical symptoms of gastroesophageal reflux.
3. The presence of symptoms suggestive of gastroesophageal reflux in patients with other abdominal or thoracic diseases.
4. The presence of dysphagia and esophageal motility disorders thought to be secondary to gastroesophageal reflux.
5. The suspicion of gastroesophageal reflux in pediatric or disabled patients who are unable to communicate their symptoms.
6. Prior to initial surgical therapy for gastroesophageal reflux.
7. The recurrence of symptoms in patients with a history of esophageal or gastric operations.

COMPARISON WITH OTHER TESTS

Twenty-four-hour esophageal pH monitoring is comparable to other diagnostic tests for gastro-

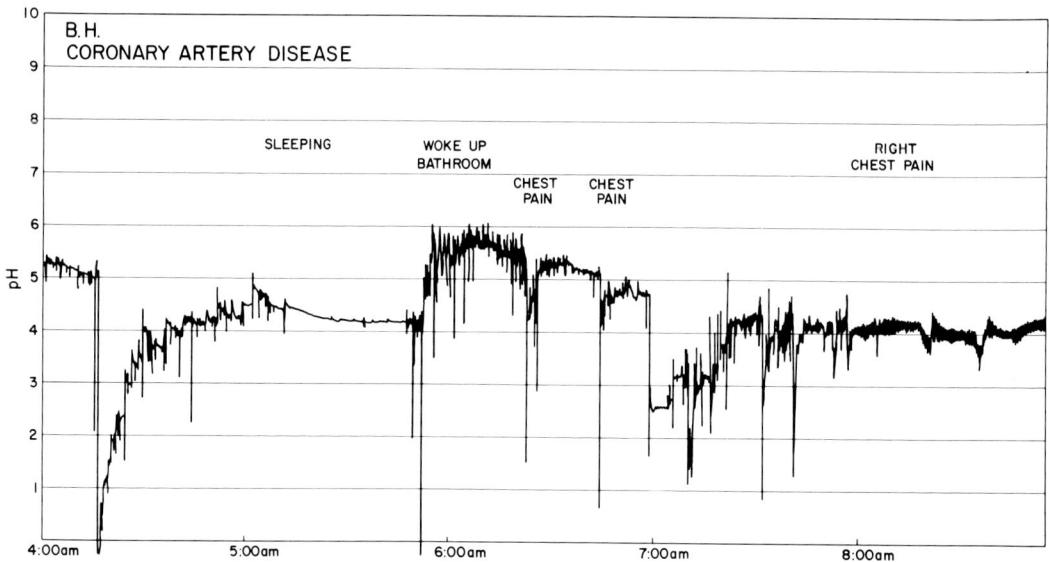

FIG. 18–5. A portion of a 24-hour pH record of a patient (B.H.) with coronary artery disease. One sees the relationship between several reflux episodes and chest pain.

esophageal reflux disease in terms of specificity, which allows one to exclude the diagnosis of a disease when it is known to be absent. The major differences among these tests are in sensitivity, which enables one to detect disease when it is known to be present[12] (Fig. 18–6). The two most popular tests, the lower esophageal sphincter pressure measurement and the standard acid reflux test, allow one to detect only 58 and 84% of reflux in symptomatic patients, respectively.

Esophagoscopy is an insensitive method of diagnosing gastroesophageal reflux because of the inconsistency among endoscopists in recognizing the subtle changes in the esophageal mucosa that are characteristic of grade I esophagitis. The relation of endoscopic findings to 24-hour esophageal pH monitoring has been reported, in a study of 199 patients with symptoms typical of reflux. Fifty-five percent of the 96 patients with normal results of endoscopic examination had positive results of the 24-hour esophageal pH test. Of 103 patients with typical symptoms and esophagitis, 90% had positive test results.[1] From these data, it can be concluded that when the results of the 24-hour pH test are normal and when no esophagitis is seen endoscopically, regardless of the presence of symptoms typical of gastroesophageal reflux, the patient's symptoms probably have another cause. Biopsy, to obtain

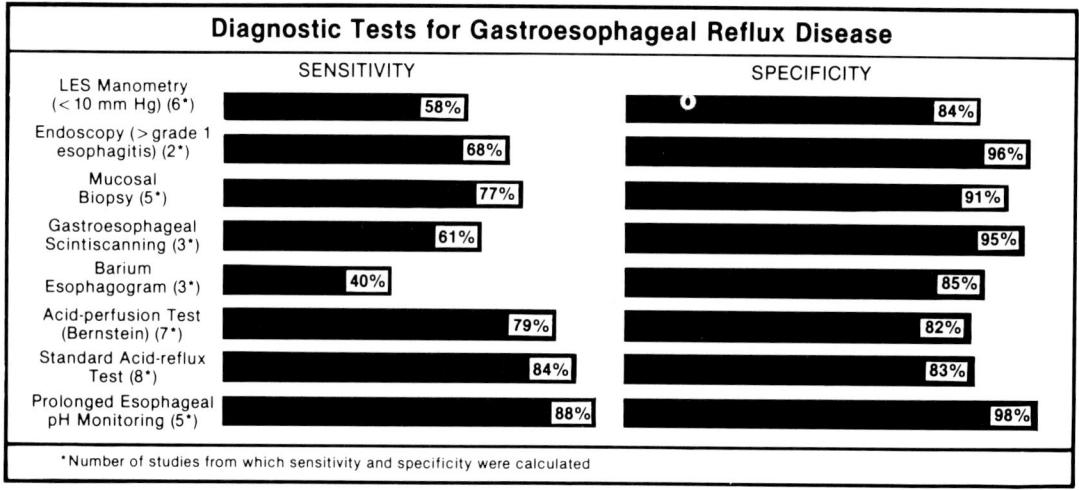

FIG. 18–6. Specificity and sensitivity of esophageal function tests. LES, Lower esophageal sphincter.

histologic evidence of esophagitis, does not enable one to detect gastroesophageal reflux more accurately than by endoscopic examination alone.

Ten percent of patients who have symptoms typical of gastroesophageal reflux and endoscopically proved esophagitis have normal results of the 24-hour pH monitoring test. This finding is disturbing until one remembers that gastroesophageal reflux, although the most common cause of esophagitis, is not the only cause of that disorder. Other causes may be alkaline reflux following vagotomy or extensive gastric resection, herpetic and monilial infections, unrecognized ingestion of caustic agents, such as drugs and vitamin C tablets, repetitive vomiting from gastrointestinal illness or long-term chemotherapy administration, radiation therapy, and smoking. Any of these forms of esophagitis may be associated with a normal 24-hour pH test.

The various esophageal function tests are compared in Figure 18–7, with respect to measurements, acceptability to patients, and sensitivity and specificity for detecting gastroesophageal reflux. Figure 18–7 suggests that prolonged esophageal pH monitoring provides the best test for identification or exclusion of gastroesophageal reflux. Prolonged esophageal pH monitoring has the greatest sensitivity and specificity of the common clinical tests for gastroesophageal reflux.[12] Because prolonged esophageal pH monitoring is the most sensitive test, the measurement of abnormal esophageal acid exposure may be used not only to confirm a diagnosis of gastroesophageal reflux in patients with symptoms suggestive of the disease, but also to diagnose the disorder in patients with atypical symptoms, such as angina-like chest pain, chronic cough, asthma, or hoarseness. Because it is the most specific test, the measurement of normal esophageal acid exposure by this method rules out gastroesophageal reflux disease as the cause of the patient's discomfort and symptoms. In a few patients who are achlorhydric, pure alkaline reflux may be responsible for the symptoms, and when appropriately interpreted the prolonged esophageal pH monitoring record may suggest this abnormality.

LIMITATIONS

Long-term esophageal pH monitoring provides extensive data on and documentation of gastroesophageal reflux. The degree and pattern of esophageal acid exposure, the acid-clearing response, and the relation of esophageal acid exposure to symptoms are comprehensively evaluated. In addition, the technique offers ease of administration and testing under near-physiologic conditions, especially when the test is performed on an ambulatory basis. The test does not, however, enable

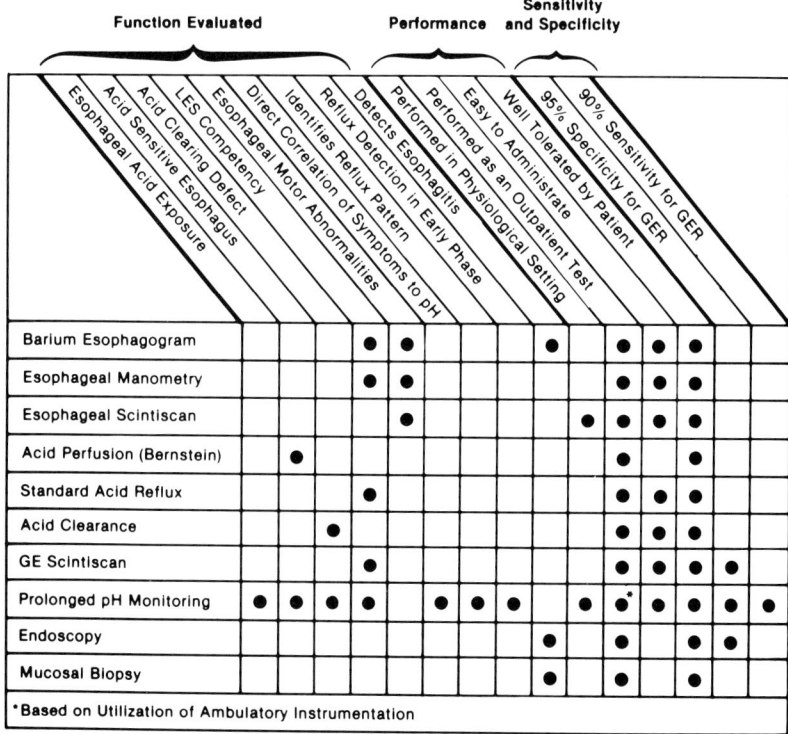

FIG. 18–7. Comparison of esophageal function tests. GER, Gastroesophageal reflux; LES, lower esophageal sphincter.

one to identify the cause of the abnormal acid exposure, such as a mechanically defective cardia, delayed gastric emptying, or an isolated motor abnormality in the body of the esophagus.[13-15]

Disorders other than Acid Reflux

One of the limitations of monitoring the esophagus for acid reflux is that abnormal alkaline reflux may go unnoticed. In the presence of an excess of acid secretion, the alkaline component, if present, is not detected. It surfaces only when the acid secretion is reduced by cimetidine therapy and may be responsible for the treatment failure in symptomatically improved patients because of continuous reflux of alkaline gastric contents through the incompetent cardia. For this reason, it is important to record normal acid pH for alkaline reflux by noting the time the pH in the esophagus exceeds 7.0 in a manner similiar for acid reflux. When abnormal alkaline exposure of the esophagus is noted, certain precautions are necessary prior to accepting the diagnosis of alkaline gastroesophageal reflux. First, alkaline changes during meals must be disregarded because the pH in the esophagus may be altered by swallowed saliva. Salivary pH usually ranges between 5.0 to 6.0, but it may increase to 7.8 during meals. Second, the patient's mouth should be examined for the presence of oral infections, which may increase salivary pH to above 7 and may result in an erroneous reading. Third, esophageal obstruction should be ruled out as a cause of the pooling and stagnation of saliva that produces bacterial overgrowth and a high alkaline pH.[16]

With simultaneous esophageal and gastric pH monitoring, one may detect alkaline gastroesophageal reflux with greater certainty because rises in intraesophageal pH to alkaline values follow rises in gastric pH to similar levels. Such a finding indicates that the alkaline material is from the stomach and not from the mouth.[17]

An esophageal stricture can reduce the amount of gastroesophageal reflux to within normal limits as measured by the 24-hour pH test. The reason is that the stricture prevents the regurgitation of gastric acid into the distal esophagus and causes the pooling of alkaline salivary secretions proximal to it. This phe-

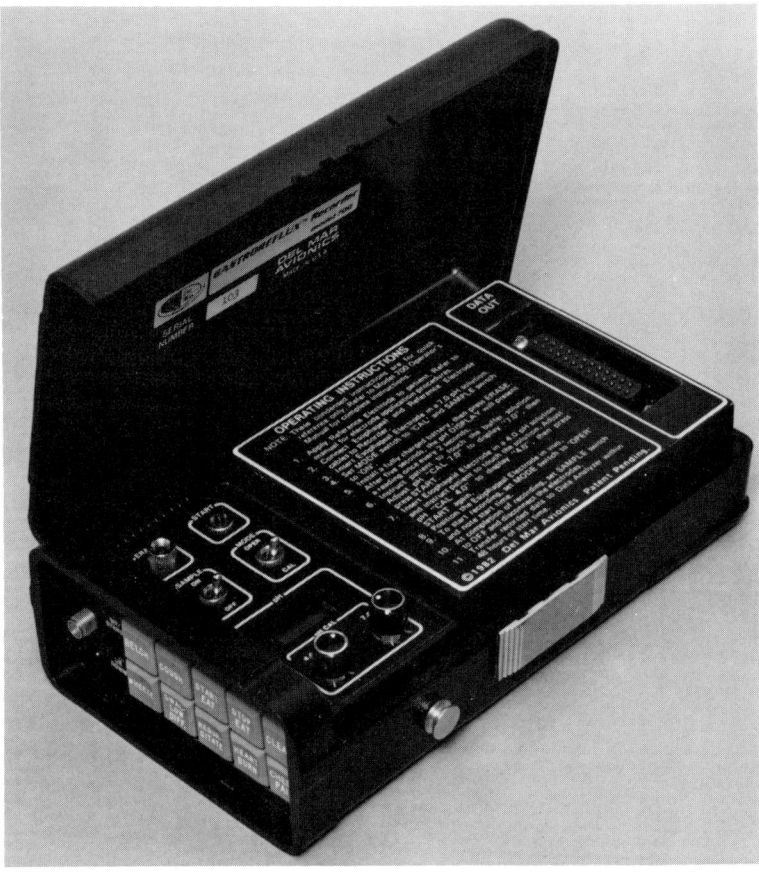

FIG. 18-8. Ambulatory unit for prolonged pH monitoring (Gastroreflux Recorder, Model 700). (Courtesy of Del Mar Avionics, Irvine, CA.)

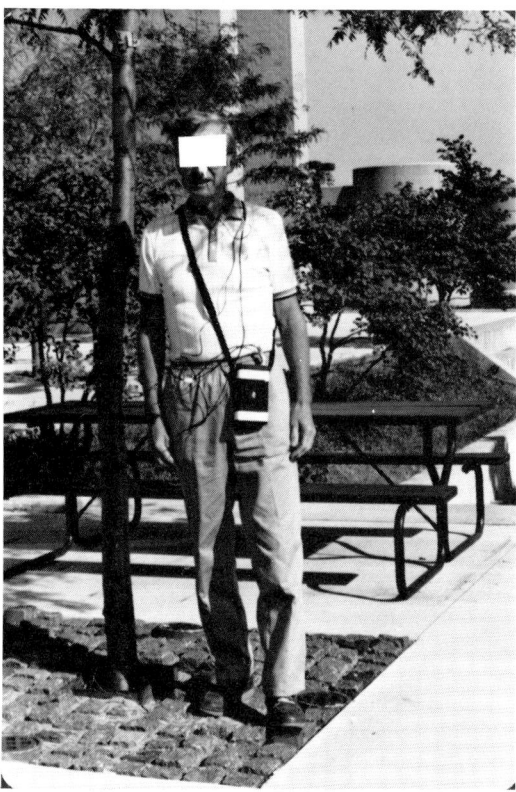

FIG. 18–9. Prolonged esophageal pH monitoring as performed on an outpatient basis.

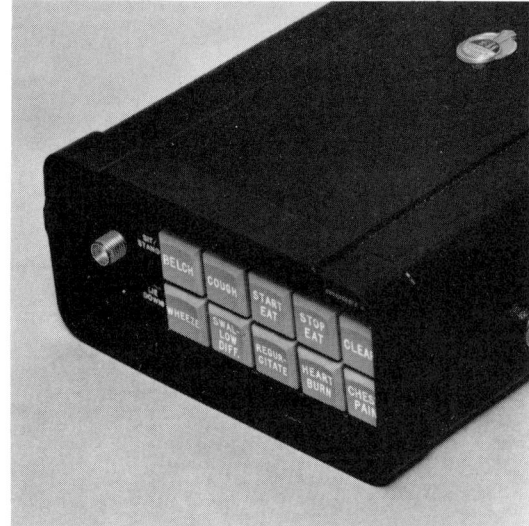

FIG. 18–10. Detail of the keyboard of the ambulatory unit shown in Figure 18–8. (Courtesy of Del Mar Avionics, Irvine, CA.)

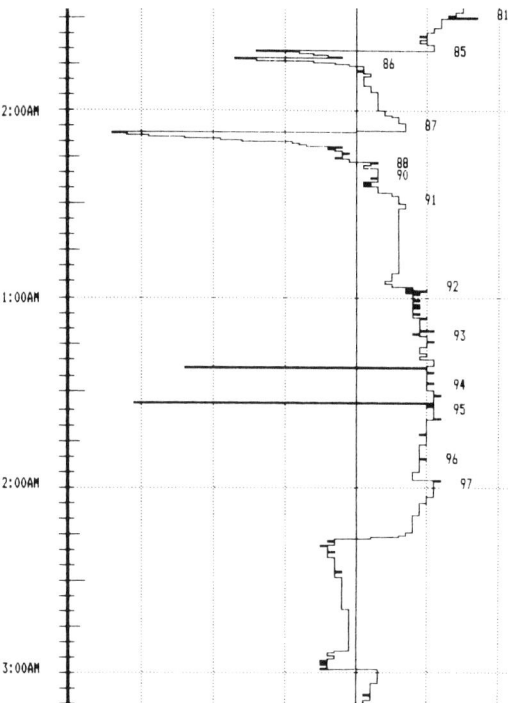

FIG. 18–11. A portion of a graphic record obtained by computer. The numbers correspond to physiologic events and symptoms entered by the patient. Each number is listed in a separate printout along with the corresponding event.

nomenon explains the observation that patients with reflux-induced strictures note a change in symptoms as the disease progresses. They initially complain of severe heartburn and regurgitation, but with the development of a stricture, these symptoms lessen, and dysphagia becomes more prominent. Dilatation of the stricture changes the results of the 24-hour pH test to abnormal if the cause is reflux and if the stomach produces acid. Should the 24-hour test results remain normal after dilatation of the stricture, the possibility of a drug-induced stricture or malignant disease should be considered.

Mandatory Co-operation

Despite its simplicity, prolonged esophageal pH monitoring requires education of the patient, if one is to obtain a meaningful record. The patient not only must record the symptoms, but also must identify precisely when the symptom occurred. As simple as it sounds, this technique has several difficulties in practice. The time lapse between experiencing the symptom and finding the pencil with which to note it on the recording paper may be significant. In the meantime, the reflux episode that caused the symptom will have passed, thereby complicating the exact timing of the symptom. Sometimes, patients

POSITION CHANGE OR SYMPTOMS	REFLUX EPISODES	TIME
	23----START	4:11 PM
14----LYING		4:12 PM
	23----STOP	4:12 PM
	24----START	4:13 PM
15----HEARTBURN		4:13 PM
16----HEARTBURN		4:19 PM
	24----STOP	4:27 PM
	25----START	4:27 PM
17----CHEST PAIN		4:30 PM
18----COUGH		4:40 PM
	25----STOP	4:41 PM
19----LYING		4:42 PM
	26----START	4:44 PM
20----VOMIT		4:44 PM
	26----STOP	4:44 PM
	27----START	4:45 PM
	27----STOP	4:46 PM
	28----START	4:48 PM
	28----STOP	4:49 PM
	29----START	4:54 PM
	29----STOP	4:54 PM
	30----START	4:56 PM
21----VOMIT		4:56 PM
	30----STOP	4:56 PM
22----SIT/STAND		4:57 PM

FIG. 18–12. Sample of computer printout listing the sequence of events recorded during the test.

```
THERE WERE 142 EPISODES WITH 12 BEING GREATER
THAN 5 MINUTES AND THE LONGEST SINGLE EPISODE
HAVING A DURATION OF 35.67 MINUTES.

PH WAS BELOW 4 FOR 13.45% OF THE TOTAL TIME,
2.53% OF THE UPRIGHT TIME AND 24.36% OF
THE SUPINE TIME.

THE SCORE WAS CALCULATED TO BE 94.74.

THE TOTAL TIME FOR THIS TEST WAS 23 HOURS
AND 18 MINUTES.
```

FIG. 18–13. Summary of the 24-hour pH monitored data elaborated by the computer.

are simply too lazy to record their symptoms, especially at night, when one must wake up, find a pencil, legibly record the symptoms, and draw a line to the pinpoint of the recorder, all in the twilight of a hospital room. Logging the symptoms and their time of occurrence in a diary and using an event marker on the recorder have not improved the accuracy of this important aspect of the 24-hour pH study.

Extensive Data Analysis

One of the difficulties of 24-hour esophageal pH monitoring, as currently performed on an inpatient basis using traditional equipment, is that generation of an enormous amount of data, which must be analyzed in a manner that indicates whether the patient has a pathologic pattern and degree of esophageal acid exposure. This laborious task requires the reading of each tracing, the counting and measurement of the duration of each reflux episode, and the calculation of the percentage of exposure to pH under 4.

APPLICATION OF SOLID STATE TECHNOLOGY

Twenty-four hour esophageal pH monitoring has been criticized for being expensive because of the requirement for hospitalization. Today, technologic advances have allowed 24-hour esophageal pH monitoring to be performed on an outpatient, ambulatory basis.[18] This development not only has omitted the need for the overnight hospital stay, but also has provided the opportunity to monitor patients in their daily setting. Comparisons between inpatient and outpatient monitoring show no statistical difference in the amount of acid reflux. Contrary to the popular belief, reflux is not more severe when the patient undergoes monitoring in the outpatient environment.

Available ambulatory pH equipment now allows one to overcome the drawbacks of the inpatient test (Fig. 18–8). The pH data are stored in the solid-state memory of a small microprocessor-based recorder worn by the patient during a routine 24-hour period (Fig. 18–9). As in the inpatient procedure, a standardized pH diet is ingested. The patient uses the keyboard of the recorder for input of physiologic data (Fig. 18–10). Recording changes in body position and eating periods are useful in identifying the reflux pattern. Symptoms are entered as they occur, without the patient's awareness of the esophageal pH level. This "blind" approach provides an unbiased record of the relation of symptoms to pH level; in contrast, patients who manually write their symptoms on a strip chart may be influenced by the knowledge of the intraesophageal pH level. The reduction in the time lag between experiencing a symptom and recording it allows for a more dependable evaluation of the relationship between symptoms and reflux episodes. The symptom keyboard also forces the patient to be concise.

When the test has been completed, the data in the recorder are transferred to an analysis system, either by direct cable connection or by telephone modem from a remote location. The analyzer computes the data and generates a complete, multipage report. In addition to the graphic record (Fig. 18–11), a sequential listing of the number and duration of reflux episodes is printed along with the recorded symptoms, for easy comparison (Fig. 18–12). A summary prints out an evaluation of the 6 components, that is, the total number of reflux episodes, the number of episodes lasting longer than 5 min, the single longest reflux episode, and the percentage of total time, upright time, and supine time during which the pH level was below 4, to give an overall score to the acid exposure (Fig. 18–13). A more precise analysis of the 6 components and overall score for all pH levels can be done with the commercially available software program ESOpHOGRAM. The pH profile generated is compared to a profile obtained from a bank of normal subjects.

REFERENCES

1. DeMeester, T.R., et al.: Technique, indications, and clinical use of 24-hour esophageal pH monitoring. J. Thorac. Cardiovasc. Surg., 97:656, 1980.
2. Winans, C.S., and Harris, L.D.: Quantification of lower esophageal sphincter competence. Gastroenterology, 51:773, 1967.
3. Johnson, L.F., and DeMeester, T.R.: Twenty-four hour pH monitoring of the distal esophagus: a quantitative measure of gastroesophageal reflux. Am. J. Gastroenterol., 62:325, 1974.
4. Johnson, L.F.: Development of the 24-hour pH monitoring systerm. In Esophageal Disorders. Pathophysiology and Therapy. Edited by T.R. DeMeester and D.B. Skinner. New York, Raven Press, 1984.
5. DeMeester, T.R., et al.: Patterns of gastroesophageal reflux in health and disease. Ann. Surg., 184:459, 1976.
6. Johnson, L.F., DeMeester, T.R., and Haggitt, R.C.: Esophageal epithelial response to gastroesophageal reflux: a quantitative study. Am. J. Dig. Dis., 23:498, 1978.
7. Johnson, L.F., and DeMeester, T.R.: Evaluation of elevation of the head of the bed, bethanechol, and antacid foam tablets on gastroesophageal reflux. Dig. Dis. Sci., 26:673, 1981.
8. Behar, J., et al.: Medical and surgical management of reflux esophagitis. N. Engl. J. Med., 292:263, 1975.
9. Pellegrini, C.A., et al.: Gastroesophageal reflux and pulmonary aspiration: incidence, functional abnormality, and results of surgical therapy. Surgery, 86:110, 1979.
10. DeMeester, T.R., et al.: Esophageal function in patients with angina-type chest pain and normal coronary angiograms. Ann. Surg., 196:488, 1982.
11. O'Sullivan, G.C., et al.: Twenty-four hour pH monitoring of esophageal function: its use in evaluation in symptomatic patients after truncal vagotomy and gastric resection or drainage. Arch. Surg., 116:581, 1981.
12. Richter, J.E., and Castell, D.O.: Gastroesophageal reflux: pathogenesis, diagnosis, and therapy. Ann. Intern. Med., 97:93, 1982.
13. DeMeester, T.R., et al.: Clinical and in vitro analysis of gastroesophageal competence: a study of the principles of antireflux surgery. Am. J. Surg., 137:39, 1979.
14. Little, A., et al.: Pathogenesis of esophagitis in patients with gastroesophageal reflux. Surgery, 88:101, 1980.
15. Joelsson, B.E., et al.: The role of the esophageal body in the antireflux mechanism. Surgery, 92:417, 1982.
16. Pellegrini, C.A., et al.: Alkaline gastroesophageal reflux. Am. J. Surg., 135:177, 1978.
17. Little, A.G., et al.: Duodenogastric reflux and reflux esophagitis. Surgery, 96:447, 1984.
18. Falor, W.H., et al.: Twenty-four hour esophageal pH monitoring by telemetry: cost effective use in outpatients. Am. J. Surg., 142:514, 1981.

19

Esophageal Motility Studies

C. Thomas Bombeck

The term "esophageal motility studies" is used loosely to describe a collection of functional studies of the esophagus designed to detect either gastroesophageal reflux or motor dysfunction in the body of the esophagus and in its sphincters. First introduced as a clinical diagnostic tool in 1952 by Code of the Mayo Clinic, motility studies have become important in the diagnosis of such conditions as achalasia and diffuse esophageal spasm. In other aspects, these studies have remained primarily a research tool and have been widely applied in attempts to explain the normal function and the failure of the lower esophageal sphincter. For more extensive information, the reader is referred to several detailed texts.[1-3]

Because methods of performing these studies are not standardized, the physician who requests such investigations must know exactly the provisions and the methods of the laboratory where the studies will be conducted. In addition, the surgeon must be aware of the normal values used in a particular laboratory and the means by which they were obtained.

For purposes of this discussion, we shall consider esophageal motility studies to include the following:

1. Manometric measurement of resting pressure through the entire esophagus, including both the upper and lower esophageal sphincters, achieved by pulling an open-tipped catheter assembly connected to external manometers by 1-cm increments from the stomach to the hypopharynx.
2. Rapid pullback measurements of the lower esophageal sphincter carried out by continuous withdrawal of a manometric catheter assembly from the stomach through the sphincter into the lower esophagus while the patient holds his breath; the pullback must be at a steady rate and may be accomplished either by hand or with a mechanical device.
3. Measurement of intragastric and intraesophageal pH at the catheter assembly tip during both pullback techniques.
4. Measurement of esophageal body and peristaltic activity at each station of the pullback technique during both dry swallows and swallows of a bolus of water.
5. Measurement of esophageal motor response to a bolus of 0.1 normal hydrochloric acid injected into the upper esophagus with the motility catheter assembly positioned in the lower body of the esophagus.
6. Measurement of the efficiency of esophageal clearing of that bolus of injected acid by determination of the number of peristaltic waves necessary to return the intraesophageal milieu to the resting pH level.
7. Measurement of esophageal body and sphincter motor response to pharmacologic agents such as pentagastrin or bethanechol.
8. Measurement of motor and sphincteric response to mechanical maneuvers such as abdominal pressure or a Valsalva or Müller maneuver.
9. Continuous recording of pH levels from a sensor placed just superior to the lower esophageal sphincter and maintained in that position for a period of 12 to 24 hours; although this determination is not truly part of the standard esophageal motility examination, it is usually carried out in conjunction with such an examination by the same laboratories. This examination may either be done in the hospital setting or while the patient goes about his daily activities; ambulatory patients carry a small recording device that determines intraesophageal pH at intervals of a few seconds (see Chapter 18, "Prolonged Esophageal pH Monitoring").

INDICATIONS

Esophageal motility studies are not routinely indicated for the investigation of every patient with esophageal symptoms. The technique of examination is time-consuming and expensive, both because of the equipment required and because of the painstaking data acquisition and interpretation. These examinations are therefore reserved for the following patients, in whom similar data can be obtained by no other means:

1. Patients with atypical chest pain in whom the diagnosis of a cardiac disorder has been excluded.
2. Patients with symptoms of gastroesophageal reflux in whom standard methods of treatment have failed or who have been shown not to have esophageal inflammation by the usual endoscopic examinations.
3. Patients whose symptoms have failed to improve following a standard operation for gastroesophageal reflux.
4. Patients in whom an antireflux operation is contemplated.
5. Patients who have radiologic or symptomatic evidence of an esophageal motility disorder.

The examination is not indicated in patients with simple symptoms of gastroesophageal reflux, and indeed, little further investigation is required in such patients, beyond obtaining a complete medical history and performing a physical examination. Such a symptom is simple heartburn or pyrosis, which is aggravated by positional change or by ingestion of acid foods and may be accompanied by frank regurgitation of gastric or duodenal content. If these patients respond satisfactorily to routine nonoperative therapy such as weight reduction, elevation of the head of the bed, administration of antacids, and avoidance of tight clothing, then no further studies will be required. In patients who have mechanical esophageal obstruction, such as caused by benign or malignant neoplasms, results of motility studies are confusing, and such tests lend nothing to therapy.

As a general rule, the studies are indicated whenever an esophageal motility derangement is suspected as a cause of symptoms and whenever definitive therapeutic intervention is planned, such as a surgical procedure. The first indication is obvious, but the second is recommended because reflux, for which the majority of such procedures are planned, may be accompanied by varying degrees of disordered esophageal motility. The "stagnant" esophagitis of achalasia may be mistaken endoscopically for reflux esophagitis, and an antireflux procedure may be then undertaken, with disastrous results. Even if the antireflux procedure is indicated, as in a patient with reflux disease, failure to recognize a concomitant motility disorder will result in failure of the operation to relieve symptoms, and the patient will be dissatisfied even though reflux has been stopped.

INTERPRETATION

A full description of the interpretation of motility findings is beyond the scope of this chapter. Such interpretation should be undertaken only by physicians skilled in these techniques. Nonetheless, a brief description of common findings in motility and other disorders is warranted. For each condition, the characteristic pressures at the lower esophageal sphincter, esophageal body, and the upper esophageal sphincter are described.

Gastroesophageal Reflux and Reflux Esophagitis

Lower esophageal sphincter zone pressures are normal in 20 to 30% of patients with symptoms of esophageal reflux, but are decreased in the remainder of these patients. In some persons, no lower esophageal sphincter pressures are detectable. The cause of the decrease in pressure is unclear. Whether the decrease is the cause or the effect of reflux is still controversial. Commonly, pressures are in the range of 5 to 10 mm Hg.

In the esophagus peristaltic pressures are normally in the range of 40 to 60 mm Hg, with ordered progression of at least 95% of contractions caudad. Spontaneous motor activity occurs in up to 30% of patients and is characterized by low-pressure, spontaneous contractions in the inflamed area of the esophagus. Acid clearance is impaired, requiring more than 12 to 15 primary peristaltic waves to clear an injected acid bolus.

Upper esophageal sphincter pressures are normal.

Achalasia

The lower esophageal sphincter has normal or elevated resting pressures, with failure to relax on swallowing. Increased postswallow contraction pressure may occur early in the disease, with no response to swallowing in the later stages. The administration of exogenous pentagastrin usually provokes hypercontraction of the lower esophageal sphincter to a much greater degree than normal.

Esophageal body pressures, which are characterized early in the disease as "vigorous achalasia," may have a motility pattern resembling that seen in diffuse spasm, with multiple nonconducted, nonprogressive, high-pressure, spontaneous contractions. Many of the swallow-provoked contractions are simultaneous, rather than progressive and are of high pressure, greater than 150 mm Hg. As the disease progresses, the esophageal body becomes increasingly sensitive to exogenous cholinergic stimulation with a variety of agents, including methacholine and bethanechol. Contraction produced by these agents is frequently accompanied by severe, substernal, crushing pain. The pain is relieved by atropine blockade.

As the disease progresses, all contraction in the esophagus is lost, and the organ becomes a flaccid, dilated, tortuous tube. Primary peristalsis is absent, and swallow provokes a simultaneous, weak, pressure response throughout the body of the esophagus (the common cavity effect). Lower esophageal sphincter pressures remain normal, but sphincter relaxation is not found.

Upper esophageal sphincter pressures usually remain normal, as does sphincter relaxation.

Mixed Collagen-Vascular Disease (Scleroderma)

All peristaltic contraction is gradually lost in the involved area of the esophagus, usually the distal third. Pressures gradually decrease, over time, until none are measurable.

Lower esophageal sphincter pressure also gradually disappears, and findings associated with reflux become prominent. Upper esophageal sphincter pressures usually remain normal.

Diffuse Esophageal Spasm

This condition shares many of the features of early achalasia, as discussed previously, but high pressures and simultaneous contractions are more frequent. These contractions account for more than 66% of induced contractions (swallows), which may be repetitive and may have pressures in excess of 300 mm Hg. The duration of esophageal contraction during these "spastic" contractions is also prolonged. High-pressure contractions are often associated with pain. Normal pressure and normally progressive contractions may also be present, either interspersed with spastic contractions or localized to the upper esophagus when the spastic contractions are localized to the lower esophagus. The upper esophagus is rarely involved with diffuse spasm while the lower esophagus retains normal motility.

Lower esophageal sphincter pressures may be normal, with normal relaxation, or they may be increased, with a prolonged post-relaxation contraction phase. This second condition has been termed "hypercontracting lower esophageal sphincter." Upper esophageal sphincter pressures and relaxation phases are normal.

Diverticular Diseases of the Esophagus

Esophageal diverticula are almost always associated with some area of spasm in the esophagus or with failure of one of the sphincters to relax normally during swallowing. Pharyngoesophageal (Zenker's) diverticulum is associated with a nonrelaxing upper esophageal sphincter in at least 50% of patients. Midesophageal diverticulum, the most common type, is associated with distal diffuse spasm, and epiphrenic diverticulum is found in patients with early achalasia, or hypercontracting lower esophageal sphincter.

All diverticular diseases of the esophagus are probably due to the relative distal obstruction produced by localized spasm with increased intraluminal esophageal pressure, both because of obstruction and because of high-pressure contractions. It also seems likely that no entity such as a "traction diverticulum" really exists and that all diverticula are of the pulsion type.

Carcinoma of the Esophagus

All obstructing lesions of the esophagus may alter motility, depending on the completeness of the obstruction and on the suddenness of its onset. No distinctive motility pattern is seen, except as the obstruction becomes complete, the esophagus dilates superior to it and is unable to close completely because of entrapped air and saliva. Contraction pressure generated anywhere along the length of the obstructed segment is therefore rapidly transmitted hydraulically through the trapped fluid and gives what appears to be a simultaneous contraction on motility examination. This common cavity effect is an artifactual finding and may mask an underlying normal peristaltic wave.

Infectious Esophageal Disease

Acute inflammatory disease of the esophagus caused by the Herpes simplex or genitalis virus or by candida may produce disordered motility similar to that found in patients with reflux-induced inflammation. The lower esophageal sphincter is usually normal, with normal relaxation, unless the disease is severe.

CONTINUOUS RECORDING OF pH

By far the most accurate method for the direct measurement of gastroesophageal reflux is the 12- to 24-hour pH study. Chapter 18 describes this technique in detail. Only the highlights of its application are presented here.

Results are usually reported in terms of the number of reflux episodes, their average duration, their longest duration, and the total percentage of time measured that the intraesophageal pH was below 4.0. The most significant measurement is the total time of low pH, with a sensitivity of 70 to 80% in patients with known reflux esophagitis. Most of those individuals have pH values below 4.0 in excess of 10% of the measured period, whereas normal persons have these values in less than 5.0% of the measured period. Although much attention has been given to the position of the patient during reflux episodes (supine or upright), the significance of this relationship is controversial, as is the relation to meals or to reflux of material of pH greater than 7.0 (alkaline reflux.)

The test is useful in confirming the cause of a patient's symptoms, especially in persons who have symptoms of reflux without demonstrable, or with ony minimal, endoscopic evidence of esophagitis. These patients are at risk of aspiration and associated pulmonary diseases, rather than esophageal damage, and so must still be aggressively treated for reflux. The test is also useful to monitor the success of any operation done to correct reflux.

Other tests of reflux, such as the standard acid reflux test (SART) or the pH pullback test (Tuttle), have much less sensitivity and specificity than the 12- or 24-hour reflux test.

MOTILITY STUDIES IN OTHER ORGANS

Variations of esophageal motility tests have been applied to the stomach, duodenum, small bowel, biliary tract, and rectum. All such tests are currently investigational in nature and are not routinely applied clinically.

REFERENCES

1. Henderson, R.D.: The Esophagus: Reflux and Primary Motor Disorders. Baltimore, Williams & Wilkins, 1980.
2. Skinner, D.B., et al.: Gastroesophageal Reflux and Hiatal Hernia. Boston, Little, Brown, 1972.
3. Vantrappen, G., and Hellemans, J.: Diseases of the Esophagus. New York, Springer, 1974.

20

Gastroduodenal Function Studies

Daniel H. Dunn ■ M. Michael Eisenberg

Gastric juice is a mixture of electrolytes, mucus, protein, and water. The composition and concentration of the various constituents of gastric juice are determined by the number and secretory capacity of the gastric cells. Parietal cells secrete hydrochloric acid and intrinsic factor. The chief cells secrete pepsinogen, which, when activated by acid exposure, is converted to a potent proteolytic enzyme, pepsin. The surface epithelial cells and mucous cells secrete an alkaline mucus. In addition, endocrine cells within the gastric mucosa secrete many different hormones. Collectively, these various exocrine and endocrine cells produce a solution that can be qualitatively and quantitatively analyzed.

Acid-secretory studies are performed to quantify one constituent of gastric juice secreted by the stomach within a specified period of time under basal and stimulated conditions. Various clinical syndromes are associated with abnormally high or low acid secretion. In the past, prior to the development of upper gastrointestinal endoscopy, gastric secretory studies were important in distinguishing between duodenal and gastric ulcers and between benign and malignant gastric ulcers. Currently, gastric-secretory studies are performed infrequently, and their clinical application is limited. Nevertheless, gastroduodenal function studies may be helpful in the evaluation of certain gastrointestinal problems. In this chapter, a review of various types of gastric function tests and their application in the management of patients is presented.

GASTRIC-ACID-SECRETORY TERMINOLOGY

The term "basal acid output" is used to refer to acid secretion during an unstimulated or resting period. The basal acid output is the sum of 4 15-min collections of gastric juice expressed in milliequivalents per hour. The peak acid output is the highest rate of gastric secretion following administration of a gastric-acid secretagogue. Specifically, it is the sum of the 2 highest 10-min collection periods or the 2 highest 15-min collection periods. The peak acid output is obtained by multiplying the sum of the 2 greatest 10-min collection periods (20 min) by 3 or the 2 greatest 15-min periods (30 min) by 2. The result is expressed in millequivalents per hour. The term "maximal acid output" is used to denote the sum of the 4 highest 15-min collection periods obtained after a given gastric-acid stimulant and expressed in millequivalents per hour.

TYPES OF TESTS

Acid-secretory testing involves the measurement of basal and stimulated acid secretion. Tests are performed by aspirating gastric content before and after the stimulation of gastric secretion. The following is a description of the test procedure.

Acid-secretory tests are usually performed in the morning because the patient must have been fasting for at least 12 hours. In addition to fasting, the patient must have abstained from any medication that may affect acid secretion for 24 hours prior to testing, such as cimetidine and pilocarpine. The procedure should be explained to the patient, including any side effects from the acid stimulus, such as histamine, which may cause flushing, dizziness, headache, and wheezing.

The patient lies on a bed or sits in a chair in a semirecumbent position. A nasogastric tube is placed into the patient's stomach. The primary consideration in the choice of nasogastric tube is the ease with which fluid may be aspirated from the stomach. A sump tube usually allows the most complete aspiration of gastric juice. Fluoroscopy facilities should be available because the position of the nasogastric tube is critical for accurate and complete aspiration of gastric juice. The tip of the tube should lie in the most dependent portion of the patient's stomach. The nasogastric tube should then be tested to ascertain patency, to determine the presence of any retained food, and to make sure that at least 90% of test fluid instilled is immediately returned. If not, the tube should be repositioned.

The patient should be in a semirecumbent position to ensure comfort, as well as to prevent any adverse reactions, such as hypotension or dizziness, that might occur with administration of the gastric secretagogue histamine or insulin. The nasogastric tube is then taped in place, and the tube is attached to a suction device. If possible, continuous suction should be used, with a sump tube. If a sump tube is not available, then intermittent suction should be used, to obtain more complete aspiration of fluid. Suction at the rate of 30 to 50 mm Hg is sufficient for aspiration.

When the patient's stomach has been completely emptied and the gastric juice thereby obtained has been discarded, gastric juice is then collected for an hour. Ten to 15-min collections are taken during the hour, and volume and titratable acid levels are recorded. The amount secreted during the first hour of collection is the basal acid secretion and is expressed as millequivalents per hour.

Stimulated acid secretion is obtained after injection of one of many different types of secretagogues. Gastric juice is then collected in 10- or 15-min intervals for 60 to 120 min. Maximal acid output and peak acid output can be determined from these collections. Each of the stimulants elicits a different response; the result is variations in the timing of peak and maximal acid output. One of the most important factors in determining the type of stimulant for testing has been the incidence of side effects. Three varieties of stimulants may be used for testing: (1) histamine, betazole, and gastrin analogues, to induce a parietal cell response; (2) hypoglycemic agents, to assess vagal innervation; and (3) secretin and calcium, to provoke gastrin release.

Testing with Histamine, Betazole, and Gastrin Analogues

In 1929, Bloomfield and Polland studied the effect of histamine on gastric secretion in man.[1] Although these workers were not the first to show the effect of histamine on acid secretion, they were the first to analyze a large number of "normal" subjects. The early use of histamine was associated with many untoward side effects, of which hypotension was the most serious; some fatalities were reported.[2,3] Antihistamines, such as diphenhydramine (Benadryl), were used to decrease some of the H_1 receptor side effects. Although these agents were effective in reducing the side effects of histamine without altering the effects on gastric secretion,[4] the antihistamines had their own side effects, such as drowsiness and headaches. Betazole, 3-β-aminoethylpyrazole (Histolog), an analogue of histamine, was found to stimulate acid secretion, similar to histamine, but with fewer side effects than histamine.[5] Betazole was used as the primary stimulus for acid secretion until pentagastrin was approved for clinical testing (Fig. 20–1). The peak acid output after betazole administration usually occurs 60 to 120 min after injection, whereas the peak response after histamine administration occurs within the first 60 min. Additionally, the 2 available forms of histamine are not equivalent in the dose response elicited. One milligram histamine base is equivalent to 1.66 mg histamine dihydrochloride, which is equal to 2.75 mg histamine acid phosphatase[6] (Table 20–1).

Pentagastrin, N-t-butyloxy-carbonyl-β-alanyl-L-tryptophyl-L-metionyl-L-aspartyl-L-phenylalanine-amide, is a potent gastric secretagogue. Pentagastrin can be given subcutaneously, intramuscularly, or intravenously. The standard dose of pentagastrin is 6 μg/kg subcutaneously or intramuscularly; the dose is the same for intravenous infusion, 6 μg/kg/hour. The maximum response is similar to that to histamine or betazole, but the peak response occurs earlier than with betazole, usually 45 to 60 min. The degree and timing of the acid response elicited by pentagastrin are the same as with human synthetic gastrin and tetragastrin.[7,8] The dosage of gastrin is 1 to 2 μg/kg subcutaneously or intramuscularly, or 0.8 μ/kg/hour by intravenous infusion. Tetragastrin can be given either subcutaneously or intramuscularly at a dose of 10 to 20 μg/kg.[9]

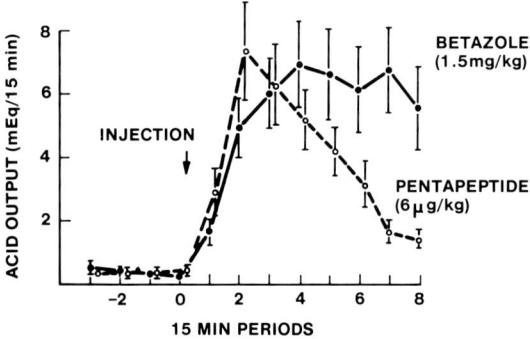

FIG. 20–1. Gastric acid output after administration of betazole (1.5 mg/kg subcutaneously) or pentapeptide (6 μg/kg subcutaneously) in 20 patients with various gastrointestinal disorders. (Adapted from Isenberg, J.I., Brooks, A.M., and Grossman, M.L.: JAMA, 206:2897, 1968.)

Table 20–1. Measurement of Maximal Acid Output After Various Stimuli in Man

Stimulant	Dose	Route	Peak Response
Histamine	40 μg/kg	subcutaneous	0–60 min
Betazole	1.7 mg/kg	intramuscular	60–120 min
	50–100 mg	intramuscular	60–120 min
Pentagastrin	6 mg/kg	subcutaneous or intramuscular	45–60 min
Insulin	0.2 μ/kg	intravenous	60 min
	0.4 μ/kg/hr	intravenous	

(Adapted from Baron, J.H.: Clinical Test of Gastric Secretion. New York, Oxford University Press, 1979, p. 55.)

The major advantage of pentagastrin, gastrin, and tetragastrin is the low incidence of side effects.[10] For this reason, pentagastrin or human synthetic gastrin is now used exclusively in most centers in preference to histamine or betazole. Transient hypotension, nausea, lightheadedness, and tachycardia may occur in a few patients; when these side effects are severe, administration of intravenous antihistamines and hydrocortisone may be helpful.[11]

Vagal Innervation Tests

In 1814, Brodie first demonstrated the importance of the vagus nerve in gastric-acid secretion.[12] In 1927, insulin was shown to be an effective stimulator of gastric-acid secretion, and later, other hypoglycemic agents such as tolbutamide and 2-deoxy-D-glucose (2-DG) were also shown to stimulate acid secretion.[13,14] The effects of insulin, tolbutamide, and 2-DG on acid secretion are multiple. Sympathetic and parasympathetic nerve stimulation plays a role in hypoglycemia-induced acid secretion.[15]

The mechanism of gastric secretion elicited by insulin is not completely understood. Although early studies indicated that the effect of insulin on acid secretion was an all-or-none phenomenon,[16] subsequent studies have shown that the gastric-secretory response to insulin is dose dependent.[17] The patient's blood glucose level is important in determining the response to insulin. Blood glucose levels of 25 to 40 mg/100 ml are associated with the greatest acid secretion, whereas levels below 15 mg/100 ml inhibit acid secretion.[18-19] Although each patient responds differently to insulin, the dose of insulin that produces the peak acid response in most individuals is 0.2 μ/kg, given as an intravenous bolus.[6] Although rapid intravenous bolus injection produces maximal acid secretion, the side effects of intravenous infusion of insulin are fewer because the blood sugar level falls more gradually. Because the response to intravenous infusion (0.1 μ/kg/hr) is similar to that of intravenous bolus injection (0.2 μ/kg), and because the incidence of untoward side effects is lower with intravenous infusion, the intravenous infusion of insulin is recommended for clinical tests.[20]

Tolbutamide is an oral hypoglycemic agent and has been used to stimulate acid secretion. Tolbutamide competes with glucose for cellular membrane transport and decreases intracellular glucose concentration. The test has not been standardized, however, and few data are available to support its routine use.[21] In contrast, 2-DG, a potent vagal stimulus, has been studied in man and in the animal laboratory.[22] This agent elicits a small but greater acid response than 0.2 μ/kg insulin. The peak response to an intravenous injection of 2-DG of 50 μg/kg occurs at 45 min, whereas the peak acid response to insulin occurs later, usually at 60 min.

The major side effect of the insulin test for completeness of vagotomy is severe hypoglycemia, which may lead to shock, coma, and death. For this reason, a physician must always be in attendance during the test. An intravenous infusion of dextrose and water should be administered during the test, and ampules of 50% glucose should be available in case the patient becomes confused or disoriented or in case a significant change occurs in the patient's vital signs. A similar hypoglycemic response may be seen following administration of 2-DG. Because 2-DG produces an intracellular glucopenia, the patient's blood sugar level is not significantly altered.[23] Therefore, administration of glucose, although recommended, may not be effective in reversing the side effects, and the use of 2-DG may consequently be potentially more dangerous than the use of insulin.

The patient should be prepared as described previously. In addition to the routine placement of a nasogastric tube and the collection of basal acid secretion, the precautions outlined earlier in this chapter should be taken when insulin is used as the gastric stimulant. After collection of basal acid secretion, 0.2 μ/kg insulin is given by rapid intravenous injection, or an intravenous infusion of 0.1 μ/kg insulin is started. Gastric secretion is collected every 15 min for 2 hours, and each 15-min sample is analyzed separately, to give a more accurate picture of the acid-secretory response to insulin. The test is then terminated, but the patient should be observed until fully recovered from the hypoglycemic effects of insulin. Blood sugar determinations must be obtained during the tests. The patient's blood sugar level should be under 50 mg/100 ml 30 min after insulin injection.[24]

Gastrin-Stimulation Tests

Calcium stimulates gastric-acid secretion; the exact mechanism for its action is still unknown, however.[25,26] The intravenous infusion of calcium, at 4 to 5 mg/kg/hour, gradually increases gastric-acid secretion, together with an increase in serum calcium levels. This test is not generally used as a gastric-acid-secretory study, but it is frequently used as a stimulus for gastric acid and gastrin release in the diagnosis of the Zollinger-Ellison syndrome.[27] The gastrin level in a normal patient may rise 50 to 100 pg/ml following calcium infusion, whereas the gastrin level may increase by threefold or fourfold in a patient with Zollinger-Ellison syndrome.

Secretin inhibits pentagastrin-stimulated acid secretion in normal subjects. The intravenous injection of 1 to 2 μ/kg secretin in patients with Zollinger-Ellison syndrome causes an immediate rise in serum gastrin to levels 3 to 5 times those of basal levels. The secretin test is easier to perform and has fewer side effects than the calcium-infusion test and is therefore the diagnostic test of choice in differentiating patients with the Zollinger-Ellison syndrome from those with hypergastrinemia of uncertain origin.

Other tests of gastric secretion include test-meal stimulation,[28-31] "tubeless" analysis,[32-36] and technetium study.[37,38] These tests are seldom used clinically today to quantify gastric-acid secretion.

APPLICATION OF GASTRIC-SECRETORY TESTING

Normal Subjects

Age, sex, body habitus, and ethnic background all affect basal and maximal acid secretion.[6] With increasing age, acid-secretory capacity decreases.[39] Oi and co-workers found that the parietal cell mass correlates well with maximal acid output, and with advancing age, the parietal cell mass diminishes, resulting in less acid production.[40] Males secreted more acid than females in virtually every early study that considered this variable. Other studies, however, have reported that this difference in acid secretion is perceived, not real, because when the acid-secretory rate is corrected for body weight, the difference between normal males and females is minimal.[41]

The effects of body habitus, weight, and height on acid secretion have been examined. Body weight has a strong correlation with acid secretion, as mentioned previously. Acid secretion is also correlated with height. In fact, Maybury and associates have formulated a secretion index based on a patient's height,[42] as follows:

$$\text{secretion index} = \log e \frac{\text{actual gastric-acid secretion} \times 100}{\text{excpected gastric-acid secretion}}$$

In this manner, a patient's acid secretion (actual gastric-acid secretion) can be compared to a normal acid-secretory response (expected gastric-acid secretion).

Most "normal" acid-secretory values have been obtained from studies conducted in the Western world. Studies of histamine-stimulated acid secretion in Indians, Chinese, and Bantus have shown that a patient's maximal acid output in these countries is approximately half that of a patient in the Western world.[43-45] The differences cannot be explained totally by a difference in body weight. Makhlouf suggested that the difference may be caused by a difference in "lean body" weight; Indian population has a greater percentage of lean body weight.[46]

Despite these important factors in determining variations in acid secretion among patients, "average" basal and maximal acid-secretory rates have been established for normal patients. The average normal basal acid output is approximately 2 meq/hour. The upper limit of normal basal acid output is less than 5 meq/hour. The average maximal acid output (histamine- or pentagastrin-stimulated) is 20 meq/hour, and the upper limits of normal are under 40 meq/hour.

Patients with Duodenal Ulcer Disease

Because 25% of patients with duodenal ulcers have acid-secretory rates "within normal limits," acid-secretory studies have been largely abandoned in the routine evaluation of these patients. Whatever the acid-secretory rate, a patient with a duodenal ulcer is secreting "too much acid." Even though such a patient may have a normal acid-secretory rate, most persons with duodenal ulcers are acid hypersecreters. In contrast, all patients with duodenal ulcer secrete some acid; the dictum "no acid, no ulcer" is therefore a reliable rule.

Baron, Grossman and colleagues, and Kirkpatrick and associates have compared acid-secretory rates in normal adult patients and in patients with duodenal ulcer.[47-49] Basal acid output was greater than 5 meq/hour in most patients with duodenal ulcer (75%), and maximal acid output averaged 40 meq/hour after histamine and pentagastrin stimulation (Table 20-2). Although the average peak acid output was higher in patients with duodenal ulcers than in the normal group, 25 to 35% of the ulcer patients were in the normal range. Duodenal ulcers are rare in patients with a maximal acid output of less than

Table 20-2. Basal and Maximal Stimulated Gastric-Acid Secretion in Normal Subjects and in Patients with Duodenal Ulcer

		Acid Output (meq/hour)			
		Normal		Duodenal ulcer	
	Sex	Mean	ULN	Mean	LV-DU
Basal	M	2.4	26.6	5.3	0.1
	F	1.3	24.1	2.9	0.1
Histamine	M	21.6	49.2	42.0	15
	F	12.3	30.2	32.0	18.8
Betazole	M	21.8	45.8	35.0	14.4
	F	16.8	40.0	30.8	13.4
Pentagastrin	M	25.0	45.0	43.0	15.0

ULN, Upper limit of normal (mean + 2SD); LV-DU, lowest value duodenal ulcer.

(Adapted from Isenberg, J.I.: Gastric secretory testing. In Gastrointestinal Disease. Edited by M.H. Sleisinger and J.S. Fordtran. Philadelphia, W.B. Saunders, 1978, p. 725.)

12 meq/hour, however. These studies point out the futility of using gastric-acid analysis in the preoperative evaluation of patients with duodenal ulcer.

Patients with Gastric Ulcer

Gastric-secretory rates of patients with gastric ulcer vary with the location of the ulcer. Gastric ulcers in the prepyloric region or in the distal antrum, the pyloric channel, are usually associated with normal or hypersecretory states. In other words, they are in the "pathophysiologic" category of peptic ulcer disease of the duodenal ulcer variety. These patients respond to therapy similar to that for duodenal ulcer disease. Similarly, patients with combined gastric and duodenal ulcers are usually also gastric-acid hypersecreters, provided the gastric ulcer is in the pyloric channel. These two groups of patients with gastric ulcer generally have a basal acid output of greater than 5 meq/hour and a maximal acid output of 40 meq/hour.

Gastric ulcers located in the fundus or proximal body of the stomach are more likely to occur in patients who are acid hyposecreters. The theories of the origin of this variety of gastric ulcer are multiple and are largely speculative. Acid-back diffusion,[50] "locus minoris resistentiae,"[40] gastric stasis,[51] and bile reflux gastritis[52] have all been proposed as primary or secondary factors in the origin of benign gastric ulcer. These patients usually have basal acid secretory rates of less than 5 meq/hour. Achlorhydria can occur in patients with "benign" gastric ulcer, but it is rare and usually necessitates operative treatment, to rule out a diagnosis of malignant disease.

Patients with Gastric Carcinoma

Patients with gastric carcinoma usually secrete less-than-normal amounts of acid. Histamine-fast achlorhydria may occur in patients with gastric carcinoma; however, only 20% of patients with gastric carcinoma are achlorhydric.[53] In contrast, 5 to 10% of patients with gastric cancer secrete more acid than average (greater than 20 meq/hour peak acid output).[54] Thus, gastric analysis as a screening diagnostic test in a patient with a possibly malignant gastric ulcer is only helpful in the presence of complete anacidity. Theoretically, any level of acid secretion may occur in patients with gastric carcinoma (Fig. 20–2).

Postvagotomy Gastric Analysis

Testing for completeness of vagotomy may be performed either during operation or postoperatively.

INTRAOPERATIVE VAGOTOMY TESTING. This type of testing, to assess the completeness of vagotomy using electrical stimulation and intragastric pressure monitoring, was first described by Burge and Bane

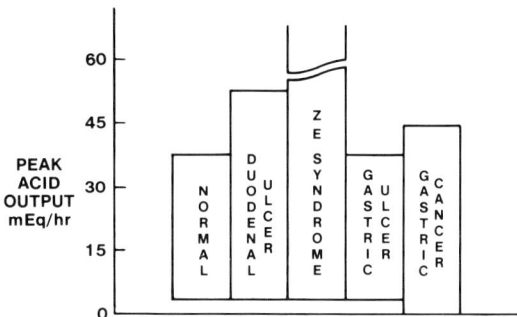

FIG. 20–2. A comparison of peak acid output in normal patients and in patients with duodenal ulcer, Zollinger-Ellison (Z-E) syndrome, gastric ulcer, or gastric cancer.

in 1958.[55,56] The equipment, additional operating time required, and the need to stimulate all vagal fibers to obtain an accurate result render this test impractical for routine use. Postoperative recurrent ulcers in patients who have undergone intraoperative testing suggest that the test is not foolproof.[2,3] Allgöwer and Perren improved the equipment and technique of Burge and Bane,[57] but the basic concept and the defects in the test remain the same, and the test has not been widely adopted.

Congo red has been used as an indicator dye to delineate mucosa that remains innervated after "complete vagotomy." Congo red is oxidized when exposed to the hydrochloric-acid-secreting mucosa, which turns the red to black. This test requires the administration of histamine, as betazole, 50 mg subcutaneously, or pentagastrin, 0.6 µg/kg/min, just prior to topical administration of Congo red. The mucosa must be visualized completely, or small areas of mucosa with persistent innervation may be missed. Transillumination of the gastric wall with an intragastric light source, to avoid gastrotomy, has been attempted, but with equivocal results.[58] Direct visualization of the gastric mucosa, by intraoperative endoscopic examination or through a gastrotomy, provides an adequate view of the gastric mucosa. Long-term clinical follow-up studies of large numbers of patients who have undergone intraoperative vagotomy testing using Congo red have not been conducted.

Several investigators have reported studies using Congo red to delineate the acid-secreting gastric mucosa from the non-acid-secreting mucosa (antrum).[59–61] The Congo red test has been used extensively, both experimentally and clinically, for antral-corpus delineation during parietal-cell vagotomy.[62,63]

The Congo red test has been largely replaced by the use of pH probes. Amdrup and Jensen used intragastric pH monitoring to mark the antral-corpus junction during parietal-cell vagotomy, with satisfactory results.[64] Johnston and Wilkinson performed parietal-cell vagotomy without the use of a pH probe for antral-corpus boundary mapping, however.[65] No discernible difference in ulcer recurrence was observed between the two groups. Grassi and co-workers and Johnson and Baxter have also used the pH probe intraoperatively with success; these workers found persistent innervation after "complete" vagotomy in 2 of 20 and in 29 of 50 vagotomies, respectively.[66,67] These workers also reported a lower ulcer recurrence rate using this technique.

In summary, intraoperative testing for completeness of vagotomy using the foregoing techniques shows a surprising number of incomplete vagotomies. These tests are simple to perform and cause no increased risk to the patient, other than the minimal increase in operative time. Whether the tests reduce the incidence of recurrent ulcer is unknown and requires longer follow-up.

POSTOPERATIVE INSULIN TEST FOR VAGOTOMY. Ulcer recurrence following operative procedures for duodenal ulcer disease is usually due to incomplete vagotomy, if vagotomy was attempted during the first procedure, or to inadequate gastric resection, if subtotal gastrectomy was performed. In the second instance, vagotomy testing is unnecessary, and operative treatment by repeated resection and added vagotomy "cures" the ulcer diathesis in 90% of patients. In patients who have ulcer recurrence after "attempted" vagotomy, tests for completeness of vagotomy may be of diagnostic and therapeutic importance in deciding on further operative intervention.

The insulin-stimulated gastric-acid-secretory test or Hollander test was first used clinically to determine the completeness of vagal denervation by Hollander in 1946.[68] He established criteria for a positive or negative test result. These criteria have been criticized and revised, primarily because of the variability in the response of postvagotomy patients to insulin. Eisenberg and associates and Hodge and colleagues have shown that insulin-induced hypoglycemia not only is a parasympathetic (vagal) stimulus, but also it may inhibit acid secretion, it may stimulate acid secretion directly by sympathetic pathways, or it may indirectly stimulate acid by release of epinephrine, which may in turn release gastrin, to cause acid secretion.[18,69]

Thus, a positive response to insulin by Hollander's criteria may not represent an incomplete vagotomy. Additionally, because the majority of patients who have positive results of Hollander tests do not develop recurrent ulcers, the test is not an accurate predictor of ulcer recurrence.[70] Gillespie and co-workers showed that the incidence of "positive" Hollander test results also increases with time up to 2 years; after then, few results convert to positive.[71]

As mentioned previously, the insulin test has been reported to cause shock, convulsions, coma, and death. For this reason, and because of the unreliability of the test in predicting ulcer recurrence, the Hollander test has been largely abandoned as a clinical test of vagal integrity. Pentagastrin stimulation and histamine stimulation following vagotomy are more common, but again, these tests are not accurate predictors of ulcer recurrence. Kronborg compared preoperative and postoperative histamine-stimulated acid-secretory responses and found that only 5% of patients with a preoperative maximal output of less than 20 meq/hour developed recurrent ulcers.[72]

CRITERIA FOR COMPLETENESS OF VAGOTOMY. Many different criteria have been used to determine the completeness of vagotomy. A basal acid output of greater than .25 meq/hour,[73] an acid output after insulin of greater than 3 times basal,[74] an acid output after insulin of 2 meq/hour,[75] an acid output after insulin of 5 meq/hour,[76] an acid output in the first and second hour after insulin administration that is higher than basal acid output,[77] and an increase in volume of gastric juice after insulin administration[78] all suggest incomplete vagotomy. Because none of these criteria alone enable one to predict ulcer recurrence, combinations of criteria have been proposed as a more accurate means of predicting incompleteness of vagotomy and possible ulcer recurrence. Hood and associates, however, did not find multiple criteria to be more accurate than a single criterion for predicting ulcer recurrence.[79]

Hollander's original criteria were based on studies performed in animals with Heidenhain (denervated) gastric pouches.[80] The qualitative changes in acid secretion after insulin administration were then applied clinically. Basal acid secretion varies sufficiently that the "reference" point for a positive Hollander test result is different for each test, thereby complicating reproducibility; moreover, other anatomic factors contribute to the unreliability of this test.[81] For example, after vagotomy and pyloroplasty, and especially after vagotomy and antrectomy, loss of acid into the intestine and reflux of alkaline juices into the stomach occur. In addition, because antrectomy involves the removal of a major source of gastrin, remaining gastric mucosa becomes far less sensitive to parasympathetic stimuli. A retained vagus nerve after antrectomy may easily be missed by the Hollander test. Therefore, the measurement of acid output by nasogastric suctioning after insulin stimulation is inaccurate. In Hollander's original studies in animals with excluded fundic pouches, neither bile reflux nor loss of acid occurred.

In summary, the Hollander test is rarely used clinically to determine completeness of vagotomy. The side effects and unreliability of the test have relegated it to the experimental laboratory, where many of the factors that contribute to the unpredictability of the test results can be controlled.

PANCREATIC POLYPEPTIDE TESTING FOR COMPLETENESS OF VAGOTOMY. Pancreatic polypeptide is secreted from the pancreas when stimulated by bombesin or insulin. Modlin and co-workers have shown experimentally that pancreatic polypeptide release after bilateral truncal vagotomy is almost completely abolished.[82] Release of this substance was decreased only slightly after unilateral vagotomy in the foregoing study. This information has not been applied clinically, but this test may become an important indicator of vagal integrity.[83]

2-DEOXY-D-GLUCOSE TESTING. The mechanism of action and the side effects of this potent vagal stimulator of acid secretion are described previously in this chapter. This substance is a stronger vagal stimulant than insulin.[84] Because the side effects of 2-DG are less predictable than those of insulin, however, it is rarely used for postvagotomy testing.

Zollinger-Ellison Syndrome

Patients with gastrin-secreting tumors usually have abnormally high basal and maximal acid-secretory rates. The basal output is usually greater than 15 meq/hour in the patient who has not undergone an operation and greater than 5 meq/hour in the patient who has undergone operation.[85] The ratio of basal to maximal acid output is greater than 60% in the majority of patients. Some patients with duodenal ulcer secrete acid at basal levels higher than 15 meq/hour,[86] and 5 to 10% of patients with duodenal ulcer have a ratio of basal to maximal acid output of greater than 60%.[87] In patients with recurrent ulceration after gastric operations, or in those with ulcers in abnormal locations such as in the jejunum or the third portion of the duodenum, gastrinoma should be suspected. All these patients should undergo measurement of serum gastrin levels.

Both resting (unstimulated) serum gastrin determinations and serum gastrin measurements after secretin or calcium stimulation are appropriate. Secretin stimulation is usually easier to perform and has fewer side effects than the calcium-infusion test. A single intravenous injection of 1 to 2 U/kg secretin normally inhibits acid secretion, but in the patient with a gastrin-secreting tumor, serum gastrin levels may double, and gastric-acid secretion may increase to near maximal levels.

Calcium gluconate infusion for 3 hours, at 4 to 5 mg/hour, elicits a marked increase in gastric-acid secretion and serum gastrin levels. This test has been shortened to a calcium "challenge," which consists of a single intravenous bolus of 2 mg/kg. Both calcium and secretin tests are accurate in the diagnosis of gastrinoma and enable one to differentiate among patients with retained antrum, duodenal ulcer, and gastrinoma.

A few other conditions with associated hypergastrinemia, with or without acid hypersecretion, may be detected by testing. These conditions are usually discernible by the patient's medical history. For example, the short-bowel syndrome, which results from massive small bowel resection, usually for secondary bowel infarction, may be associated with hypergastrinemia and gastric-acid hypersecretion. Renal failure causes an abnormal clearance of gastrin and elevated serum gastrin levels; however, gastric-acid hypersecretion is usually not present. Thus, the differentiation of these clinical entities from Zollinger-Ellison syndrome is straightforward.

REFERENCES

1. Bloomfield, A.L., and Polland, W.C.: The diagnostic value of studies of gastric secretion. JAMA, *92*:1508, 1929.
2. Decker, G.A.G., and Myburgh, J.A.: A fatality during the Hollander insulin test. S. Afr. Med. J., *43*:869, 1969.
3. Blum, N.I., Mayora, N.G., and Kalser, M.M.: "Augmented" gastric analysis: a word of caution. JAMA, *191*:339, 1965.
4. Sangster, W., Grossman, M.I., and Ivy, A.C.: The effect of two new histamine antagonists (Benadryl and Compound 63) on histamine stimulated gastric secretion of the dog. Gastroenterology, *6*:436, 1946.
5. Rosiere, C.E., and Grossman, M.I.: Analog of histamine that stimulates gastric acid secretion without other actions of histamine, Science, *113*:651, 1951.
6. Baron, J.H.: Clinical Tests of Gastric Secretion. New York, Oxford University Press, 1979.
7. Baron, J.H.: Timing of peak acid output after pentagastrin. Gastroenterology, *56*:641, 1969.
8. Konturek, S.J., and Lankoz, J.: Pentapeptide infusion test. Scand. J. Gastroenterol., *2*:112, 1967.
9. Konturek, S.J., and Krol, W.: The influence of gastrin related peptides on HCl secretion in man and in cats with gastric fistulas and Heidenhain pouches. Gastroenterologia, *106*:281, 1966.
10. Multicentre Study: Intramuscular pentagastrin compared with other stimuli as tests of gastric secretion. Lancet, *1*:341, 1969.
11. McCloy, R.F., and Baron, J.H.: Acute reaction to pentagastrin. Lancet, *1*:548, 1977.
12. Brodie, B.C.: Experiments and observations in the influence of the nerves of the eighth path on the secretion of the stomach. Philos. Trans., *104*:102, 1814.
13. Weiss, A., and Sciales, W.J.: The effect of tolbutamide on human basal gastric secretion. Ann. Intern. Med., *55*:406, 1961.
14. Eisenberg, M.M., Emas, G.S., and Grossman, M.I.: Comparison of the effect of 2-deoxy-D-glucose and insulin on gastric acid secretion in dogs. Surgery, *60*:111, 1966.
15. Christensen, K.C., and Stadil, F.: Effect of epinephrine and norepinephrine on gastrin release and gastric secretion of acid in man. Scand. J. Gastroenterol., *11 (Suppl. 37)*:87, 1976.
16. Hollander, F., Jemerin, E.E., and Weinstein, V.: An insulin test for differentiating vagal from non vagal stomach pouches. Fed. Proc., *1*:116, 1942.

17. Baron, J.H.: Dose response relationships of insulin hypoglycemia and gastric acid in man. Gut, 11:826, 1970.
18. Eisenberg, M.M., et al.: Insulin inhibition of gastric secretion. J. Surg. Res., 3:479, 1963.
19. Spencer, J.: Inhibition of gastric secretion by insulin. Scand. J. Gastroenterol., 8 (Suppl. 21):1, 1973.
20. Farooz, O., and Isenberg, J.I.: Effect of continuous intravenous infusion of insulin versus rapid intravenous injection or insulin or gastric acid secretion in man. Gastroenterology, 68:683, 1975.
21. Aylett, P.: Effects of tolbutamide upon gastric secretion and emptying. Br. Med. J., 1:1464, 1965.
22. Eisenberg, M.M., Emas, G.S., and Grossman, M.I.: Comparison of the effect of 2-deoxy-D-glucose and insulin on gastric acid secretion in dogs. Surgery, 60:111, 1966.
23. Hirschowitz, B.I., and Sachs, G.: Vagal gastric secretory stimulus by 2-deoxy-D-glucose. Am. J. Physiol., 209:452, 1965.
24. Demand, H.A., Gross, H.U., and Berg, G.: Effects of continuous insulin infusions on unstimulated human gastric secretion. Part I. Inter-relations between insulin dosage, blood sugar, and gastric secretory changes. Gastroenterology, 54:1038, 1968.
25. Hall, W.H., Brandoli, H., and Read, R.C.: Effect of calcium infusions on serum calcium and gastric acid secretion. Digestion, 14:389, 1976.
26. Barreros, R.F.: Calcium and gastric secretion. Gastroenterology, 64:1168, 1973.
27. Basso, N., and Passaro, E.: Calcium-stimulated gastric secretion in the Zollinger-Ellison syndrome. Arch. Surg., 101:399, 1970.
28. Fordtran, J.S., and Walsh, J.H.: Gastric acid secretion rate and buffer content of the stomach after eating: results in normal subjects and in patients with duodenal ulcer. J. Clin. Invest., 52:645, 1973.
29. Isenberg, J.I.: Gastric secretory testing. In Gastrointestinal Disease. Edited by M.H. Sleisinger and J.S. Fordtran. Philadelphia, W.B. Saunders, 1978.
30. Malagaleda, J.R., et al.: Measurement of gastric functions during digestion of ordinary solid meals in man. Gastroenterology, 70:203, 1976.
31. George, J.D.: New clinical method for measuring the rate of gastric emptying: the double sampling test meal. Gut, 9:237, 1968.
32. Marks, I.N., and Shay, H.: Augmented histamine test, Ewold test and Diagnex test. Am. J. Dig. Dis., 5:1, 1960.
33. Bock, O.A.A., and Witts, L.J.: Tubeless gastric analysis with Azure A and betazole hydrochloride. Br. Med. J., 2:665, 1961.
34. Christiansen, P.M.: The Azur-A method as a screening test of gastric acid secretion. Scand. J. Gastroenterol., 1:9, 1966.
35. Beal, C.B., and Brown, J.E.: A rapid screening test for gastric achlorhydria. Am. J. Dig. Dis., 13:113, 1968.
36. Knapton, P.J., Hawkins, C.F., and Whitehead, T.P.: Tubeless gastric analysis: trial of the Gastro test. Lencet, 1:439, 1964.
37. Jewett, T.C., Jr., Duszynski, D.O., and Allen, J.E.: The visualization of Meckel's diverticulum with ^{99m}Tc pertechnetate. Surgery, 68:567, 1970.
38. Chaudhuri, T.K., et al.: Radioisotope scan—a possible aid in differentiating retained gastric antrum from Zollinger-Ellison syndrome in patients with recurrent peptic ulcer. Gastroenterology, 65:697, 1973.
39. Bloomfield, A.L., and Keefer, C.S.: Gastric acidity: relation to various factors such as age and physical fitness. J. Clin. Invest., 5:285, 1928.
40. Oi, M., Oshida, K., and Sugimura, S.: The location of gastric ulcer. Gastroenterology, 36:45, 1959.
41. Baron, J.H.: Lean body mass, gastric acid and peptic ulcer. Gut, 10:637, 1969.
42. Maybury, N.K., Faber, R.G., and Hobsley, M.: Postvagotomy insulin test: improved predictability of ulcer recurrence after corrections for height and collection errors. Gut, 18:449, 1977.
43. Goyal, R.K., Gupta, P.S., and Chuttam, H.K.: Gastric acid secretion in Indians with particular reference to the ratio of basal to maximal acid output. Gut, 7:619, 1966.
44. Varma, R.A.: Peptic ulcer in developing countries. In After Vagotomy. Edited by J.A. Williams and A.G. Cox. London, Royce, 1969.
45. Lissoos, I., Hunt, J., and Stein, A.: The augmented histamine test in the South African Bantu. S. Afr. Med. J., 42:1336, 1968.
46. Makhlouf, G.M.: The highest effective dose of histamine for gastric acid secretion. Gastroenterology, 57:766, 1969.
47. Baron, J.H.: Gastric function tests. In Chronic Duodenal Ulcer. Edited by C. Wastell. London, Butterworth, 1972.
48. Grossman, M.I., Kirsner, J.B., and Gillespie, T.E.: Basal and histolog-stimulated gastric secretion in control subjects and in patients with peptic ulcer or gastric cancer. Gastroenterology, 45:14, 1963.
49. Kirkpatrick, J.R., et al.: The short pentagastrin test in the investigation of gastric disease. Gut, 10:760, 1969.
50. Ivey, K.J., and Clifton, J.A.: Back diffusion of hydrogen ions across gastric mucosa of patients with gastric ulcer and rheumatoid arthritis. Br. Med. J., 1:16, 1974.
51. Dragstedt, L.R.: Is gastric ulcer due to hyperfunction or dysfunction of the gastric antrum? Surg. Gynecol. Obstet., 97:517, 1953.
52. Delaney, J.P., et al.: Gastric ulcer and regurgitation gastritis. Gut, 11:715, 1970.
53. Gilbertsen, V.A., and Knatterund, G.L.: Gastric analysis as a screening measure for cancer of the stomach. Cancer, 20:217, 1967.
54. Fischermann, K., Beck, I., and Andersen, B.: Diagnostic value of the augmented histamine test in cancer of the upper part of the stomach. Scand. J. Gastroenterol., 4:517, 1969.
55. Burge, H.W., and Bane, J.R.: Method of testing for complete nerve section during vagotomy. Br. Med. J., 1:615, 1958.
56. Burge, H. (Ed.): Incomplete nerve section—tests for completeness. In Vagotomy. Baltimore, Williams & Wilkins, 1964.
57. Allgöwer, M., and Perreu, S.: Comments concerning intra-operative electro-test for completeness of vagotomy. Prog. Surg., 8:69, 1970.
58. Moe, R.E., and Klopper, P.J.: Demonstration of the functional anatomy of the canine gastric antrum. II. Operative techniques not requiring gastrotomy. Am. J. Surg., 111:80, 1966.
59. Kronborg, O.: Assessment of complete vagotomy. Surg. Clin. North Am., 56:1421, 1976.
60. Asinazi, Y., et al.: Clinical aspects of amyloid Congo red binding. Isr. J. Med. Sci., 3:572, 1967.
61. Lowicki, R., and Littlefield, J.B.: An experimental method of precisely defining the dimension of the gastric antrum. Surg. Forum, 12:308, 1961.
62. Kragelund, E., et al.: Pentapeptide and insulin stimulated gastric acid secretion in patients with gastric

ulcer before and after precise antrectomy. Ann. Surg., 176:659, 1972.
63. Kusakari, K., et al.: An endoscopic test for completeness of vagotomy. Arch. Surg., 105:386, 1972.
64. Amdrup, E., and Jensen, H.E.: Selective vagotomy of the parietal cell mass preserving innervation of the undrained antrum: a preliminary report of results in patients with duodenal ulcer. Gastroenterology, 59:522, 1970.
65. Johnston, D., and Wilkinson, A.R.: Highly selective vagotomy without a drainage procedure in the treatment of duodenal ulcer. Br. J. Surg., 57:289, 1970.
66. Grassi, G., et al.: Variations in secretion during gastric resection for duodenal ulcer. Chir. Gastroenterol., 5:318, 1971.
67. Johnson, A.G., and Baxter, H.K.: Where is your vagotomy incomplete? Observations on operative technique. Br. J. Surg., 64:583, 1977.
68. Hollander, F.: The insulin test for the presence of intact nerve fibers after vagal operations for peptic ulcer. Gastroenterology, 7:607, 1946.
69. Hodge, A.J., Masarei, J.R., and Catchpole, B.N.: The role of the sympathetic nervous system in hypoglycemia-stimulated gastric secretion. Gut, 13:134, 1972.
70. Kronborg, O.: The value of the insulin test in predicting recurrence after vagotomy and drainage for duodenal ulcer. Scand. J. Gastroenterol., 6:471, 1971.
71. Gillespie, G., et al.: The long term stability of the insulin test. Gastroenterology, 58:625, 1970.
72. Kronborg, O.: Influence of the number of parietal cells on risk of recurrence after truncal vagotomy and drainage for duodenal ulcer. Scand. J. Gastroenterol., 7:423, 1972.
73. Gillespie, G., Gillespie, I.E., and Kay, A.W.: An analysis of the insulin test after vagotomy using single and multiple criteria. Gut, 9:470, 1968.
74. Gillespie, G., et al.: Analysis of basal acid secretion and its relation to the insulin response in normal and duodenal ulcer subjects: new criterion for the insulin test. Gastroenterology, 62:903, 1972.
75. Bank, S., Marks, J.N., and Louw, J.H.: Histamine and insulin stimulated gastric acid secretion after selective and truncal vagotomy. Gut, 8:36, 1967.
76. Clark, C.G., and Murray, J.G.: The Burge test for complete vagotomy. J.R. Coll Surg. Edinb., 8:212, 1963.
77. Bitsch, V., et al.: Gastric secretory patterns before and after vagotomy. Lancet, 1:1288, 1966.
78. Waddell, W.R.: The acid secretory response to histamine and insulin hypoglycemia after various operations on the stomach. Surgery, 42:652, 1957.
79. Hood, J.M., et al.: Predictive value of perioperative gastric acid tests. Gut, 17:998, 1976.
80. Jemerin, E.E., Hollander, F., and Weinstein, V.: A comparison of insulin and food as stimuli for the differentiation of vagal and non-vagal gastric pouches. Gastroenterology, 1:500, 1942.
81. Saik, R.P.: Vagotomy Testing. Mount Kisco, NY, Futura Publishing, 1983.
82. Modlin, I.M., Lamers, C.B., and Jaffe, B.M.: Evidence of cholingeric dependence of pancreatic polypeptide (PP) release by bombesin—a possible application. Surgery, 88:75, 1980.
83. Schwartz, T.W.: Pancreatic polypeptide: a hormone under vagal control. Gastroenterology, 85:1411, 1983.
84. Emas, S., and Borg, J.: Stimulation of gastric acid secretion by insulin and 2-deoxy-D-glucose in duodenal ulcer patients. Digestion 7:44, 1972.
85. Thompson, J.C., et al.: Zollinger-Ellison syndrome. Natural history and experience with diagnosis and treatment. Surg. Gynecol. Obstet., 140:721, 1975.
86. Bernades, P., et al.: Discriminative interest of the study of basal acid secretion and pepsin acid correlation in Zollinger-Ellison syndrome and peptic ulcer. Digestion, 9:1, 1973.
87. Isenberg, J.I., Brooks, A.M., and Grossman, M.I.: Pentagastrin versus betazole as a stimulant of gastric secretion. JAMA, 206:2897, 1968.

21

Vascular Laboratory Tests in Peripheral Vascular Disease

Michael C. Dalsing ▪ John V. White ▪ James S. T. Yao

During the last decade, the vascular laboratory has become a vital part of the diagnostic division of many medical centers. Most such laboratory tests are designed to evaluate vascular problems. These disorders include occlusive diseases of the upper and lower extremities, acute deep-venous thrombosis, chronic venous insufficiency, and cerebrovascular disease. The purpose of this chapter is to view the tests in current use in the vascular laboratory and to describe the advantages and shortcomings of each test.

INDIRECT BLOOD PRESSURE MEASUREMENT

Systemic arterial blood pressure is a parameter of cardiovascular function that depends largely on cardiac output and systemic vascular resistance. Indirect measurement of blood pressure, using a sphygmomanometer and stethoscope, is based on the principle that arterial blood flow within a vessel ceases when external pressure on that vessel exceeds systolic pressure, the maximal driving force. Flow through the vessel resumes when external pressure decreases below systolic pressure. This return of flow, detected by auscultation using a Doppler probe or a stethoscope, can be used as the end point for systolic pressure measurement. For diastolic pressure, the point at which sounds disappear is often used as the index for diastolic blood pressure.

Indications

The indirect determination of systemic blood pressure, usually at the brachial level, is the fundamental physiologic test in routine evaluation of the patient. As a general parameter of cardiovascular function, this determination is helpful in the diagnosis and treatment of disorders causing hypertension or hypotension. Aortic valvular abnormalities, coarctation of the aorta, and subclavian or axillary artery disease can be detected by bilateral brachial pressure measurement. For the lower extremities, indirect pressure measurements at the thigh, calf, and ankle levels are useful in establishing the diagnosis of occlusive arterial disease.

Technique

The patient should be comfortably positioned in a quiet environment, with all clothing removed from the limb chosen for the pressure measurement. The vessel auscultated should be at approximately the level of the left ventricle. If the patient is seated, then the arm should be supported on a surface of the appropriate height.

The cuff must contain an air bladder whose width is 40% of the circumference of the midpoint of the limb. Use of a narrower bladder results in falsely high recordings, whereas use of a wider bladder yields falsely low pressures. The length of the bladder should be 80% of the circumference. In the average adult, a cuff containing an air bladder 12 to 14 cm wide and 35 to 40 cm long is adequate. The cuff must be positioned such that the bladder is directly over the artery to be compressed. For the brachial artery, the cuff should be placed 25 cm superior to the antecubital fossa, with the bladder centered on the medial aspect of the arm.

A preliminary determination of the systolic pressure is made by palpating the radial artery and by inflating the cuff until the pulse disappears. Prior to auscultation, the brachial pulse should be palpated inferior to the cuff, to determine the point of auscultation. The bell stethoscope is placed over this point with enough pressure to ensure contact. The bladder is inflated to 30 mm Hg above the palpated systolic pressure and is then deflated at a rate of 2 to 3 mm Hg/sec. A more rapid deflation yields falsely low systolic pressures. The first return of clear, tapping sounds represents the systolic pressure. The point at which these sounds disappear represents the diastolic pressure.[1,2]

The size of the bladder influences the level of pressure; cuff sizes recommended by the American Heart Association are listed in Table 21–1. Other conditions, such as shock or obesity, may also affect the accuracy of indirect pressure measurement. Falsely high blood pressures are often obtained in patients with obese arms if the standard-sized bladder is used.[3] To eliminate this problem, a standard cuff should be applied to the patient's forearm, rather than to the upper arm, and blood pressure should be determined by auscultation over the radial artery.

Interpretation

When correctly performed, sphygmomanometry yields five distinctly audible phases of blood flow. The first phase is the initial return of faint, but clear, tapping sounds, which increase in intensity as cuff pressure slowly decreases. The level of pressure at which these sounds first appear is the systolic blood pressure. These sounds develop a murmur or swishing quality, which marks phase two. During phase three, the auscultatory sounds become more intense. As the cuff pressure is further reduced, an abrupt muffling produces a soft, blowing sound. The level of pressure at which this muffling begins correlates best with diastolic pressure in children. The fifth and final phase of sphygmomanometry is marked by the disappearance of sounds. The point of disappearance provides the best index of diastolic pressure in adults.

If the cardiac rhythm is irregular, accurate determination of indirect blood pressure may be difficult. For patients with atrial fibrillation, the systolic pressure should be recorded as the average of a series of readings of the appearance of the first sound, and the diastolic pressure should be recorded as the average of the fourth and fifth phases.[1]

Diagnostic Efficacy

The accuracy of auscultatory measurements of arterial blood pressure is controversial. Studies by Ragan and Bordley,[4] London and London,[5] and others have reported strong correlation of indirect and direct measurements of both systolic and diastolic arterial pressure, with mean differences no greater than 10 mm Hg. Other investigations, such as those of Van Bergan[6] and Bruner and co-workers,[7] have documented a more variable correlation.

Because variations in methods affect these studies, actual sensitivities of auscultatory pressure measurements are difficult to establish. The ease with which a large amount of clinical information is obtained from the application of auscultatory blood pressure determination makes it an important screening and diagnostic tool, however.

Acceptance by Patients

Because of increasing public awareness of hypertension and because of the ease of testing, most patients accept and expect auscultatory blood pressure determination as a part of each clinical evaluation.

DIRECT BLOOD PRESSURE MEASUREMENT

Direct pressure measurements are obtained by inserting a needle or catheter into the vascular system. This instrument is coupled to an internal or external transducer.[8,9] Modern transducers are simply mechanical electrical converters made of a stiff diaphragm that moves slightly during transmitted catheter pressure changes.[8] Because the diaphragm is part of an electrical circuit, movement varies electrical resistance, capacitance, or inductance.[8] Therefore, mechanical energy is converted to electrical energy. When the electrical signal is passed through a preamplifier and amplifier, a recorder or cathode-ray tube can display rapidly changing pressures visually.[10] Most current monitors contain the preamplifier, amplifier, and recorder in

Table 21–1. Recommended Bladder Dimensions for Blood-Pressure Cuffs

Arm Circumference at Midpoint* (cm)	Cuff Name	Bladder Width (cm)	Bladder Length (cm)
5–7.5	Newborn	3	5
7.5–13	Infant	5	8
13–20	Child	8	13
17–26	Small adult	11	17
24–32	Adult	13	24
32–42	Large adult	17	32
42–50†	Thigh	20	42

*Midpoint of arm is defined as half the distance from the acromion to the olecranon.
†In persons with large limbs, the indirect blood pressure should be measured in the leg or forearm.

(From Kirkendall, W.M., et al.: Recommendations for human blood pressure determination by sphygmomanometers. Subcommittee of the American Heart Association Postgraduate Education Committee. Circulation, 62:1146A, 1980. By permission of the American Heart Association.)

one unit. A computerized recorder provides a numeric (digital) display.

Indications

Direct arterial blood pressure measurements are indicated when rapidly changing blood pressure is of concern or when an arterial line is available for continuous blood-gas monitoring.[11,12] These measurements are often taken in the operating room, recovery room, or intensive care unit for close monitoring of changes in blood pressure. For vascular surgeons, direct recording of arterial pressure from the common femoral artery may be necessary to determine the hemodynamic significance of an angiographic stenosis of the iliac artery.

Technique

The catheter for direct pressure measurements must be placed percutaneously or by standard cutdown technique. The radial, ulnar, brachial, femoral, dorsalis pedis, and superficial temporal arteries have all been used.[11] Careful suture or taped attachment of the catheter to the patient is mandatory, to prevent inadvertent removal and bleeding.

The tubing used to connect the catheter to the flush system and the transducer must be of proper size, stiff, short, and firmly attached to the patient, to prevent movement artifact, decreased frequency, or dampening.[8,13,14] A flushing system, using continuous or intermittent injection of heparinized saline solution through the catheter and connecting tubing, is necessary to prevent clotting and to remove air bubbles. The use of stopcocks must be minimized because of inherent problems with air trapping and small lumen size.[12,14] If an external transducer is used for monitoring, it must be positioned at the level of the catheter, to offset gravitational and hydrostatic forces.

Transducers must have a natural frequency of at least 24 Hz to be acceptable for a wide range of clinical situations.[8,12,15] Air bubbles are more compressible than fluid, and their presence dampens the readings.[10,12-14] Small air bubbles change the system's frequency, with possible overshoot.[14] Therefore, all air bubbles in the system must be removed. The transducer and recorder must be zeroed and calibrated for meaningful data generation. Cleanliness and sterility of the catheter, flushing system, and transducers decrease the incidence of septic problems.

Damage to the vessel by catheter insertion may result in pseudoaneurysm formation, intimal flap, thrombosis, emboli, or sepsis.[10,16-18] Death is a rare complication with proper medical care, however, and ischemic tissue loss is only sporadically reported.[19]

Some controversy exists regarding central, consisting of aortoiliac, femoral, or axillary artery, catheter placement, as opposed to more peripheral arterial placement.[18] In a patient in extreme shock central arterial pressure may be the only reliable or obtainable pressure, and it must be measured. Otherwise, in most patients, placement of the catheter in a peripheral artery seems acceptable and has a lower incidence of complications. The more proximal the catheter placement, the more at risk is the extremity.

Besides use in monitoring, direct arterial pressure recording is useful in the determination of the hemodynamic significance of iliac artery stenosis.[20] This measurement is often made by placing the catheter in the patient's femoral artery and by recording pressure changes that occur during pharmacologically induced vasodilatation. Moreover, recording of intra-arterial pressure is useful at the time of percutaneous balloon dilatation of stenotic lesions of the iliac artery.

Interpretation

The blood pressure pulse has a typical appearance. Systolic pressure is the maximal pressure generated in the vascular system by ventricular systole. Diastolic pressure is the lowest intravascular pressure at the end of ventricular diastole. Mean pressure is the integral area under the curve and is generally one-third of the pulse pressure added to diastolic pressure. It can be obtained directly from direct arterial pressure monitoring by mechanical or electrical dampening. The pulse pressure is the difference between systolic and diastolic pressures. In general, the upstroke of the curve is the result of ventricular pressure and flow generation. As ventricular blood flow begins to decrease, runoff flow exceeds volume input, and the curve starts a gentle decline. With aortic valve closure, forward flow stops, coronary flow increases, and the sinus of Valsalva becomes distended. Continued runoff occurs, generating the dicrotic notch. Finally, a gentle downward curve of peripheral runoff into multiple capacitance vessels is noted, until the next ventricular systole. Factors affecting any of these components of the pressure curve may change its appearance. Systolic peak pressure depends more strongly on cardiac ability to generate flow and pressure, whereas diastolic pressure is influenced more strongly by peripheral resistance and aortic valve closure.[10,16,21]

Although detailed interpretation of the blood pressure curve, with reasons for abnormal generation, is not possible in this chapter, a few facts should be considered. Blood pressure is equal to cardiac stroke volume multiplied by heart rate, multiplied by total peripheral resistance. That blood pressure changes directly with abnormalities in these three variables helps to explain the change and to suggest possible management of the patient. Systolic blood pressure may be elevated in patients with hypermetabolic states that increase the stroke volume and heart rate, such as thyrotoxicosis. Diastolic blood pressure may be elevated in hypertension or in other states of increased total peripheral resistance. Similarly, the pulse pressure may change in patients with states such as cardiac tamponade, hypovolemic shock, or aortic valve malfunction, with a variation noted in the dicrotic notch.[11,16,21] Coupled with the electrocardiogram, simultaneous blood pressure measurements can determine the instantaneous effectiveness of each heartbeat, a determination that may be useful in the management of such problems as premature ventricular contractions. Trends in blood pressure are more important than sporadic determinations in an adequate evaluation of the patient's well-being.

For direct femoral artery pressure recording to determine the adequacy of inflow, both resting (baseline) pressure and pressure changes after vasodilatation. (exercise or drug-induced) are used for assessment.[22-25] The percentage of change in femoral-brachial pressure index (% FBI) is then calclated at maximum vasodilatation.[25] Most studies consider reductions in the percentage of change (%Δ) of the FBI of up to 15% as normal, of 15% to 18% as borderline, and of greater than 18% as abnormal.[22-25] Using a reduction in the percentage of change in FBI of 15% as determined by the receiver-operator curve, Flanigan and colleagues found that papaverine-induced vasodilatation accurately identified subcritical aortoiliac stenosis, with no false-positive results.[25]

Diagnostic Efficacy

Considering all the mechanical factors that may contribute to an error, as well as the controversy regarding central versus peripheral monitoring, specific direct measurement may be ±95% accurate.[2,10,13] This rate of accuracy is probably no better than that of indirect measurement; however, the direct-catheter method has two other benefits.[26] It gives a continuous recording, to enable one to correct rapid trends, and it allows one to obtain repeated blood-gas measurements.

DOPPLER ULTRASOUND

A piezoelectric crystal vibrates under the influence of an electric field and radiates energy in the form of sound waves. Such a crystal also changes dimension when it is hit by a moving sound wave, and it develops a voltage across the crystal. These properties allow the crystal to generate and also to detect sound waves. The waves emanating from the crystal are in the ultrasonic frequency spectrum of 1 to 10 megacycles per second or megaHertz, usually expressed as MHz, and they do not harm living tissue.

The Doppler effect is the apparent change in frequency by movement. This effect is exemplified most commonly by the sound frequency change in a train whistle as the train moves away from a stationary listener.

Doppler instruments are based on the Doppler effect and on the properties of the piezoelectric crystal. Generated ultrasonic waves penetrate the tissue and are backscattered by moving red blood cells. The Doppler shift in frequency between the transmitted and the reflected sound is proportional to the blood velocity. This shift is expressed mathematically as follows:

change in frequency (Doppler shift) = $2 fv \cos \theta / C$

where f is the frequency of the incident sound beam, v is velocity, θ is the angle of the incident sound beam to the vessel examined (applicable below 60°), and C is the velocity of sound in tissue.

Because sound beam frequency, the angle of incidence, and the velocity of the sound in tissue are considered constant, the frequency shift is proportional to the blood flow velocity.[27]

Two types of Doppler instruments are available: continuous-wave and pulsed-wave devices. The continuous-wave Doppler uses one piezoelectric crystal to generate sound waves continuously and an adjacent crystal to sample the backscattered sounds. The backscattered sound is mixed with the transmitted frequency to form an audible sound proportional to blood-flow velocity.[28] Two types of voltage converters process the sounds for either nondirectional or directional analog recording. The directional velocity meters introduce a 90° phase-shift network prior to flow detection, which adds to or subtracts from the Doppler shift.[27] The wave of forward and reverse components may be displayed on a single-channel recorder or as 2 separate waveforms.

The pulsed Doppler instrument uses the same crystal to generate and to receive sound waves.[28] An electric gating system examines sounds returning at different times, thereby measuring flow velocity at a given tissue depth. This instrument samples small intraluminal areas of blood velocity, rather than complete cross-sectional areas, as does the continuous-wave Doppler device.

Indications

Doppler ultrasound is useful in evaluating occlusive arterial disease of the upper and lower extremities, including disorders of the large arteries and the small peripheral arteries, such as digital and penile vessels. In addition, Doppler ultrasound may provide information useful in the evaluation of patients with acute deep-venous thrombosis and with chronic venous insufficiency. New developments with microprocessors have made it possible to image flow within an artery. This technique, called ultrasonic arteriography, is useful in assessing the carotid artery. Further, flow-velocity signals may be recorded and subjected to frequency spectral analysis, to detect flow abnormalities.

Techniques and Technical Pitfalls

The arterial testing techniques for lower limb, upper limb, digital, or penile pressure measurement involve the continuous-wave Doppler and an appropriately sized sphygmomanometry cuff.[27,29,30] The Doppler transducer is positioned over the artery to be examined at an angle of 60° and is coupled to the skin with a water-soluble gel. Examination is often conducted with the patient in the supine position, after a period of rest. A zero-crossing frequency-to-voltage converter creates an analog waveform depicting systolic and diastolic flows. A sonogram of the entire frequency spectrum can be generated by real-time, time-compression, or fast-Fourier transforming techniques for quantitative analysis.[31] Most quantitative analysis is applied to femoral-artery recording, and it has been used to determine the adequacy of inflow to the aortoiliac segment.[32-34]

The vessels examined in the lower extremity are the femoral, popliteal, posterior tibial, and dorsalis pedis, or the lateral tarsal and the digital arteries. For recording of lower limb pressure, the bladder cuff should be 20% wider than the diameter of the patient's limb. Table 21–2 outlines current cuff sizes used in most vascular laboratories.

In stress testing by treadmill exercise, the patient walks on a treadmill at 4 km/hour, or on a 12% grade at 2.5 km/hour, for 5 min or until the patient must stop because of leg pain.[28] The patient then resumes the supine position, and brachial and ankle pressures are taken every minute until they reach baseline level (10 to 15 min). If treadmill exercise testing is not possible, the alternate stress test is by reactive hyperemia. The blood-pressure cuff is inflated to 50 mm Hg above the systolic pressure for 5 min, and ankle and brachial pressures are recorded at 1-min intervals after deflation of the cuff until the baseline level is reached.

Examination of the upper extremity involves the subclavian, axillary, brachial, radial, and ulnar arteries, as well as the digital vessels. Positional changes, such as military position, hyperabduction, and Adson maneuver, are used to determine the presence of the thoracic outlet syndrome.[35]

The major pitfalls in arterial study are improper cuff size, which results in high readings if the cuff is too narrow or vice versa, and calcified vessels that resist compression, such as in diabetic patients.[29,36] Improper positioning of the Doppler probe, defective equipment, or external arterial compression may also lead to unreliable results.

For venous examination, the Doppler transducer is placed over the femoral, popliteal, and posterior tibial veins and is held at an angle of approximately 60°. A strip-chart recorder notes the change during respiration (spontaneous) or during augmentation maneuvers (Valsalva maneuver or calf and thigh compression).[37,38] The upper extremity can be evaluated with similar maneuvers. This test is used to determine acute occlusive thrombosis. Bilateral evaluation is critical. Reverse flow on standing, during inspiration, or with tourniquet localization can be determined for evaluation of valvular incompetence using the directional Doppler probe with the patient upright and holding on to a rail to ensure leg relaxation.[37,38]

The major technical pitfall in venous examination is the inability to evaluate the infrapopliteal veins, the profunda femoris vein, or the hypogastric veins. One cannot distinguish between external compression and luminal occlusion by thrombus. Right-sided heart failure, with the resultant retrograde pulsation, can cause problems in interpretation. The technician must have a gentle hand, to prevent external compression of blood vessels.

Supraorbital Doppler arterial examination for indirect evaluation of the internal carotid artery has been supplanted by other techniques and is not discussed here. Doppler examination of the carotid artery now centers around direct evaluation of the accessible extracranial vessels, especially the bifurcation of the carotid artery. Flow velocity or spectral frequency analysis from the carotid artery can be used to distinguish among occluded, stenotic, or normal vessels.[39-41] Auditory interpretation by a skilled technician can also be used in the interpretation of stenosis.[42]

The examination is performed with the patient supine and resting, and the cervical area is exposed. A pencil probe with acoustic-gel interface is placed anterior to the sternocleidomastoid, and the maximal

Table 21–2. Cuff Sizes Currently Used in the Vascular Laboratory

Location	Cuff Width (cm)
Ankle	12
Calf	12
High thigh	20
Low thigh	20
Finger or toe	2.5
Penis	2.5

signal is obtained. A paper strip-recorder measures zero baseline and the pulse waveform for several cardiac cycles. A similar reading from the brachial artery is recorded at the point of highest systolic pressure. With B-mode localization of the internal and common carotid arteries, sound recordings from these locations may be analyzed.[39,43]

The carotid Doppler examination has limitations. Nonstenotic ulcerative lesions are missed. Hematoma, scar tissue, and calcified plaque interfere with generated transmission. Diagnostic error results from improper probe placement, with less-than-maximal tracings. Any condition causing an altered rate of strength of systolic ejection changes the carotid waveform; such disorders include hyper- or hypothyroidism, cardiac failure, and anemia.

Flow imaging or ultrasonic angiography can be generated by continuous-wave or pulsed-wave Doppler devices.[44,45] All such studies are performed with the patient in the supine position, with the head turned about 30° away from the side of examination. The continuous-wave system samples the flow pattern of all vessels in its path, using a storage oscilloscope to form a visible image, to record velocity waveforms at specific locations, and to tape signals for auditory analysis. The addition of directional components can be used to eliminate the venous flow. Unlike the pulsed Doppler technique, the continuous-wave system does not allow one to study specific points in the tissue, and therefore, external flows may cause confusion. A microcomputer may be added to generate colors, to show decreased or turbulent flow at specific areas.[44] This procedure may eliminate the problem of transverse vessel analysis. Again, small ulcerating lesions are missed.

The pulsed-Doppler (Hokanson) device, by using gates to pick only reflected sound during a certain time interval, enables one to study the flow at different tissue depths.[45,46] A flow map that may be filmed is generated, both in the longitudinal and in the transverse direction (Fig. 21–1). Auditory interpretation is also used. Technical problems include differentiation of the external from the internal carotid artery, especially in patients with total occlusion of one or the other, the presence of calcification, which inhibits sound transmission, and the need for expertise in auditory interpretation. Lesions smaller than 1 mm may be difficult to find.

Interpretation

In arterial examination, velocity waveforms should be triphasic, with a diastolic reverse flow, to be absolutely normal. Once arteriosclerotic changes occur, turbulence is seen at the peak or descending forward-flow phase. The reverse flow is progressively lost from stenosis to complete occlusion.[27,36,38,47] In patients with stenosis, the systolic waveforms flatten and broaden, becoming nonpulsatile with occlusion (Fig. 21–2).

Quantitative analysis of the waveform by spectral analysis compares the peak-to-peak wave excursion to envelope height over the entire cardiac cycle. This is the pulsatile index[48] or PI. The PI is normal above 6.0 in the common femoral artery and increases more distally. Therefore, in patients with distal occlusion, the PI (proximal)-to-PI (distal), or damping factor (DF), should be greater than 1. This spectral analysis is free of velocity scatter under the systolic curve if no turbulence is present. Filling in suggests the diagnosis of stenotic or occlusive lesions.[49] If one adds this interpretation to the se-

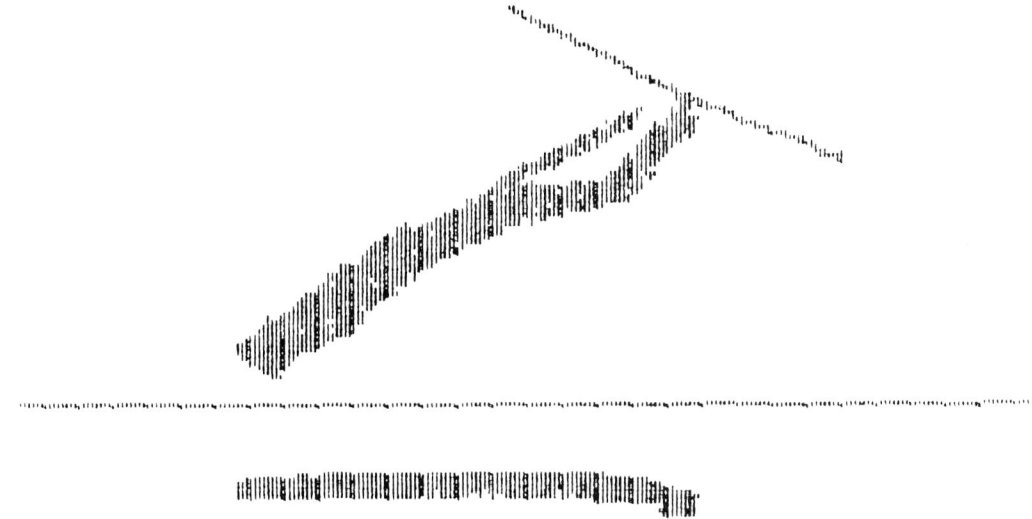

FIG. 21–1. Example of ultrasonic arteriography of the carotid artery obtained by the pulsed Doppler technique.

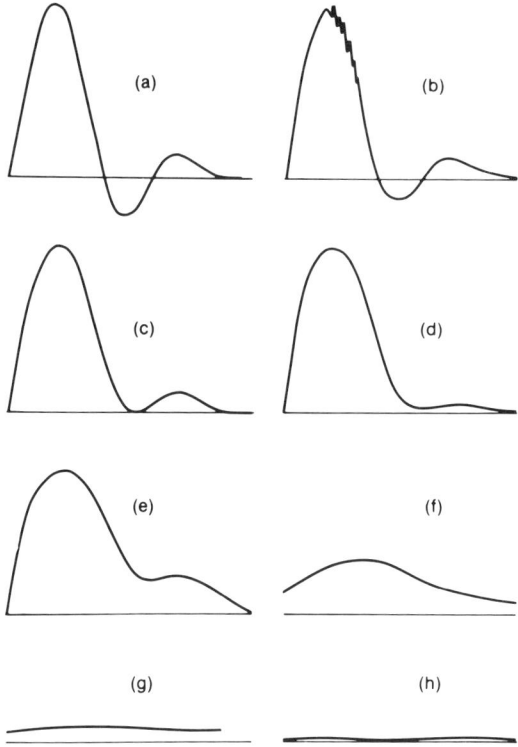

FIG. 21–2. Various shapes of flow-velocity waveforms, from normal (a) to total occlusion (h). The blood-flow-velocity waveform becomes progressively dampened with increasing arterial stenosis. (From Johnston, K.W., et al.: Methods for obtaining, processing, and quantifying Doppler blood velocity waveforms. In Investigation of Vascular Disorders. Edited by A.N. Nicolaides and J.S.T. Yao. New York, Churchill Livingstone, 1981.)

quential pressures, a clear picture of the anatomic structures may be determined.

The measure of comparative pressures by Doppler ultrasound is a simple means of evaluating occlusion. Lower leg pressures are higher than arm pressures. When comparing lower-extremity to brachial pressures, the ratio should be greater than or equal to 1 in normal patients; a lower ratio suggests stenotic disease.[27–29] Diabetic or other patients with calcified vessels are an exception because these vessels are not compressible, and therefore, the ratios are not useful for interpretation. Patients with intermittent claudication generally have a pressure index (ankle-brachial) of 0.5 to 0.7. Patients with rest pain or other severe ischemic symptoms generally have a ratio of 0.3 or less.[28,29] The normal toe-brachial pressure is 0.85 or greater. Asymptomatic patients have a ratio greater than 0.5, those with claudication have a ratio ranging from 0.2 to 0.5, and patients with severe ischemia often have a ratio of less than 0.2. A penile-brachial ratio of less than 0.6 is consistent with vasculogenic impotence.[30]

The absolute pressure can be helpful in determining segmental occlusions, both in the upper and in the lower extremity, as suggested by the pressure index results. A pressure level under 40 mg Hg is often associated with limb-threatening ischemia.[50,51] As one observes pressures from low thigh to ankle, a 30-mm Hg pressure drop indicates a severe stenotic or occlusive process. Therefore, if one observes a 30-mm Hg pressure drop from the low thigh to the calf and a flattening of the waveform with lack of reverse flow, a popliteal occlusion is probably present.

Because stress testing should result in vasodilation and increased flow, a normal examination consists of an elevation, or no decrease in, ankle pressure after 5 min of walking. If a decrease is noted, then a proximal, hemodynamically significant lesion is present.[28,29,52] One other general rule should be kept in mind: the greater the number of serial stenotic lesions, the lower the ankle-brachial ratio.

Study of the upper extremity has shown that a 15-mm Hg segmental drop in pressure is significant. Ischemic indices are greater than or equal to 0.9 for normal patients, average 0.6 for patients with exertional pain, and are 0.3 for those with severe ischemia.[53] A delay longer than 20 mm/sec in the onset of systolic flow is present in patients with unilateral subclavian artery stenosis when the brachial arteries are monitored.[54] Distal fingertip ischemia is suggested by a 30-mm Hg wrist-to-digit difference, or a 15-mm Hg finger-to-finger difference.[28]

The ultrasonic Doppler examination for acute venous thrombosis is normal if flow has respiratory variation and augments with foot or calf pressure. Loss of respiratory variation suggests an acute occlusion proximally, and loss of foot or calf augmentation (increased flow) suggests obstruction between the Doppler probe and the site of compression.[37,38]

The Doppler examination for venous insufficiency allows one to detect venous valve incompetence. Femoral venous valve incompetence is shown by reverse flow on standing or abdominal compression. With a below-knee tourniquet to occlude the greater and lesser saphenous veins, popliteal valve incompetence is suggested by reverse flow on release of compression,[28,37,38] as well as by to-and-fro fluctuation on calf-muscle compression. To-and-fro fluctuations are heard over incompetent perforating veins.

Pulse waveforms from the common carotid artery can be analyzed by flow velocity or frequency analysis. The resistance index equals the peak-systolic flow level divided by the difference between peak-systolic and diastolic levels. Normal patients have a range of 0.55 to 0.75.[41] High-grade stenosis or occlusion is suggested by a ratio greater than 0.75.

Other researchers have found the 2 systolic peaks to be useful in analysis. A primary-to-secondary-peak ratio of less than 1.5 in either vessel suggests significant bifurcation disease.[55]

Rutherford and Kreutzer analyzed the waveform by computer and found 9 variables that gave substantial information in predicting disease.[40] Five of these variables gave the most information and were used with co-efficients generated from computer analysis to make classification equations; these variables are peak-systolic velocity, end-diastolic velocity, peak-diastolic velocity, systolic peak width at midheight, and systolic acceleration. Analysis in each case requires computer interfacing.

Frequency spectral analysis can be quantitatively evaluated by observing 3 simple variables. The first is the peak-systolic velocity. Frequency less than 3.5 kHz suggests stenosis of under 50%, frequency greater than 4.0 kHz is associated with stenosis of greater than 50%, and the midrange is the gray area. Second is the spectral broadening or filling in of the systolic area. The more turbulence (stenosis), the more filling in is observed. Finally, the diastolic flow shows no reversal, except in patients with high-grade stenosis or occlusion, in those with valvular heart disease, and in some normal young people. The more hemodynamically significant the lesion, the greater the diastolic flow elevation, finally reaching more than 4 kHz, which signifies severe stenosis. Table 21–3 shows the flow velocity value suggested by Zierler and co-workers to grade the degree of stenosis.[56]

The continuous-wave Doppler device provides a flow map of the carotid bifurcation that suggests stenosis by a higher pitch and a more turbulent signal.[45,46] The pulsed-Doppler technique, as modified by Sumner and associates, generates cross-sectional and lateral views of the vessel based on flow signals, which are interpreted as stenotic or not, and enables one to calculate the percentage of stenosis.[46] A diameter and area histogram can be generated to indicate relative stenosis. Audible signals are interpreted by the technician on a 0-to-4 scale, with 3 and 4 suggesting stenosis of greater than 40%.

Diagnostic Efficacy

The ultrasonic Doppler vascular examination provides an accurate and effective method of documenting the presence and extent of vascular disease. Assessment of the lower extremity is most reliable with measurement of segmental pressures, calculation of the ankle-brachial index, inspection of flow-velocity waveforms, and, for selected patients, treadmill testing. The most accurate information is provided by the ankle-brachial index.

Ouriel and Zarins evaluated the usefulness of the absolute ankle pressure, the brachial-ankle pressure gradient, and the ankle-brachial index in predicting the presence or absence of arterial disease.[57] In a study of 260 limbs with angiographically documented peripheral vascular disease and of 68 normal limbs, these investigators found the ankle-brachial index had a 94% sensitivity and a 99% specificity for the presence of disease and a 100% specificity for the absence of significant arterial occlusive disease (Fig. 21–3). Evaluation of these parameters as predictors of limb viability showed the absolute ankle pressure to be the best determinant of limb survival. Using a minimum ankle pressure of 60 mm Hg as the lowest value for viability, 86% of viable and 77% of nonviable limbs were correctly identified. The accuracy of these indices is diminished in the presence of heavily calcified vessels, which yield falsely elevated results. For these patients, correlation of flow-velocity waveforms with

Table 21–3. Categories of Internal Carotid Artery Disease

Category	Common Carotid Artery	Internal Carotid Artery
Normal	"Normal contour"*	No or minimal spectral broadening in decelerating phase of systole; window still present
Minimal disease (1–15%)	"Abnormal contour"†	Minimal or even "no" spectral broadening in decelerating phase of systole; clear window
Moderate disease (16–49%)		Spectral broadening throughout systole; no window; systolic peak <4 kHz
Severe disease (50–99%)		Systolic peak >4 kHz; increased diastolic flow; marked spectral broadening
Occlusion	Flow to 0 or reversed	No signal

*The first zero slope after systole occurs below the midslope.
†The first zero slope after systole occurs above the midslope.

(From Zierler, R.E., Roederer, G.O., and Strandness, D.E.: The use of frequency spectral analysis in carotid artery surgery. In Cerebrovascular Insufficiency. Edited by J.J. Bergan and J.S.T. Yao. New York, Grune & Stratton, 1983, p. 137. Used with permission.)

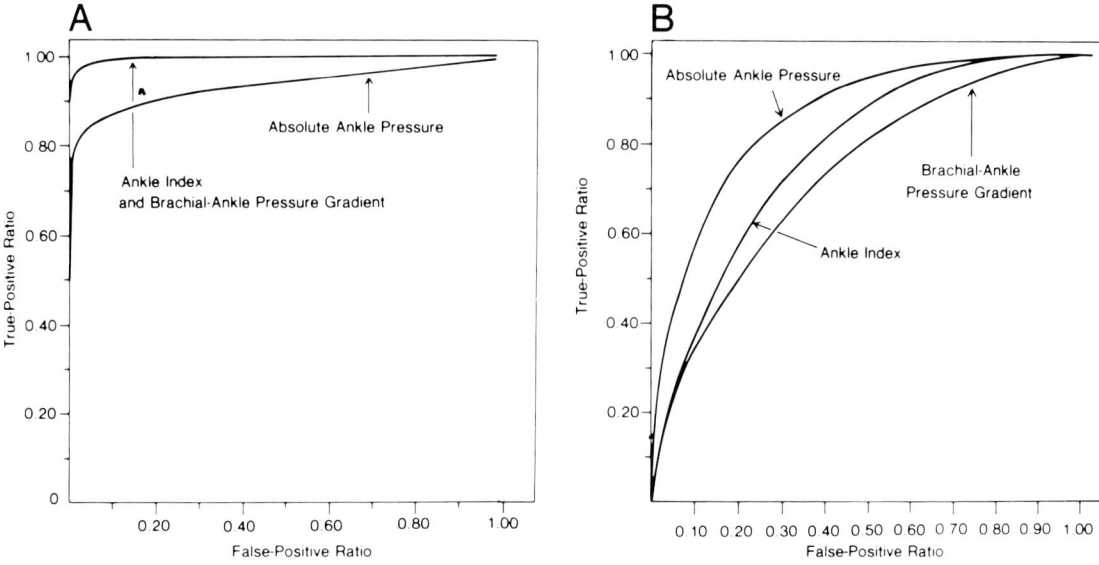

FIG. 21–3. Receiver-operator characteristic (ROC) curves illustrating absolute ankle pressure, ankle index to discriminate between normal and arteriographically diseased limbs *(A)* and between viable and nonviable limbs *(B)*. (From Ouriel, K., and Zarins, C.K.: Doppler ankle pressure: an evaluation of three methods of expression. Arch. Surg., *117*:1297, 1982. Used with permission of the American Medical Association.)

segmental pressures provides a better assessment of arterial occlusive disease.

Treadmill testing is an adjunctive method of demonstrating hemodynamically significant peripheral vascular disease in patients with claudication whose resting ankle-brachial index is in the normal range. This form of testing has been shown by Ouriel and Zarins to have a sensitivity and specificity greater than 95%.[57] Sequential examinations may vary, however, and postexercise pressures may differ as much as 24% in the more symptomatic leg and 15% in the more normal limb; this test is therefore less reliable for routine follow-up examinations.[58]

Toe pressures, though also variable on sequential testing, can enhance the interpretation of the Doppler examination of the lower extremity by providing an assessment of flow through the small end arteries of the foot. Carter and Lezack found that toe pressures were abnormal in 74% of limbs with angiographically documented arterial stenoses and in 97% of those with arterial occlusions.[59] These many facets of the lower extremity evaluation combine to produce an accurate anatomic and hemodynamic description of the arterial tree.

Many noninvasive tests are currently available for evaluation of the carotid artery. Frequency spectral analysis of carotid artery flow patterns, using a pulsed-Doppler system, provides an accurate way to evaluate the carotid artery. Blackshear and Strandness used this method of detection to study 17 vessels with minimal disease and 45 vessels with occlusive disease, as determined by angiography.[60] Computer-generated frequency spectral analysis correctly identified 76% of vessels with minimal disease and 89% with documented occlusive disease. This method of evaluation also proved accurate in the presence of bilateral disease. Using computer-assisted multidiscriminant analysis of pulse waveforms, Rutherford, Hiatt, and Kreutzer achieved an accuracy rate of 100% in identifying occluded, stenotic, and normal carotid arteries.[61] Of stenotic lesions, sensitivity in the discrimination of significant from noncritical stenoses was 82%. Although these methods of analysis are accurate, they fail to enable one to identify the contribution of the internal and external carotid arteries to the altered frequency spectrum and the flow-velocity waveform.

Ultrasonic arteriography, with recent technical improvements, has become an acceptable diagnostic tool. An overall accuracy rate of greater than 70% has been reported by many authors. Sensitivity of greater than 90% for critical stenoses has been documented.[60] This technique is limited because poorly visualized areas, such as those shadowed by calcific plaque, are depicted as stenotic, and specificity is thereby reduced. Moreover, this technique does not allow one to detect ulcerating plaque. As with B-mode scanning, ultrasonic arteriography can be coupled with frequency spectral analysis to enhance accuracy to greater than 90%.

The noninvasive detection of occlusive disease of the carotid artery continues to improve. None of the many available methods are completely accurate. Although a selected combination of diagnostic techniques may improve accuracy, as noted previously, overall specificity and cost-effectiveness decline as each additional test is added.

Doppler ultrasound is also useful for evaluation of the venous system. The venous Doppler examination of the lower extremity for the detection of deep-venous thrombosis has an overall accuracy rate of 88%, with an average false-positive rate of 12% and an average false-negative rate of 12%.[62,63] This method of testing is more effective in proximal thrombosis; the rate of accuracy is 92% in patients with iliofemoral venous occlusion. In a comparison of Doppler examination with venography in the diagnosis of deep-venous thrombosis occurring inferior to the knee, the noninvasive test had a sensitivity of 95% and a specificity of 85%, for an overall accuracy rate of 88%.

The directional Doppler assessment of chronic venous insufficiency can be accomplished with an accuracy rate of 92%. This method of examination permits the localization of insufficiency to the greater or lesser saphenous systems or the deep venous system. The ease and reliability with which this test can be performed make it the screening test of choice in the outpatient setting.[90]

FLUID-FILLED PLETHYSMOGRAPHY

The principle of oculoplethysmography is the recording of phasic eye-volume change produced by pulsatile blood flow.[64] The ophthalmic artery, a branch of the internal carotid artery, is the major blood supply to the eye, and therefore, pulse delays noted in the eye correlate with delayed blood flow to the internal carotid artery. Plastic eyecups are placed on the sclera and are connected by a fluid-filled system to a sensitive pressure transducer for eye-pulse recording. As the globe expands with each arterial pulse, the cornea is drawn away from the cup, to exert a negative pressure, which is recorded. Simultaneous contralateral eye and ear lobe pulses are recorded, to determine delay.

Indications

Oculoplethysmography is used to determine carotid artery stenosis in symptomatic patients or in asymptomatic patients with bruits.[68,85]

Technique and Technical Pitfalls

The patient sits, leaning forward, and focuses on a stationary object to decrease eye movement. Anesthetic agents allow eyecup application bilaterally to the cornea with 45-mm Hg negative suction. Prior to placement, the corneal cups are filled with saline solution. Suction is equalized between the 2 eyes, and a pressure transducer is connected to a paper strip-chart recorder with differential output that can simultaneously record the eye pulses. Generally, the recorder is calibrated at 2.5 mm vertical deflection/ 1 mm Hg at 100 mm/sec. A photoelectric transducer records ear pulses simultaneously, to allow display of 3 pulse waveforms with differential eye output (fourth line) together.[27] The technique is simple, safe, and rapid to perform, requiring under 5 min in cooperative subjects. The eyecups are switched, and a new tracing is made, to delete mechanical error.

Patients who blink continuously may pose a problem. Because of the application of anesthetic eyedrops, patients must be instructed not to rub their eyes or otherwise traumatize them during the period of decreased sensation.[65]

Interpretation

Comparison is made of pulse arrival times in the right and left eyes, using the ear pulse as the reference point. The differential line is a machine-generated waveform amplifying right and left eye differences by subtracting the respective amplitudes and multiplying by two. In patients with no pulse delay, no variable change is noted, and a straight line is formed. Using the tracing, one makes two pseudobaselines by drawing a line between the last peak and the first pulse rise (total outflow). Deviation of the differential line from these pseudobaselines suggests pulse delay. Moreover, a visual delay in the pulse is a significant indicator of pulse delay, and the differential study may not be necessary. Computer-generated pulse-delay determinations have also become available.

Diagnostic Efficacy

Oculoplethysmography combined with carotid phonoangiography has been reported to be an accurate determinant of significant carotid artery stenosis, that is, stenosis of 40 to 60%, in 90% of patients.[66–69] We have found such accuracy only in patients with stenosis that is greater than 60%.[70] Several investigators have found that carotid phonoangiography adds little to the diagnostic accuracy of oculoplethysmography.[69,70,71] Furthermore, when oculoplethysmograms were analyzed alone in patients with carotid lesions with 50% stenosis or greater, the false-negative response was 40 to 50%.[71,72] Keagy and associates noted a similar problem in comparing the results of the foregoing methods with angiographic findings.[73] Based on these observations, the useful place of oculoplethysmography in evaluation of the carotid artery remains controversial.

AIR-FILLED PLETHYSMOGRAPHY

Air-filled plethysmography measures the change in air pressure produced by a corresponding change in volume of the part examined. The air may be enclosed in a cuff that encircles the volume-changing organ (phleborrheograph or pulse-volume recorder) or in a cup to attach to the globe of the eye (oculopneumoplethysmograph). The pressure change is directly proportional to the change in volume. By various manipulations, one may analyze abnormal venous outflow, differential eye pressures, or arterial pulse pressures.

Indications

Phleborrheography is used to determine the presence of acute venous thrombosis. The pulse-volume recorder is clinically useful in evaluating arterial occlusive disease. This recorder enables one to assess claudication, rest pain, and the patient's ability to heal in the presence of ischemic disease, and it helps to pinpoint the level of anatomic abnormality. This technique has been used in patients with lower- and upper-extremity arterial occlusive disease, as well as in those with vasospastic, compressive, and malformation-induced vascular diseases. Oculopneumoplethysmography aids in the evaluation of carotid stenotic disease.

Techniques and Technical Pitfalls

The phleborrheogram consists of a polygraph (paper-strip recorder), a volumetric transducer, in which the diaphragm moves with the slightest pressure change, and a series of 6 sphygmomanometric-type cuffs. The chest cuff records respiratory movements; the remaining cuffs are placed on the low thigh, below the knee, on the midleg, and on the ankle and the foot. The last 2 cuffs may be used to record volume change or to apply pressure to the leg or foot. The cuffs are inflated automatically with volume to a pressure of 10 mm Hg, and removal of 0.2 ml air allows calibration of a 2-cm deflection on the polygraph in each cuff. The change in pressure during respiration is first noted. The second run allows 3 100-mm Hg pulses to the foot cuff, with pressure measurement in the remaining cuffs, to observe a change in baseline. The final run is generated with 3 50-mm Hg pressure pulses to the ankle cuff, with all remaining cuffs measuring pressure changes.[74]

The major pitfall of phleborrheography is technical error. The technician must recognize abnormal patterns, and the patient must have the knee flexed or the thigh extended, or else must be in the decubitus position to obtain a true picture of the problem without external, nonpathologic compression.[74,75] False-negative results may be caused by calf-vein thrombosis, partial occlusions, or occlusions with large collateral vessels; such results also occur in patients receiving mechanical respiration.[74,76] External venous compression must be ruled out clinically.

The pulse-volume recorder is a neoprene bladder with Velcro straps of varying sizes, to accommodate various anatomic positions, even a digit.[77] The cuff is positioned on the extremity such that 75 ± 10 ml air cause a 65-mm Hg pressure in the cuff, as measured by a pressure-sensitive diaphragm transducer. The changes in pressure are recorded on a paper printer and are compared to changes in limb volume caused by arterial inflow. Usually, a 1-mm Hg pressure change corresponds to a 20-mm Hg deflection on the recorder. Pressures return at systole and become maximal in amplitude with diastole. Present machines may have Doppler and other sophisticated attachments.

Pitfalls of the pulse-volume recorder are improper cuff placement and machine calibration error. Sources of external arterial compression must be eliminated.

Oculopneumoplethysmography basically measures ophthalmic artery pressure based on the principle that ocular suction can eliminate ocular pulsations when the ophthalmic artery pressure is exceeded. The system has a vacuum, 500-mm Hg maximum, with rapid deployment and precision for steady, continuous scleral suction through the ocular eyecups. Three pressure-sensitive transducers and a 4-channel paper recorder measure a simultaneous bilateral eye-pressure wave, the vacuum applied, and an electrocardiographic tracing. The eyecups, in addition to applying suction, measure pressure change caused by the varying volume of sclera present in the eyecups during arterial pulsations. Ophthalmic anesthetic agents are applied to decrease eye movement. With the patient looking straight ahead, both eyecups are applied to the outer canthus, and a foot pedal activates the maximal volume. Temporary vision loss may happen at this moment, and the patient should be made aware of this possibility.

Because technical manipulation is minimal, technical errors are uncommon. Protection from eye abrasion must be explained to the patient because of the local anesthetic. A few patients have developed subconjunctival erythema or hematoma requiring no special treatment.[78] Carotid-artery compression, to study collateral blood flow, must be done low in the neck, to prevent the formation of emboli.[79] This study is contraindicated in patients with certain conditions, such as eye trauma, previous eye operation, acute conjunctivitis, glaucoma, a history of retinal detachment, or lens transplantation. Hypertensive patients with intraocular pressure greater than 130 to 140 mm Hg are difficult to evaluate because 140 mm Hg seems to be the maximal intraocular pressure possible with the present machinery.[80] Bilateral carotid stenosis or subclavian disease may complicate the interpretation of this study.

Interpretation

Two components are evaluated in the interpretation of the phleborrheogram: venous obstruction and collateralization, as observed by respiratory wave patterns.[74] A normal study shows adequate respiratory movement in each individual leg tracing, no change in the baseline of any cuff during foot compression, and a drop in baseline of about 3 cm in the foot cuff during ankle compression, with a minor drop in the more proximal calf cuff caused by the brisk movement of blood toward the heart. Obstruction is signified by a rise in the cuff baseline after compression because of the increased volume of blood distal to the obstruction after forceful movement.

Some generalizations may be made about the phleborrheograph. Obstruction without respiratory waves often signifies an acute process, and exaggerated respiratory waves indicate a more chronic problem. The lack of respiratory waves and the rise in baseline venous pressure are always distal to the point of venous obstruction in the leg.

The pulse-volume recorder, although based on a different principle from Doppler ultrasound, is used much in the same manner. The maximal pulse-volume recorder amplitude at the ankle, as well as the ratio between this value and the maximal brachial amplitude, are calculated.[77,81] Pulse-contour changes indicative of arterial occlusive disease are rounding and delay in the peak, a decrease in the rise and fall of the limbs, and an absence of a reflected diastolic wave. Raines classifies the pulse-volume recorder readings on a 1-to-5 grading basis in which 1 represents adequate amplitude and dicrotic notch, 2 represents adequate and no dicrotic notch, 3 indicates moderately decreased amplitude, 4 indicates severely decreased, but pulsatile, amplitude, and 5 is a flat nonpulsatile tracing.[77] Grades 4 and 5 indicate significant occlusive disease. When patients with occlusive disease exercise, the amplitude of the pulse decreases, rather than increases, as in normal subjects.[81] Vasospastic and compressive diseases are confirmed if cooling in ice water or anatomically exaggerated motions result in pressure changes; pulse-contour changes indicate occlusive disease.

Interpretation of the oculopneumoplethysmogram requires the tracing, a calibrated rule for comparing applied suction to corresponding intraocular pressure, and the value of the highest brachial artery pressure. If the pulse is present at maximal vacuum, then the intraocular pressure will be regarded as greater than 140 mm Hg. Otherwise, the pressure is measured at the point at which the pulse first returns. Test results are abnormal if the difference between the 2 tracings is 5 mm Hg or greater; such a finding suggests the presence of stenosis on the side with the lower pressure. Bilateral stenosis is suggested by an ocular-to-brachial artery pressure ratio of less than 0.6.[78,80]

Diagnostic Efficacy

With adequate training in the reading of the phleborrheogram, the correct diagnosis of deep-vein thrombosis is obtained in approximately 93% of patients.[29,74] False-negative results average approximately 9%, and the rate of false-positive results is approximately 4%. The major problem appears to be in the diagnosis of infrapopliteal nonocclusive venous thrombosis. One study has shown an incidence of pulmonary emboli of 0.2% in patients with a negative phleborrheogram; this finding indicates the reliability of this noninvasive test.[83]

Several studies have found that oculopneumoplethysmography is approximately 92% accurate in defining significant carotid-artery disease, when compared to angiographic stenosis.[78,80,82,84] Although carotid-artery compression is not a routine part of the screening process in most noninvasive-study laboratories, it may be a useful addition to oculopneumoplethysmography in determining collateral blood flow in patients who may need carotid interruption for tumor or other reasons. Again, oculopneumoplethysmography is not sensitive to ulcerative, nonstenotic lesions. As with fluid-filled oculoplethysmography, only high-grade stenosis, greater than 75%, is detectable. The oculopneumoplethysmogram is therefore unsuitable for screening purposes.

STRAIN-GAUGE PLETHYSMOGRAPHY

Strain-gauge plethysomography is a method of measuring limb volume based on the principle that a thin, mercury-filled Silastic tube (strain gauge) displays measurable changes in electrical resistance with small changes in its length. The electrical resistance, detected with a Wheatstone-bridge circuit, can be amplified and displayed continuously on a strip-chart recorder. By applying a strain gauge around the limb, small variations in limb circumference can be measured. Because the length of the limb remains constant, its volume varies directly with the circumference according to the following equations:

$$C = \pi \cdot r^2, \text{ and } V = \pi \cdot r^2 \cdot L$$

where C is the circumference, r is the radius, V is the volume, L is length, and π is the constant π. Because the mass of the limb remains constant, changes in circumference reflect changes in limb blood content that result from arterial inflow and venous reflux.[85–87]

Indications

Strain-gauge plethysmography may be useful in determining muscle and skin blood flow, for pulse registration of the digits, and for recording limb blood pressure. The technique has also been used to detect deep-venous thrombosis and to evaluate the functional status of patients with chronic venous insufficiency. For the detection of arterial occlusive disease, strain-gauge plethysmography has generally been replaced by noninvasive methods of pressure measurement because of the cumbersome nature of the technique and because of the wide range of skin and muscle flow values in both normal subjects and in patients with arterial occlusive disease.

Technique and Technical Pitfalls

Evaluation of the lower extremity for venous occlusion is performed with the patient in the supine position, with the limb slightly flexed at the knee and elevated on a pillow to the level of the right atrium. Leg veins must be emptied prior to cuff inflation, to determine the change in calf volume accurately. This procedure is accomplished by elevating the patient's leg above the level of the right atrium for several minutes before beginning the examination. The strain gauge is applied around the calf at its widest point. The length of the gauge should be about 90% of the calf's circumference. The gauge should be applied with a small amount of stretch, but not so tight that it occludes venous flow. A wide, tapered pneumatic cuff is placed around the thigh, to provide uniform venous occlusion when the cuff is inflated.

Current plethysmographs provide electrical standardization with a signal indicating a 1% change in volume. After standardization, the pneumatic cuff is rapidly inflated to 50 mm Hg, to occlude the underlying veins without reducing arterial inflow. Failure to inflate the thigh cuff rapidly yields erroneous measurement of small changes in calf volume.

After cuff inflation, calf volume increases rapidly at first, and then more slowly as the venous capacitance vessels distend and as the contained venous volume increases. When the venous pressure exceeds 50 mm Hg, usually in 2 to 3 min, venous outflow returns, and calf expansion ceases. Once maximal expansion has been achieved and a steady-state venous outflow is established, the cuff is rapidly deflated. The maximal venous outflow occurs during the first second after cuff deflation, and the rate of decrease is directly proportional to venous outflow. Therefore, slow cuff deflation produces a recording showing an erroneously slow rate of venous outflow.

When venous pressures have returned to the baseline level, the patient's leg veins may once again be emptied by elevation, and the test may be repeated. Because sequential testing may cause stretching of venous capacitance vessels, however, venous volume may increase with each subsequent cuff inflation.

The evaluation of a patient with suspected chronic venous insufficiency can be performed in 2 ways. The first method requires that the patient be placed in the supine position, with the leg to be tested elevated slightly above the heart but below the level of the right atrium. A narrow pneumatic cuff is placed around the patient's proximal thigh, and a wide tapered cuff is placed around the distal thigh. When the limb is completely relaxed, the proximal thigh cuff is inflated to 300 mm Hg, to occlude blood flow to and from the leg completely. After a brief pause to allow venous pressures within the leg to equilibrate, the distal thigh cuff is rapidly inflated to 50 mm Hg to force blood distally. In the normal patient, venous valves prevent the distal displacement of venous blood. In the patient with incompetent valves, retrograde flow of blood into the calf is experienced. This retrograde flow is reflected in an increased cuff circumference recorded by the strain gauge.

The second method for determining the presence of incompetent venous valves uses the strain gauge to record venous refilling times. One places an appropriately sized strain gauge around the widest portion of the patient's calf, and the patient stands erect against a wall. The plethysmograph is standardized and zeroed at this point, to indicate normal calf volume. The patient is asked to raise the heel rapidly five times, to empty the calf veins through the muscle pump, and then to return to the standing position. The time required for the calf volume to return to the pre-exercise level is recorded as the venous refilling time. Because calculations are based on the time from cessation of exercise to the return to baseline, the plethysmograph should be mechanically zeroed to record all phases of the examination on the strip chart. To avoid hyperemia and increased arterial inflow during sequential testing, mechanical compression of the calf can be substituted for exercise.

For pulse registration, the strain gauge is simply applied to the patient's index finger or big toe. The pulse tracing thus obtained can be analyzed, or it may be used as the end point for recording lower-limb pressure.

Interpretation

In the presence of deep-venous thrombosis, fewer capacitance veins are available. Therefore, when the superficial veins are occluded with a tourniquet, the increase in venous and calf volume is smaller. In the normal patient, calf volume usually increases 2 to 3%. In the presence of deep-venous thrombosis, however, this increase is less than 2%. For similar reasons, the maximal venous outflow is decreased in patients with venous thrombosis.

With the currently available electrically calibrated plethysmograph, an internal standard is used to indicate a 1% change in volume. This change can be displayed graphically in divisions. The strip-chart recorder displays the rise in calf volume. The percentage of change can be calculated according to the following equation:

maximal venous outflow
$$= \frac{\text{slope (divisions/min)}}{\text{divisions/1\% volume change}}$$

The 2-sec venous outflow is calculated as follows:

2-sec venous outflow
$$= \frac{(\text{division fall/2 sec}) \times 30 \text{ sec}}{\text{divisions/1\% volume change}}$$

The maximal venous outflow is reduced in the presence of deep-venous thrombosis. Barnes and co-workers reported normal values to be in the range of 20 ml/100 ml/min; values were in the range of 91 ml/100 ml/min in the presence of deep-venous thrombosis (45 ± 18 ml/100 ml/min mean).[88] This reduction in venous outflow is not specific for deep-venous thrombosis, however. Any cause of increased venous resistance, such as extrinsic compression from tumors or obliterative phlebitis, is reflected in a reduced maximal venous outflow.

The calculations used for the interpretation of strain-gauge plethysmography in patients with chronic venous insufficiency are the same as those for maximal venous outflow. These calculations indicate venous reflux flow, for which the upper limit of normal is 6 ml/100 ml/min.[89] The mean reflux flow in patients with secondary venous insufficiency is 13 ± 7 ml/100 ml/min. Following exercise, the average time required to return to baseline calf volume is 22 ± 7 seconds. In patients with primary venous insufficiency, mean refilling time is 7 ± 3 seconds, and in those with secondary venous insufficiency, the value is 7 ± 2 seconds.

Diagnostic Efficacy

Standard values for these tests have not been uniformly established. Using a maximal venous outflow value of 20 ml/100 ml/min as the cutoff point between normal and abnormal, Barnes and colleagues found a 91% sensitivity and an 88% accuracy for determining the presence of deep-venous thrombosis.[90] The sensitivity and accuracy of the strain-gauge plethysmograph in the detection of chronic venous insufficiency have not been established.

Acceptance by Patients

Because of the noninvasive nature of this test and the minimal amount of effort required by the patient, strain-gauge plethysmography is readily accepted by patients. Performed under calm and comfortable conditions, this test can be accomplished in less than an hour with minimal discomfort to the patient.

PHOTOPLETHYSMOGRAPHY

Photoplethysmography is a method of detecting chronic venous insufficiency by assessing the venous refilling time of an extremity. Venous refilling, a function of arterial inflow and venous reflux, governs the blood content of the cutaneous capillary beds before, during, and after exercise. Changes in venous refilling time can be detected with a photoplethysmograph, which consists of a transducer, an amplifier, and a strip-chart recorder. When the transducer is in contact with the skin, it emits an impulse of infrared light into the underlying tissue. The light backscattered by the blood in the capillary beds is received by an adjacent photodetector. After filtering, the reflected signal is amplified, is DC-coupled, and is displayed as a continuous line on the strip-chart recorder. A shift from the baseline indicates a change in the blood content of the cutaneous capillary beds.[91,92] Although this method does not enable one to measure the exact amount of venous flow directly, photoplethysmography can provide quantitative information about venous reflux by recording the change in cutaneous capillary blood content before and after exercise.

Indications

Photoplethysmography is most useful in the evaluation of the lower extremity for chronic venous insufficiency. By performing the test with selective tourniquets, one may differentiate primary from secondary venous insufficiency.[91] Although one may assess the pulsatile flow within the capillary beds by means of photoplethysmography, the technique is not of clinical value in the arterial evaluation of the extremity.

Technique and Technical Pitfalls

The test is performed with the patient seated, with feet dependent but not weight bearing. The transducer is fixed to the skin with double-stick tape in an area that will not be affected by joint motion. The most common area is the skin just superior to the medial malleolus; however, any representative area of skin may be used. The site chosen should permit complete and constant transducer contact. One should avoid areas of ulceration or those with a large underlying varix or artery.

Once the transducer is attached, a baseline measurement is made, and the recorder is mechanically zeroed. When a stable baseline has been established, a preliminary examination is done by asking the patient to dorsiflex and plantarflex the foot rapidly five times, and then to relax completely. Venous pressure falls during exercise. The nadir of the pressure tracing must be evident on the recorder. In normal patients, the change in venous pressure may be great and may fall below the lower limit of the recorder. This problem can be corrected by adjusting the mechanical gain and zero level of the baseline, to obtain a complete tracing within the boundaries of the recorder. Conversely, patients with severe venous insufficiency may display a minimal fall in venous pressure during exercise. Increasing the mechanical gain in these patients exaggerates and helps one to identify the changes in venous pressure.

The final phase of the test, that of venous recovery, is often rapid in patients with severe venous insufficiency and reflux and is best displayed with a chart speed of 5 mm/sec. Because recovery times in normal patients may be slow, a chart speed of 1 mm/sec facilitates interpretation.

Once the zero, gain, and chart speed have been adjusted to permit a complete and reproducible examination, three to five examinations, consisting of the baseline test, exercise with five rapid plantar flexion and dorsiflexion movements of the foot, and resting recovery should be performed. To differentiate primary from secondary venous insufficiency, a narrow tourniquet is placed around the thigh and is inflated to 50 mm Hg to occlude the greater saphenous system, and the tests are repeated. Finally, the tourniquet should be moved down to the proximal calf and should be reinflated to occlude the lesser saphenous system, and the test should be performed again.

Interpretation

In the normal limb, venous pressure falls rapidly during exercise because of the muscle pump emptying the veins. On cessation of exercise, the veins gradually refill through arterial inflow. In the presence of venous insufficiency, however, the efficiency of the muscle pump is reduced. This change is reflected in a smaller drop in venous pressure during exercise and, therefore, a more rapid return of venous pressure. The end point of the photoplethysmogram is the return of stable venous pressure after exercise. This refilling time forms the basis for the measurement (Fig. 21–4). The recovery baseline begins at the level of venous pressure that remains stable for at least 5 sec, or a peak overshoot of this level. The initial pre-exercise baseline is used only to establish a mechanical zero, and not to calculate the test result. The value of the photoplethysmogram is calculated by determining the time required to re-establish a stable venous pressure after the cessation of exercise. The values of the 3 tests are averaged, for an overall result.[93]

A venous refilling time of 23 sec or more is normal, whereas a refilling time of less than 20 sec suggests venous insufficiency. Patients with postphlebitic syndrome often have a venous recovery time of less than 15 sec. A prolongation of venous recovery time over 23 sec by inflation of the thigh cuff indicates valvular incompetency of the greater saphenous system (Fig. 21–5), whereas normalization of the recovery time with inflation of the calf tourniquet implies incompetence of the lesser saphenous system. Failure of either tourniquet test to produce a venous recovery time within the normal range indicates valvular incompetence of the deep venous system.[93,94]

Diagnostic Efficacy

Studies that have simultaneously measured photoplethysmographic venous recovery and direct venous pressure have found a significant correlation between the 2 techniques. In a comparative study of photoplethysmography and venous pressure by Abramowitz and colleagues, 338 paired measurements were made in 14 varicose, 25 postphlebitic, and 24 normal limbs.[95] The correlation co-efficient was 0.989, with only 3 false-positive results and 1 false-negative result. Although direct venous pressure measurements remain the standard for the diagnosis of chronic venous insufficiency, photoplethysmography provides an excellent, reliable, and noninvasive method of determining venous pressure.

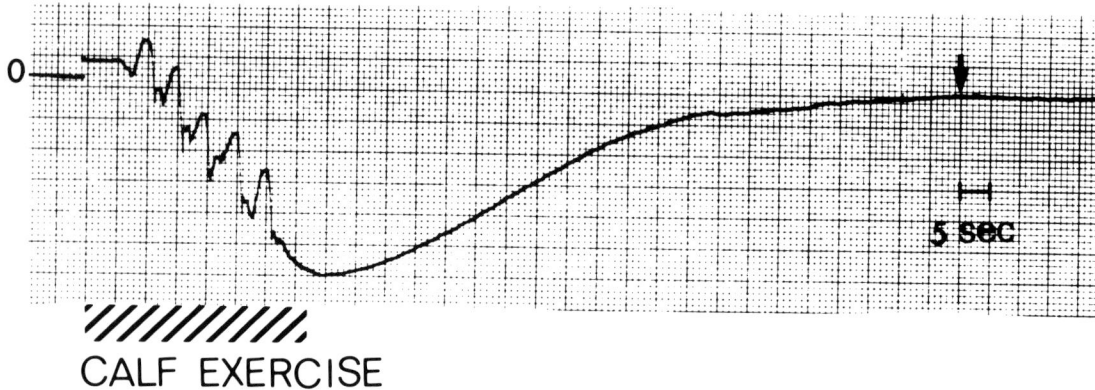

FIG. 21-4. Example of venous refilling time following calf muscle exercise.

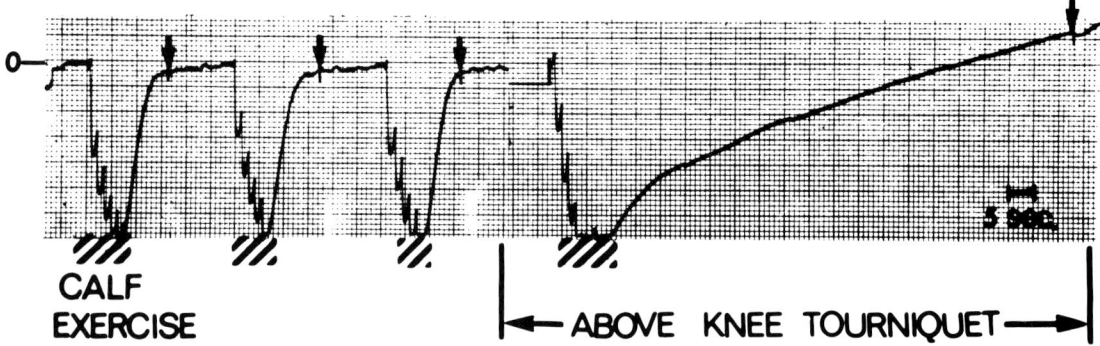

FIG. 21-5. Recording of venous refilling time in a patient with long saphenous vein varicosities and incompetence. The venous refilling time is normalized after application of a thigh tourniquet inflated to 50 mm Hg. The photoplethysmographic tourniquet test accurately predicted the response to long saphenous vein stripping. (From Flinn, W.R., et al.: The use of photoplethysmography in the assessment of chronic venous insufficiency. In Practical Noninvasive Vascular Diagnosis. Edited by R.F. Kempczinski and J.S.T. Yao. Chicago, Year Book Medical Publishers, 1982.)

Acceptance by Patients

Because of the minimal amount of exertion required by the patient, and because of the noninvasive nature of the examination, most patients readily accept photoplethysmography.

IMPEDANCE PLETHYSMOGRAPHY

Impedance plethysmography is based on Ohm's law (voltage = current × resistance). Because blood is the path of least resistance (impedance) in the body, a constant current results in a decrease in voltage between two reference points as the blood content (volume) of a limb increases, and vice versa.[27] Based on this relationship, the relative amount and rate of blood entering or leaving an extremity can be determined.

Indications

This noninvasive study is most useful in evaluating patients with clinically suspected deep-venous thrombosis.

Technique and Technical Pitfalls

The patient lies on his back, with the leg to be examined externally rotated, muscles fully relaxed, knee slightly bent, and with the calf elevated approximately 30° above heart level. A large thigh cuff is loosely placed around the patient's lower thigh. Conductive jelly coats the 4 electrodes, 2 per strip, placed around the patient's calf. The 2 strip electrodes are placed approximately 10 cm apart.[96] A constant current is generated, and the thigh cuff is inflated to 45 or 70 cm H_2O for 45 or 120 sec, and then is rapidly deflated.[97,98] The changes in voltage corresponding to impedance changes (limb volume changes) are constantly recorded on a paper-strip recorder.

Many conditions other than deep-venous thrombosis may result in a positive test response. External compression with decreased venous outflow is not distinguishable from internal occlusion. Improper muscle relaxation of pregnancy may produce false-positive results.[99,100] Causes of decreased internal venous flow, such as valvular or congestive cardiac disease and chronic venous disease, may result in a positive response to impedance plethysmography in patients who do not have acute thrombosis.[101,102] Arterial inflow abnormalities may also affect venous outflow studies.[97] Most of these problems can be eliminated by careful clinical correlation. False-negative results from nonocclusive venous disease are seen most commonly in the calf with multiple channels for venous drainage, or with collateral-circulation generation in patients with proximal acute venous thrombosis.[102,103] Nonocclusive proximal thrombosis may not be detectable.[102-104]

Interpretation

Figure 21-6 is an example of a paper-strip impedance plethysmogram showing venous capacitance, which is the percentage of increase of the calf volume with cuff inflation, and maximal venous outflow, which is the percentage of decrease in venous volume during the 3 min immediately following thigh cuff release. Venous capacitance is recorded when the plateau of the impedance curve has been reached. Because the capacitance and outflow are compared for analysis, no actual expression of impedance or voltage change need be calibrated. The technician merely counts the number of small boxes for venous capacitance, and for maximal venous outflow, plots the result on a nomogram, as suggested by Wheeler and Anderson (Fig. 21-7).[97] Repeat studies done after exercise, after warming, or at a higher cuff pressure, such as 70 cm H_2O, are employed in patients with borderline test results.

Limbs with values above the regression line are normal; those with values below the line are abnormal and suggest acute venous thrombosis.[97]

Diagnostic Efficiency

Impedance plethysmography has been compared with venography.[98,101-105] If results are above the solid white line, the physician may be 90+% sure that acute venous thrombosis is not an immediate threat. Similarly, if results continually fall below the solid dark line, only 3% of patients will have a normal venogram, and treatment without venography is indicated. Results plotted in the gray zone are unpredictable, however, and the percentage of deep-venous thrombosis of the calf is high; in these patients, venography may be the next appropriate diagnostic step. Deep-venous thrombosis of the calf, the test's major failure, is underdiagnosed in 25% of patients with a normal impedance plethysmogram. Therefore, to be more certain of therapy, venography may be indicated for patients with normal or borderline results of impedance plethysmography. Others have suggested repeating impedance plethysmography a day or so later, to ensure that the disease has not progressed and thus to omit the need for venography. Clinically, such an approach has been successful for at least one group of investigators.[106]

The addition of Doppler ultrasound or [125]iodine fibrinogen testing to the impedance plethysmogram may add sensitivity by showing calf thrombi and by eliminating cardiac abnormalities from consideration.[102,107,108] Several investigators have suggested algorithms whereby a positive test result in both

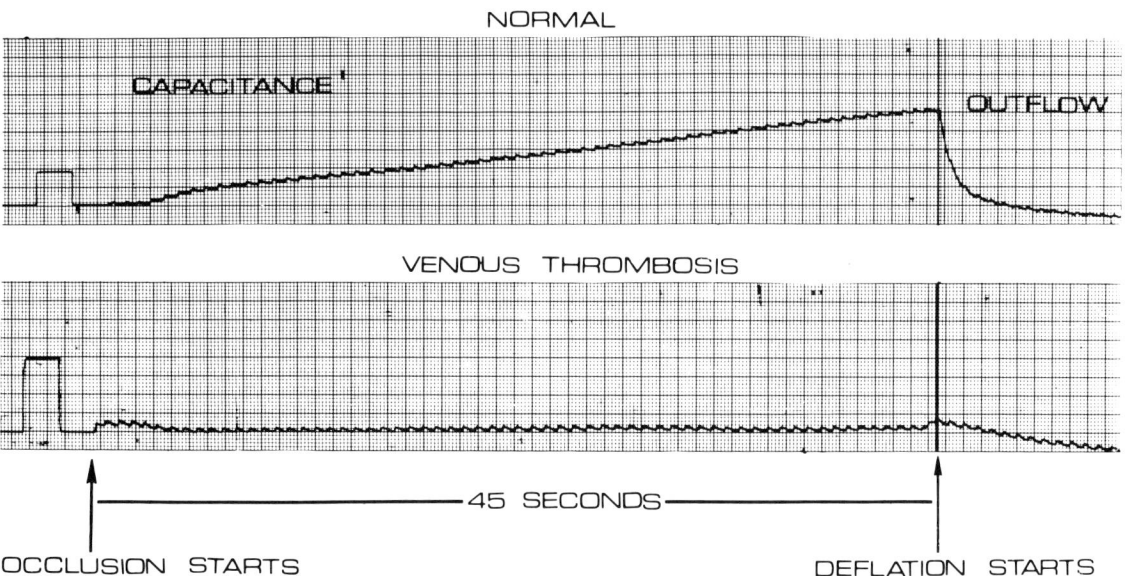

FIG. 21-6. Strip-chart recording of venous capacitance and outflow by cuff-occlusive impedance plethysmography. In patients with venous thrombosis, both capacitance and outflow are decreased.

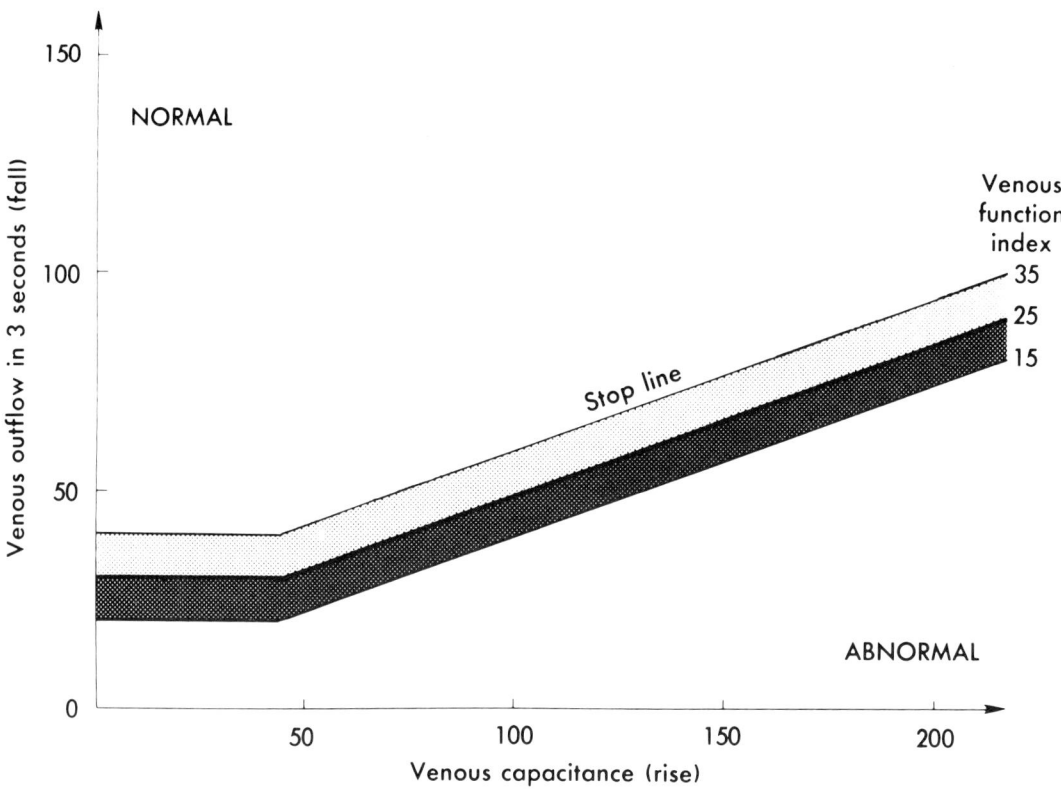

FIG. 21–7. Modified nomogram for cuff-occlusive impedance plethysmography. The venous function index is calculated by plotting the results of impedance plethysmography on a graph of venous capacitance and venous outflow. (From Wheeler, H.B., and Anderson, F.A., Jr.: Impedance phlebography: the diagnosis of venous thrombosis by occlusive impedance plethysmography. *In* Noninvasive Diagnostic Techniques in Vascular Disease. 2nd Ed. Edited by E.F. Bernstein. St. Louis, C.V. Mosby, 1982.)

studies indicates treatment for deep-venous thrombosis, a negative dual test result indicates no further treatment, and disagreement between the two tests indicates venography.[28,101,102] More than 90% of patients are treated correctly by this method, which is biased in favor of treatment in questionable cases.

Acceptance by Patients

The patient is in a comfortable position for the test. The test itself is quick and usually causes no pain. Therefore, patients readily accept the procedure, and repeat studies are well tolerated.

REFERENCES

1. Kirkendall, W.M., et al.: Recommendations for human blood pressure determination by sphygmomanometers: Subcommittee of the American Heart Association Postgraduate Education Committee. Hypertension, 3:509A, 1981.
2. Bruner, J.M.R., et al.: Comparison of direct and indirect methods of measuring arterial blood pressure. Part I. Med. Instrum., 15:11, 1981.
3. Nielsen, P.E., and Jannicke, H.: The accuracy of auscultatory measurement of arm blood pressure in very obese subjects. Acta Med. Scand., 195:403, 1974.
4. Regan, C., and Bordley, J.: The accuracy of clinical measurements of arterial blood pressure, with a note on the auscultatory gap. Bull. Johns Hopkins Hosp., 69:504, 1941.
5. London, S.B., and London, R.E.: Comparison of indirect pressure measurements (Korotkoff) with simultaneous brachial artery pressure distal to the cuff. Adv. Intern. Med., 13:127, 1967.
6. Van Bergan, F.H.: Comparison of indirect and direct methods of measuring arterial blood pressure. Circulation, 10:481, 1954.
7. Bruner, J.M.R., et al.: Comparison of direct and indirect methods of measuring arterial blood pressure. Part III. Med. Instrum., 15:182, 1981.
8. Geddes, L.S.: The Direct and Indirect Measurement of Blood Pressure. Chicago, Year Book Medical Publishers, 1970, p. 9.
9. Cromwell, L., et al.: Medical Instrumentation for Health Care. Englewood Cliffs, NJ, Prentice-Hall, 1976, p. 158.
10. Bruner, J.M.: Handbook of Blood Pressure Monitoring. Littleton, MA, PSG Publishing, 1978, pp. 49 and 101.
11. Fragen, R.J.: Arterial catheterization and maintenance of indwelling arterial lines. Critical Care for Surgical Patients. Edited by J.M. Beal. Toronto, MacMillan Publishing, 1982, p. 91.
12. Saidman, L.J., and Smith, N.T.: Monitoring in Anesthesia. New York, John Wiley & Sons, 1978, p. 66.

13. Gravenstein, J.S., and Paulni, D.A.: Monitoring Practice in Clinical Anesthesia. Philadelphia, J.B. Lippincott, 1982, pp. 37 and 291.
14. Rothe, C.F., and Kim, K.C.: Measuring systolic arterial blood pressure. Crit. Care Med., 8:683, 1980.
15. Gardner, R.M.: Direct blood pressure measurement dynamics response requirements. Anesthesiology, 54:227, 1981.
16. Behnia, R.: Blood pressure control. In Critical Care for Surgical Patients. Edited by J.M. Beal. Toronto, MacMillan Publishing, 1982, p. 563.
17. Slogoff, S., Keab, A.S., and Arlund, C.: On the safety of radial artery cannulation. Anesthesiology, 59:42, 1983.
18. Soderstrom, C.A., et al.: Superiority of the femoral artery in monitoring. Am. J. Surg., 144:309, 1982.
19. Cannon, B.W., and Meshier, W.M.: Extremity amputation following radial artery cannulation in a patient with hyperlipoproteinemia type V. Anesthesiology, 56:222, 1982.
20. Udoff, E.J., et al.: Hemodynamic significance of iliac artery stenosis: pressure measurement during angiography. Radiology, 132:289, 1979.
21. O'Rourke, M.F.: The arterial pulse in health and disease. Am. Heart J., 82:687, 1971.
22. Moore, W.S., and Hall, A.D.: Unrecognized aorto-iliac stenosis: a physiologic approach to the diagnosis. Arch. Surg., 103:633, 1971.
23. Barber, G.G., et al.: Hemodynamic assessment of the aorto-iliac segment: a prospective study. Can. J. Surg., 23:542, 1980.
24. Quin, R.O., Evans, D.H., and Bell, P.R.F.: Haemodynamic assessment of the aorto-iliac segment. J. Cardiovasc. Surg., 16:586, 1975.
25. Flanigan, D.P., et al.: Hemodynamic evaluation of the aortoiliac system based on pharmacologic vasodilatation. Surgery, 93:709, 1983.
26. Zsigmoid, E.K.: Intra-arterial blood pressure measurements. (Editorial.) JAMA, 245:703, 1981.
27. Dean, R.H., and Yao, J.S.T.: Hemodynamic measurements in peripheral vascular disease. Curr. Probl. Surg., 13:5, 1976.
28. Pearce, W.H., Yao, J.S.T., and Bergan, J.J.: Noninvasive vascular diagnostic testing. Curr. Probl. Surg., 8:460, 1983.
29. Yao, J.S.T.: New techniques in objective arterial evaluation. Arch. Surg., 106:600, 1973.
30. Queral, L.A., et al.: Pelvic hemodynamics after aortoiliac reconstruction. Surgery, 86:799, 1979.
31. Johnson, K.W., et al.: Methods of obtaining, processing, and quantifying Doppler blood velocity waveforms. In Investigation of Vascular Disorders. Edited by A.N. Nicolaides and J.S.T. Yao. New York, Churchill Livingstone, 1981, p. 532.
32. Bone, G.E.: The relationship between aortoiliac hemodynamics and femoral pulsatility index. J. Surg. Res., 32:228, 1982.
33. Baird, R.N., et al.: Upstream stenosis: its diagnosis by Doppler signals from the femoral artery. Arch. Surg., 115:316, 1980.
34. Flanigan, D.P., et al.: Hemodynamic and arteriographic evaluation of femoral pulsatility index. J. Surg. Res., 32:234, 1982.
35. Stallworth, J.M., Quinn, G.H., and Aiken, A.F.: Is rib resection necessary for relief of thoracic outlet syndrome? Ann. Surg., 185:581, 1977.
36. Yao, J.S.T., and Takaki, H.S.: Noninvasive techniques of measuring lower limb arterial pressure. In Noninvasive Diagnostic Techniques in Vascular Disease. 2nd Ed. Edited by E.F. Bernstein. St. Louis, C.V. Mosby, 1982, p. 50.
37. Yao, J.S.T., and Blackburn, D.: Doppler venous survey. In Practical Noninvasive Vascular Diagnosis. Edited by R.F. Kempczinski and J.S.T. Yao. Chicago, Year Book Medical Publishers, 1982, p. 263.
38. Barnes, R.W.: Doppler ultrasonic diagnosis of venous disease. In Noninvasive Diagnostic Techniques in Vascular Disease. Edited by E.F. Bernstein. St. Louis, C.V. Mosby, 1982, p. 452.
39. Blackshear, W.M., Jr., et al.: Carotid artery velocity patterns in normal and stenotic vessels. Stroke, 11:67, 1980.
40. Rutherford, R.B., and Kreutzer, E.W.: Doppler ultrasound techniques in the assessment of extracranial arterial occlusive disease. In Investigation of Vascular Disorders. Edited by A.N. Nicolaides and J.S.T. Yao. New York, Churchill Livingstone, 1981, p. 139.
41. Plainol, T., and Pourcelot, L.: Doppler effect study of the carotid circulation. In Ultrasonics in Medicine. Edited by M. De Vlieger, D.N. White, and V.W. McGreedy. New York, American Elsevier Publishing, 1975, p. 67.
42. Barnes, R.W., Nix, L., and Rittgers, S.E.: Audible interpretation of carotid Doppler signals: an improved technique to define carotid artery disease. Arch. Surg., 116:1185, 1981.
43. Roederer, G.O., et al.: Ultrasonic duplex scanning of extracranial carotid arteries: improved accuracy using new features from the common carotid artery. J. Cardiovasc. Ultrasonogr., 1:373, 1982.
44. White, D.N.: Color-coded Doppler carotid imaging. In Noninvasive Diagnostic Techniques in Vascular Disease. 2nd Ed. Edited by E.F. Bernstein. St. Louis, C.V. Mosby, 1982, p. 258.
45. Hokanson, D.E., et al.: Ultrasonic arteriography: a new approach to arterial visualization. Biomed. Eng. (Lond.), 6:420, 1971.
46. Sumner, D.S., Russell, J.B., and Miles, R.D.: Pulsed-Doppler arteriography and computer assisted imaging of the carotid bifurcation. In Cerebrovascular Insufficiency. Edited by J.J. Bergan and J.S.T. Yao. New York, Grune & Stratton, 1983, p. 115.
47. Nicolaides, A.N., and Angelides, N.S.: Waveform index and resistance pattern using directional Doppler, ultrasound, and zero crossing detector. In Investigation of Vascular Disorders. Edited by A.N. Nicolaides and J.S.T. Yao. New York, Churchill Livingstone, 1981, p. 291.
48. Johnson, K.W., et al.: Quantitative analysis of Doppler blood flow velocity recording using pulsatile index. In Investigation of Vascular Disorders. Edited by A.N. Nicolaides and J.S.T. Yao. New York, Churchill Livingstone, 1981, p. 274.
49. Felix, W.R., Jr., et al.: Pulsed Doppler ultrasound detection of flow disturbances in arteriosclerosis. J. Clin. Ultrasound, 4:275, 1976.
50. Carter, S.A.: The relationship of distal systolic pressures to healing of skin lesions in limbs with arterial occlusive disease, with special reference to diabetes mellitus. Scand. J. Clin. Lab. Invest., 31(Suppl. 128):239, 1973.
51. Verta, M.J., et al.: Forefoot perfusion pressure and minor amputation for gangrene. Surgery, 80:729, 1976.
52. Johnson, W.C.: Doppler ankle pressure and reactive hyperemia in the diagnosis of arterial insufficiency. J. Surg. Res., 18:177, 1975.
53. Gross, W.S., et al.: Chronic upper extremity arterial

54. Berguer, R., Higgins, F.T., and Nelson, R.: Noninvasive diagnosis of reversal of vertebral artery blood flow. N. Engl. J. Med., 302:1349, 1980.
55. Gosling, R.G., and King, D.H.: Processing arterial Doppler signals for clinical data. In Handbook of Clinical Ultrasound. Edited by M. De Vlieger, et al. New York, John Wiley & Sons, 1978, p. 613.
56. Zierler, R.E., Roederer, G.O., and Strandness, D.E.: The use of frequency spectral analysis in carotid artery surgery. In Cerebrovascular Insufficiency. Edited by J.J. Bergan and J.S.T. Yao. New York, Grune & Stratton, 1983, p. 137.
57. Ouriel, K., and Zarins, C.K.: Doppler ankle pressure. Arch. Surg., 117:1297, 1982.
58. Clyne, C.A.C., Tripolitis, A., and Jamieson, C.W.: The reproducibility of the treadmill walking test for claudication. Surg. Gynecol. Obstet., 149:727, 1979.
59. Carter, S.A., and Lezack, J.O.: Digital systolic pressures in the lower limb in arterial disease. Circulation, 43:905, 1971.
60. Blackshear, W.M., and Strandness, D.E., Jr.: Angiographic imaging by ultrasound compared with indirect methods. In Investigation of Vascular Disorders. Edited by A.N. Nicolaides and J.S.T. Yao. New York, Churchill Livingstone, 1981, p. 165.
61. Rutherford, R.B., Hiatt, W.R., and Kreutzer, E.W.: The use of velocity waveform analysis in the diagnosis of carotid artery occlusive disease. Surgery, 82:695, 1977.
62. Sumner, D.S.: Diagnosis of deep venous thrombosis by Doppler ultrasound. In Investigation of Vascular Disorders. Edited by A.N. Nicolaides and J.S.T. Yao. New York, Churchill Livingstone, 1981, p. 377.
63. Nicolaides, A.N., Fernandes e Fernandes, J., and Zimmerman, H.: Doppler ultrasound in the investigation of venous insufficiency. In Investigation of Vascular Disorders. Edited by A.N. Nicolaides and J.S.T. Yao. New York, Churchill Livingstone, 1981, p. 478.
64. Kartchner, M.M., and McRae, L.P.: Noninvasive detection and evaluation of stroke-prone patients. Angiology, 28:750, 1977.
65. McRae, L.P., and Kartchner, M.M.: Oculoplethysmography: timed comparison of ocular pulses and carotid phonoangiography. In Noninvasive Diagnostic Techniques in Vascular Disease. Edited by E.F. Bernstein. 2nd Ed. St. Louis, C.V. Mosby, 1982, p. 87.
66. Kartchner, M.M., et al.: Oculoplethysmography: an adjunct to arteriography in the diagnosis of extracranial carotid occlusive disease. Am. J. Surg., 132:728, 1976.
67. Kartchner, M.M., and McRae, L.P.: Carotid phonoangiography and oculoplethysmography. In Investigation of Vascular Disorders. Edited by A.N. Nicolaides and J.S.T. Yao. New York, Churchill Livingstone, 1981, p. 91.
68. Archie, J.P., Posey, P.H., and Goodson, D.S.: Accuracy of digitalized differential pulse timing oculoplethysmography. Surg. Gynecol. Obstet., 152:259, 1981.
69. Ginsberg, M.G., Greenwood, S.A., and Goldberg, N.E.: Noninvasive diagnosis of extracranial cerebrovascular disease: oculoplethysmography, phonoangiography and directional Doppler ultrasonography. Neurology, 29:623, 1979.
70. Gross, W.S., et al.: Comparison of noninvasive diagnostic techniques in carotid artery occlusive disease. Surgery, 82:271, 1977.
71. Blackshear, W.M., et al.: A prospective evaluation of oculoplethysmography and carotid phonoangiography. Surg. Gynecol. Obstet., 148:201, 1979.
72. Pearce, W.H., et al.: Direct and indirect tests for carotid artery lesions. In Cerebrovascular Insufficiency. Edited by J.J. Bergan and J.S.T. Yao. New York, Grune & Stratton, 1973, p. 179.
73. Keagy, B.A., et al.: Oculoplethysmography/phonoangiography. Arch. Surg., 115:1199, 1980.
74. Cranley, J.J.: Diagnosis of deep venous thrombosis of the lower extremity by phleborrheography. In Noninvasive Diagnostic Techniques in Vascular Disease. Edited by E.F. Bernstein. 2nd Ed. St. Louis, C.V. Mosby, 1982, p. 459.
75. Didolkar, S.M., Koontz, C., and Schimberg, P.I.: Phleborrheography in pregnancy. Obstet. Gynecol., 61:363, 1983.
76. Classen, J.N., Richardson, J.B., and Koontz, C.: A three year experience with phleborrheography. Ann. Surg., 195:800, 1982.
77. Raines, J.K.: The pulse volume recorder in peripheral arterial disease. In Noninvasive Diagnostic Techniques in Vascular Disease. 2nd Ed. Edited by E.F. Bernstein. St. Louis, C.V. Mosby, 1982, p. 360.
78. Baker, J.D., and Machleder, H.I.: Oculopneumoplethysmography. In Investigation of Vascular Disorders. Edited by A.N. Nicolaides and J.S.T. Yao. New York, Churchill Livingstone, 1981, p. 121.
79. Gee, W., Oller, D.W., and Wylie, E.J.: Noninvasive diagnosis of carotid occlusion by ocular pneumoplethysmography. Stroke, 7:18, 1976.
80. Dix, D., et al.: Diagnosis of carotid stenosis in the hypertensive patient using ocular pneumoplethysmography at 500 mm Hg vacuum. Bruit, 12:171, 1983.
81. Darling, R.C., et al.: Quantitative sequential pulse volume recorder: a clinical tool. Surgery, 72:873, 1972.
82. Gee, W.: Ocular pneumoplethysmography (OPG-Gee). In Practical Noninvasive Vascular Diagnosis. Edited by R.F. Kempczinski and J.S.T. Yao. Chicago, Year Book Medical Publishers, 1982, p. 167.
83. Stallworth, J.M., Plank, G.W., and Home, J.B.: Negative phleborrheography. Arch. Surg., 116:795, 1981.
84. Gee, W., Mehigan, J.T., and Wylie, E.J.: Measurement of collateral cerebral hemispheric blood pressure by ocular pneumoplethysmography. Am. J. Surg., 130:121, 1975.
85. Rutherford, R.B., Lowenstein, D.H., and Klein, M.F.: Combining sequential systolic pressures and plethysmography in diagnosis of arterial occlusive disease of the legs. Am. J. Surg., 138:211, 1979.
86. Whitney, R.J.: The measurement of volume changes in human limbs. J. Physiol. (Lond.), 121:1, 1953.
87. Sigdell, J.E.: A critical review of the theory of the mercury strain-gauge plethysmograph. Med. Biol. Eng., 7:365, 1969.
88. Barnes, R.W., et al.: Detection of deep venous thrombosis with an automatic electrically calibrated strain-gauge plethysmograph. Surgery, 82:219, 1977.
89. Barnes, R.W., et al.: Noninvasive quantitation of venous reflux in the post-phlebitic syndrome. Surg. Gynecol. Obstet., 136:769, 1973.
90. Barnes, R.W., Ross, E.A., and Strandness, D.E.: Differentiation of primary from secondary varicose veins by Doppler ultrasound and strain-gauge plethysmography. Surg. Gynecol. Obstet., 141:207, 1975.

91. Holm, V.S.E.: A simple plethysmographic method for differentiating primary from secondary varicose veins. Surg. Gynecol. Obstet., 143:609, 1976.
92. Barnes, R.W., and Yao, J.S.T.: Photoplethysmography in chronic venous insufficiency. In Noninvasive Diagnostic Techniques in Vascular Disease. 2nd Ed. Edited by E.F. Bernstein. St. Louis, C.V. Mosby, 1982, p. 514.
93. Flinn, W.R., et al.: The use of photoplethysmography in the assessment of chronic venous insufficiency. In Practical Noninvasive Vascular Diagnosis. Edited by R.F. Kempczinski and J.S.T. Yao. Chicago, Year Book Medical Publishers, 1982, p. 323.
94. Flinn, W.R., et al.: Photoplethysmography in the assessment of chronic venous insufficiency. In Investigation of Vascular Disorders. Edited by A.N. Nicolaides and J.S.T. Yao. New York, Churchill Livingstone, 1981, p. 516.
95. Abramowitz, H.B., et al.: The use of photoplethysmography in the assessment of venous insufficiency: a comparison to venous pressure measurements. Surgery, 86:434, 1979.
96. Wheeler, H.B., et al.: Occlusive impedance phlebography: a diagnostic procedure for venous thrombosis and pulmonary embolism. Prog. Cardiovasc. Dis., 17:199, 1974.
97. Wheeler, H.B., and Anderson, F.A.: Impedance phlebography: the diagnosis of venous thrombosis by occlusive impedance plethysmography. In Noninvasive Diagnostic Techniques in Vascular Disease. 2nd Ed. Edited by E.F. Bernstein. St. Louis, C.V. Mosby, 1982, p. 482.
98. Hull, R., et al.: Impedance plethysmography: the relationship between venous filling and sensitivity and specificity for proximal vein thrombosis. Circulation, 58:898, 1978.
99. Baker, J.D.: Position artifacts in occlusive impedance phlebography (plethysmography). Am. J. Surg., 136:181, 1978.
100. Clarke-Pearson, D.L., and Jelovsek, F.R.: Alterations on occlusive cuff impedance plethysmography results in the obstetric patient. Surgery, 89:594, 1981.
101. Flanigan, D.P., Miles, C., and Nicolaides, A.N.: Impedance plethysmography. In Investigation of Vascular Disorders. Edited by A.N. Nicolaides, and J.S.T. Yao. New York, Churchill Livingstone, 1981, p. 403.
102. Flanigan, D.P., et al.: Vascular laboratory diagnosis of clinically suspected acute deep-vein thrombosis. Lancet, 2:331, 1978.
103. Young, A.E., et al.: Impedance plethysymography: its limitation as a substitute for phlebography. Cardiovasc. Radiol., 1:233, 1978.
104. Benedict, K.T., Wheeler, H.B., and Patwardham, N.A.: Impedance plethysmography: correlation with contrast venography. Diagn. Radiol., 125:695, 1977.
105. Hull, R., et al.: Impedance plethysmography using the occlusive cuff technique in the diagnosis of venous thrombosis. Circulation, 53:696, 1976.
106. Wheeler, H.B., et al.: Suspected deep vein thrombosis: management by impedance plethysmography. Arch. Surg., 117:1206, 1982.
107. Moser, K.M., Brach, B.B., and Dolan, G.F.: Clinically suspected deep venous thrombosis of the lower extremities. JAMA, 237:2195, 1977.
108. Hull, R., et al.: Replacement of venography in suspected venous thrombosis by impedance plethysmography and ^{125}I-fibrinogen leg scanning. Ann. Intern. Med., 94:12, 1981.

Acknowledgement. This work was supported in part by the Conrad Jobst Foundation, the Seabury Foundation, and the Northwestern Vascular Foundation.

22

Fine-Needle Abdominal Aspiration

Gregory P. Lewis ■ Peter L. Cooperberg

Percutaneous imaged-guided fine-needle aspiration techniques allow accurate, rapid, economical, and safe diagnosis of many neoplastic and non-neoplastic abdominal disorders. Application of these techniques frequently shortens the diagnostic interval and enables one to avoid unnecessary, expensive, or more invasive diagnostic procedures. Percutaneous fine-needle aspiration often allows specific medical or surgical therapy to be applied in a direct and timely manner. The clinician should be aware of the applications of these techniques, their limitations, and their possible, but rare, complications.

Fine-needle aspiration cytology was introduced by Martin and Ellis in 1930 and was subsequently applied by workers in Scandinavia, who refined the techniques and developed a large and diverse clinical experience.[1-5] Acceptance in North America has been slow, in part because of a skeptical medical community long accustomed to surgical biopsy and because of a shortage of cytopathologists.[6] The use of fine-needle imaged-guided aspiration cytology is rapidly evolving and is gaining acceptance. This trend should continue as a result of increased sophistication and understanding of both the imaging techniques and cytologic interpretation. Considerable experience with fine-needle aspiration cytology in patients with carcinoma of the breast, head, and neck has shown the utility, high rate of accuracy, and histologic concordance of this procedure.[7-10]

In this chapter, we discuss the indications for fine-needle aspiration, the costs, time, and safety of this technique, the technical considerations, and the cytopathologic results.

INDICATIONS

Although specific diagnoses are frequently suspected on the basis of the patient's medical history and imaging characteristics, the institution of specific therapy or the estimation of prognosis ultimately depends on histologic or cytologic confirmation. As imaging technology improves diagnostic detection, fine-needle aspiration allows cytologic specificity to be applied to the detected abnormality. Nearly every abdominal site has been successfully aspirated (Table 22–1). Most procedures involve the liver, pancreas, lymph nodes, and fluid collections. The overall accuracy rate for abdominal aspirations approaches 90% (Tables 22–2 to 22–4).

Sensitivity is greatest for lesions of the liver and lymph nodes involved with metastatic adenocarcinoma. Imaged-guided aspiration of malignant disease of the liver has a sensitivity exceeding 90% in most series (see Table 22–2). Sensitivity is lower for cancer of the pancreas. Table 22–3 shows the results of multiple reports of patients with proved carcinoma of the pancreas. The sensitivity of fine-needle abdominal aspiration in these reports was 76% (Fig. 22–1). Although this sensitivity may seem low, it reflects the difficulty in obtaining adequate histologic material in patients with pancreatic carcinoma. In 84 patients with carcinoma of the pancreas who underwent diagnostic laparotomy, only 61 (73%) had positive results of biopsy during the initial operation.[11] One patient required a third operation before histologic diagnosis was established. In a total of 438 patients undergoing pancreatic fine-needle abdominal aspiration, 3 complications (0.66%) occurred: 1 patient experienced an exacerbation of pancreatitis, and 2 patients had pain. No fistulas, pseudocysts, or infections were reported. The sensitivity of fine-needle aspiration for retroperitoneal malignant disease is almost 90% (Table 22–4). The success rate for imaged-guided aspiration of abdominal fluid collections approaches 100% (Table 22–5).

Ureteral obstruction following treatment for malignant abdominal disease often requires laparotomy for diagnosis. In four of five patients with ureteral obstruction following treatment for malignant abdominal tumors, fine-needle abdominal imaged-guided aspiration showed malignant rather than benign disease.[12]

Abnormalities of the spleen have been aspirated under the guidance of imaging techniques.[13] The safety of this procedure has been established; over a thousand blind punctures have been performed

Table 22–1. Indications for Abdominal Image-Guided Aspiration

General Indications	Specific Lesion or Situation
Suspected solid tumors	Focal liver lesion
	Focal splenic lesion
	Pancreatic mass
	Lymphadenopathy
	Abdominal masses
	Staging of recurrent or known malignant tumor
	Distinction between lymphoma and metastatic carcinoma
	Distinction between recurrent malignant tumor and new primary tumor
	Renal mass in selected cases only
	Ureteral stricture in patients with malignant disease
	Doubtful lesion seen on other studies (equivocal lymphangiogram)
Fluid collections	Abscess
	Hematoma
	Urinoma
	Bile collection
	Lymphocele
	Renal cyst
	Pancreatic pseudocyst

with the fine-needle technique without complications.[14]

Renal aspiration is usually undertaken to evaluate cysts for possible malignancy. Because most solid renal masses are hypernephromas, which require surgical removal, such masses are not routinely aspirated. If one suspects the presence of a benign solid lesion or a metastatic lesion to the kidney, then biopsy may be useful.

Detection of metastatic lymph node involvement in a patient with a known primary tumor may enable one to avoid staging laparotomy, may suggest alterations in the clinical stage of the tumor or in the patient's therapy, or may even allow one to identify a new primary tumor.[15–17]

ECONOMIC FACTORS

Significant economic savings result from shortening the diagnostic interval and avoiding unnecessary tests, hospitalizations, and procedures. Mitty and associates estimated cost savings of $169,800 in 53 patients with pancreatic carcinoma who avoided surgical exploration as a result of radiologic staging and cytologic diagnosis.[18] Ho and colleagues found that fine-needle abdominal aspiration rendered an operation unnecessary in 24% (12/51) of their patients.[19] Schwerk and Schmitz-Moorman found that liver aspirations altered therapy or diagnostic plans in 21% (11/51) of patients with malignant disease.[20]

RAPIDITY OF DIAGNOSIS

The value of obtaining cytologic information in 30 min should not be underestimated for both clinical planning and addressing patients' fears. A diagnosis can provide early information, to allow a patient to begin the adjustment to a medical condition. Hospitalization for diagnosis may be minimized in patients with metastatic disease, and functional time outside a hospital setting may be maximized. A positive cytologic diagnosis can reduce operating time in patients who require a surgical procedure by eliminating the need for intraoperative biopsy and frozen sections.

SAFETY OF THE PROCEDURE

The relative safety of any procedure must be known if intelligent decisions are to be made about its application and possible alternatives. The safety of fine-needle abdominal aspiration can be considered in two respects: needle-produced trauma and local or systemic dissemination of tumor. Considerable clinical and experimental data are available for evaluation of both these issues.

Animal experiments have failed to show a significant rate of traumatic complications of fine-needle abdominal aspirations.[21,22] No complications or worsening of induced acute pancreatitis in a porcine model were noted after fine-needle pancreatic aspirations.[22] Clinical experience has been similar to animal experiments. Surgeons performing operations after fine-needle aspirations cannot usually identify the site of puncture. Occasionally, small punctate petechiae or asymptomatic hematomas are seen.[23,24] The frequent course of the needle through bowel or stomach is without reported clinical

Table 22–2. Fine-Needle Aspiration in Malignant Tumors of Liver

Authors	Year	Imaging Method	Number of Patients	Overall Accuracy	Sensitivity	Specificity
Johansen and Svendsen[a]	1978	Radionuclide scanning	83	96% (80/83)	94% (51/54)	100% (29/29)
Zornoza and co-workers[b]	1980	Computed tomography, ultrasound, angiography	36	83% (30/36)	67% (12/18)	100% (18/18)
Schwerk and Schmitz-Moorman[c]	1981	Ultrasound	60	91.6% (55/60)	92.2% (47/51)	88.9% (8/9)
Montali and co-workers[d]	1982	Ultrasound	126	94% (119/126)	92% (85/92)	100% (34/34)
Sundaram and co-workers[e]	1982	Computed tomography	88	99% (87/88)	98.8% (83/84)	100% (4/4)
Totals:			393	94% (371/393)	93% (278/299)	96% (93/94)

[a]Johansen, P., and Svendsen, K.N.: Scan-guided fine needle aspiration biopsy in malignant hepatic disease. Acta Cytol., 22:292, 1978.
[b]Zornoza, J., et al.: Biopsy of the liver. AJR, 134:331, 1980.
[c]Schwerk, W.B., Schmitz, Moorman, P.: Ultrasonically guided fine needle biopsies in neoplastic liver disease. Cancer, 48:1469, 1981.
[d]Montali, G., et al.: Fine-needle aspiration biopsy of liver focal lesions ultrasonically guided with a real-time probe. Report on 126 cases. Br. J. Radiol., 55:717, 1982.
[e]Sundaram, M., et al.: Utility of CT-guided abdominal aspiration procedures. AJR, 139:1111, 1982.

Table 22-3. Percutaneous Fine-Needle Aspiration Biopsy of Pancreatic Neoplasms

Authors	Year	Imaging Method	No. of Patients	No. of Positive Results No. of Proved Malignant Neoplasms	Sensitivity (%)	False-Positive Results
Smith and co-workers[a]	1975	Ultrasound	7	5/6	83	0
Hancke and co-workers[b]	1975	Ultrasound	25	17/21	81	0
Tylen and co-workers[c]	1876	Angiography	29	22/29	76	0
Evander and co-workers[d]	1977	Percutaneous transhepatic-cholangiography, angiography	88	31/52	60	0
Goldman and co-workers[e]	1977	Ultrasound, fluoroscopy	13	6/11	54	0
Ho and co-workers[f]	1977	Fluoroscopy, endoscopic retrograde cholangiopanocreatography	9	7/8	87	0
Goldstein and Zornoza[g]	1978	Ultrasound, computed tomography, fluoroscopy	34	20/31	65	0
Holm and co-workers[h]	1978	Ultrasound	90	43/53	81	0
Tao and co-workers[i]	1978	Endoscopic retrograde cholangiopancreatography, angiography	34	24/26	92.3	0
Yamanaka and Kimura[j]	1979	Ultrasound	28	19/22	86	0
Mitty and co-workers[k]	1981	Ultrasound, fluoroscopy	53	37/43	86	0
Kolm and co-workers[l]	1981	Computed tomography	15	10/11	90	0
Sundaram and co-workers[m]	1982	Computed tomography	28	11/16	69	0
Totals:			453	253/329	76	0

[a]Smith, E.H., et al.: Percutaneous aspiration biopsy of the pancreas under ultrasonic guidance. N. Engl. J. Med., 292:825, 1975.
[b]Hancke, S., Holm, H.H.J., and Koch, F.: Ultrasonically guided percutaneous fine needle biopsy of the pancreas. Surg. Gynecol. Obstet., 140:361, 1975.
[c]Tylén, V., et al.: Percutaneous biopsy of carcinoma of the pancreas guided by angiography. Surg. Gynecol. Obstet., 142:737, 1976.
[d]Evander, A., et al.: Percutaneous cytodiagnosis of carcinoma of the pancreas and bile duct. Ann. Surg., 188:90, 1977.
[e]Goldman, M.L., et al.: Preoperative diagnosis of pancreatic carcinoma by percutaneous aspiration biopsy. Dig. Dis. Sci., 22:1076, 1977.
[f]Ho, C., et al.: Percutaneous fine needle aspiration biopsy of the pancreas following endoscopic retrograde cholangiopancreatography. Radiology, 125:351, 1977.
[g]Goldstein, H.M., and Zornoza, J.: Percutaneous fine needle aspiration biopsy of pancreatic masses. Dig. Dis. Sci., 23:840, 1978.
[h]Holm, H.H., et al.: Ultrasonically guided percutaneous puncture. Radiol. Clin. North Am., 13:493, 1975.
[i]Tao, L., et al.: Percutaneous fine needle aspiration biopsy of the pancreas. Acta Cytol., 22:215, 1978.
[j]Yamanaka, T., and Kimura, K.: Differential diagnosis of pancreatic mass lesion with percutaneous fine-needle aspiration biopsy under ultrasonic guidance. Dig. Dis. Sci., 24:694, 1979.
[k]Mitty, H.A., Efremidis, S.C., and Yeh, H.C.: Impact of fine needle biopsy on management of patients with carcinoma of the pancreas. AJR, 137:1119, 1981.
[l]Kolms, M.D., Bernacki, E.G., Jr, and Schwab, R.: Diagnosis of pancreatic lesions by percutaneous aspiration biopsy. Acta Cytol., 25:675, 1981.
[m]Sundaram, M., et al.: Utility of CT-guided abdominal aspiration procedures. AJR, 139:1111, 1982.

Table 22-4. Fine-Needle Retroperitoneal Lymph Node Aspiration for Malignant Tumors

Authors	Year	Imaging Method	Number of Patients	Overall Accuracy	Sensitivity	Specificity
Zornoza and co-workers[a]	1977	Fluoro	72	82% (59/72)	76% (43/56)	100% (16/16)
Göthlin and MacIntosh[b]	1979	Fluoro	132		97% (64/66)	98% (59/60)
Bonfiglio and co-workers[c]	1979	Fluoro	47		84% (11/13)	100%
Dunnick and co-workers[d]	1980	Fluoro	6		100 (5/5)	100% (1/1)
Sundaram and co-workers[e]	1982	CT	32	87.5%	100%	100%
Totals:			289		89.6% (147/164)	

[a]Zornoza, J., et al.: Fine-needle aspiration biopsy of retroperitoneal lymphoceles and abdominal masses: an updated report. Radiology, 125:87, 1977.
[b]Göthlin, J.H., and MacIntosh, P.K.: Interventional radiology in the assessment of the retroperitoneal lymph nodes. Radiol. Clin., North Am., 17:461, 1979.
[c]Bonfiglio, T.A., et al.: Fine needle aspiration cytopathology of retroperitoneal lymph nodes in the evaluation of metastatic disease. Acta Cytol., 23:126, 1979.
[d]Dunnick, N.R., et al.: Percutaneous aspiration of retroperitoneal lymph nodes in ovarian cancer. AJR, 135:109, 1980.
[e]Sundaram, M., et al.: Utility of CT-guided abdominal aspiration procedures. AJR, 139:1111, 1982.

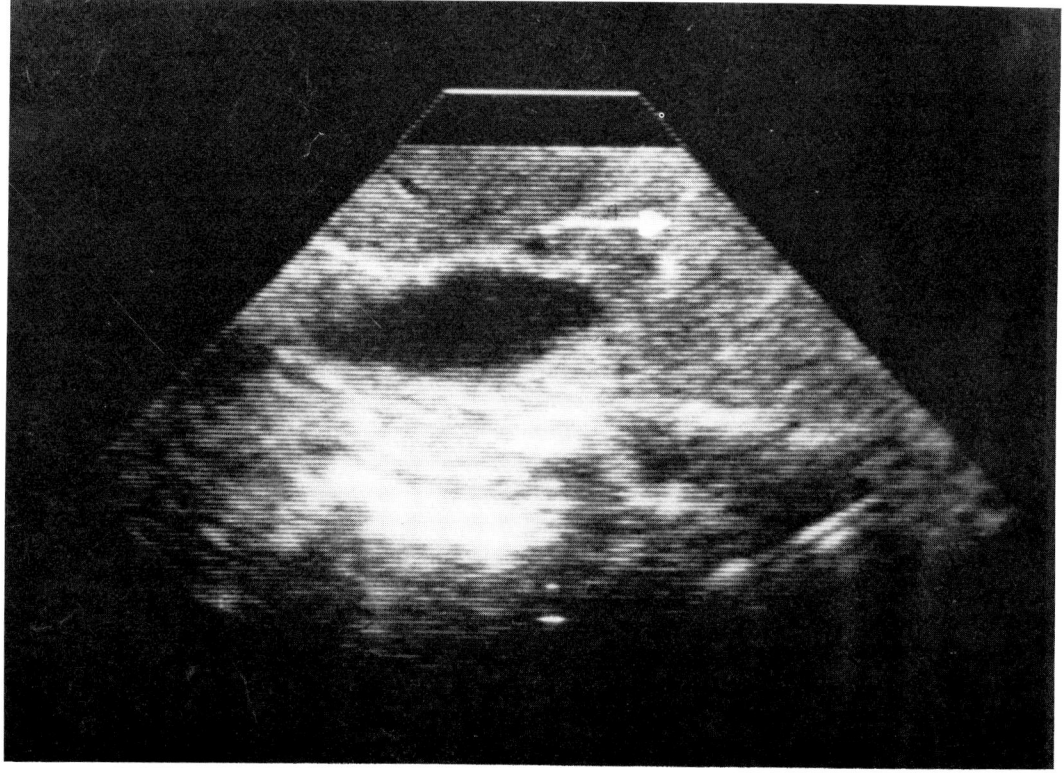

FIG. 22-1. Longitudinal real-time sonogram of a common bile duct obstructed by a pancreatic mass. The arrow shows the aspirating needle in the mass, which was determined cytologically to be an adenocarcinoma.

Table 22-5. Image-guided Aspiration of Abdominal Fluid Collections

Authors	Year	Number of Patients	Overall Accuracy (%)	Sensitivity	Specificity (%)
Sundaram and co-workers[a]	1982	30	100	100 (30/30)	100
Holm and Kristensen[b]	1980	72	—	95% (69/72)	—
Totals:		102		97% (99/102)	

[a]Sundaram, M., et al.: Utility of CT-guided abdominal aspiration procedures. AJR, *139*:1111, 1982.
[b]Holm, H.H., and Kristensen, J.K. (Eds.): Ultrasonically Guided Puncture Technique. Philadelphia, W.B. Saunders, 1980.

complication. Fine aspiration needles are smaller in diameter than the suture needles used in abdominal operations.[24,25]

A literature review of complications in 11,700 patients who underwent fine-needle abdominal aspirations showed 1 aspiration-related death from necrotizing pancreatitis, for a mortality rate of 0.008%.[26] Major complications occurred in 6 patients (0.05%): 2 had bile peritonitis, 2 had tumor seeding along the needle tract, 1 had intrahepatic hematoma, and 1 had peritonitis after aspiration of an abscess caused by a retained surgical sponge. Forty-eight minor complications were reported (0.49%). No other procedure that allows cytologic or histologic examination, including endoscopy, laparoscopy, and laparotomy, has a higher margin of safety or can be performed more rapidly (Table 22-6). In patients with medical conditions precluding open biopsy who require a diagnosis before beginning therapy, fine-needle imaged-guided aspirations may usually be safely performed.

We routinely perform aspirations in outpatients without preparation. Contraindications to fine-needle aspiration are few. Major bleeding diathesis, suspected echinococcal cyst, ovarian lesions, and vascular abnormalities are the main contraindications to aspiration. We do not routinely check blood-clotting parameters unless the patient's clinical status or medical history suggests a major abnormality. The risk of anaphylaxis and the availability of serologic tests make puncture of echinococcal cysts unnecessary. Ovarian cytologic features are difficult to evaluate accurately, and as a result, the value of aspiration is limited. Vascular lesions, such as liver hemangiomas, have been inadvertently punctured without consequence, but their diagnosis cannot be

Table 22-6. Diagnostic Procedures and Associated Morbidity and Mortality Rates

Procedure	Complication Rate (%)	Mortality Rate (%)
Fine-needle abdominal aspirations[a]	0.55	0.008
Fiberoptic endoscopy[b]	0.1–0.2	0.014–0.065
Colonoscopy with polypectomy[b]	1.9–4.9	0.09
Laparoscopy and biopsy in malignant liver disease[c]	1	0.03
Endoscopic retrograde cholangiopancreatography, in experienced hands[b]	2–5	0.001–0.2
Percutaneous renal biopsy[d,e]	5–8	0.1
Liver cutting-needle biopsy[f,g,h]	5.9	0.1–0.17
Renal cyst exploration[i,j]	15.6–30	1–2

[a]Livraghi, T., et al.: Risk in fine-needle abdominal biopsy. JCU, *11*:77, 1983.
[b]Shalmir, M., and Schuman, B.C.: Complications of fiberoptic endoscopy. Gastrointest. Endosc., *26*:86, 1980.
[c]Lightdale, C.J.: Laparoscopy and biopsy in malignant liver disease. Cancer, *50*:2672, 1982.
[d]Slotkin, E.A., and Madsen, P.D.: Complications of renal biopsy: incidence in 5000 reported cases. J. Urol., *87*:13, 1962.
[e]Diaz-Buxo, J.A., and Donadio, J.V., Jr.: Complications of percutaneous renal biopsy: an analysis of 1,000 consecutive biopsies. Clin. Nephrol., *4*:223, 1975.
[f]Perrault, P., et al.: Liver biopsy: complications in 1,000 inpatients and outpatients. Gastroenterology, *74*:103, 1978.
[g]Terry, R.: Risks of needle biopsy of the liver. Br. Med. J., *1*:1102, 1952.
[h]Stauffer, M.H.: Needle biopsy of the liver. Surg. Clin. North Am., *47*:851, 1967.
[i]Stanisic, T.H., Badcock, J.R., and Grayhack, J.T.: Morbidity and mortality of renal exploration for cyst. Surg. Gynecol. Obstet., *145*:733, 1977.
[j]Kropp, K.A., et al.: Morbidity and mortality of renal exploration for cyst. Surg. Gynecol. Obstet., *125*:803, 1967.

established by aspiration. Nonetheless, although fine-needle aspiration cytology has a record of exceptional safety, it should not be applied unless clinically indicated.

The issue of tumor dissemination by fine-needle abdominal aspiration biopsy is frequently addressed emotionally rather than objectively. Fine-needle abdominal aspiration can theoretically result in local or systemic dissemination of tumor. The biopsy procedure could disseminate malignant cells through blood or lymphatic channels. Engzell and co-workers investigated this possibility in rabbits with metastatic popliteal lymph nodes that underwent biopsy while venous blood and lymph were collected; no evidence of biopsy-induced vascular or lymphatic spread was found.[27]

Local dissemination of malignant cells by biopsy is uncommon in frequently performed procedures, which use a large needle, such as prostate biopsies. Through 1973, only 6 cases of prostatic cancer needle-tract seeding following percutaneous biopsy has been reported in the world literature,[28] despite the use of large, coring biopsy needles with up to 12 times the cross-sectional area of a 23-gauge needle and, presumably, a greater risk of dissemination. Engzell and colleagues reviewed the records of 157 patients with pleomorphic adenoma of the major salivary glands, 469 patients with prostatic carcinoma, and 656 patients with cervical lymph node metastases, all of whom underwent diagnosis with fine-needle aspiration.[27] The follow-up period lasted at least 10 years, 5 years or until death, and 5 years, respectively. No evidence of needle-tract seeding was found.

Two instances of tumor seeding along the tract of a fine abdominal needle have been reported in the world literature.[29,30] Both occurred in patients with pancreatic carcinoma, one of whom underwent biopsy ten times. In neither of these patients did the seeding apparently alter prognosis.

Does fine needle aspiration biopsy alter survival rates? At least 2 reported studies have addressed this issue. Berg and Robbins compared 370 patients with breast cancer who had aspiration biopsy with 370 carefully matched control subjects, with a total of 15 years of follow-up.[31] The patients who had undergone aspiration had slightly better outcomes although not statistically significant. Von Schreeb and associates compared 5-year survival rates in 77 patients operated on for renal carcinoma following puncture and contrast injection with 73 matched control patients who did not undergo puncture.[32] No difference in survival rates was observed.

TECHNIQUE

The techniques of fine-needle-aspiration cytologic study have changed little since their introduction.

The use of image-guidance systems allows the extension of aspiration techniques to deep, nonpalpable abnormalities. A fine needle, 20 to 23 gauge, is placed in the area of abnormality using an imaging-guidance system. The stylet is removed, and the needle is turned and moved 1 to 2 cm back and forth through the area of abnormality several times to dislodge the cellular material while applying suction with a 10- to 20-ml syringe. The cytologic sample usually remains within the needle. Suction is released prior to withdrawal of the needle from the lesion, to minimize the aspiration of cells into the needle tract or into the syringe where removal is difficult. The needle is then transferred to an air-filled syringe to express the cells onto glass slides for fixation.

Tissue fragments can be collected for cell blocks, and a suspension from saline rinsings of the needle can be collected. The slides are fixed in 95% alcohol and are stained with Papanicolaou's or, occasionally, special stains. Two to 3 samples are obtained initially. The diagnostic yield increases with the number of samples, up to 4 to 5 aspirations, but not beyond this number. Ferrucci and co-workers showed that positive cytologic results were obtained on the first pass in 75% of patients with abnormalities and by the third aspiration in 95% of patients with abnormalities.[33] One or 2 samples may be obtained initially if it appears likely that results will be positive, with the provision that if results of the initial examination are negative in 15 to 20 min, a repeat aspiration will be immediately obtained to reduce the incidence of inadequate sampling.

Fine-needle abdominal aspiration is well tolerated by the majority of patients. We have found that the administration of a local anesthetic agent frequently causes more pain than unanesthetized aspiration. Rarely does pain require analgesics or does it persist beyond the immediate postaspiration period. In a series of 107 patients who underwent fine-needle lymph node aspiration, 41 patients reported no pain, 46 patients had slight pain equivalent to a venipuncture, 3 had moderate pain, and 17 patients reported tenderness at the abdominal wall puncture site the following day.[34] Others have noted that only approximately 20% of patients experience pain at the time of the actual biopsy.[21]

Fine-needle abdominal aspirations have been successfully performed using a diversity of planar and cross-sectional imaging methods, including fluoroscopy, ultrasound, and computed tomography (Tables 22-2 to 22-5). The choice of an imaging method should be governed by considerations of availability, accuracy, flexibility, and cost. Generally, one should use the simplest, most flexible, and most economical method that displays the abnormality adequately for aspiration. Accurate localization is

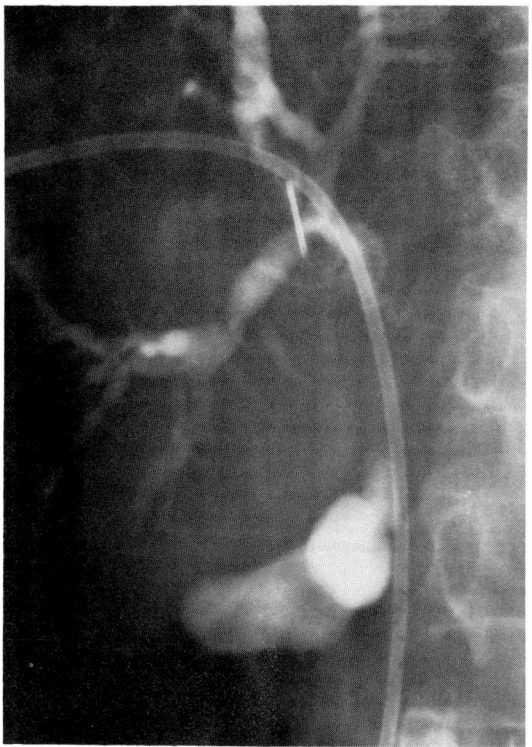

FIG. 22-2. Fluoroscopy-guided successful aspiration of a Klatskin tumor. Note the needle in the obstructing lesion.

required for successful needle aspiration. Table 22-7 tabulates some of the features, advantages, and disadvantages of each system. Fluoroscopy and ultrasound should be used for the majority of cases because of their availability, cost, and flexibility (Fig. 22-2). Because of its cost and because of considerations of time, computed tomography is indicated only when the other methods fail to show the location of the lesion accurately (Fig. 22-3).

CYTOLOGIC RESULTS

A skilled cytopathologist and a capable cytology technician are required for optimal results. Cytologic examination begins with a review of the pertinent clinical information, the suspected diagnosis, differential considerations, and the site of aspiration. Cytologic criteria of malignancy are well described.[35]

False-positive diagnoses are rare. In the case of breast carcinoma, for which more comparative data are available, Zajdela and colleagues reported the results of both histologic and cytologic examination in 2772 breast masses.[7] In only 3 cases (0.3%) were false-positive cytologic diagnoses made. Histologic false-positive diagnoses are also made from samples prepared in a traditional way and, more frequently, from frozen sections. Some pathologists are uneasy about making diagnoses from cytologic specimens and prefer histologic specimens; however, cytologic examination may be more accurate than corresponding histologic study. Cytologic touch samples of liver biopsy cores allow a higher percentage of positive diagnoses of metastatic disease than histologic specimens.[36,37] Cytologic and histologic examinations together have a higher diagnostic yield than when either study is done separately.[38]

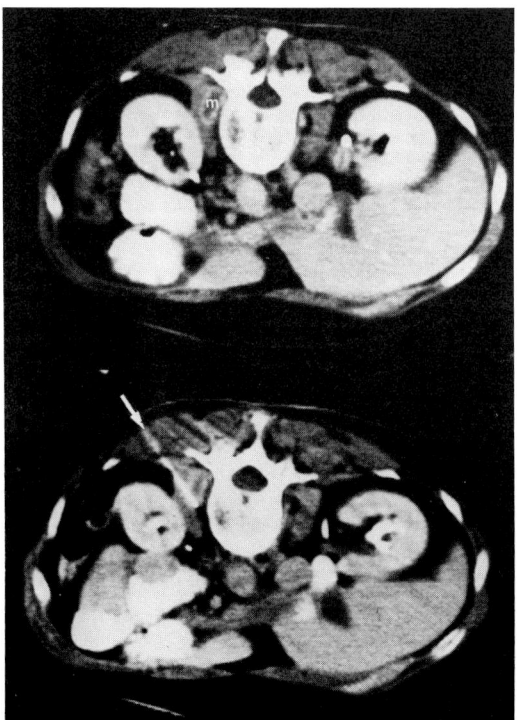

FIG. 22-3. Computed tomographic scan shows a left psoas lesion (A, m); aspiration revealed a psoas abscess. B, The arrow indicates the needle in the area of abnormality.

Table 22-7.

Imaging Method	Advantages	Disadvantages	Applications
Fluoroscopy	Low cost Ready availability Ease of use	Radiation exposure Contrast material needed to visualize most abnormalities Necessity for vertical needle direction	Transhepatic cholangiography Endoscopic retrograde cholangiopancreatography Angiography Barium studies Lymphangiography Intravenous pyelography, retrograde urography
Ultrasound	Low cost Ready availability Multiple planes of display Nonionizing radiation No need for contrast material Ease of use	View obscured by gas, wounds, appliances Documentation of needle location difficult	Study of entire abdomen
Computed tomography	Precise cross-sectional display Documentation of needle location possible Identification of small or deep abnormalities possible Unhindered by gas, wounds, appliances Determination of tissue vascularity possible	Cumbersome apparatus Time-consuming procedure High cost Co-operation of the patient required Radiation exposure Limited scanning planes Limited availability	Study of entire abdomen

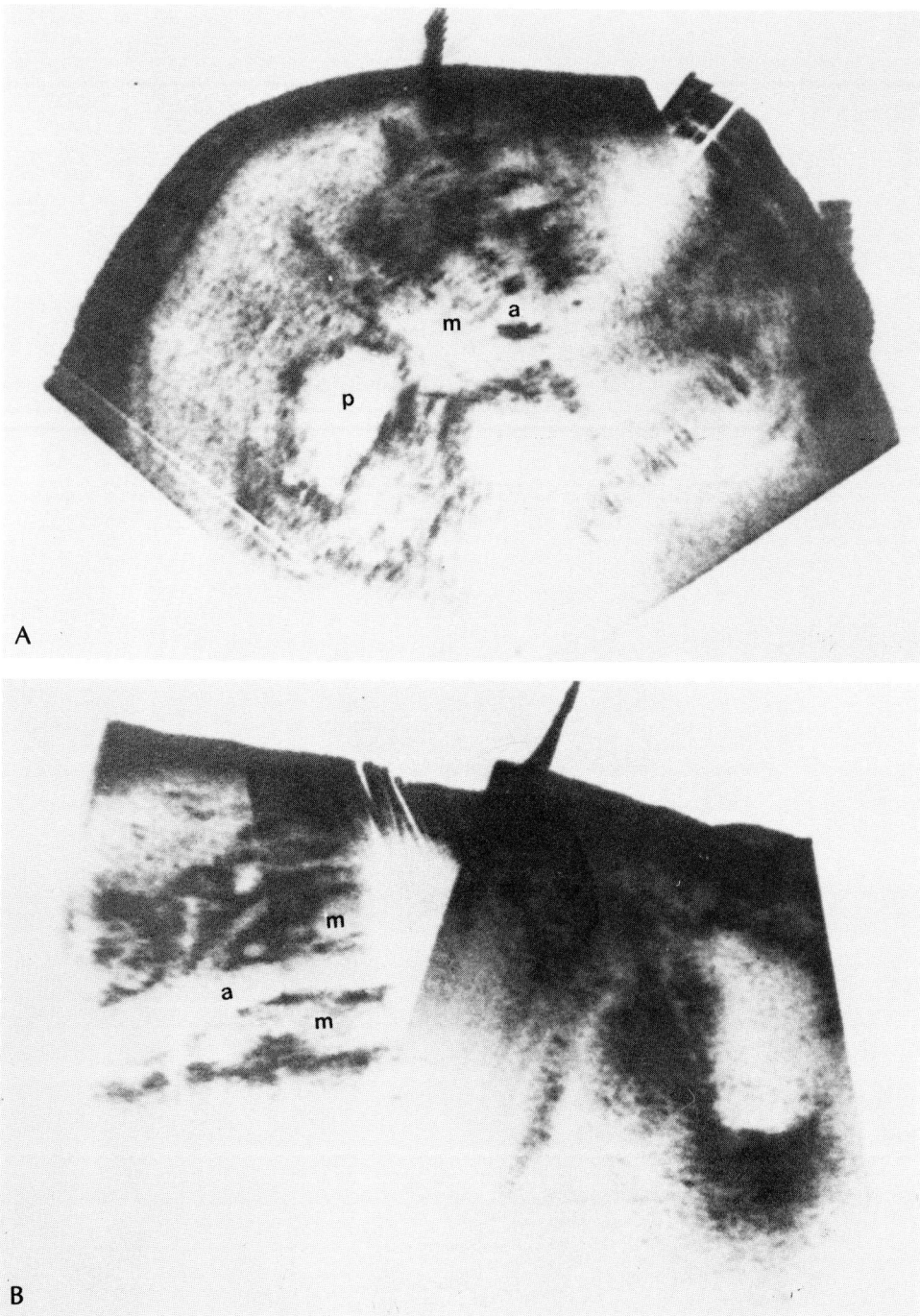

FIG. 22–4. Transverse (A) and longitudinal (B) static sonograms showing para-aortic adenopathy (m). Aspiration showed lymphoma, and the presence of a Reed-Sternberg cell allowed further subtyping as a Hodgkin's lymphoma. a, Aorta.

This observation has led to the development of several cutting needles that allow retrieval of small histologic fragments in addition to cytologic samples, even though the external diameter of these needles is no larger than 20 or 22 gauge. Abdominal aspirations performed with a fine, cutting-type needle (Greene) resulted in a 7% increase of positive diagnoses in 150 patients and an overall accuracy rate of 85%.[39] No significant increased risk appears to result from the use of these needles. Image-guided aspiration has obvious advantages over "blind" techniques. Conn and Yesner showed a 20% rate of recovery in patients with minimal metastatic liver disease who underwent blind liver biopsy.[40] A similar group of patients with minimal liver involvement who underwent biopsy under computed-tomographic guidance had an 86% recovery rate.[41]

Cytologic cellular yields in malignant disease are highest with cellular tumors that have reduced cellular cohesiveness, such as adenocarcinoma, melanoma, and squamous carcinoma. The cellularity of solid mesodermal tumors such as sarcomas may be reduced by the cohesiveness of the stromal cells. Use of a large, cutting-type needle, 18 to 20 gauge, may facilitate sampling of these tumors.

The diagnosis of lymphoma by cytologic examination may be difficult. If the cells are anaplastic, such as in histiocytic lymphoma, the diagnosis may be simple (Fig. 22-4). If the cells are well differentiated, however, histologic examination will be necessary to evaluate cellular architecture. Zornoza and co-workers investigated the results of 48 patients with proved lymphoma who underwent fine-needle image-guided aspiration.[42] The overall sensitivity rate was 58%. The sensitivity for aspiration of lymphomatous masses was 77% (17/22), whereas lymph node sensitivity was only 28% (4/14). If lymphoma is suspected by clinical or cytologic data, then open biopsy is recommended. Fine-needle aspiration is justified in retroperitoneal lymph nodes, especially in patients without splenomegaly. Patients with metastatic adenocarcinoma or with histiocytic lymphoma may have retroperitoneal lymph node involvement and may be spared the further morbidity and discomfort of an open biopsy procedure.

Cytologically, one cannot distinguish among adenocarcinomas from different primary sites, such as primary tumors of the pancreas or colon. At times, however, specific diagnoses are possible. Zornoza reported a definite cytologic diagnosis in 27 of 37 patients with unknown primary malignant tumors and abdominal masses (73%).[43] Although a negative result makes the possibility of malignant disease less likely, it does not exclude the diagnosis of neoplasm. A negative result may help one to select repeat biopsy, open biopsy, or additional diagnostic procedures. Cytology is not competitive with histology, but is complementary and useful because of its high diagnostic yield and low risk.

Fine-needle image-guided abdominal aspiration allows cytologic specificity to be applied to nonpalpable abdominal abnormalities. Use of these techniques frequently results in substantial cost and time savings while offering a margin of safety greater than that of alternate methods.

REFERENCES

1. Martin, H.E., and Ellis, E.B.: Biopsy by needle puncture and aspiration. Ann. Surg., 92:169, 1930.
2. Lundquist, A.F.: Fine needle aspiration biopsy of the liver: applications in clinical diagnosis and investigation. Acta Med. Scand. (Suppl.), 520:1, 1971.
3. Lundquist, A.: Fine-needle aspiration biopsy for cytodiagnosis of malignant tumor in the liver. Acta Med. Scand., 188:465, 1970.
4. Söderström, N.: Fine Needle Aspiration Biopsy. New York, Grune & Stratton, 1966.
5. Zajicek, J.: Aspiration Biopsy Cytology. Parts 1 and 2. White Plains, NY, S. Karger, 1979, p. 1974.
6. Fox, C.H.: Innovation in medical diagnosis—the Scandinavian curiosity. Lancet, 1:1387, 1979.
7. Zajdela, A., et al.: The value of aspiration cytology in the diagnosis of breast cancer: experience at the Foundation Curie. Cancer, 33:499, 1975.
8. Frable, W.J.: Thin needle aspiration biopsy: a personal experience with 469 cases. Am. J. Clin. Pathol., 65:168, 1976.
9. Young, J.E., Archibald, S.D., and Shier, K.J.: Needle aspiration cytologic biopsy of head and neck masses. Am. J. Surg., 142:484, 1981.
10. Franzén, S., and Zajicek, J.: Aspiration biopsy in diagnosis of palpable lesions of the breast: critical review of 3,479 consecutive biopsies. Acta Radiol. Oncol. Radiat. Phys. Biol., 8:241, 1968.
11. Gudjonsson, B., Livstone, E.M., and Spiro, H.M.: Cancer of the pancreas: diagnostic accuracy and survival statistics. Cancer, 42:2494, 1978.
12. Freiman, D.B., et al.: Thin needle biopsy in the diagnosis of ureteral obstruction with malignancy. Cancer, 42:714, 1978.
13. Solbiati, L., et al.: Focal lesions in the spleen. AJR, 140:59, 1983.
14. Söderström, N.: How to use cytodiagnostic spleen puncture. Acta Med. Scand., 199:1, 1976.
15. Bonfiglio, T.A., et al.: Fine needle aspiration cytopathology of retroperitoneal lymph nodes in the evaluation of metastatic disease. Acta Cytol., 23:126, 1979.
16. Dunnick, N.R., et al.: Percutaneous aspiration of retroperitoneal lymph nodes in ovarian cancer. AJR, 135:109, 1980.
17. Mennemeyer, R., Bartha, M., and Kidd, C.R.: Diagnostic cytology and electron microscopy of fine needle aspirates of retroperitoneal lymph nodes in the diagnosis of metastatic pelvic neoplasms. Acta Cytol., 23:370, 1979.
18. Mitty, H.A., Efremidis, S.C., and Yeh, H.C.: Impact of fine needle biopsy on management of patients with carcinoma of the pancreas. AJR, 137:1119, 1981.
19. Ho, C.S., Tao, L.C., and McLoughlin, M.J.: Percutaneous fine-needle aspiration biopsy of intra-abdominal masses. Can. Med. Assoc. J., 119:1311, 1978.
20. Schwerk, W.B., and Schmitz-Moorman, P.: Ultrason-

ically guided fine needle biopsies in neoplastic liver disease. Cancer, 48:1469, 1981.
21. Goldstein, H.M., and Zornoza, J.: Percutaneous fine needle aspiration biopsy of pancreatic masses. Dig. Dis. Sci., 23:840, 1978.
22. Coel, M.N., and Niwayama, G.: Safety of percutaneous fine needle biopsy of mass lesions affecting the hepatobiliary tract. Acta Radiol. [Diagn.] (Stockh.), 22:549, 1981.
23. Goldman, M.L., et al.: Preoperative diagnosis of pancreatic carcinoma by percutaneous aspiration biopsy. Dig. Dis. Sci., 22:1076, 1977.
24. Holm, H.H., et al.: Ultrasonically guided percutaneous puncture. Radiol. Clin. North Am., 3:493, 1975.
25. Tao, L., et al.: Percutaneous fine needle aspiration biopsy of the pancreas. Acta Cytol., 22:215, 1978.
26. Livraghi, T., et al.: Risk in fine-needle abdominal biopsy. JCU, 11:77, 1983.
27. Engzell, V., et al.: Investigation on tumor spread in connection with aspiration biopsy. Acta Radiol. Oncol. Radiat. Phys. Biol., 10:385, 1971.
28. Desai, S.G., and Woodruff, L.M.: Carcinoma of prostate—local extension following perineal needle biopsy. Urology, 3:87, 1974.
29. Smith, F.P., et al.: Cutaneous seeding of pancreatic cancer by skinny-needle aspiration biopsy. Arch. Intern. Med., 140:855, 1980.
30. Ferrucci, J.T. Jr., et al.: Malignant seeding of the tract after thin-needle aspiration biopsy. Radiology, 130:345, 1979.
31. Berg, J.W., and Robbins, G.F.: A late look at the safety of aspiration biopsy. Cancer, 15:826, 1962.
32. Von Schreeb, T., et al.: Renal adenocarcinoma: is there a risk of spreading tumor cells in diagnostic puncture? Scand. J. Urol. Nephrol., 1:270, 1967.
33. Ferrucci, J.T., Jr., et al.: Diagnosis of abdominal malignancy by radiologic fine needle aspiration biopsy. AJR, 134:323, 1980.
34. Göthlin, J.: Percutaneous transperitoneal fluoroscopy-guided fine needle biopsy of lymph nodes. Acta Radiol. [Diagn.] (Stockh.), 20:660, 1979.
35. Koss, L.G.: Diagnostic Cytology and Its Histopathologic Basis. 3rd Ed. Vols. 1 and 2. Philadelphia, J.B. Lippincott, 1979.
36. Carney, C.N.: Clinical cytology of the liver. Acta Cytol., 19:244, 1975.
37. Sherlock, P., Young, Y.S., and Koss, L.G.: Cytologic diagnosis of cancer from aspirated material obtained at liver biopsy. Am. J. Dig. Dis., 12:396, 1967.
38. Grossman, E., et al.: Cytological examination as an adjunct to liver biopsy in the diagnosis of hepatic metastases. Gastroenterology, 62:56, 1972.
39. Wittenberg, J., et al.: Percutaneous core biopsy of abdominal tumors using 22 gauge needles. AJR, 139:75, 1982.
40. Conn, H.D., and Yesner, R.: A re-evaluation of needle biopsy in the diagnosis of metastatic cancer of the liver. Ann. Intern. Med., 59:53, 1963.
41. Haaga, J.R., and Vanek, J.: Computed tomographic guided liver biopsy using the Menghini needle. Radiology, 133:405, 1979.
42. Zornoza, J., et al.: Percutaneous needle biopsy in abdominal lymphoma. AJR, 136:97, 1981.
43. Zornoza, J.: Percutaneous Needle Biopsy. Baltimore, Williams & Wilkins, 1981, p. 133.

23

Clinical Magnetic Resonance Imaging

G.M. Bydder

Magnetic Resonance Imaging (MRI) is the latest major addition to medical imaging technology. The majority of patients have been examined with research-prototype imaging machines, which have usually been located in factories or other clinically disadvantageous sites. The examinations have generally been slow, and clinical evaluation has run in parallel with machine development. These machines were designed to study the possibility of clinically useful MRI the form it should take. Because these machines were not designed for routine clinical use, the criteria used to assess the value of established imaging techniques in clinical use can only be applied to MRI in a general sense. Many applications, such as flow studies, ^{23}sodium (^{23}Na) imaging, combined ^{31}phosphorus (^{31}P)) spectroscopy and imaging, and the use of paramagnetic contrast agents, have been shown to be feasible in phantom experiments and in animals, but these applications have not yet been assessed in clinical practice.

In spite of these difficulties, it appears likely that, in future, this technique will play a significant role in neurologic diagnosis and possibly in other areas as well. Therefore, some knowledge of the basic principles and diagnostic capability of MRI may soon become relevant in clinical practice.

HISTORICAL DEVELOPMENT

In MRI, some atomic nuclei respond to the application of particular magnetic fields by emitting or absorbing electromagnetic radiation. This phenomenon was first demonstrated by Bloch and Purcell and their colleagues in 1946.[1,2] The variation in this electromagnetic absorption or emission with frequency can be viewed as a spectrum (Fig. 23–1). The frequency and intensity of the peaks of the spectrum reflect nuclear and molecular interaction, and the technique has proved valuable in analytic chemistry over the past three decades.

The medical application of this technique was pioneered by Erik Odeblad, a Swedish physicist. In an extensive body of work beginning in the 1950s, he and his associates used MRI spectroscopy to

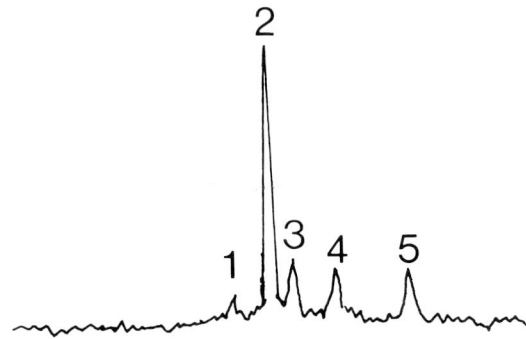

FIG. 23–1. ^{31}Phosphorus spectrum of muscle. The peaks correspond to the presence of inorganic phosphate (1), phosphocreatine (2), adenosine triphosphate (ATP) (3, 4, and 5).

study the properties of human red cells, cervical mucus, vaginal epithelial cells, myometrium, human milk, saliva, gingival tissues, tissues and fluids of the eye, and cells during ovulation.[3–10] Later in vitro work with spectroscopy by Damadian in 1971 and by Weisman and co-workers in 1972 showed an increase in the relaxation tissue of tumors in animals,[11,12] a finding also demonstrated in humans by Parrish and colleagues in 1974.[13]

A proposal for an imaging system was filed as a patent by Damadian in 1972,[14] but the first published MRI image was produced by Lauterbur in 1973.[15] Human in vivo images were published in 1977 by Mansfield and Maudsley,[16] by Damadian and co-workers,[17] and by Hinshaw and associates,[18] and in vivo MRI images showing pathologic features were published by Hawkes and colleagues in 1980.[19]

Since then, about a dozen groups have become involved in the evaluation of MRI systems.[19–30] Initial emphasis was placed on imaging of the brain, but studies of other organ systems have also been performed, and some general indication of the potential of MRI is possible.

INSTRUMENTATION

All MRI machines are constructed around a large magnet that provides a uniform, static magnetic

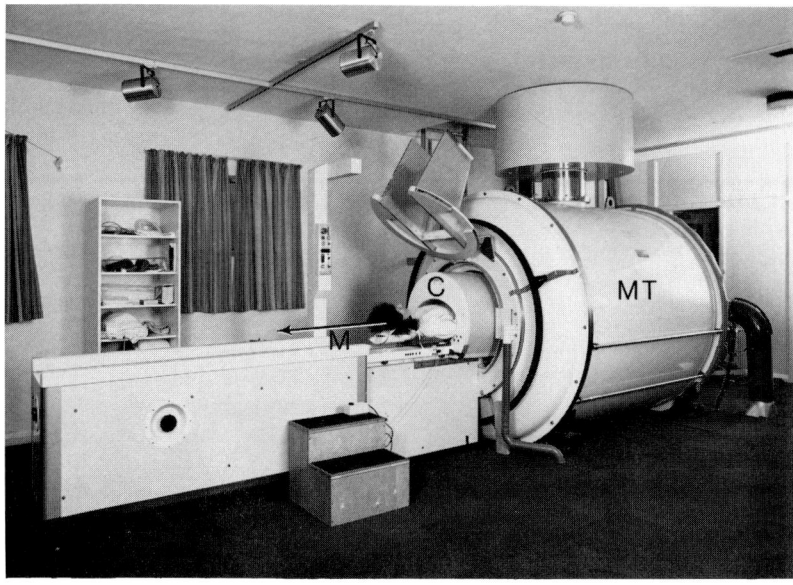

FIG. 23–2. A magnetic resonance imaging machine. The machine is constructed around a large cryomagnet (MT). The patient is slid into the bore of this machine and is surrounded by a transmitter and receiver coil (C). The magnet induces a net proton magnetization (M) in the patient.

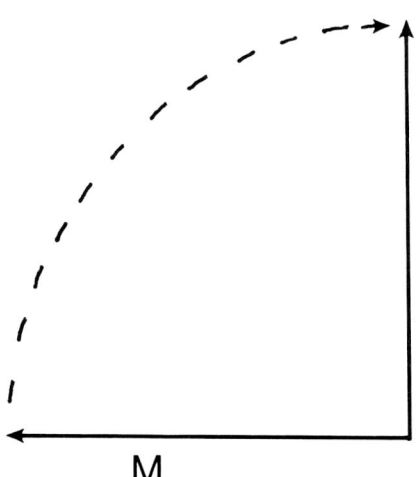

FIG. 23–3. Rotation of the magnetization (M). Magnetic pulses are used to rotate the proton magnetization (M) into the transverse plane; it then recovers or relaxes back to its original orientation and magnitude.

field. In the presence of this field, protons behave like tiny bar magnets. Their magnetization is aligned with the static magnetic field, to produce a net proton magnetization in the long axis of the patient (Fig. 23–2). Additional magnetic pulses are applied by means of a coil surrounding the patient. These pulses are used to rotate the nuclear magnetization, following which it recovers or relaxes back to its original position. For example, a so-called 90° pulse can be used to rotate the nuclear magnetization through 90° (Fig. 23–3). Following this rotation, the component of the magnetization in the long axis of the patient recovers from zero to its original amplitude in an exponential way. This recovery is called longitudinal or spin-lattice relaxation and is characterized by the time constant T_1. Relaxation of the magnetization in the transverse direction back to its original value of zero is termed transverse relaxation, or spin-spin relaxation, and is characterized by the time constant T_2. As the magnetization changes, it induces an electrical signal in a receiver coil that surrounds the patient. The electrical signal detected by this coil after such a 90° pulse is known as the free induction decay (FID); this signal is used to reconstruct the image.

Longitudinal relaxation (T_1) depends on the interaction of protons with surrounding nuclei and molecules (the "lattice"), whereas transverse relaxation depends on the interaction of protons with each other. Both T_1 and T_2 are sensitive indices of the local nuclear and molecular environment. By using a variety of pulse sequences, it is possible to produce images with varying dependence on proton density (ρ), T_1, and T_2. Several common pulse sequences designed for this purpose are summarized in Table 23–1. More detailed descriptions of MRI systems are available elsewhere.[31,32]

HAZARDS

Possible hazards associated with MRI include the static magnetic field, the heating effects from the radiofrequency pulses, and the induced currents

Table 23–1. Dependence of Pixel Values on ρ, T_1, and T_2 with Different Magnetic Pulse Sequences*

Pulse Sequence	Image Parameters		
	ρ	T_1	T_2
Repeated Free Induction Decay (RFID)	proportional to ρ	reduced if T_1 is long	
Inversion-Recovery (IR)	proportional to ρ	decreases as T_1 increases	
Spin-Echo (SE)	proportional to ρ	reduced if T_1 is long	increases as T_2 increases

*The principal image parameters for each sequence are shown in the boxes.

from changing magnetic fields.[33,34] The National Radiological Protection Board in Britain and the Bureau of Radiation Health in the United States have issued guidelines designed to exclude these possible hazards, and present systems operate well within these guidelines. No adverse effects have so far been reported, except a 3 to 4% incidence of claustrophobia.

NORMAL ANATOMIC FEATURES

Proton-density-dependent repeated free induction decay (RFID) images (Table 23–1) show little gray-white matter contrast, although flowing blood is readily seen and is highlighted when the scan cycle is shortened (Fig. 23–4).

T_1-dependent inversion-recovery (IR) images display a high level of gray-white matter contrast and enables one to see white matter from the central areas to the subcortical regions of the brain (Fig. 23–5). IR scans show more anatomic detail than images produced by computed tomography (CT) and have been used as reference scans. The gray-white matter interface on these scans is a source of partial volume effects, but this interface also produces a series of anatomic landmarks that are of value in localizing lesions and in assessing mass effects.

Spin-echo (SE) images have much poorer gray-white matter contrast than IR images (Fig. 23–5). Contrast in these images becomes more obvious as the scan cycle is lengthened, although the images become noisier. In addition, cerebrospinal fluid (CSF), which appears darker than brain tissue with a short scan cycle, becomes lighter when the cycle is lengthened.

The anatomic features of the brain on RFID and SE scans are similar to those seen on CT scans, but more detail is seen toward the apex of the skull, at the base of the brain, and in the posterior fossa, because of the absence of bone artifact and partial volume effects from bone. No signal is seen from cortical bone, although bone marrow and the scalp are clearly visible.

In the body, RFID images show less contrast than IR images, but they demonstrate flow effects. IR images show anatomic detail in a manner similar to that of radiographic CT scans, although with a lower level of spatial resolution and a degree of blurring caused by respiratory motion.

The lack of bone artifact is valuable in demonstrating the spinal cord. The heart can be visualized, and gating to the cardiac cycle is simple. The liver has a short T_1, as does subcutaneous fat, whereas the spleen has a long T_1. Renal cortex and medulla can be seen without the use of contrast agents.

DISORDERS OF THE BRAIN

Such disorders include vascular disease, disease of white matter, cerebral tumors, and neurologic disorders in children.

Vascular Disease of the Brain

Cerebral infarction produces an increase in T_1 and T_2 and a loss of gray-white matter contrast on IR scans.[35,36] One may also see a small associated mass effect with large areas of infarction. MRI is of most value in showing brain-stem and cerebellar infarction, in which abnormalities on CT scans are frequently obscured by the presence of artifact from bone (Fig. 23–6). For similar reasons, peripheral infarction over the hemispheres of the brain may be seen on MRI scans when it is not shown on CT images.

Scans of patients with acute intracerebral hemorrhage display a short T_1 and a long T_2. In addition, central areas of liquefaction or clot dissolution are seen.[35-37] Hemorrhages evolve and may eventually leave residual cysts. During these changes, T_1 and T_2 increase. Both the medial and lateral margins of subdural hemorrhages are seen unobscured by

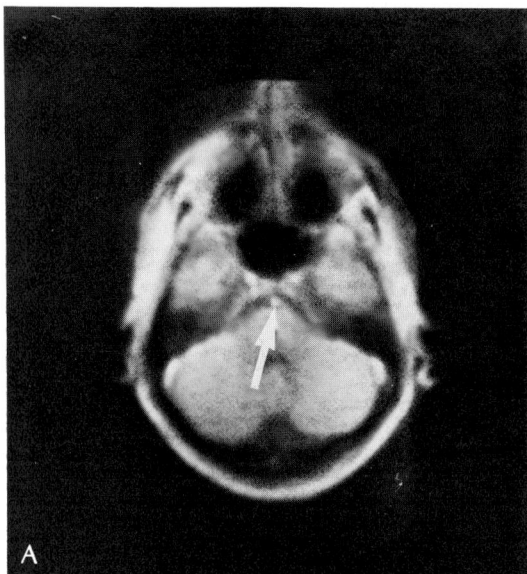

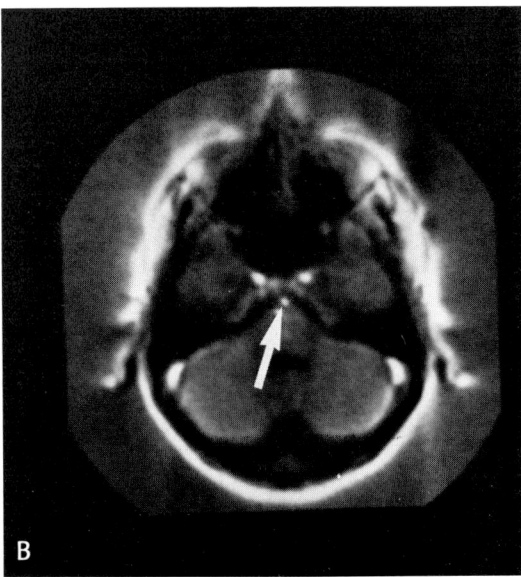

FIG. 23–4. Normal brain; normal repeated free induction decay (RFID) *(A)* and short-cycle RFID *(B)* scan. Decreasing the length of the scan cycle highlights blood flowing in the internal carotid and basilar (arrows) arteries.

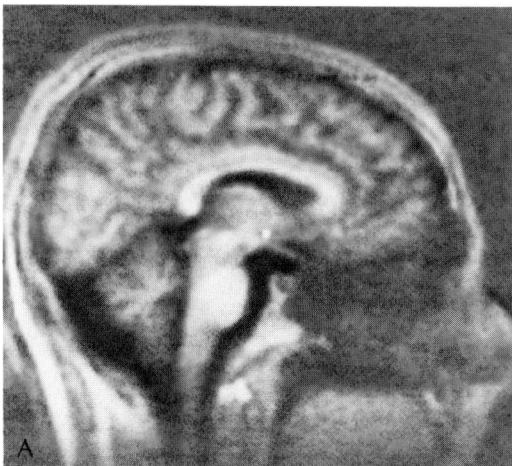

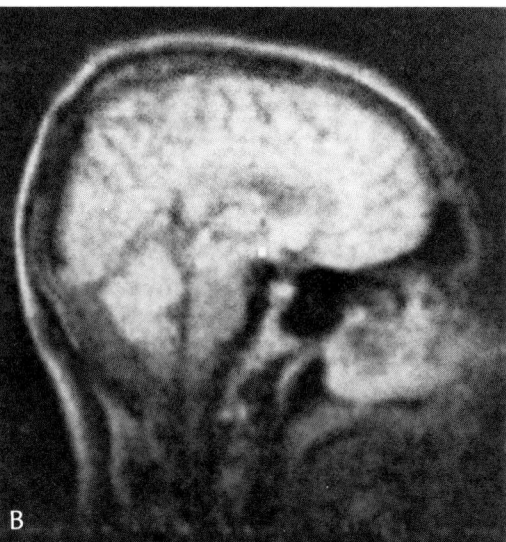

FIG. 23–5. Normal brain; sagittal inversion-recovery (IR) *(A)* and spin-echo (SE) *(B)* scans. A high level of gray-white matter contrast is seen on the IR scan (A), but much less contrast is seen on the SE scan (B).

bone (Fig. 23–7). In addition, mass effects are clearly visible because of the series of gray-white matter interfaces present on the IR scans.

Aneurysms may either display a light (short T_1) area caused by the presence of clotted blood or a dark area as a consequence of blood flow.[38] The resolution of MRI scanners is insufficient to provide the detail generally required for surgical treatment of aneurysms.

Scans of arteriovenous malformations display a loss of gray-white matter contrast, but in addition, rapid RFID scans may be used to highlight blood flowing into the area of interest. Occlusions of major vessels can be shown by the failure of vessels to display this response.[39] Although it is not yet possible to quantify blood flow, a variety of techniques designed for this purpose are being developed.

White-Matter Disease of the Brain

The lesions of multiple sclerosis are clearly shown by MRI.[40,41] They are characteristically periventricular and have an increased T_1 and T_2 (Fig. 23–8). Small lesions and lesions in the posterior fossa are frequently shown on MRI scans when they are not evident on CT scans.

In patients with leukodystrophy, the abnormal

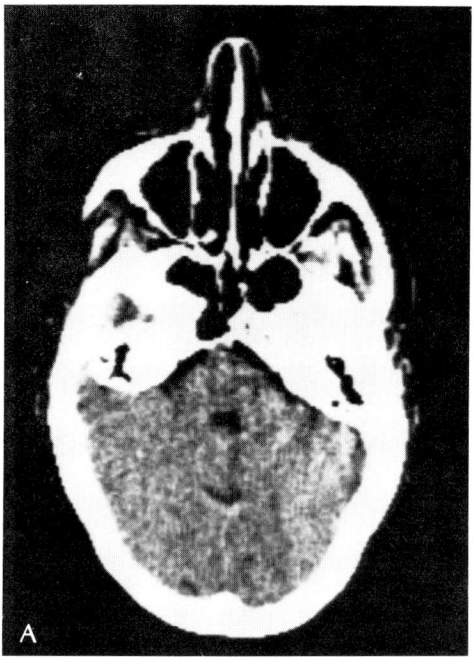
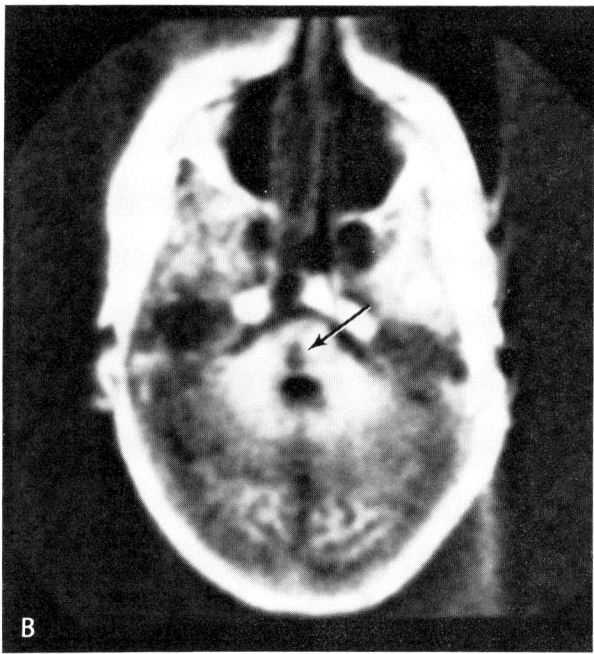

FIG. 23-6. Brain stem infarction; contrast-enhanced computed tomographic (A) and inversion-recovery (IR) (B) scans. The infarct (arrow) is only seen on the IR scan.

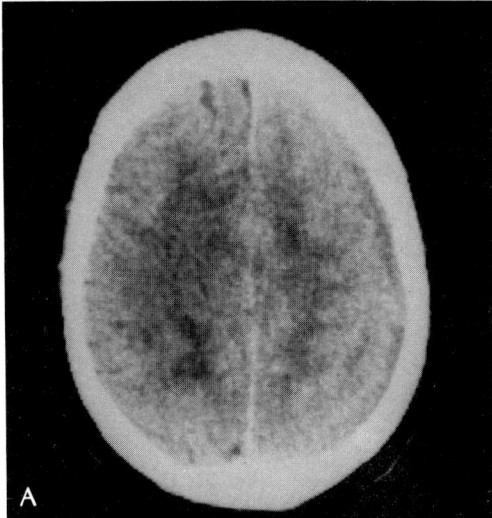

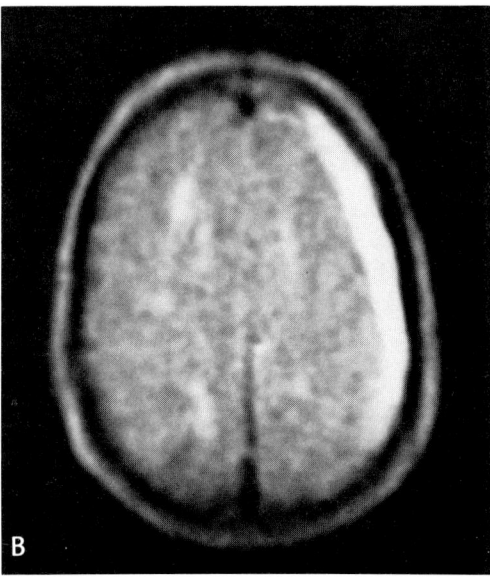

FIG. 23–7. Subdural hematoma; contrast-enhanced computed tomographic (A) and spin-echo (SE) (B) scans. The subdural hematoma has a long T_2, giving a light appearance on the magnetic resonance scan (B).

white matter is highlighted on the MRI scans because of its increased relaxation time. The characteristic distribution of lesions around the posterior lateral ventricles has been seen in adrenoleukodystrophy, together with loss of gray-white matter contrast in the adjacent occipital lobes. Binswanger's disease is another condition in which abnormal white matter is seen in relation to the ventricular system.

Radiation-induced damage also predominates in white matter and is frequently more extensive than appears on CT scans. Such damage often occurs within the radiation fields, but it may also be periventricular.

Cerebral Tumors

In vitro studies of human cerebral tumors in 1974 showed an increase in T_1 and T_2.[13] The first cerebral tumors were shown in vivo in 1980.[19] Tumors generally show an increase in T_1 and T_2 (Figs. 23–9 and 23–10), although tumors without an increase in T_1 have been described.[26] Lipid-containing tumors may also have a short T_1, as does recent hemorrhage into a tumor.

Scans of edema show an increase in T_1 and T_2 and, in a proportion of cases, it may be difficult to define the margin between tumor and edema. In these instances, contrast-enhanced CT may be superior to MRI. The development of MRI contrast agents to mark blood-brain-barrier breakdown is now in progress and may be important in resolving this problem.

Mass effects are clearly visible on IR scans, particularly in the sagittal and coronal imaging planes. Because periventricular edema is well seen on SE images (Fig. 23–11), this technique may be of value in distinguishing ventricular enlargement due to obstructive hydrocephalus from that due to cerebral atrophy.

The response of patients with tumors to therapeutic measures is yet to be studied, but much interest surrounds the possibility that direct measurements of T_1 and T_2 may be valuable in assessing therapeutic response.

Pediatric Neurologic Disease

The high level of gray-white matter contrast available with IR sequences provides a basis for the demonstration of the normal process of myelination in infants in vivo.[42] A rapid phase of myelination occurs in the first 2 years of life and is followed by a slower phase extending into the second decade. Delays in this development are seen following intraventricular hemorrhage and a variety of other conditions (Fig. 23–12).

Periventricular edema is also clearly visible in children. Cerebral tumors, hydrocephalus infarction, and infective changes have all been seen on MRI scans. Although ultrasonic imaging is free of hazard, it is limited by the closure of the fontanelles. In older infants, CT is used, but the lack of risk with MRI is potentially a major advantage over CT.

HEART LESIONS

Repeated FID images, which largely reflect proton density, show little contrast between blood and myocardium, but these structures are clearly distinguished using the IR sequence (Fig. 23–13). In volunteers, differences have been seen in the spin-

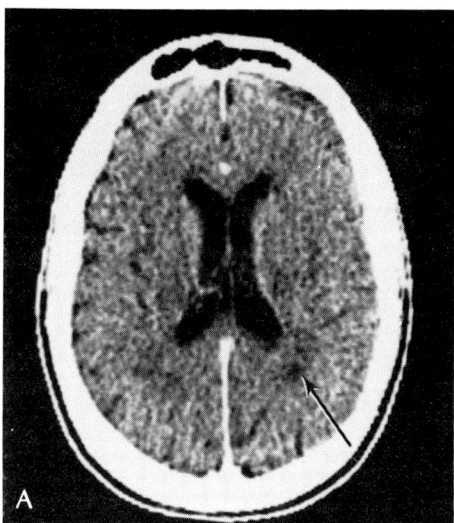 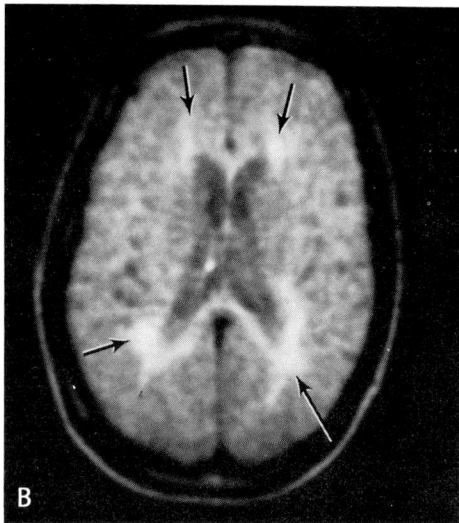

FIG. 23–8. Multiple sclerosis; contrast-enhanced computed tomographic (CT) *(A)* and spin-echo (SE) *(B)* scans. A single lesion is seen on the CT scan (arrow). This lesion is also seen on *B* (large arrow); additional lesions are only seen on *B* (small arrows).

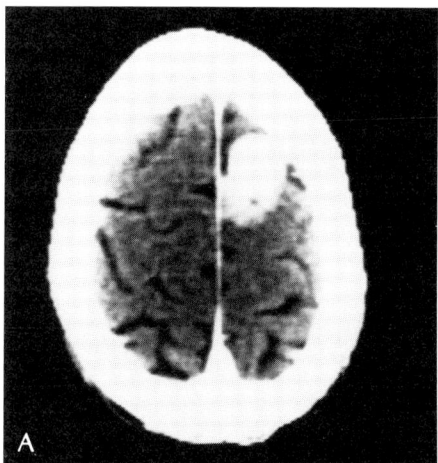

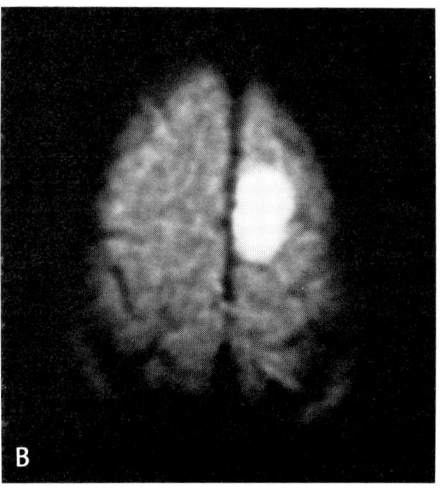

FIG. 23–9. Meningioma; contrast-enhanced computed tomographic (CT) *(A)* and spin-echo (SE) *(B)* scans. The tumor is well seen on both scans.

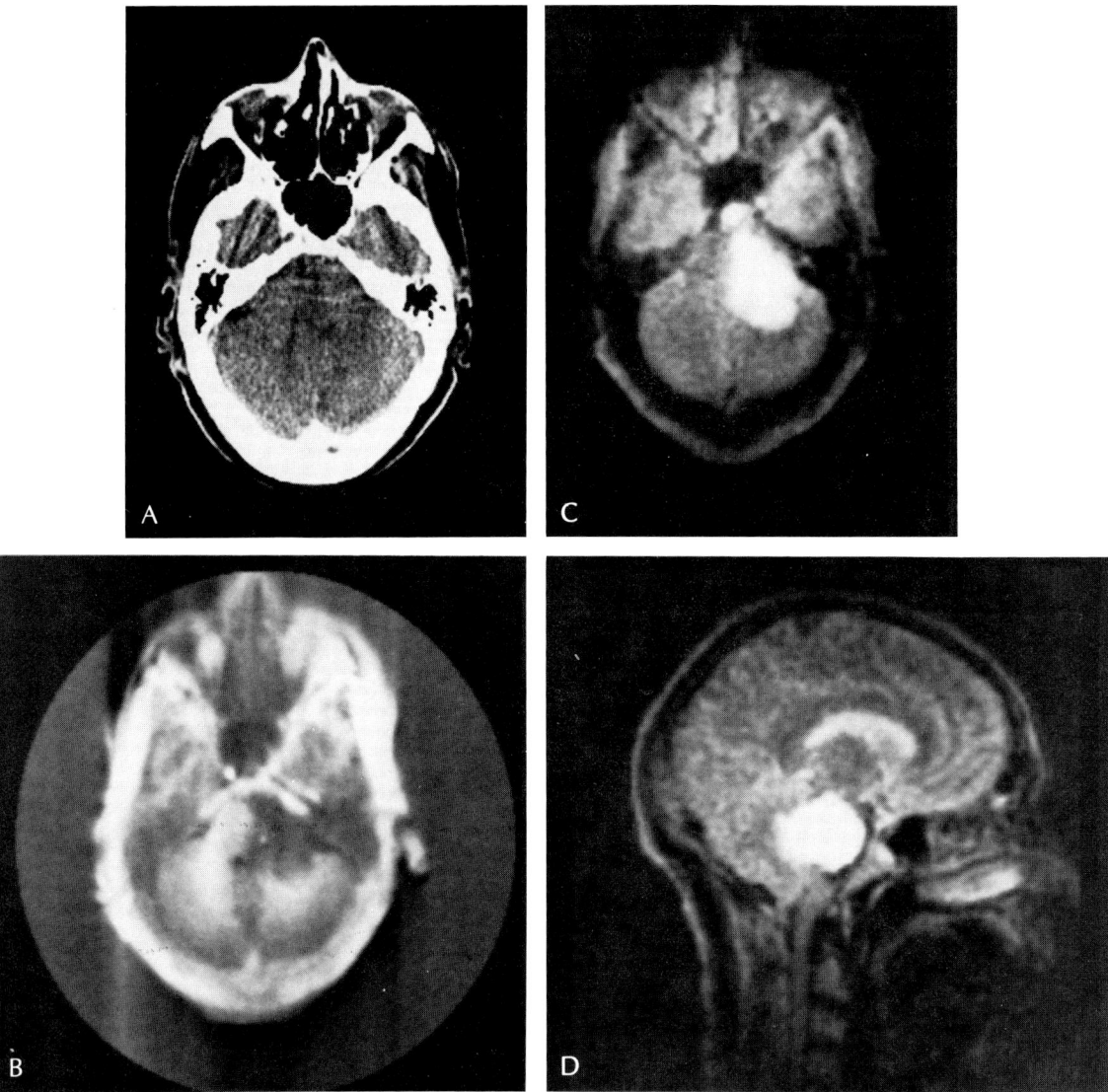

FIG. 23–10. Intrinsic tumor of the brainstem; contrast-enhanced computer tomographic *(A)*, inversion-recovery *(B)*, spin-echo *(C)*, and sagittal spin-echo *(D)* scans. An ill-defined low attenuation area and some displacement of the fourth ventricle are seen in *A*. Tumor within the left pons and cerebellum is well demonstrated on the magnetic resonance scans *(B* to *D)*.

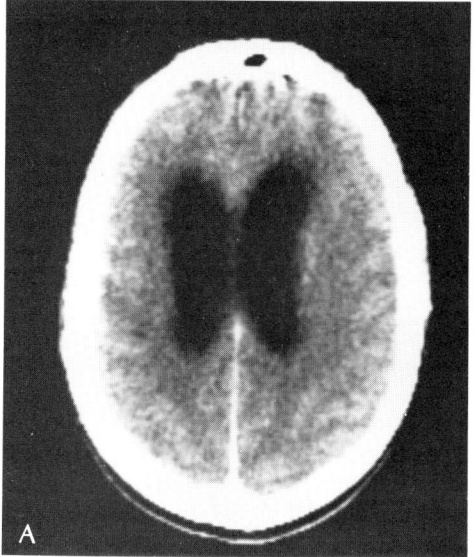
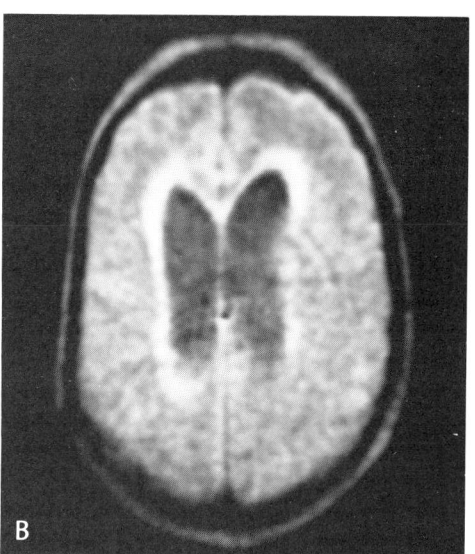

FIG. 23–11. Hydrocephalus; contrast-enhanced computed tomographic (A) and spin-echo (B) scans. Periventricular edema (light appearance) is well displayed on B.

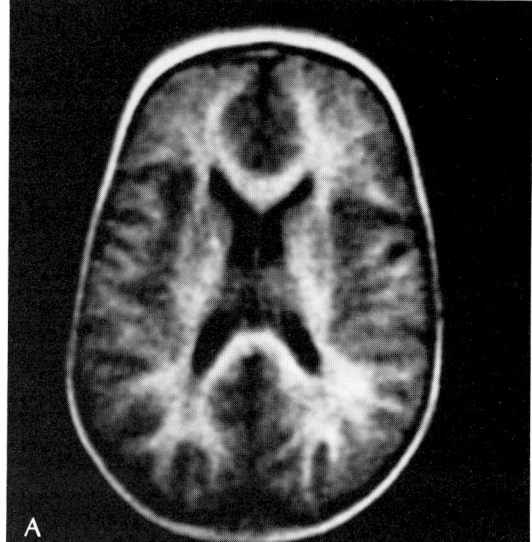
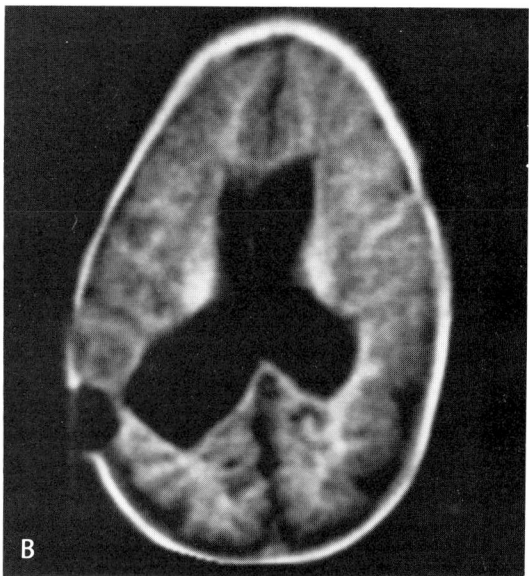

FIG. 23–12. Normal infant aged 20 months (A) and hydrocephalus following intraventricular hemorrhage in an infant aged 30 months (B); inversion-recovery scans. The level of myelination is less in the older infant (B). The semicircular ventricular shunt artifact is noted at the margin of the brain in B.

lattice relaxation time of blood in the left and right ventricular cavities on inhaling 100% oxygen; this change may be due to the paramagnetic effect of molecular oxygen in increasing the rate of relaxation. Whether this phenomenon will have clinical importance remains to be seen.

Experimental infarction produced by occlusion of the left anterior descending artery can be seen (Fig. 23–14). In patients, abnormal ventricular contours have been seen in ventricular hypertrophy and hypertrophic obstructive cardiomyopathy.[43]

Gating of the MRI image can be performed using the peripheral pulse with a pressure transducer or the electrocardiogram. It is difficult to ensure that the electrocardiographic leads do not interfere with the image, but this combined MRI-electrocardiographic technique improves the quality of the image (Fig. 23–15).

The sensitivity of the MRI images to changes in flow is of value both in showing obstruction or occlusion of vessels and in visualizing atheromatous plaque in major vessels.[44] As with cardiac imaging, the clinical usefulness of this remains to be determined.

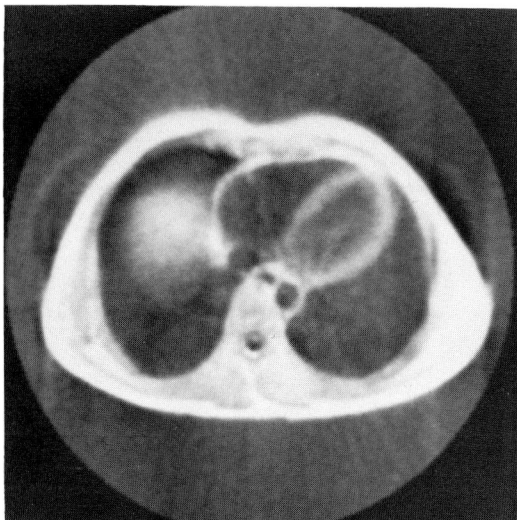

FIG. 23–13. Normal heart (ungated); inversion-recovery scan. The blood and myocardium are clearly distinguished.

The development of Echoplanar imaging by Mansfield and others offers the potential of real-time imaging of the heart. Data acquisition only requires milliseconds, and the process can be repeated rapidly.[45] Initial results have been obtained in animals, and the spatial resolution has been limited, but the technique is improving.

Imaging with ^{23}Na enables the heart margins to be defined, although most of the signal is obtained from surrounding blood.[46] In infarction or other conditions, however, the extracellular fluid component of the disease process may well be highlighted against the low signal from the surrounding normal heart. Again, results have so far only been obtained in animals.

ABDOMINAL DISORDERS

In spite of blurring caused by respiratory movement during the 2- to 4-min scan time, the high level of soft tissue contrast on IR images enables one to see the liver clearly. Intrahepatic blood vessels and bile ducts appear dark against the gray or normal liver parenchyma.

In a study of 30 patients, Smith and associates compared MRI favorably with isotope scanning and ultrasonography and first drew attention to the value of T_1 in the diagnosis of liver disease.[47]

From the initial experience of my colleagues and myself with 32 patients, focal disease is well seen on both CT and MRI scans, although the diagnosis of a hepatic infarct was only correctly recognized with MRI in 1 patient, and an area of focal atrophy was only seen with MRI in another.[48]

Metastases are clearly visible on CT and MRI scans (Fig. 23–16), and studies by Moss and co-workers on metastases have shown a sensitivity similar to that of CT.[49]

In diffuse disease, the pattern is more varied. In patients with steatosis, CT is usually diagnostic, whereas IR scans show no change. This feature may be of value in distinguishing focal fatty infiltration from tumor, which may be a problem with CT.

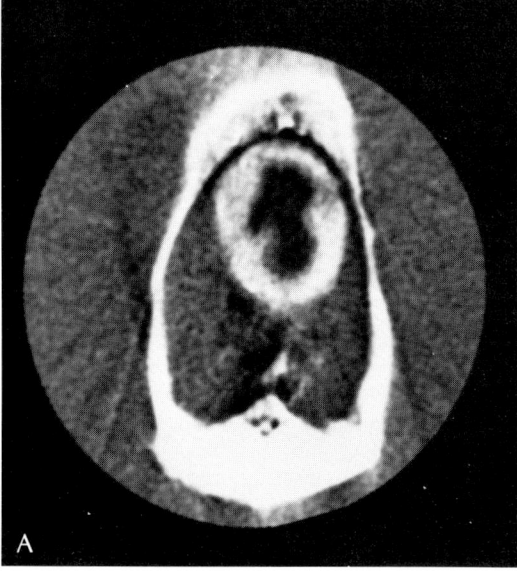 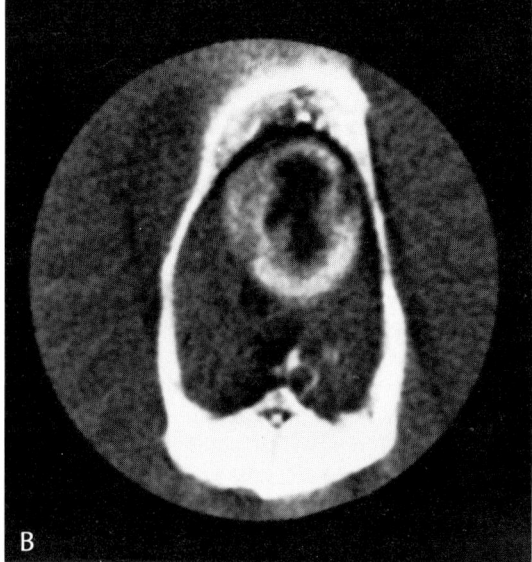

FIG. 23–14. Experimental infarction in the dog before *(A)* and after *(B)* occlusion of the left anterior descending artery (ungated); inversion-recovery scans. Evidence of infarction is seen as a dark area (long T_1) at the anterolateral margin of the left ventricle *(B)*.

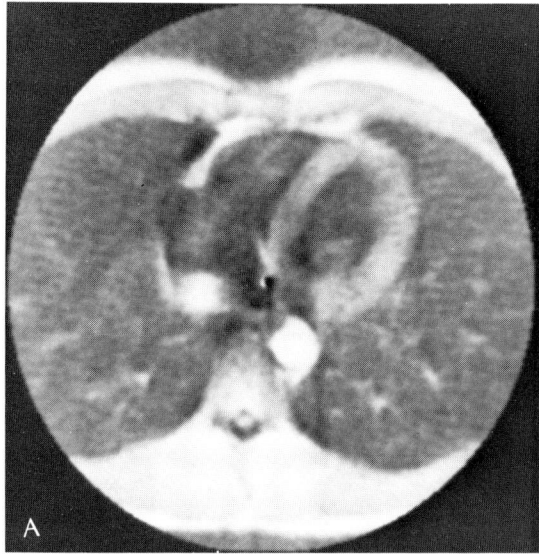 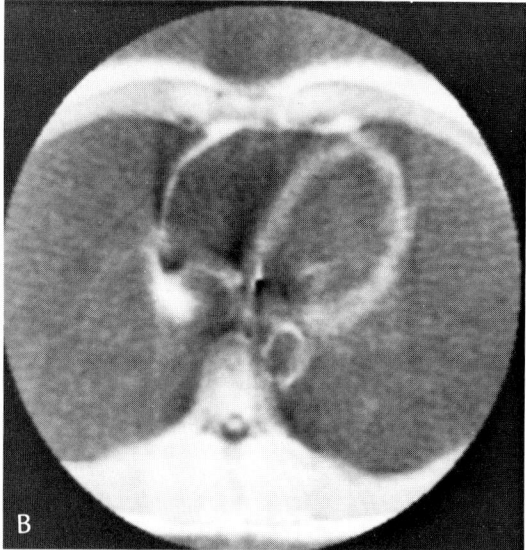

FIG. 23–15. Normal heart (electrocardiogram, gated) in systole *(A)* and in diastole *(B)*; inversion-recovery scans. The change in ventricular contour is well shown.

In other conditions, information of varying specificity is contributed by both CT and MRI.

Cirrhosis is of particular interest. In addition to the morphologic abnormalities, which are similar on CT and MRI scans, T_1 is prolonged to varying degrees (Fig. 23–17). Exceptions to this pattern may be found in forms of cirrhosis in which excessive copper, which is paramagnetic, is accumulated, such as primary biliary cirrhosis.

Overall, in patients with liver disease, T_1 values are a sensitive but nonspecific diagnostic parameter; T_1 is shortened in diseases associated with excessive copper or iron, which is also paramagnetic, and is lengthened in a variety of conditions, including infectious hepatitis and chronic active hepatitis. SE images are also valuable. Although the use of T_1 and T_2 measurements offers some additional information, the changes are usually not specific.

RETROPERITONEAL AND PELVIC DISORDERS

The pancreas has a T_1 value similar to that of liver, and disease processes such as tumor and pancreatitis have the effect of lengthening this parameter.[50,51] As a result of these conditions, the pancreas may be difficult to visualize because its relaxation time becomes similar to that of adjacent fluid-filled loops of bowel. I have used diluted oral ferric chloride solution in volunteers to label bowel, but more work will be required, to ascertain whether MRI has a useful role in showing diffuse and focal disease within the pancreas. High-resolution images, which may be obtained by increasing the gradient fields, are useful in imaging small structures such as the adrenal gland. The images are usually noisy, but better quality may be obtained by increasing the scan time. The adrenal cortex and medulla may possibly be visible with MRI.[52]

The most striking feature about the kidney images is the differentiation of cortex and medulla seen with the IR sequence. Perirenal fat is clearly seen around the kidney. In a patient with renal failure due to chronic glomerulonephritis, the MRI scan displayed both shrunken kidneys and loss of the cortical margin, whereas a well-defined cortical rim was seen on the patient's transplanted kidney. Focal changes in tumors and cysts have been observed with MRI,[53,54] but these conditions are clearly seen with other techniques. If MRI is to have a specific role in renal disease, it will probably be in diffuse parenchymal disease, rather than in focal diseases that are already well shown by existing techniques. Other diseases in the retroperitoneum may appear as on a CT scan.

COMPARISON WITH OTHER TECHNIQUES

Undoubtedly, CT was a major stimulus for the development of MRI imaging, but it has also provided a standard for assessment of MRI and is likely to be its main competition. Although one-to-one image comparison of the two techniques has been valuable in assessing the potential of MRI and in image interpretation, comprehensive assessment of the role of MRI in relation to CT and other techniques in routine diagnostic use is not yet possible.

Many basic questions about MRI machine design remain unanswered. For example, the static mag-

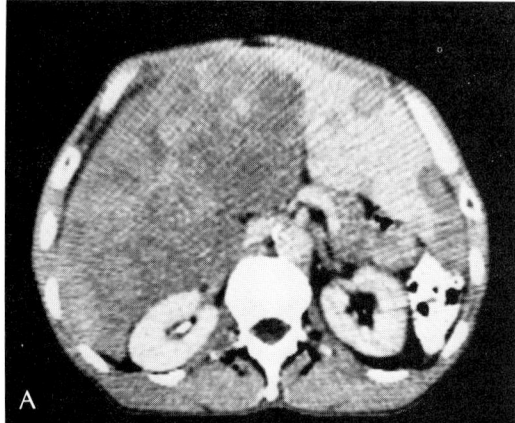

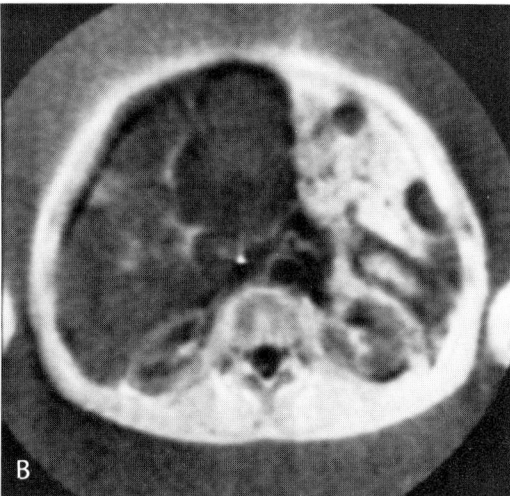

FIG. 23–16. Multiple liver metastases; contrast-enhanced computed tomographic *(A)* and inversion-recovery (IR) *(B)* scans. The IR image is blurred, but it shows the multiple metastases with greater contrast than A.

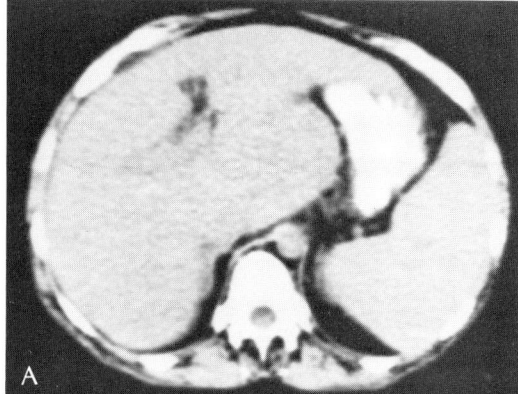

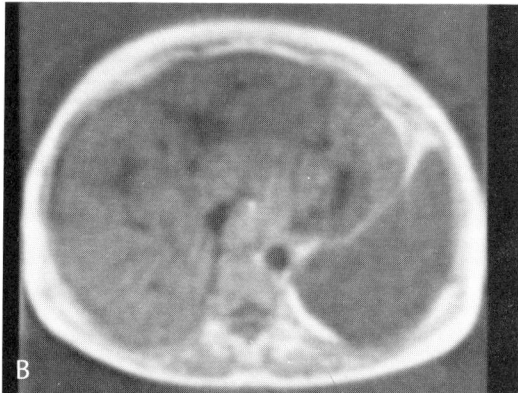

FIG. 23–17. *A* and *B*, Cirrhosis of the liver; inversion-recovery (IR) scans. The liver appears abnormally dark.

nets may be permanent, resistive, or cryogenic, with many possibilities within these categories. Although from a theoretic point of view, the magnetic field provided by these different types of magnets may be identical, from a practical point of view, the problems are different. Permanent magnets require no power and have a closely confined magnetic field, but they may be heavy, and they require precise temperature control. Resistive magnets are cheaper than cryomagnets, but they are less stable. Cryomagnets are expensive and require supplies of liquid nitrogen and helium, as well as familiarity with low-temperature physics on the part of the operators.

The indications for MRI are also uncertain. I provide a limited diagnostic service for patients with conditions of the posterior fossa, with suspected disease of white matter, and with a limited number of other cerebral conditions, but I regard the use of MRI elsewhere in the body as a research tool. With more experience, the indications for MRI may increase.

The requirements for personnel reflect the state of development of MRI. The majority of MRI machines now functioning in the world are supported by the research teams of physicists and engineers who designed and built them. Similarly, they are operated by technicians and radiologists with a research orientation, and the cost of each examination, if calculated, would be high. These features reflect research and development realities more than any intrinsic features about the technique, however.

FUTURE DEVELOPMENTS

Little doubt exists that improvements in MRI image quality will continue in the next few years, although probably at a slower rate than over the past several years. In particular, increased spatial resolution in the body may result in a significant role for MRI.

Other nuclei besides protons are also of interest,

and Hilal and associates successfully imaged ^{23}Na in rats following experimental cerebral infarction.[55] Although the natural abundance of ^{23}Na in the body is much less than that of protons, the relative changes in concentration in diseases such as infarction are much greater, so this technique may have clinical implications. ^{31}P is another nucleus of interest in this context, but it has not yet been successfully imaged. ^{19}Fluorine (^{19}F) images of gaseous fluorocarbons in the lung have been demonstrated, and ^{19}F may prove useful in the form of contrast agents.

Much interest surrounds the development of paramagnetic contrast agents and, in particular, the use of so-called spin-labels such as the nitroxide-stable free radicals. These substances shorten T_1 and T_2 and can potentially be attached to a wide range of chemicals or metabolites. The studies of these agents in animals by Brasch and associates appear promising,[56] but time will be required to assess their toxicity before clinical use is contemplated.

Another field of interest has been the possibility of obtaining clinically useful images and ^{31}P spectra on the same machine. This technique requires the use of a high magnetic field, such as 15 kilogauss. At these fields, it is anticipated that radiofrequency absorption may become a problem with larger objects and more complex sequences. The high field also restricts the choice of magnet to cryogenic systems and increases the expense. Although the clinical advantages of such a system are uncertain, research in this direction is being actively pursued at several centers.

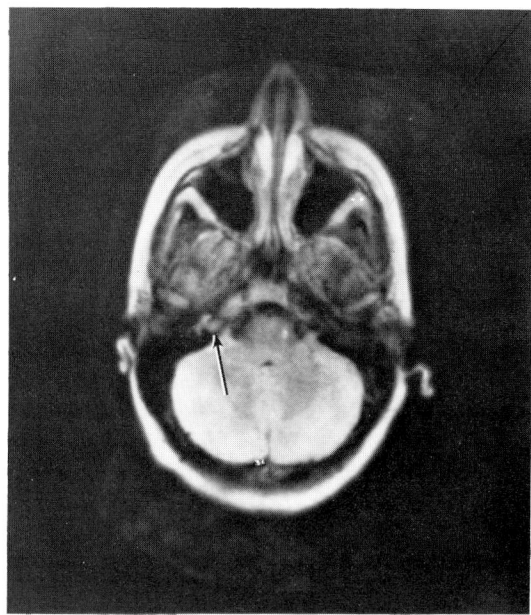

FIG. 23–19. Acoustic neuroma; spin-echo scan. The intracanalicular tumor (arrow) is well defined.

Although most MRI machines cost $1 million or more, the possibility of producing much cheaper machines is attracting interest. Resistive and permanent magnets are cheaper than the cryomagnets that are most frequently used, and the cost of computers is decreasing. X-ray tubes, solid-state detectors, and moving gantries are not required for MRI machines. A high-quality resistive-magnet machine for general use may therefore be a realistic possibility and would alter the whole basis for assessing the cost-effectiveness of this technique.

Over the last year, significant advances have occurred in MRI. Image quality has improved, and many operators now use a 256 × 256 matrix rather than 128 × 128, with a resultant improvement in resolution (Fig. 23–18).

Further advances in contrast-agent development have occurred; the emphasis now is on gadolinium-chelates. Clinical trials are expected soon.

The diagnosis of acoustic neuroma has become a preferred application for MRI (Fig. 23–19), and the recognition of posterior fossa tumors is generally better with MRI than CT.[57]

More detailed experience with scanning of the brain in children has also suggested that this may be a major use for MRI.[58] Many more clinical sites are under study, and much more experience is likely to accumulate soon.

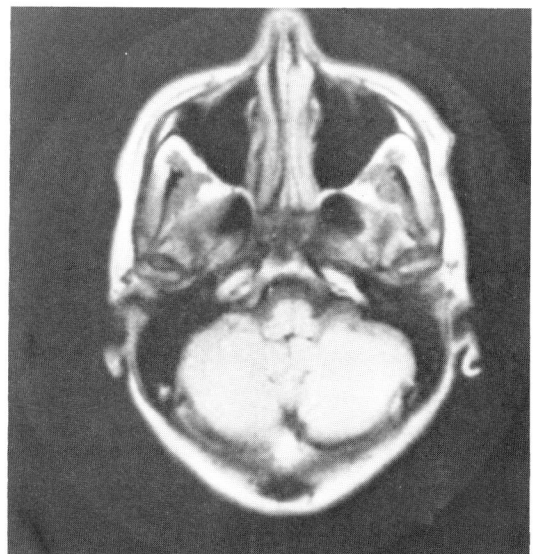

FIG. 23–18. Normal brain at the level of the upper medulla; spin-echo scan. The anatomic features are clearly defined.

ACKNOWLEDGEMENTS

I am grateful to Dr. Ian Young and his team from Picker International and the General Electric Company who designed and built the MRI machine from which all the foregoing images were obtained.

REFERENCES

1. Bloch, F., Hansen, W.W., and Packard, M.E.: Nuclear induction. Phys. Rev., 70:460, 1946.
2. Purcell, E.M., Torrey, H.C., and Pound, R.V.: Resonance absorption by nuclear magnetic movements in a solid. Phys. Rev., 69:37, 1946.
3. Odeblad, E., and Lindstrom, G.: Some preliminary observations on the proton magnetic resonance in biologic samples. Acta Radiol., 43:469, 1955.
4. Odeblad, E., Bhan, B.H., and Lindstrom, G.: Proton magnetic resonances of human red blood cells in heavy water exchange experiments. Arch. Biochem. Biophys., 63:221, 1956.
5. Odeblad, E., and Bryhn, U.: Proton magnetic resonance of human cervical mucus during the menstrual cycle. Acta Radiol., 47:315, 1957.
6. Odeblad, E.: Studies on vaginal contents and cells with proton magnetic resonance. Ann. N.Y. Acad. Sci., 83:189, 1959.
7. Huggert, A., and Odeblad, E.: Proton magnetic resonance studies of some tissues and fluids of the eye. Acta Ophthalmol., 37:93, 1959.
8. Forsbland, G., Odeblad, E., and Bergstand, A.: Proton magnetic resonance of human gingival tissue. Acta Odontol. Scand., 20:121, 1962.
9. Odeblad, E., and Lugelman-Sundberg, A.: Proton magnetic resonance studies on the structure of water in the myometrium. Acta Obstet. Gynecol. Scand., 44:117, 1965.
10. Odeblad, E.: Micro-NMR in high permanent magnetic fields. Acta Obstet. Gynecol. Scand. 45 (Suppl. 2):1, 1966.
11. Damadian, R.: Tumor detection by nuclear magnetic resonance. Science, 171:1151, 1971.
12. Weisman, I.D., et al.: Recognition of cancer in vivo by nuclear magnetic resonance. Science, 179:1288, 1972.
13. Parrish, R.G., et al.: Proton relaxation rates of water in brain and brain tumor. Science, 183:438, 1974.
14. Damadian, R.: Apparatus and method for detecting cancer in tissue. United States Patent No. 3789832. Filed March, 1982.
15. Lauterbur, P.C.: Image formation by induced local interactions: examples employing NMR. Nature, 242:190, 1973.
16. Mansfield, P., and Maudsley, A.A.: Medical imaging by NMR. Br. J. Radiol., 60:188, 1977.
17. Damadian, R., Goldsmith, M., and Minkoff, L.: NMR in Cancer. XVI. Fonar image of the live human body. Physiol. Chem. Phys., 9:97, 1977.
18. Hinshaw, W.S., Bottomley, P.A., and Holland, G.N.: Radiographic thin section image of the human wrist by nuclear magnetic resonance. Nature, 270:722, 1977.
19. Hawkes, R.C., et al.: NMR tomography of the brain: a preliminary clinical assessment with demonstration of pathology. J. Comput. Assist. Tomogr., 4:577, 1980.
20. Mallard, J.: The noes have it! Do they? Br. J. Radiol., 54:831, 1981.
21. Doyle, F.H., et al.: Imaging of the brain by nuclear magnetic resonance. Lancet, 2:53, 1981.
22. Zeitler, E., and Schwierer, G.: NMR clinical results. Nuremburg. In Nuclear Magnetic Resonance (NMR) Imaging. Edited by C.L. Partain et al. Philadelphia, W.B. Saunders, 1983, p. 267.
23. Luiten, A.L., et al.: Clinical results of NMR imaging. In NMR Imaging. Edited by R.L. Witcofski, N. Karstaedt, and C.L. Partain. Winston-Salem, N.C., Bowman Gray School of Medicine of Wake Forest University, 1982, p. 133.
24. Kaufman, B.: NMR imaging of the pituitary. Paper presented at the Clinical NMR Symposium, Cleveland, September 7 to 9, 1982.
25. Buananno, F.S., et al.: Clinical relevance of two different nuclear magnetic (NMR) approaches to imaging of a low grade astrocytoma. J. Comput. Assist. Tomogr., 6:529, 1982.
26. Weinstein, M.A., et al.: NMR—comparison of inversion recovery, saturation recovery and T_1-measurements in the brain and spine. J. Comput. Assist. Tomogr., 7:181, 1983.
27. Brant-Zawadski, M., et al.: Nuclear magnetic resonance of cerebral abnormalities: comparison with computed tomography. In Program and Book of Abstracts. First Annual Meeting of the Society of Magnetic Resonance in Medicine, Boston, 1982, p. 23.
28. Huk, W., and Loeffler, W.: NMR clinical results erlangen. In Nuclear Magnetic Resonance (NMR) Imaging. Edited by C.L. Partain et al.: Philadelphia, W.B. Saunders, 1983, p. 276.
29. Maudsley, A.A., et al.: Multinuclear NMR imaging. Paper presented at the First Annual Meeting of the Society of Magnetic Resonance in Medicine, Boston, August 16 to 18, 1982.
30. Sepponen, R.E., and Sepponen, J.T.: Repeated FID sequence in pituitary tumor diagnosis: a case report. Mag. Res. Med., 1:81, 1984.
31. Pykett, I.L., et al.: Principles of nuclear magnetic resonance imaging. Radiology, 143:157, 1982.
32. Bradley, W.G., and Tostetan, H.: Basic physics of NMR. In Nuclear Magnetic Resonance Imaging in Medicine. Edited by L. Kaufman, L.E. Crooks, and A.R. Marquis. Tokyo, Igaku-Shoin, 1982, p. 11.
33. Budinger, T.F.: Nuclear magnetic health effects. J. Comput. Assist. Tomogr., 5:800, 1981.
34. Saunders, R.D.: Biological hazards of NMR. In NMR Imaging. Edited by R.L. Witcofski, N. Karstaedt, and C.L. Partain. Winston-Salem, NC, Bowman Gray School of Medicine of Wake Forest University, 1982, p. 65.
35. Bailes, D.R., et al.: NMR imaging of the brain using spin-echo sequences. Clin. Radiol., 33:395, 1982.
36. Bydder, G.M., et al.: Clinical NMR imaging of the brain. AJR, 139:216, 1982.
37. Alfidi, R.J., et al.: Preliminary experimental results in humans and animals with a superconducting, whole-body nuclear magnetic resonance scanner. Radiology, 143:175, 1982.
38. Doyle, F.H., et al.: Imaging of the brain by nuclear magnetic resonance. Lancet, 1:53, 1981.
39. Bydder, G.M., et al.: NMR imaging of the posterior fossa: 50 cases. Clin. Radiol., 34:173, 1983.
40. Young, I.R., et al.: Nuclear magnetic resonance imaging of the brain in multiple sclerosis. Lancet, 2:1063, 1981.
41. Buonanno, F.S., et al.: Proton NMR imaging of normal and abnormal brain experimental and clinical observations. In NMR Imaging. Edited by R.L. Witcofski, N. Karstaedt, and C.L. Partain, Winston-Salem, NC, Bowman Gray School of Medicine of Wake Forest University, 1982, p. 147.
42. Levene, M.I., et al.: Nuclear magnetic resonance (NMR) imaging of the brain in children. Br. Med. J., 285:774, 1982.
43. Steiner, R.E.: The Hammersmith clinical experiments

with nuclear magnetic resonance. Clin. Radiol., 34:13, 1983.
44. Kaufman, L., et al.: Evaluation of NMR imaging for detection and qualification of obstructions in vessels. Invest. Radiol., 17:554, 1982.
45. Ordidge, R.J., et al.: Real time movie images by NMR. Br. J. Radiol., 55:729, 1982.
46. Delayre, J.L., et al.: Gated sodium-23 nuclear magnetic resonance images of an isolated perfused working rat heart. Science, 212:935, 1981.
47. Smith, F.W., et al.: Nuclear magnetic resonance tomographic imaging in liver disease. Lancet, 1:963, 1981.
48. Doyle, F.H., et al.: Nuclear magnetic resonance (NMR) imaging of the liver. AJR, 138:193, 1982.
49. Moss, A.A., et al.: NMR scanning of hepatic tumors: evaluation of various imaging techniques. Mag. Res. Med., 1:83, 1984.
50. Young, I.R., et al.: Initial clinical evaluation of a whole-body NMR tomograph. J. Comput. Assist. Tomogr., 6:1, 1982.
51. Smith, F.W., et al.: Nuclear magnetic resonance imaging of the pancreas. Radiology, 142:677, 1982.
52. Moon, K.L., et al.: NMR imaging of the adrenal gland: a preliminary report. Presented at the Radiological Society of North America Annual Meeting, Chicago, December 2, 1982.
53. Smith, F.W., et al.: Renal cyst or tumor—differentiation by whole-body nuclear magnetic resonance imaging. Diag. Imaging, 50:61, 1981.
54. Hricak, H., et al.: NMR imaging of the kidney. Mag. Res. Med., 1:83, 1984.
55. Hilal, S.K., et al.: Multinuclear NMR imaging in vivo. Paper presented at the Radiological Society of North America Annual Meeting, Chicago, November 29, 1982.
56. Brasch, R.C., et al.: Evaluation of nitroxide stable free radicals for contrast enhancement in NMR imaging. Paper presented at the First Annual Meeting of the Society of Magnetic Resonance in Medicine, Boston, August 16 to 18, 1982.
57. Bydder, G.M., et al.: NMR imaging of the posterior fossa: 50 cases. Clin. Radiol., 34:173, 1983.
58. Johnson, M.A., et al.: Clinical NMR imaging of the brain in children: normal and neurologic disease. AJNR 4:1013, 1983.

SUGGESTED READING

Gadian, D.G.: Nuclear Magnetic Resonance and Its Applications to Living Systems. Oxford, Clarendon Press, 1982.

Kaufman, L., Crooks, L.E., and Margulis, A.R. (Eds.): Nuclear Magnetic Resonance Imaging in Medicine. New York, Igaku-Shoin, 1981.

Partain, C.L., et al. (Eds.): Nuclear Magnetic Resonance Imaging. Philadelphia, W.B. Saunders, 1983.

Index

Page numbers followed by "f" indicate figures; page numbers followed by "t" indicate tables.

A mode ultrasound, 59, 60f, 61
A wave
  pulmonary artery wedge pressure, 333
  right atrial pressure, 330, 331f
  right ventricular pressure, 332, 332f
Abdomen
  abscess
    CT localization for percutaneous drainage, 149
    percutaneous drainage, 149
    radionuclide imaging in localization, 120, 120f, 121f
    ultrasound for, 84
  angiography, 167, 169-174
    adrenal gland, 174
    in gastrointestinal bleeding, 170, 172-174
    kidney, 172-174
    liver and portal system, 167, 169-170
    pancreas, 170, 171f
  CT of, 138-146
    abscess, 145
    adrenal glands, 143
    biliary tract, 140
    gastrointestinal tract, 141-142
    kidney, 142
    liver, 138-140
    pancreas, 140-141
    for percutaneous drainage, 149
    retroperitoneal lymph nodes, 143-144
    in trauma, 145-146, 174
  fine-needle aspiration, 401-411
    accuracy, 401, 403-405t, 408, 411
    complications, 402, 406-407, 406t
    contraindications, 406-407
    cytologic results, 408, 411
    imaging methods used with, 403-405t, 407-408, 408f, 409t
    indications, 401-402, 402t
    rapidity of diagnosis by, 402
    safety, 402, 406-407
    sites successfully studied, 401, 402t
    survival influenced by, 407
    technique, 407-408, 408f, 409t
    tumor dissemination by, 407
  fluid collections in, fine-needle aspiration cytology for, 401, 406t
  magnetic resonance imaging of, 422-423, 424f
  plain film of, 54-56f, 55, 57
    bowel gas patterns, 54f, 55
    indications for, 57
    in nephrolithiasis, 56f, 57
    in pneumoperitoneum 55, 55f
    positioning of patient for, 54f, 55
    technique, 55, 57
  trauma
    in chest stab wound, 297
    CT compared with angiography in, 174
    decision to perform surgical exploration, 293
    gunshot wounds, 296-297
    hemoperitoneum, 290
    injuries associated with, 294
    liver injury, 290
    minilaparoscopy in, 289-291, 289f
      complications, 291
      results, 291
    organ perforation, 290
    paracentesis in, 283, 293-297
      indications, 293-294
    penetrating injury, 290
    peritoneal lavage in, 283, 289-290, 293-297
      in blunt injury, 293-294
      contraindications, 295-296
      criteria for positive results, 294-295
      in penetrating injury, 296-297
    in pregnancy, 295
    splenic injury, 290
    stab wounds, 297
  ultrasound, 79-92
    adrenal glands, 85, 88f
    common bile duct, 79-81, 81f
    gallbladder, 79, 80f
    kidney, 84-85, 86-87f
    left upper quadrant mass, 83-84
    liver, 81-82, 82f
    needle puncture guidance by, 88, 91-92, 92f
    pancreas 82-83, 83f
    retroperitoneum, 85, 88, 90-91f
    spleen, 83-84, 84f
    testes, 85, 89f
Abdominal lavage, 283. See also Peritoneal lavage
Abscess
  abdominal
    CT in, 145
    subphrenic, 84
    ultrasound for, 84
  percutaneous drainage
    CT localization, 149
    technical considerations, 149
  radionuclide imaging in localization, 120
Achalasia, esophageal motility studies in, 366-367
Acid-base balance, arterial blood gases in evaluation, 305-306, 306f
Acid-secretory testing, 369-375. See also Stomach, acid-secretory testing

Acoustic neuroma, magnetic resonance imaging in, 425, 425f
Adhesions, peritoneal, 230, 233f
Adrenal gland
    angiography, 174
    CT of, 143, 143f
    masses, imaging methods for, 174
    metastases to, 143
    tumors, CT of, 143
    ultrasound, 85, 88f
Age, electrocardiogram related to, 311
Airway obstruction, flow volume loops in, 303, 305, 305f
Allergic reactions
    to contrast media, 153
    in excretory urography, 245, 247
Alzheimer's disease, CT findings, 134
Anemia, cardiac catheterization in, 328
Anesthesia
    in gastrointestinal endoscopy, 270-271
    in laparoscopy, 285-286
Aneurysm
    aortic, 163-165
        ultrasound, 88, 90f
    of hepatic artery, 169
    innominate artery, 165
    intracranial
        cerebral angiography in, 158-159, 158f, 159f
        congenital, 158
        magnetic resonance imaging in, 416
    subclavian artery, 165
Angiocardiography, 334-335
    equipment, 335
Angiodysplasia of colon, 172, 174f
    colonoscopy in, 277
Angiography, 153-179
    in abdominal trauma, 174
    of adrenal gland, 174
    aortography, 162-166. *See also* Aortography
    balloon catheters in, 155
    balloon occlusion arteriography, 176, 179f
    biplane filming in, 154
    in bone tumors, 176-177
    bronchial, 166, 166f
    cardiac output determined by, 338
    carotid, 155-158
    catheterization technique, 154
    cerebral, 158-162
    of chest, 162-167
    complications, 153-154, 154t
    digital subtraction, 155
        in aorta rupture, 164
        aortography, 162, 163f
        in carotid artery evaluation, 156, 156f
        comparison with conventional angiography, 155
        procedure, 155
        in pulmonary embolism, 167
    extracranial, 155-158
    of gastrointestinal tract, 170, 172, 172-174f
    of head and neck, 155-162
    of inferior vena cava, 177-178
    of liver and portal circulation, 167, 169-170, 169f
    multiple sequential exposures during, 154
    pancreatic, 170, 171f
    in pelvic trauma, 175
    in peripheral vascular disease, 175-176, 178-179f
    pulmonary, 166-167
    renal, 172-174
    selective injection of vasoconstrictor or vasodilator in, 154
    spinal, 158
    of superior vena cava, 178
    technique, 154-155
    ultrasonic, 383, 384, 384f
        diagnostic efficacy of, 388
    venography, 177-178, 179f
Ankle injuries, radiography in, 37f, 38f, 41
Ankle-brachial index, in Doppler ultrasound, 385, 386-387, 387f
Anterior communicating artery aneurysm, 158, 158f
Anticoagulants, cardiac catheterization danger with, 329
Aorta
    abdominal, ultrasound, 85, 88
    aneurysm
        aortography in, 163-165
        arteriosclerosis, 164
        congenital, 164-165
        CT in, 136
        mycotic and syphilitic, 164
        thoracic, 163-165
        traumatic, 164, 164f
        true versus false, 163
        ultrasound, 88, 90f
    coarctation, aortography in, 163
    dissection, 165-166
        classification, 165, 165f
        CT in, 136, 137f
    pressure waveforms in, 333, 335f
        in aortic stenosis, 333, 336f
    pseudocoarctation, 163
Aortic arch
    angiography, 156
        in subclavian steal phenomenon, 157
    congenital anomalies detected by aortography, 162-163, 163f
    right, 162
Aortic regurgitation
    hemodynamic measurements in, 333, 337f
    left ventricular hypertrophy in, 318, 319f
Aortic stenosis
    hemodynamic measurements in, 333, 336f
    left atrial abnormality in, 318
    left ventricular hypertrophy in, 318, 319f
Aortic valve
    cardiac catheterization evaluation of, 340
    echocardiographic evaluation, 75, 76f, 77f
Aortography, 162-166
    in aortic aneurysm, 163-165
    in aortic arch congenital anomalies, 162-163, 163f
    in coarctation and pseudocoarctation, 163
    in dissecting hematoma, 165-166
    procedure, 162
    in renovascular hypertension, 172, 175f
    subtraction technique, 162, 163f
    in Takayasu's arteritis, 166
Arrhythmias
    blood pressure determination in, 380
    Swan-Ganz catheters causing, 351
Arterial blood gases
    in preoperative patient, 306
    in pulmonary evaluation, 305-306
Arteries
    blood pressure measurement in
        direct, 380-382
        indirect, 379-380
    peripheral
        occlusive disease, Doppler ultrasound in, 382-383, 385
        pressure waveforms in, 333
    stenosis, Doppler ultrasound in, 384, 385f
Arteriography. *See also* Angiography

balloon occlusion, 176, 179f
bronchial, 166, 166f
catheterization in, 154
extracranial, 155-158
in peripheral vascular disease, 175-176, 178-179f
preventing hematoma or thrombosis after, 153
Arteriovenous fistula, traumatic, 175, 176f
Arteriovenous malformation
  in brain, 159, 160f
    CT of, 133, 133f
    magnetic resonance imaging in, 416
  brain scan in, 100
  pulmonary, angiography in, 167
Arteritis
  cerebral arteries, 159
  Takayasu's, 159-160, 166
Arthritis, bone scan in, 113, 116f
Aschoff-Rokitansky sinuses, 195f, 197
Ascites, laparoscopy in, 287-288
Aspiration, pulmonary, of barium sulfate, 214
Aspiration biopsy
  in abdomen, 401-411
    accuracy, 401, 403-405t, 408, 411
    in adenocarcinoma, 411
    complications, 402, 406-407, 406t
    contraindications, 406-407
    cost savings, 402
    cytologic results, 408, 411
    imaging methods used with, 403-405t, 407-408, 408f, 409t
    indications, 401-402, 402t
    in lymphoma, 410f, 411
    rapidity of diagnosis by, 402
    safety, 402, 406-407
    sites successfully studied, 401, 402t
    survival influenced by, 407
    technique, 407-408, 408f, 409t
    tumor dissemination by, 407
    ultrasound guidance in, 88, 91-92, 92f
  CT localization in, 148-149
  of lung, 257
  needles in, 148-149
Asthma, gastroesophageal reflux related to symptoms of, 356-357, 357f
Atherosclerosis
  aortic aneurysm due to, 164
  ulcerated carotid plaque, 157, 157f
Atrial abnormalities
  left, 313, 314f, 315
  right, 313, 314f
Atrial fibrillation
  blood pressure determination in, 380
  in mitral valve disease, 317-318
Atrial pressures, normal waveforms, 330-331, 331f
Attenuation, of x-rays, 4
Avascular necrosis, bone scan in, 113, 116f

Back, radiography, 18-27f, 33, 37-39
Balloon catheters
  in angiography, 155
  Swan-Ganz, 343-344, 344f
Balloon occlusion
  arteriography, 176, 179f
  of pulmonary artery, in preoperative evaluation of pneumonectomy patient, 307-308
Barium enema, 230-231, 234-237
  basics of interpretation, 235-236
  complications, 214
  diagnostic efficacy, 236-237
  in diverticular disease, 235, 236f
  indications, 230
  in intestinal obstruction, 229, 231f
  perforation in, 214
  preparation of patient for, 230
  single- versus double-contrast examination, 230-231, 234f
    choice of method, 236-237
  small bowel examination by, 227, 229
  technical problems in, 231, 235
  ultrasound of pelvis compared with, 93-94
Barium sulfate
  complications, 214
  in gastrointestinal studies, 213-214
  pulmonary aspiration, 214
Basilar artery aneurysm, 159, 159f
Betazole, in acid-secretory testing, 370, 370f
Bile leakage, after percutaneous transhepatic cholangiography, 200
Biliary tract
  atresia, radionuclide scanning for, 80-81
  carcinoma of bile duct, 201f
  common bile duct
    ERCP visualization, 204, 205-209f, 210
    stricture, 210
    ultrasound, 79-81, 81f
  CT of, 140, 140f
  dilatation, CT role, 140, 140f
  endoscopy, indications, 268
  luminal contrast studies, 183-210
    endoscopic retrograde cholangiopancreatography, 202-210
    intravenous cholangiography, 198
    oral cholecystography, 183-198
    percutaneous transhepatic cholangiography, 199-202
  obstruction
    CT role, 140, 140f
    ERCP compared with percutaneous transhepatic cholangiography in, 205, 209
    in percutaneous transhepatic cholangiography, 201-202, 202-204f
    ultrasound for, 80, 81f
  radionuclide imaging, 108f, 108-109
  ultrasound, 79-81, 81f
Binswanger's disease, magnetic resonance imaging in, 418
Biopsy
  CT in, 148-149
  by laparoscopy, 287, 288
  needle. See also Aspiration biopsy
    fine-needle aspiration in abdomen, 401-411. See also Aspiration biopsy
    ultrasonic guidance for, 88, 91-92, 92f
    of lung, 257
  pleura, 257-258
Biplane filming, in angiography, 154
Bladder
  cancer, CT in, 144
  cystometrography, 252, 253f, 254
  cystoscopy, 243-244
  in excretory urography, 245, 248f
  neurogenic, cystometrography for, 252, 254
  outlet obstruction, uroflow studies, 252, 253f
  retrograde cystography, 248-249
  traumatic perforation, 248-249
Bleomycin, radionuclide labeling in imaging soft tissue neoplasms, 124
Blood flow, Doppler ultrasound for, 63
Blood gases. See Arterial blood gases

Blood pressure
  direct measurement, 380-382
    diagnostic efficacy, 382
    indications, 381
    interpretation, 381-382
    technique, 381
    transducers used in, 380-381
  indirect measurement, 379-380
    diagnostic efficacy, 380
    indications, 379
    interpretation, 380
    patient acceptance, 380
    technique, 379-380
  pulse pressure, 381-382
  stroke volume, heart rate, and total peripheral resistance related to, 381-382
Blow-out fracture, 16f, 17f
Bone
  arteriography, 176-177
  CT of, 148
  Paget's disease, bone scan in, 113, 114f
  radionuclide imaging, 111-113
    in benign bone neoplasms, 113, 114f
    in fractures, 113, 115f
    in joint disease, 113, 116f
    in metastatic disease, 111-113, 113f
    normal findings, 112, 112f
    in osteomyelitis, 113, 115f
    physiologic basis, 111
    procedure, 112
  tumors
    angiography in, 176-177
    bone scan in, 113, 114f
Bone marrow, radionuclide imaging, 119-120
  indications, 119
  interpretation, 119-120
  procedure, 119
Brachial artery
  approach in cardiac catheterization, 329-330
    complications, 341
  in blood pressure measurement, 379
  pressure waveforms in, 333
Brachiocephalic arteritis, 159-160
Brain
  abscess
    brain scan in, 100
    comparison of CT with brain scan in, 101
    CT in, 133-134
  arteriovenous malformations in, 159, 160f
  CT of, 133, 133f
  magnetic resonance imaging in, 416
  atrophy, CT in, 134, 134f
  cerebral angiography, 158-162. See also Cerebral angiography
  CT of, 132-134, 132-134f
    anatomic structures, 128, 129f
  cysts, brain scan in, 100
  difficulties in ultrasonography, 64
  hemorrhage in, magnetic resonance imaging in, 415-416, 418f
  magnetic resonance imaging of, 415-418
    cerebral edema, 418, 421f
    myelination in infant, 418, 421f
    normal anatomy, 415, 416f, 425
    tumors, 418, 419-421f, 425, 425f
    vascular disease, 415-416, 417f
    white-matter disease, 416, 418, 419f
  metastases to, CT of, 132-133, 132f
  radionuclide imaging, 98-102
    in abscesses and cysts, 100
    in cerebrovascular accident, 99-100, 100f
    cisternography, 101-102, 101f, 102f
    CT compared with, 100-101
    indications, 98
    normal findings, 99, 99f
    procedure, 99
    in subdural hematoma 100, 100f
    in tumors, 99, 99f
  tumors. See Brain tumors
Brain stem
  infarction, magnetic resonance imaging in, 415, 417f
  tumors, magnetic resonance imaging in, 420f
Brain tumors
  angiography in, 160, 161f, 162, 162f
  brain scan in, 99, 99f
  comparison of CT with brain scan in, 100-101
  CT in, 131-133, 132f
Breast
  cancer, bone scan in, 112, 113f
  fine-needle aspiration cytology, accuracy, 408
  mammography, 6
  mass
    solid versus cystic, 74
    ultrasound evaluation, 72-73f, 74
  ultrasonography, 69, 72-73f, 74
    mammography compared with, 69, 74
    after mass discovered by xeromammography, 73f, 74
  xeroradiography, 6
Bremstrahlung, 3, 3f
Bronchial arteriography, 166, 166f
  embolization therapy in, 166, 166f
Bronchogenic cyst, 136, 136f
Bronchography, 257
Bronchoscopy, 256-257
  indications, 256
  technique, 256-257

C wave, 331, 331f
Calcifications, intracranial, on CT, 128
Calcium
  gastrin stimulation by, 371, 375
  parathyroid gland and, 67-68
Calculi
  kidney. See Kidney, calculi
  ureteral, ureteropyeloscopy in removal, 244
Camera, scintillation, 97-98
Cancer
  abdominal fine-needle aspiration cytology for, 401-411
    accuracy, 401, 403-405t, 408, 411
    complications, 402, 406-407, 406t
    contraindications, 406-407
    sites successfully studied, 401, 402t
    tumor dissemination in, 407
  radiation producing, 8
Carbon monoxide single-breath test, 306
Cardiac care unit, Swan-Ganz catheter in, 344-345, 345-347f
Cardiac catheterization, 327-341
  angiocardiography, 334-335
  in anticoagulated patient, 329
  cardiac output measurements, 335-338, 338f
  choice of approach, 329-330
  complications, 340-341
  contraindications, 328-329
  in electrophysiologic studies, 340
  equipment in, 329
  hemodynamic measurements in, 330-334

normal and abnormal pressure waveforms, 330-334, 331-338f
    technique, 330
  historical background, 327
  in hypertension, 328
  indications, 327-328
    assessment of surgical results, 328
    cardiomyopathy, 328
    clear diagnosis in medical or surgical patient, 327
    follow-up of myocardial infarction, 328
    unexplained chest pain, 327-328
  intracardiac shunts assessed by, 338-339
  in myocardial infarction, 329
  preparation and premedication for, 340
  protocol for, 340
  in research, 328
  Swan-Ganz catheter in, 344, 345f
  valvular evaluation by, 340
  in vascular resistance calculation, 339-340
  in ventricular arrhythmias, 328
Cardiac output, measurement, 335-338, 338f
  angiographic method, 338
  dye-dilution method, 337-338, 338f
  Fick oxygen method, 335-337
  Swan-Ganz catheter in determination, 348, 349f
Cardiomyopathy
  congestive, electrocardiogram in, 320
  echocardiography in, 75
  hypertrophic obstructive
    electrocardiogram in, 320
    hemodynamic measurements in, 334
  radionuclide imaging in, 118
Carotid angiography, 155-158
  digital subtraction technique, 156, 156f
  indications, 156
  procedure, 155-156
  in stenosis, 156, 157f
  in ulcerated atherosclerotic plaque, 157, 157f
  in vascular malformations, 159, 160f
  in vascular tumors, 157-158
Carotid artery(ies)
  Doppler ultrasound evaluation of, 383-384, 384f, 386, 386t
  frequency spectral analysis of, 387-388
  occlusive disease, 159
  oculoplethysmography study of, 388-389
  stenosis, 156, 157f
    oculoplethysmography in, 388-389
    oculopneumoplethysmography in, 389, 390
  tumors, 157-158
  ulcerated atherosclerotic plaque, 157, 157f
  ultrasonography, 69, 70-71f
Carotid cavernous aneurysm, 159
Catheter(s)
  in angiography, 154-155
  complications in angiography, 153
  Swan-Ganz, 343-344, 344f. See also Swan-Ganz catheter
Catheterization
  cardiac, 327-341. See also Cardiac catheterization
  percutaneous, in angiography, 154
  superselective, 154
Cavernous carotid aneurysm, 159
Cerebral angiography, 158-162
  in aneurysms, 158-159, 158f, 159f
  in brain tumors, 160, 161f, 162, 162f
  indications, 158
  in occlusive disease, 159
  procedure, 158
  in vascular malformations, 158, 159

  in vasculitis, 159-160
Cerebral artery
  occlusive disease, 159
  vasculitis, 159-160
Cerebral edema, in head injury, 130
Cerebral infarction
  CT in, 133
  magnetic resonance imaging in, 415
Cerebrospinal fluid
  CT evaluation of spaces, 134, 134f
  leaks, radionuclide cisternography in, 102
  radionuclide cisternography study of dynamics, 101-102, 101f, 102f
Cerebrovascular accident
  brain scan in, 99-100, 100f
  comparison of CT with brain scan in, 101
Cervical spine. See Spine, cervical
Chest
  angiography, 162-167
    aortography, 162-166
    bronchial arteriography, 166
    pulmonary, 166-167
  CT of, 134-138
    anatomic structures, 134, 135f, 136
    hilum, 137
    lung, 137-138, 138f
    mediastinum, 136-137, 136f
    pleura and chest wall, 138
  rationale and selection of diagnostic procedures in, 255-261
    bronchography, 257
    bronchoscopy, 256-257
    diffuse lung disease, 260
    focal lung lesions, 259-260
    laryngoscopy, 255-256
    mediastinal and hilar masses, 260-261
    mediastinoscopy, 258-259
    needle aspiration, 257
    pleural biopsy, 257-258
    pleural effusion, 260
    thoracentesis, 258
    thoracoscopy, 259
  stab wounds, abdominal injury in, 297
  ultrasound, 69, 72-73f, 74-75, 76-78f, 79. See also Echocardiography
Chest pain
  cardiac catheterization in evaluation, 327-328
  esophageal motility studies in, 366
  esophageal pH monitoring in evaluation of, 356-357, 358f
Chest wall, CT of, 138, 138f
Chest x-ray, 43-53
  in acute abdominal series, 55
  in aorta dissecting hematoma, 165
  in aorta rupture, 164
  apical view, 46f, 47
  fluoroscopically positioned spot films, 47, 48-49f
  indications for, 43, 45
  interpretation errors, 51, 51-53f
  lateral decubitus view, 45, 46f, 47, 47f, 48f
  lateral view, 45, 46f, 47f
  mobile units for, 50-51, 50f
  oblique view, 46f, 47
  optimal position on, 43, 44f
  posteroanterior, 43, 44f
  in preoperative period, 45
  projections
    accessory, 45, 47, 49, 46-49f
    routine, 43, 44f
  in pulmonary embolism, 166

Chest x-ray *(Continued)*
  radiation dose in, 10t
  in screening, 45
  tomography, 49-50, 49f
Children
  colonoscopy in, 277
  demyelination in, magnetic resonance imaging for, 418, 421f
  fractures in, comparative x-rays, 31f, 40
  Swan-Ganz catheter in, 345
Cholangiocarcinoma, ERCP in, 207f, 210
Cholangiography
  intravenous, 198
  percutaneous transhepatic, 199-202
    bile leakage in, 200
    complications, 200-201
    contraindications, 200
    ERCP compared with in biliary obstruction, 205, 209
    hemorrhage after, 200
    indications, 200
    interpretation, 201-202
    in pancreatic cancer, 201, 202-203f
    technique, 199-200
    time required for procedure, 202
Cholangiopancreatography, endoscopic retrograde, 202-210
  of common bile duct, 204, 205-208f
  complications, 209
  contraindications, 209
  indications, 203-205, 209, 268
  interpretation, 209-210
  pancreatitis after, 209
  percutaneous transhepatic cholangiography compared with, 205, 209
  in postcholecystectomy syndrome, 204, 205-206f
  sepsis after, 209
  technique, 202-203
Cholangitis, sclerosing, ERCP in, 207f, 210
Cholecystectomy, postcholecystectomy syndrome, 204, 205-206f
Cholecystitis
  laparoscopic examination, 287
  radionuclide imaging in, 108-109, 109f
  ultrasound versus radionuclide imaging in, 79
Cholecystography, oral, 183-198
  cholecystokinin administration in, 191, 197
  factors determining opacification, 183
  filling defects in gallbladder on, 194f, 197f, 198
  gallstones on, 186-189f, 197-198
  interpretation, 191, 197-198
  nonbiliary causes of nonvisualization, 185, 185f
  normal studies, 184-186f
  technique, 183, 185, 187-189f, 191
Cholecystokinin, in oral cholecystography, 191, 197
Cholelithiasis. *See* Gallstones
Cholesterolosis, of gallbladder, 194f, 197
Chromosomal abnormalities, radiation causing, 8
Circadian rhythm, electrocardiogram effects, 312
Circle of Willis, aneurysms at, 158
Cirrhosis of liver. *See* Liver, cirrhosis
Cisternography, radionuclide, 101-102, 101f, 102f
  in CSF leaks, 102
  in hydrocephalus, 101-102, 102f
  in ventriculoperitoneal shunt patency evaluation, 102, 102f
Coagulation disorder, and percutaneous transhepatic cholangiography, 200
Colitis
  colonoscopy in, 276-277
  Crohn's, radiographic appearance, 235, 237f
  ischemic
    colonoscopy in, 277
    sigmoidoscopy in, 279
  radiation-induced, colonoscopy in, 277
  ulcerative, radiographic appearance, 235, 236f
Colon
  angiodysplasia, 172, 174f
    colonoscopy in, 277
  cancer
    barium enema in, 235-236
      diagnostic efficacy, 236, 237
    colonoscopy in, 275-276
      in surveillance, 278
    screening with sigmoidoscopy, 280
  diverticulitis, 235, 236f
  filling defects, 235-236, 237f
  idiopathic ileus or pseudo-obstruction, colonoscopic decompression in, 278
  inflammatory diseases, 235
  obstruction, after barium enema, 214
  polyps, 235-236, 237f
    colonoscopy in
      in diagnosis, 275-276
      in removal of polyps, 277-278
    diagnostic efficacy of barium enema, 236-237
  radiographic contrast studies, 230-231, 234-237. *See also* Barium enema
  stricture, colonoscopy in, 277
  vascular anomalies, colonoscopy in, 277
Colonoscopy, 275-278
  in colon cancer, 275-276
    in surveillance, 278
  contraindications, 278
  in decompression of colon in Ogilvie's syndrome, 278
  in diverticular disease, 277
  indications for, 275-278
    diagnostic, 275-277, 276t
    in surveillance, 276t, 278
    therapeutic, 276t, 277-278
  in inflammatory bowel disease, 276-277
  intraoperative, 277
  in ischemic colitis, 277
  pediatric, 277
  polypectomy by, 277-278
  preparation of patient for, 275
  reduction of cecal volvulus by, 278
  removal of foreign body by, 278
  in stricture, 277
    periodic studies to exclude cancer, 278
  technique, 275
  time-consuming factors, 278
  in unexplained rectal bleeding, 277
  in vascular anomalies, 277
Common bile duct. *See under* Biliary tract
Compton scattering, 4, 4f
Computed tomography. *See* Tomography, computed
Computers
  in acid-base analysis, 305-306
  in electrocardiogram interpretation, 312
  in esophageal pH monitoring, 361-362f, 362-363
  in heart radionuclide imaging, 115, 117f, 118
Congo red test, of vagotomy efficacy, 373
Conn's syndrome, CT in, 143
Consent, for laparoscopy, 284
Contrast agents
  in angiocardiography, 335
    complications, 341
  barium sulfate, 213-214
    complications, 153-154, 154t
  in CT
    in abdominal trauma, 145-146

in head scan, 128
in echocardiography, 75, 79
in gastrointestinal studies, 213-214
water-soluble, 214
Coronary angiography. *See also* Cardiac catheterization
contraindications, 328-329
indications, 327-328
Coronary artery bypass surgery, cardiac catheterization after, 328
Coronary artery disease
electrocardiogram in, 322
radionuclide heart imaging in, 114-116, 117f, 118
Coronary artery spasm, electrocardiogram in, 322
Cost
of spirometry, 303, 304t
of Swan-Ganz catheter, 351
Craniotomy, ultrasound in, 65
Crohn's colitis
colonoscopy in, 276-277
radiographic appearance, 235, 237f
CT number, 127, 127t
CT scan. *See* Tomography, computed
Cystic duct
obstruction, oral cholecystogram in, 185, 190-192f
radionuclide imaging of, 108-109, 109f
Cystography, retrograde, 248-249
complications, 249
indications, 248
technique, 248-249
Cystometrography, 252, 253f, 254
complications, 252, 254
interpretation, 254
technique, 252
Cystoscopy, 243-244
complications, 243-244
indications, 243
technique, 243
Cystourethrography, voiding, 251-252
complications, 251-252
indications, 251
technique, 251

Deep vein thrombosis. *See* Thrombosis, deep vein
Dementia, CT in, 134
2-Deoxyglucose, gastric secretion elicited by, 371
for vagotomy efficacy, 374-375
Diet, in esophageal pH monitoring, 353, 354t
Diffusion capacity, 306
Digital subtraction angiography, 155. *See also under* Angiography, digital subtraction
Digitalis toxicity, cardiac catheterization in, 328-329
Diphosphonate, technetium-99m labeling in imaging soft tissue neoplasms, 124
Disc herniation, CT evaluation, 146-147, 147f
Diverticular disease
barium enema in, 235, 236f
colonoscopy in, 277
sigmoidoscopy in, 279
Doppler effect, 382
Doppler shift, 382
Doppler ultrasound, 63, 382-388
angiography generated by, 383, 384, 384f
diagnostic efficacy of, 388
ankle-brachial index, 385, 386-387, 387f
of arteries, 383
of carotid artery, 383-384, 384f
continuous-wave, 382, 384
cuff sizes used in, 383t
diagnostic efficacy, 386-388

frequency spectral analysis, 386, 387-388
indications for, 382-383
instruments in, 382
interpretation, 384-386
pressure index, 382, 385
pulsed-wave, 382, 384
resistance index, 385-386
techniques and technical pitfalls, 383-384
toe pressures in, 387
of veins, 383
Duodenum
cancer, radiographic appearance, 226
endoscopy
complications, 272
indications, 268
technique, 271
perforation, after endoscopy, 272
radiography of, 219, 222-227
basics of interpretation, 224, 226
diagnostic efficacy, 226-227
indications, 219
patient preparation for, 219
single- versus double-contrast examination, 219, 222-223f, 224, 224f, 226-227
technical problems, 224
ulcer
acid-secretion testing in, 372-373, 372t
endoscopy in, 268
radiographic appearance, 224, 227f
diagnostic efficacy, 227, 228f
Dye-dilution method for cardiac output, 337-338, 338f
Dysphagia, endoscopy in, 267

Echinococcus cyst, fine-needle aspiration of, 406
Echocardiography, 74-75, 76-78f, 79
conditions interfering with, 74
contractility of heart walls evaluated by, 75
contrast agents used with, 75, 79
M-mode method, 63
real-time compared with, 74
in pericardial effusion, 75
technique and views used in, 74-75
in tumors of heart, 75
valves demonstrated by, 75
in ventricular hypertrophy, 75
Echoencephalogram, 65, 66f
Elbow fractures, radiography in, 32f, 41
Electrocardiogram, 311-324
age influence on, 311
in chronic obstructive pulmonary disease, 317
computers in interpretation, 312
in coronary spasm, 322
diurnal variations, 312-313
intracavitary via Swan-Ganz catheter, 348
left atrial abnormality, 313, 314f, 315
left ventricular hypertrophy, 315, 315f
in mitral regurgitation, 318, 320
in mitral valve prolapse, 320
in myocardial infarction, 320, 321f, 322
normal study, 311f
P wave, 313, 313f
in pericardial effusion, 320
in pericarditis, 320, 321f
physiologic variables, 312
in pre-excitation syndrome, 322, 323f, 324
in pulmonary embolism, 317, 318f
race and, 312
right atrial abnormality, 313, 314f
right ventricular hypertrophy, 315-317, 316f

Electrocardiogram *(Continued)*
  sex influence on, 311-312
  technical variations in, 312
  variables in interpretation, 311-313
  in ventricular aneurysm, 322
  weight and height influence on, 312
Electrophysiologic studies, 340
Embolization therapy, in bronchial arteriography, 166, 166f
Endoscopes
  esophagogastroduodenoscope, 264
  fiberoptic, 263-265
  historical background, 263
  new developments, 266
  pediatric, 265
  rigid esophagoscope, 264
  side-viewing versus end-viewing, 265-266
  television camera in, 263-264
Endoscopic retrograde cholangiopancreatography, 202-210. *See also under* Cholangiopancreatography, endoscopic retrograde
Endoscopy
  of biliary tract, 268
  bronchoscopy, 256-257
  colonoscopy, 275-278. *See also* Colonoscopy
  of duodenum, 268
  endoscopic retrograde cholangiopancreatography, 202-210
  of esophagus, 267
  of gastrointestinal tract
    in chemical trauma, 270
    esophagus, 267
    for foreign body, 270
    laboratory for, 266
    lower, 275-280
      colonoscopy, 275-278. *See also* Colonoscopy
      flexible fiberoptic sigmoidoscopy, 278-280
    after myocardial infarction, 269-270
    in perforation, 270
    perforation after, 271-272
    upper, 263-272
      in bleeding, 268-269
      complications, 271-272
      contraindications, 269-270
      examination technique, 271
      failure to find existing lesion, 271, 272
      historical aspects, 263-264
      indications, 266-269
      instruments in, 264-266
      lesions commonly diagnosed, 272
      preparation of patient for, 270-271
  laryngoscopy, 255-256
  of pancreas, 268. *See also* Cholangiopancreatography, endoscopic retrograde
  sigmoidoscopy, 278-280
  specialization in, 266
  of stomach, 267-268
  of urinary tract
    cystoscopy, 243-244
    ureteropyeloscopy, 244
Enteroclysis, 227, 230f
  diagnostic efficacy, 230
  technical problems, 229
Epididymitis, radionuclide imaging in, 122, 122f
Epidural hematoma, 130, 131f
Equipment
  in angiocardiography, 335
  in cardiac catheterization, 329
  in Doppler ultrasound, 382
  in gastrointestinal radiography, 213
  in gastrointestinal upper endoscopy, 264-266
  in laparoscopy, 284, 285f, 289f
  in magnetic resonance imaging, 413-414, 414f, 423-424
ERCP. *See* Cholangiopancreatography, endoscopic retrograde
Esophageal sphincter, lower. *See* Lower esophageal sphincter
Esophagitis
  gastroesophageal reflux related to, 356
  infectious, motility studies in, 367
  radiographic detection, 219
  reflux, esophageal motility studies in, 366
Esophagogastroduodenoscope, 264
Esophagoscope, rigid, 264
Esophagoscopy
  esophageal pH monitoring compared with, 358-359
  technique, 271
Esophagus
  body pressures
    in achalasia, 366
    in gastroesophageal reflux, 366
  cancer
    motility studies in, 367
    radiographic detection, 219
  diffuse spasm, motility studies in, 367
  diverticula
    endoscopy in, 267
    motility studies in, 367
  endoscopy
    after chemical injury, 270
    indications, 267
    instruments, 264-266
    perforation complicating, 272
    technique, 271
  lesions protruding into lumen, 219, 221f
  motility studies, 365-368
    in achalasia, 366-367
    in diffuse esophageal spasm, 367
    in esophageal cancer, 367
    in esophageal diverticula, 367
    in esophagitis, 366
    indications for, 365-366
    in infectious esophagitis, 367
    interpretation, 366-367
    manometric measurements of pressures within esophagus, 365
    pullback measurements of lower esophageal sphincter, 365
    in scleroderma, 367
    tests included in, 365
  narrowing, 219, 220f
  perforation, radiographic evaluation, 215
  pH monitoring, 353-363
    acid reflux in, 353, 355f
    alkaline reflux in, 353
    in chest pain, 357, 358f
    comparison with other tests, 357-359, 358f, 359f
    computers in, 361-362f, 362-363
    diet during, 353, 354t
    esophagoscopy compared with, 358-359
    extensive data analysis required in, 362
    in gastroesophageal reflux, 367-368
    indications for, 357
    instructions to patient in, 353, 354t
    limitations, 359-362
    mandatory co-operation required in, 361-362
    normal values, 353, 355, 355t
    on outpatient, 361f, 362

relation of symptoms to reflux determined by, 356-357, 357f
solid state technology applied to, 362-363
specificity and sensitivity of, 358, 358f
technique, 353-355, 354t, 355f
radiographic examination, 215-219
diagnostic efficacy, 219
interpretation, 219
mucosal relief films, 215, 218f, 219
patient preparation for, 215
single- versus double-contrast examination, 215, 216f
technical problems with, 215, 219
stricture, gastroesophageal reflux in, 360-361
varices. See Gastroesophageal varices
vascular ring compressing, 162-163
Zenker's diverticulum, endoscopy danger in, 267
Exercise
hemodynamic measurements after, 334
myocardial thallium imaging after, 116, 118, 118f
Expiratory reserve volume, 299, 300f
Extremities
Doppler ultrasound of arteries of, 382-388
fluoroscopy, 39
plethysmography of, 388-396
air-filled, 389-390
fluid-filled, 388-389
impedance, 394-396
photo, 392-394
strain-gauge, 390-392
radiography, 28f-40f, 39-41
high-resolution magnification, 28f, 39-40
indications and limitations, 40-41
in nontraumatic conditions, 41
techniques, 39-40
in trauma, 40-41
xeroradiography, 28f, 40
tomography, 39
trauma
angiography in, 175, 176f
radiography in, 40-41
venography, 177

Facial bones, radiography
in inflammatory and neoplastic disease, 33
in trauma, 16-17f, 27
views, 13, 14f
Fallopian tubes, laparoscopic examination, 287
Fat, ultrasound image degraded by, 64-65
Femoral artery
approach in cardiac catheterization, 329, 330
complications, 341
arteriography in peripheral vascular disease, 176, 178f
pressure waveforms in, 333
Femoral-brachial pressure index, 382
interpretation in arterial disease, 385
Fetus, ultrasound evaluation, 93f, 94
Fever, cardiac catheterization in, 328
Fick oxygen method, 335-337
Fluorine, as nucleus in magnetic resonance imaging, 425
Fluoroscopy
of bones and joints, 39
in fine-needle abdominal aspiration, 408f, 409t
image reception in, 6
Foot injury, radiography in, 41
Forced expiratory spirogram, 301-302, 302f
Forearm fractures, radiography in, 30f, 31f, 40
Foreign body, in gastrointestinal tract
colonoscopy removal, 278

endoscopy, 270
Fractures
bone scan in, 113, 115f
Jefferson burst, 22f
radiography in, 40-41
comparative views in children, 31f, 40
two-views, 29f
of ring and ring-like structures, 29f, 40
thoracic spinal compression, 22f, 23f
vascular injury with, 175, 177f
Functional residual capacity, 299, 301, 304t

Gallbladder. See also Biliary tract
adenomyomatosis, 191, 193f
Aschoff-Rokitansky sinuses, 195f, 197
carcinoma, oral cholecystography in, 197f, 198
cholesterolosis, 194f, 197
comparison of imaging methods, 183
CT of, 140
developmental variations in position, 191, 196f, 197
hyperplastic cholecystoses, 193-195f, 197
laparoscopic examination, 287
oral cholecystography for, 183-198
in percutaneous transhepatic cholangiography, 201
phrygian cap, 195f
postcholecystectomy syndrome, 204, 205-206f
radionuclide imaging, 108f, 108-109, 183
ultrasound, 61, 62f, 79, 80f
Gallium scanning
in abscess localization, 120, 120f, 121f
of kidney, 110-111, 111f
of lung, 106-107, 106f
in lymphoma 123f, 124
in tumors, 106-107
Gallstones
CT in, 140
Mercedes Benz sign, 196f, 198
on oral cholecystography, 186-189f, 197-198
in percutaneous transhepatic cholangiography, 201, 201f, 202f
ultrasound for, 62f, 79, 80f
Gamma rays, 7-8, 97. See also Radiation; Radionuclide imaging
Gastric juice
basal acid output, 369
composition, 369
hypoglycemic agents stimulating, 371
insulin stimulating, 371
maximal acid output, 369
peak acid output, 369
in peptic ulcer disease, 372-373, 372f
stimulants of secretion, 370, 370t
in stomach cancer, 373, 373f
in stomach ulcer, 373
types of secretory tests, 369-370. See also Stomach, acid-secretory testing
Gastrin
in acid-secretory testing, 370-371, 370t
conditions associated with increased levels, 375
stimulation tests, 371-372
in Zollinger-Ellison syndrome, 371-372, 375
Gastrocamera, 263-264
Gastroesophageal reflux
alkaline, 360
esophageal motility studies in, 366
esophageal pH monitoring in, 353-363, 367-368. See also Esophagus, pH monitoring
in esophageal stricture, 360-361
esophagitis related to, 356

Gastroesophageal reflux *(Continued)*
  lower esophageal sphincter pressure in, 366
  patterns of abnormality, 356, 356f
  physiologic versus pathologic, 355, 355f
  radionuclide imaging in, 120-121, 121f
  symptoms related to, 356-357, 357f
  upright versus supine, 356
Gastroesophageal varices
  interventional angiography in, 170
  radiography of, 215, 216f
Gastrointestinal bleeding
  angiography in, 170
  lower, colonoscopy in control, 278
  radionuclide imaging in, 121, 121f
  upper, endoscopy in, 268-269
Gastrointestinal tract
  acid-secretory testing, 369-375. *See also under*
    Stomach
  angiography of, 170, 172, 172-174f
  bleeding from. *See* Gastrointestinal bleeding
  caliber changes, 215
  CT of, 141-142
  endoscopy
    lower tract, 275-280
    upper tract, 263-272
  esophageal motility studies, 365-368
  esophageal pH monitoring, 353-363
  filling defects, 215
  gastroduodenal function studies, 369-375
  luminal contrast studies, 213-237. *See also under*
    specific organ
    contrast agents in, 213-214
    equipment, cost and radiation risk, 213
    interpretative principles, 214-215
  obstruction, radiographic evaluation, 229, 231f
  pathologic alterations affecting, 214-215
  perforation
    endoscopy causing, 271-272
    endoscopy danger in, 270
    in trauma, 290
  projecting lesions, 215
  radionuclide imaging, 120-122
    in bleeding, 121, 121f, 170
    in Meckel's diverticulum, 122, 122f
Gastroscopy
  complications, 272
  failure to find existing lesion, 272
  fiberoptic, 263
  historical development, 263
  indications, 267-268
  technique, 271
Genetic disorders, radiation causing, 8
Glioblastoma
  angiography in, 160, 162f
  CT in, 132, 132f
Glomus jugulare tumor, 157-158
Glucose, gastric secretion related to, 371
Gray, 7
Gray-scale imaging, 60f, 61
Gunshot wounds
  abdominal, 296-297
  laparoscopy in, 290
  peritoneal lavage in, 296-297

Hand
  magnification radiography, 28f
  trauma, radiography in, 33f, 34f, 41
  xeroradiography, 28f
Head
  angiography of, 155-162
    cerebral, 158-162
    extracranial, 155-158
    indications, 156
    procedure, 155-156
  CT of, 128-134
    anatomic structures, 128, 129f
    in arteriovenous malformations, 133, 133f
    in brain abscess, 133-134
    in brain tumor, 131-133, 132f
    in cerebral infarction, 133
    in hydrocephalus, 134, 134f
    in subarachnoid hemorrhage, 133
    in trauma, 128, 130-131, 130f, 131f
  radiography, 13-19, 27, 33
    indications and limitations, 15, 15-18f, 19, 27, 33
    technique, 13-15
  trauma. *See* Head trauma
  ultrasonography, 65, 66f
    in craniotomy surgery, 65
    in infants, 65, 66f
Head trauma
  CT in, 128, 130-131, 130f, 131f
    brain parenchymal injury, 130-131, 130f
    epidural hematoma, 130, 131f
    subdural hematoma, 130, 130f, 131f
  facial injury, 16-17f, 27
  paracentesis and abdominal lavage in, 293
  skull x-ray in, 15, 15f, 19, 27
Heart
  echocardiography, 74-75, 76-78f, 79. *See also*
    Echocardiography
  function studies, 311-351
    cardiac catheterization, 327-341. *See also* Cardiac
      catheterization
    electrocardiography, 311-324. *See also*
      Electrocardiogram
    hemodynamic monitoring, 343-351
    hemodynamic measurements in cardiac
      catheterization, 330-334
  magnetic resonance imaging of, 418, 421-422
    blood-myocardium contrast, 418, 421, 422f
    experimental infarction, 421, 422f
    gated imaging, 421, 423f
  radionuclide imaging, 113-118
    in coronary artery disease, 114-116, 117f, 118
    gated scans, 115, 117f
    hot spot scanning, 114-115
      interpretation, 115, 117f
    perfusion scan, 115
      in exercise stress test, 116, 118, 118f
      interpretation, 115-116, 117f
      tomographic cuts for interpretation, 115, 117f
    procedure, 114-115
    wall motion studies
      interpretation, 117f, 118
      procedure, 115
  tumors, echocardiography for, 75
  ultrasound. *See* Echocardiography
  ventricular hypertrophy demonstrated by
    echocardiography, 75
  wall motion evaluation by echocardiography, 75
Heart failure, cardiac catheterization in, 328
Heart valves, echocardiography for, 75, 76f, 77f
Helium, closed-circuit dilution method for lung volumes,
  299
Hemangioma
  CT of, 148
  liver, 138-139
Hemodynamic monitoring, 343-351. *See also* Swan-
  Ganz catheter

flow-directed catheters in, 343-344, 344f. *See also* Swan-Ganz catheter
  measurement in cardiac catheterization, 330-334
    normal and abnormal pressure waveforms, 330-334, 331-338f
    technique, 330
Hemoperitoneum, 290
Hepatic artery
  aneurysm, 169
  angiography, 167, 169-170
Hepatic veins, studies in portal hypertension, 169
Hepatoma, angiography in, 169, 169f
Hepatomegaly, liver scan in, 107
Hilum, CT of, 137
Hip
  aseptic necrosis, bone scan in, 113, 116f
  trauma, radiography in, 34f, 41
Histamine, in acid-secretory testing, 370, 370f
Hoarseness, laryngoscopy for, 256
Hodgkin's disease, CT versus lymphangiography in, 144
Hollander test, of vagotomy efficacy, 374-375
Hollinger endoscope, 264
Hounsfield units, in CT of various body structures, 127, 127t
Hydrocephalus
  CT in, 134, 134f
  magnetic resonance imaging in, 421f
  radionuclide cisternography in, 101-102, 102f
Hypertension
  cardiac catheterization in, 328
  renovascular, 172, 175f
Hypoglycemia, gastric secretion elicited by, 371
Hypoglycemic agents, gastric secretion elicited by, 371
Hypokalemia, cardiac catheterization in, 328-329

Idiopathic hypertrophic subaortic stenosis, echocardiography in, 75
Ileum, barium enema evaluation, 227, 229
Iliac artery stenosis, direct blood pressure recording in evaluation of, 381
Imaging
  with fine-needle aspiration of abdomen, 403-405t, 407-408, 408f, 409t
  radiologic physics, technique and radiobiology, 3-10
Impedance plethysmography, 394-396
Indocyanine green
  in cardiac output measurement, 337-338, 338f
  in intracardiac shunt assessment, 339
Infants, echoencephalogram in, 65, 66f
Inferior vena cava, venography, 177-178
Inflammatory bowel disease
  colonoscopy in, 276-277
  in evaluation for cancer, 278
  sigmoidoscopy in, 279
Innominate artery aneurysm, 165
Inspiratory reserve volume, 299, 300f
Insulin, gastric secretion elicited by, 371
  for vagotomy efficacy, 374-375
Insulinoma, angiography in, 170, 171f
Intensifying screens, 6
Intervertebral discs, CT evaluation, 146-147, 147f
Intestinal obstruction, radiographic contrast studies, 229, 231f
Intracranial hemorrhage
  epidural, 130, 131f
  intracerebral, 130
  subdural, 130, 130f, 131f
Inversion recovery, 415, 415t, 416f

Iodinated contrast agents
  complications, 214
  in excretory urography, 245
  in gastrointestinal studies, 214

Jackson endoscope, 264
Jaundice
  obstructive
    CT role in, 140
    percutaneous transhepatic cholangiography in diagnostic workup, 200
    ultrasound evaluation of common bile duct, 79-81, 81f
Jefferson burst fracture, 22f
Joint effusion, radiography in, 40f, 41

Kidney
  angiography, 172-174
  calculi
    abdominal x-ray in, 55, 56f, 57
    ultrasound in, 85, 87f
  cancer, CT of, 142, 142f
  CT of, 142, 142f
  cysts
    CT of, 142, 142f
    puncture, 85
  excretory urography, 245, 246f
  failure, cardiac catheterization in, 329
  fine-needle aspiration cytology, 402
  magnetic resonance imaging of, 423
  mass, ultrasound for, 85, 86f
  obstruction. *See* Urinary obstruction
  radionuclide imaging, 109-111
    in glomerulonephritis, 110-111, 111f
    in kidney transplantation, 110, 111f
    physiology underlying, 109
    procedure, 109-110
    renal blood flow interpretation, 109-110, 110f
  retrograde pyelography in, 247-248
  transplantation, radionuclide imaging in, 110, 111f
  trauma
    arteriography in, 174
    CT in, 146, 173-174
    ultrasound, 84-85, 86-87f
    in newborn, 85, 87f
Klatsken tumor, ERCP in, 207f
Knee trauma, radiography in, 35-37f, 41
KUB, 55, 57

Laparoscopy (diagnostic), 283-291
  in abdominal trauma, 289-291
    complications, 291
    hemoperitoneum, 290
    results, 291
  anesthesia in, 285-286
  in ascites, 287-288
  complications, 288, 288t
  conditions requiring special precautions, 284
  contraindications, 284
  fallopian tube examination, 287
  gallbladder examination, 287
  indications, 283-284
  information for patients, 284
  insertion of examining trocar, 286
  insertion of second trocar, 286
  instrumentation in, 284, 285f, 289f
  liver examination, 286-287
    biopsy, 287, 288
    comparison with other methods, 288

Laparoscopy (diagnostic) *(Continued)*
 minilaparoscopy, in abdominal trauma, 289-291
 nonoperative alternatives, 283
 pneumoperitoneum in, 286
 preparation of instruments, 286
 preparation of patients, 284-285
 puncture site, 286
 results, 289, 289t
 single-puncture versus dual-puncture approach, 284, 285f
 spleen examination, 287
 technique, 286-287
 termination of procedure, 287
Laparotomy, decision-making in abdominal trauma
 laparoscopy in, 283-291
 peritoneal lavage in, 293-297
Laryngoscopy, 255-256
 direct versus indirect, 255-256
 indications, 255, 256
 technique, 255-256
Lavage, abdominal. *See* Peritoneal lavage
Left atrium
 left atrial abnormality
  in aortic valve disease, 318
  electrocardiogram in, 313, 314f, 315
  in mitral valve disease, 317-318
 pressure waveforms, 331, 331f
Left ventricle
 pressure waveforms, 333, 334f
  in mitral regurgitation, 334, 338f
  in mitral stenosis, 333, 337f
 radionuclide imaging for, 115, 117f, 118
 wall motion studies, radionuclide imaging in, 114
Left ventricular failure, cardiac catheterization in, 328
Left ventricular hypertrophy
 in aortic valve disease, 318, 319f
 electrocardiogram in, 315, 315f
 in mitral regurgitation, 318, 320
Leukemia, radiation producing, 8
Leukocytes, radioactive labeling in abscess localization, 120
Leukodystrophy, magnetic resonance imaging in, 416, 418
Lipoma
 CT of, 148
 cystic lesions distinguished from, 136, 136f
Liposarcoma, CT of, 148
Liver
 abscess, radionuclide imaging of, 120, 121f
 angiography, 167, 169-170, 169f
 biopsy
  fine-needle aspiration cytology, 401, 403t, 408, 411
  by laparoscopy, 287, 288
 cirrhosis
  CT in, 140
  liver scan in, 107f, 108
  magnetic resonance imaging in, 423, 424f
 CT of, 138-140
  benign lesions, 138-139
  cirrhosis, 140
  fatty infiltration, 139-140, 139f
  malignant lesions, 139, 139f
  normal anatomy, 138, 139f
 cyst, CT of, 138
 fatty infiltration, CT in, 139-140, 139f
 hemangioma, 167, 169f
  CT of, 138-139
 hepatomegaly, liver scan in, 107
 laparoscopic examination, 286-287
  comparison with other methods, 288
 magnetic resonance imaging of, 422-423, 424f

metastases to
 angiography in, 167, 169
 CT in, 139, 139f
 liver scan in, 107f, 108
 magnetic resonance imaging of, 422, 424f
neoplasms
 angiography in, 167, 169
 CT in, 139
 fine-needle aspiration cytology in, 403t, 408, 411
 percutaneous transhepatic cholangiography, 199-202. *See also* Cholangiography, percutaneous transhepatic
 radionuclide imaging, 107-108
  comparison with other techniques, 108
  interpretation, 107-108, 107f
  procedure, 107
  uses, 107
 trauma, laparoscopy in, 290
 ultrasound, 81-82, 82f
  bile ducts 80, 81f
Lower esophageal sphincter
 in achalasia, 366
 in diffuse esophageal spasm, 367
 in gastroesophageal reflux, 366
 measurements in esophageal motility studies, 365
 pressure measurement, 358, 358f
 in scleroderma, 367
Lown-Ganong-Levine syndrome, electrocardiogram in, 323f, 324
Lung
 arteriovenous malformations in, 167
 biopsy
  choice of method in various disease states, 259-261
  needle aspiration, 257
  thoracoscopy in, 259
 bronchography, 257
 bronchoscopy, 256-257
 cancer
  bronchoscopy in, 256
  CT evaluation, 137-138
   in staging, 137, 138f
  gallium scan in, 106
  operability, 307-308
  rationale and selection of diagnostic procedures for, 259-260
  resectability, 307
 chronic obstructive disease
  electrocardiogram in, 317
  flow volume loops in, 303, 305f
  forced expiratory flow in, 301
  gastrointestinal endoscopy in, 270
  preoperative pulmonary preparation in, 308
 CT of, 137-138
  anatomic structures, 135f, 136
 diffuse disease, rationale and selection of diagnostic procedures, 260
 diffusion capacity, 306
 focal lesion, 259-260
 function tests, 299-308. *See also* Pulmonary function tests
 nodule
  CT evaluation, 137
  fluoroscopically positioned spot films in 47, 48f, 49f
  tomography of, 49, 50
 oxygen arteriovenous difference across, 336-337
 radionuclide imaging, 104-108
  gallium scanning, 106-107, 106f
  in preoperative evaluation of pneumonectomy patient, 307
  in pulmonary embolism, 166-167

ventilation-perfusion study, 104-106, 105f, 106f
resection, preoperative evaluation, 307-308
restrictive disease
   flow volume loops in, 303, 305f
   forced expiratory spirogram in, 301
right ventricular hypertrophy in disorders of, 317
small airway disease, tests for, 306-307
ventilation-perfusion scans, in preoperative evaluation
      of pneumonectomy patient, 307
volumes, 299, 300f, 301, 304t
x-rays, 43-53. *See also* Chest x-ray
Lymph nodes
   mediastinal, mediastinoscopy in evaluation, 258-259
   para-aortic
      comparison of lymphangiography with CT for, 144
      CT of, 143-144, 144f
      radionuclide imaging of, 123f, 124
Lymphadenopathy
   hilar, CT in, 137
   mediastinal, CT in, 136-137
   retroperitoneal
      CT, lymphangiography and ultrasound interactions
         in, 88
      ultrasound for, 88, 91f
Lymphangiography
   CT of para-aortic lymph nodes compared with, 144
   in retroperitoneal lymphadenopathy, 88
Lymphoma
   CT versus lymphangiography in, 144
   fine-needle aspiration cytology, 410f, 411

M mode ultrasound, 63
Macruz index, 313
Magnet, in magnetic resonance imaging, 423-424
Magnetic resonance imaging, 413-425
   of abdomen, 422-423, 424f
   in acoustic neuroma, 425, 425f
   of brain, 415-418
      cerebral edema, 418, 421f
      myelination in infant, 418, 421f
      normal anatomy, 415, 416f, 425
      tumors, 418, 419-421f, 425, 425f
      vascular disease, 415-416, 417f
      white-matter disease, 416, 418, 419f
   comparison with other techniques, 423-424
   future developments in, 424-425
   hazards in, 414-415
   of heart, 418, 421-422
   historical development, 413
   indications, 424
   instrumentation in, 413-414, 414f
   inversion recovery images, 415, 415t, 416f
   of kidney, 423
   of liver, 422-423, 424f
   magnets used in, 423-424
   normal anatomic features on, 415, 416f
   nuclei used in, 424-425
   of pancreas, 423
   relaxation times in, 414, 414f
   repeated free induction delay, 415, 415t
   of retroperitoneum, 423
   spin-echo images, 415, 415t, 416f
Mahaim fibers, 324
Mammography
   ultrasound compared with, 69, 74
   xeroradiography compared with, 6
Mandible, radiography, 15, 15f
Maximum voluntary ventilation, 302, 304t
Meckel's diverticulum, radionuclide imaging of, 122, 122f

Mediastinoscopy, 258-259
   complications, 258
   diagnostic efficacy, 259
   indications, 258-259
   technique, 258
Mediastinum
   CT of, 136-137
      lipomatous versus cystic lesions, 136f
      lymphadenopathy, 136-137
      masses, 136, 138f
      vascular anomalies and aneurysms, 136, 137f
   masses, rationale and selection of diagnostic methods
      for, 260-261
Meningioma
   angiography in, 160, 161f
   brain scan in, 99, 100
   CT of, 132, 132f
   magnetic resonance imaging in, 419f
Meningitis, brain scan in, 100
Mercedes Benz sign, 196f, 198
Mesenteric artery, superior, arteriography in
      gastrointestinal bleeding, 170
Metastases
   bone scan for, 112-113, 113f
   liver scan for, 107f, 108
Metrizamide-enhanced CT, for spinal cord, 146, 146f
Minilaparoscopy, in abdominal trauma, 289-291, 289f
Mitral regurgitation
   electrocardiogram in, 318, 320
   hemodynamic measurements in, 334, 338f
Mitral stenosis
   echocardiography in, 75
   hemodynamic measurements in, 333, 337f
   left atrial abnormality in, 317
   pulmonary vascular resistance calculation in, 339-340
Mitral valve
   cardiac catheterization evaluation of, 340
   echocardiographic evaluation, 75, 76f, 77f
Mitral valve prolapse
   echocardiography in, 75
   electrocardiogram in, 320
Mobile radiography. *See* Portable x-rays
Morris index, 313
Multiple sclerosis, magnetic resonance imaging in, 416, 419f
Muscle, phosphorus spectrum under magnetic field, 413f
Musculoskeletal system, CT of, 148
Myelography
   CT with, 146-147, 146f, 147f
   in disc herniation, 147, 147f
   in obstructing spine lesion, 147
Myocardial infarction
   acute, recent and old, 322
   cardiac catheterization in, 328, 329
   electrocardiogram in, 320, 321f, 322
   endoscopy after, 269-270
   location in heart wall, 322
   magnetic resonance imaging in, 421, 422f
   radionuclide heart imaging in, 114-116, 117f
   site of, 322
   Swan-Ganz catheter in, 345, 345f, 347f
Myocardial thallium imaging, 115
   in exercise stress test, 116, 118, 118f
   interpretation, 115-116, 117f
   tomographic cuts for interpretation, 115, 117f

Nasogastric intubation, in acid-secretory testing, 369-370
Nasopharynx, angiofibroma, 157-158

Neck
    spine. See Spine, cervical
    ultrasound, 65-69, 67-68f, 70f
        carotid arteries, 69, 70-71f
        parathyroid, 68-69, 68f
        thyroid, 66-67, 67f
Needle
    in aspiration biopsy, 148-149
    in percutaneous transhepatic cholangiography, 199-200
Needle aspiration biopsy
    in abdomen, 401-411. See also Aspiration biopsy
        ultrasound guidance in, 88, 91-92, 92f
    CT localization in, 148-149
    of lung, 257
        indications, 257
        technique, 257
    needles in, 148-149
Neoplasms. See Cancer; and under specific disorder
Nephrotomography, 245, 246f
Neurosonography, 65, 66f
Newborn, kidney ultrasound in, 85, 87f
Nitrogen-washout method, in lung volume determination, 299, 301
Nuclear magnetic resonance. See Magnetic resonance imaging

Obstetrics, ultrasound in, 93f, 94
Oculoplethysmography, 388-389
Oculopneumoplethysmography, 389-390
Ogilvie's syndrome, colonscopic decompression of colon in, 278
Operability, 307-308
Ophthalmic artery
    oculoplethysmography for, 388
    oculopneumoplethysmography for, 389-390
Oral cholecystography. See Cholecystography, oral
Orbit, blow-out fracture
    radiography, 16f
    tomography, 17f
Osteogenic sarcoma, bone scan in, 112
Osteoid osteoma, tomography in, 26f
Osteomyelitis, tomography in, 27f
Oxygen, arteriovenous difference across lung, 336-337
Oxygen consumption, Fick method of measurement, 335-337

P pulmonale, 313, 314f
P wave, 313, 313f, 314f
Pacemakers, Swan-Ganz catheter in placement, 348, 350f
Paget's disease of bone, bone scan in, 113, 114f
Pancreas
    cancer
        CT in, 140f, 141
        ERCP in, 208f
        fine-needle aspiration cytology in, 404t
        islet cell tumors compared with ductal carcinoma, 170
        in percutaneous transhepatic cholangiography, 201, 202-203f
        ultrasound in, 83
    CT of, 140-141
        in malignant lesions, 140f, 141
        normal anatomy, 140-141, 141f
    endoscopic retrograde cholangiopancreatography for, 202-210. See also Cholangiopancreatography, endoscopic retrograde
    fine-needle aspiration cytology, accuracy, 401, 404t
    islet cell tumors, angiography, 170, 171f
    magnetic resonance imaging of, 423
    polypeptide secretion tests after vagotomy, 375
    pseudocyst
        CT in, 141, 141f
        endoscopic retrograde pancreatography of, 205f
        percutaneous drainage, 149
        ultrasound for, 82, 83f
    ultrasound, 82-83, 83f
Pancreatic angiography, 170, 171f
Pancreatic duct
    ERCP visualization of, 205-208f, 210
    stricture, 210
Pancreatitis
    chronic, ERCP in, 208f
    CT in, 141, 141f
    after ERCP, 209
    ultrasound in, 82, 83f
Pancreatography, endoscopic retrograde, 202-210. See also under Cholangiopancreatography
Papillary muscle dysfunction, Swan-Ganz catheterization in, 346f
Paracentesis. See also Peritoneal lavage
    in abdominal trauma, 293-297
        in blunt injury, 293-294
        in penetrating injury, 296-297
        peritoneal lavage compared with, 295
        technique, 294
    diagnostic use, 283
Paranasal sinuses
    air-fluid levels in, 15f, 19
    radiography, 13, 14f, 15, 15f
        in inflammatory and neoplastic disease, 17f, 18f, 33
        in sinusitis, 17f
Parathyroid gland
    adenoma 68-69, 68f
    and calcium metabolism, 67-68
    ultrasound, 68-69, 68f
Pediatric colonoscopy, 277
Pediatric endoscopes, 265
Pelvis
    abscess in
        CT localization for percutaneous drainage, 149
        percutaneous drainage, 149
        radionuclide imaging in localization, 120
    angiography of, 175
    cancer, CT in, 144-145
    comparison between ultrasound and CT for, 144
    CT of, 144-146
        in abscess, 145
        in malignancy, 144-145
        normal anatomy, 144, 145f
        in trauma, 145-146
    trauma
        angiography in, 175
        danger of decompression of hematoma by laparotomy, 295-296
        gunshot wounds, 296-297
        hemorrhage in, 295-296
        peritoneal lavage in, 295-296
        radiography in, 34f, 41
    ultrasound, 92-94, 93f
Peptic ulcer disease
    acid-secretion testing in, 372-373, 372t
    endoscopy in, 268
    radiographic appearance, 224, 227f
        diagnostic efficacy, 227
    vagotomy in
        criteria for completeness, 374-375
        2-deoxy-glucose testing, 375

intraoperative testing for efficacy, 373-374
pancreatic polypeptide testing, 375
postoperative insulin test, 374
tests after, 373-375
Percutaneous drainage, CT localization in, 149
Percutaneous transhepatic cholangiography, 199-202.
    See also Cholangiography, percutaneous
    transhepatic
Pericardial effusion
    echocardiography for, 75
    electrocardiogram in, 320
Pericarditis, electrocardiogram in, 320, 321f
Peripheral vascular disease, angiography in, 175-176,
    178-179f
Peritoneal lavage, in abdominal trauma, 283, 289-290,
    293-297
    adhesions influence on results, 295
    in altered levels of consciousness, 293
    in blunt injury, 293-294
    contraindications, 295-296
    criteria for positive results, 294-295
    in equivocal abdominal findings, 293
    in gunshot wounds, 296-297
    open versus closed method, 294, 295
    in patient undergoing surgery for nonabdominal
        trauma, 294
    in pelvic fracture, 295-296
    in penetrating injury, 296-297
    in pregnancy, 295
    in stab sounds, 297
    with surgical scars, 295
    technique, 294
Peritoneum
    hemoperitoneum in abdominal trauma, 283, 290
    laparoscopic examination, 287
    lavage, 293-297. See also Peritoneal lavage
    paracentesis, 293-294. See also Paracentesis
pH
    esophageal monitoring, 353-363. See also
        Esophagus, pH monitoring
    stomach measures after vagotomy, 373-374
Pharynx, radiographic examination, 215, 219
Pheochromocytoma
    angiography, 174
    CT of, 143
Phleborrheography, 389
    diagnostic efficacy, 390
    interpretation, 390
    technique, 389
Phosphor, 6
Phosphorus, spectrum in muscle magnetic imaging, 413f
Photoelectric reaction, 4
Photoplethysmography, 392-394
    diagnostic efficacy, 393
    indications, 392-393
    interpretation, 393, 394f
    technique and technical pitfalls, 393
Piezoelectric crystal, 382
Plethysmography
    air-filled, 389-390
    fluid-filled, 388-389
    impedance, 394-396
    in lung volume determination, 301
    oculoplethysmography, 388-389
    photo, 392-394
    strain-gauge, 390-392
Pleura
    biopsy, 257-258
        thoracoscopy in, 259
    CT of, 138

Pleural effusion
    lateral decubitus chest film for, 47, 47f, 48f
    pleural biopsy in, 257-258
    rationale and selection of diagnostic methods for, 260
    thoracentesis in, 258
Pneumonectomy
    evaluation prior to, 307-308
    operability, 307-308
Pneumonia, gallium scan in, 106
Pneumoperitoneum
    abdominal x-rays in, 55, 55f
    in laparoscopy, 286
Pneumotachometers, 302-303
Popliteal artery, arteriography in peripheral vascular
    disease, 176
Portable x-rays
    chest, 50-51, 50f
    interpretation of, 50-51
    limitations in, 50
Portal hypertension, angiography in, 169
Portal venous system, angiography, 169-170
Positron-emission transaxial tomography, 98
Postcholecystectomy syndrome, 204, 205-206f
Pre-excitation syndrome, 322, 323f, 324
Pregnancy
    peritoneal lavage in abdominal trauma in, 295
    radiation effects in, 10
Preoperative period
    arterial blood gas analysis in, 306
    chest x-ray in, 45
    in lung resection, 307-308
    pulmonary function tests, 299-308. See also
        Pulmonary function tests
Pressure index, 382
    interpretation in arterial disease, 385
Proctosigmoidoscopy, 278-280
Pulmonary angiography, 166-167
    complications, 166
    in congenital anomalies, 167
    procedure, 167
    in pulmonary embolism, 166-167, 168f
Pulmonary artery
    balloon occlusion in preoperative evaluation of
        pneumonectomy patient, 307-308
    end-diastolic pressure, 332, 332f
    Swan-Ganz catheter in determination, 348
    infarction with Swan-Ganz catheter, 351
    left, aberrant, 163
    perforation with Swan-Ganz catheter, 351
    pressure waveforms, 332-333, 332-333f
    Swan-Ganz catheter insertion in, 345-348. See also
        Swan-Ganz catheter
    wedge pressure, 332-333, 333f. See also Swan-Ganz
        catheter
        in aortic regurgitation, 333, 337f
        in mitral regurgitation, 334, 338f
        in mitral stenosis, 333, 337f
        Swan-Ganz catheter in determination, 348
Pulmonary embolism
    angiography in, 166-167, 168f
    chest x-ray in, 166
    digital subtraction angiography in, 167
    electrocardiogram in, 317, 318f
    lung scanning for, 104-106, 105f, 106f
Pulmonary function tests, 299-308
    arterial blood gases, 305-306
    costs, 303, 304t
    diffusion capacity, 306
    factors influencing results, 303
    flow volume loops, 303, 304t, 305, 305f

Pulmonary function tests *(Continued)*
  forced expiratory spirogram, 301-302, 304t
  forced vital capacity, 301-302, 302f
  gas exchange, 305-306
  indications, 299, 304t
  in lung resection patient, 307-308
  lung volumes and capacities, 299, 300f, 301, 304t
    dynamic, 299, 300f
    static, 299, 301
  maximum voluntary ventilation, 302, 304t
  normal values for, 303, 304t
  pneumotachometers in, 302-303
  in preoperative patient with chronic lung disease, 299
  in small airway disease, 306-307
  spirometers in, 300f, 302
  technical aspects of spirometry, 302-303
  of ventilation, 301-305
  ventilatory reserve, 308
Pulmonary sling, 163
Pulmonary vascular resistance
  abnormalities, 339-340
  calculation, 339
Pulse pressure, 381-382
Pyelography, retrograde, 247-248
  complications, 248
  indications, 247
  in obstruction, 248
  technique, 247

Race, electrocardiogram related to, 312
Rad, 7
Radiation. *See also* X-rays
  absorbed dose, 7
  biologic effects, 7-8, 10
  cancer and leukemia due to, 8
  chromosomal abnormalities and genetic effects, 8
  exposure, 7
    in CT, 127-128
    in gastrointestinal radiography, 213
    limits, 7, 10t
  Gray, 7
  measurement, 7
  permissible exposure limits, 10, 10t
  in pregnant woman, 10
  protection from, 7-8, 10
Radiation beam restrictors, 5f
Radiation colitis, colonoscopy in, 277
Radiation enteritis, 229-230, 232f
Radiation-induced proctosigmoiditis, sigmoidoscopy in, 279-280
Radiation-induced white matter disease, magnetic resonance imaging in, 418
Radiocolloid
  in bone marrow imaging, 119
  in spleen imaging, 118-119
Radiography
  of abdomen, 54-57. *See also* Abdomen, plain film of
  in ankle injury, 37f, 38f, 41
  of back, 18-27f, 33, 37-39
  body-section, 6-7. *See also* Magnetic resonance imaging; Tomography
  of chest, 43-53. *See also* Chest x-ray
  CT, 127-149. *See also* Tomography, computed
  in elbow fractures, 32f, 41
  equipment for cardiac catheterization, 329
  errors in interpretation, 51, 51-53f
  of extremities, 28f-40f, 39-41
    high-resolution magnification, 28f, 39-40
    indications and limitations, 40-41
    techniques, 39-40
  xeroradiography, 28f, 40
  of gastrointestinal tract, 213-237
    barium enema, 230-231, 234-237
    colon, 230-231, 234-237
    contrast agents in, 213-214
    enteroclysis, 227, 230f
    equipment, cost and radiation risk, 213
    interpretative principles, 214-215
    mesenteric small bowel, 227, 229-230
    pharynx and esophagus, 215-219
    stomach and duodenum, 219, 222-227
    upper gastrointestinal series, 219, 222-227
  in hand injury, 33f, 34f, 41
  of head, 13-19, 27, 33
    face, 13, 14f, 15, 15f
    indications and limitations, 15, 15-18f, 19, 27, 33
    mandible, 15, 15f
    paranasal sinuses, 13, 14f, 15, 15f
    skull films, 13. *See also* Skull x-ray
  in knee trauma, 35-37f, 41
  in pelvic and hip trauma, 34f, 41
  of pharynx and esophagus, 215-219
  in shoulder injuries, 31f, 32f, 40-41
  of skeleton, 13-41
  of stomach and duodenum, 219, 222-227
  in wrist injury, 33f, 34f, 41
Radiology
  contrast and edge perception in, 6, 8f
  dose of radiation in various examinations, 10t
  intensifying screens in, 6
  physics, 3-5
  quality related to dose, 6
  See also Radiation; X-rays; and under specific examination
Radionuclide, 97
Radionuclide imaging, 97-124
  in abscess localization, 120
  agents used in, 97
  of biliary tract, 108-109
  of bone, 111-113
  of bone marrow, 119-120
  of brain, 98-102
  of gallbladder, 108-109
    other imaging methods compared with, 183
  of gastrointestinal tract, 120-122
  of heart, 113-118
  instruments in, 97-98
    scintillation camera, 97-98
    tomographic systems, 98
  of kidney, 109-111
  of liver, 107-108
  of lung, 104-107
  in lymphoma, 123f, 124
  principles, 97-98
  procedures, 98
  of salivary glands, 122-123
  of scrotum, 122, 122f
  of soft tissue neoplasms, 123f, 124
  of spleen, 118-119
  of stomach, 120-122
  of thyroid, 102-104
  of vascular system, 123-124
Real-time ultrasound, 61, 62f, 63
Rectum
  colonoscopy in bleeding evaluation, 277
  sigmoidoscopy, 278-280
Relaxation times, 414, 414f
Renal angiography, 172-174
  in cysts and tumors, 172-173, 175f
  indications, 172

in renal vascular disorders, 172, 175f
  in trauma, 174
  venography, 173
Renal blood flow, radionuclide imaging for, 109-110, 110f
Renal cell carcinoma
  angiography in, 172-173, 175f
  CT in, 142, 142f, 173
Renal failure, cardiac catheterization in, 329
Renal venography, 173
Renovascular hypertension, 172, 175f
Resectability, 307
Resistance, vascular, cardiac catheterization in calculation of, 339-340
Resistance index, Doppler ultrasound studies, 385-386
Resolution
  in digital subtraction angiography, 155
  in ultrasound, 63
Retroperitoneum
  fine-needle aspiration cytology, 401, 405t
  hemorrhage, CT in, 146
  lymph nodes of, 143-144
    CT compared with lymphangiography, 144
    ultrasound for, 88, 91f
  magnetic resonance imaging of, 423
  tumors, ultrasound for, 88
  ultrasound, 85, 88, 90-91f
Rhinorrhea, CSF, radionuclide cisternography in, 102
Right atrium
  pressure waveforms, 330-331, 331f
  right atrial abnormality on electrocardiogram, 313, 314f
Right ventricle
  hypertrophy, electrocardiogram in, 315-317, 316f
  infarction, Swan-Ganz catheterization in, 347f
  pressure waveforms, 331-332, 332f
Roentgen, 7

Salivary glands, radionuclide imaging, 122-123
Sarcoidosis, gallium lung scan in, 106, 106f
Scattered radiation, of x-rays, 4-5
Scintillation camera, 97-98
Scleroderma, esophageal motility studies in, 367
Screening
  chest x-ray in, 45
  sigmoidoscopy in, 280
Scrotum, radionuclide imaging, 122, 122f
Secretin test, 371-372, 375
Seldinger technique
  in angiography, 154
  in percutaneous drainage of abscess, 149
Sepsis
  cholangitis, 209
  after ERCP, 209
  pancreatic, 209
  after percutaneous transhepatic cholangiography, 200
Sex, electrocardiogram related to, 311-312
Shoulder fractures, radiography in, 31f, 32f, 40-41
Shunts, intracardiac, cardiac catheterization in assessment, 338-339
Sigmoidoscopy, 278-280
  advances in equipment, 278-279
  contraindications, 280
  derotation of volvulus by, 280
  in diverticular disease, 279
  indications, 279-280, 279t
  in inflammatory bowel disease, 279
  in ischemic colitis, 279
  limitations, 280
  office screening procedures, 280
  preparation of patient for, 279
  in radiation-induced proctosigmoiditis, 279-280
  for redundant sigmoid colon, 279
  in stricture, 280
  in surveillance, 280
  technique, 279
  therapeutic uses, 280
Single-photon-emission computed tomography, 98
Sinuses. See Paranasal sinuses
Sinusitis, radiography of paranasal sinuses in, 17f
Skeleton, radiography of, 13-41. See also under Radiography
Skull fracture
  depressed, 14f
  epidural hematoma associated with, 130
Skull x-ray
  in depressed skull fracture, 14f
  in hospital department versus as portable film, 19, 27
  indications and limitations, 15, 15f, 19, 27
  in osteomyelitis and metastasis, 27
  technique, 13
  in unconscious patient, 19, 27
  views in, 13, 14f
Small intestine
  Crohn's disease, radiographic contrast studies, 229, 232f
  metastatic disease involving, 230, 233f
  peritoneal adhesions involving, 230, 233f
  radiation-induced injury, 229-230, 232f
  radiography of, 227, 229-230
    basics of interpretation, 229-230
    diagnostic efficacy, 230
    direct injection of barium, 227
    indications, 227
    peroral examination, 227
    preparation of patient for, 227
    retrograde studies, 227, 229
    technical problems, 229
Smoking, pulmonary function tests influenced by, 301-302
Sodium, as nucleus in magnetic resonance imaging, 424-425
Soft-tissue tumors
  CT in, 148
  radionuclide imaging, 123f, 124
Sphygmomanometer, 379-380, 380t
Spin-echo images, 415, 415t, 416f
Spinal angiography, 158
Spinal cord, CT of, 146, 146f
Spine
  cervical
    immobilization before radiography, 33
    radiography
      flexion and extension views, 21f, 37
      posterior arches, 20f
      swimmer's view, 20f, 33
      traction for visualization of cervicothoracic junction, 19f, 33
      in trauma, 19-22f, 33, 37-38
      in unconscious head trauma patient, 19, 27
      views, 18f, 33
    tomography, 22f, 24-27f, 33, 37-39
    trauma, 19-22f, 33, 37-38
  CT of, 146-147
  difficulties in ultrasonography, 64, 64f
  disc herniation, CT evaluation, 146-147, 147f
  lumbosacral, radiography
    in trauma, 23f, 38
    views, 33

Spine (Continued)
  obstructive lesions, 147
  radiography, 18-27f, 33, 37-39
    indications and limitations, 33, 37-39
    in nontraumatic conditions, 38-39
    technique, 33
  stenosis, CT in, 147
  thoracic
    compression fracture, 22f, 23f
    radiography
      in trauma, 22f, 38
      views, 33
  trauma to
    cervical portion, 19-22f, 33, 37-38
    CT in, 147
    lumbosacral portion, 23f, 38
    thoracic portion, 22f, 38
Spirometers, 300f, 302
Spirometry
  costs, 303, 304t
  forced expiratory, 301-302, 302f
  in lung volume determination, 299, 300f, 301
  maximum voluntary ventilation, 302
  technical aspects, 302-303
Spleen
  fine-needle aspiration cytology, 401-402
  laparoscopic examination, 287
  radionuclide imaging, 118-119
    indications, 119
    in infarct, 119
    procedure, 119
  size determination, 119
  trauma
    CT in, 146
    laparoscopy in, 290
  ultrasound, 83-84, 84f
Splenomegaly, causes, 119
Stab wounds
  abdominal, 297
  peritoneal lavage in, 297
Stomach
  acid-secretory testing, 369-375
    applications, 372-375
    with 2-deoxyglucose, 371, 375
    in duodenal ulcer, 372-373, 372t
    gastrin analogues in, 370-371, 370t
    gastrin stimulation, 371-372, 375
    histamine analogues in, 370, 370f
    with insulin, 371, 374-375
    nasogastric tube in, 369-370
    in normal subject, 372
    secretin test, 371-372, 375
    secretion index, 372
    stimulant secretagogues for, 370, 370t
    in stomach cancer, 373, 373f
    in stomach ulcer, 373
    technique, 369-370
    with tolbutamide, 371
    vagal innervation in, 371
    after vagotomy, 373-375
    in Zollinger-Ellison syndrome, 375
  basal acid output, 369
  cancer
    acid-secretion testing in, 373, 373f
    endoscopy in, 268
    radiographic appearance, 224, 226, 228f
      diagnostic efficacy, 226-227
  composition of gastric juice, 369
  endoscopy
    complications, 272
    failure to find existing lesion, 272
    fiberoptic, 263
    historical development, 263
    indications, 267-268
    technique, 271
  function studies, 369-375
  gastrocamera for, 263-264
  maximal acid output, 369
  peak acid output, 369
  perforation, after endoscopy, 272
  polyp, radiographic appearance, 224, 228f
  radiography, 219, 222-227
    basics of interpretation, 224, 226
    diagnostic efficacy, 226-227
    indications, 219
    patient preparation for, 219
    in postoperative period, 224
    single- versus double-contrast examination, 219, 222-223f, 224, 224f
      diagnostic efficacy, 226-227
    technical problems, 224
  radionuclide imaging, 120-122
    gastric emptying, 121
    in gastroesophageal reflux, 120-121, 121f
    in Meckel's diverticulum, 122, 122f
  ulcer
    acid-secretion testing in, 373
    endoscopy in, 268
    radiographic appearance, 224, 225-226f
      diagnostic efficacy, 226-227
Stroke, brain scan in, 99-100, 100f
Subarachnoid hemorrhage
  aneurysm rupture in, 159
  CT in, 133
Subclavian artery
  aneurysm, 165
  left, aberrant, 162
  right, aberrant, 162, 163f
Subclavian steal phenomenon, 157
Subdural hematoma
  acute, 130, 130f
  brain scan in, 100, 100f
  chronic, 130, 131f
  comparison of CT with brain scan in, 101
  CT in, 130, 130f, 131f
Subphrenic abscess, radionuclide imaging of, 120f
Subtraction techniques, angiography, 155. See also under Angiography, digital subtraction
Superior vena cava
  obstruction, vascular radionuclide imaging in 123-124, 123f
  venography, 178
Swan-Ganz catheter, 343-344, 344f
  arrhythmias due to, 351
  balloon rupture, 348
  in cardiac care unit, 344-345, 345-347f
  in cardiac catheterization, 344, 345f
  in cardiac output determination, 348, 349f
  complications, 348, 351
  cost, 351
  indications for, 344-345
  in infants and children, 345
  in intracavitary electrocardiography, 348
  knotting of catheter, 351
  pressures measured by, 348
  pulmonary artery infarction or rupture due to, 351
  in surgical patient, 345
  technique for insertion, 345-348
  in temporary pacemaker placement, 348, 350f
  uses and interpretation, 348
Syphilis, aortic aneurysm in, 164

Systemic vascular resistance
  abnormalities, 339
  calculation, 339
Technetium-99m, 97. *See also* Radionuclide imaging
Television camera, in gastroscope, 263-264
Testes
  cancer, retroperitoneal lymphadenopathy in, 88, 91f
  radionuclide imaging, 122, 122f
  torsion
    epididymitis distinguished from, 122, 122f
    radionuclide imaging in, 122, 122f
  ultrasound, 85, 89f
Thallium myocardial imaging, 115
  in exercise stress test, 116, 118, 118f
  interpretation, 115-116, 117f
  tomographic cuts for interpretation, 115, 117f
Thermodilution, in cardiac output determination, 348, 349f
Thoracentesis, 258
Thoracoscopy, 259
Thorax. *See* Chest
Thrombophlebitis, venography in, 177, 179f
Thrombosis, deep vein
  air-filled plethysmography in, 389, 390
  combination of diagnostic studies for, 395-396
  impedance plethysmography in, 394-396, 395f, 396f
  strain-gauge plethysmography in, 391, 392
  venography in, 177, 179f
Thymoma, CT findings, 136, 138f
Thyroid gland
  cancer
    radionuclide imaging in, 104, 104f
    screening persons at risk, 104
  nodule
    radionuclide imaging in, 102, 103, 103f, 104
    ultrasound evaluation, 66-67, 67f
  radionuclide scanning, 102-104
    in cancer, 104, 104f
    indications, 102
    in metastases, 104
    nonfunctioning nodule, 103, 103f
    normal findings, 103, 103f
    procedure, 102-103
    in screening persons at risk for cancer, 104
    in thyroiditis, 103-104, 103f
    uptake study, 103-104
  ultrasound, 66-67, 67f
Tibia, neoplasms, tomography in, 39f
Tidal volume, 299, 300f
Toe pressure, in Doppler ultrasound, 387
Tolbutamide, gastric secretion elicited by, 371
Tomography
  computed, 127-149
    of abdomen, 138-146
      abscess, 145
      adrenal glands, 143
      biliary tract, 140
      gastrointestinal tract, 141-142
      kidney, 142
      liver, 138-140
      pancreas, 140-141
      retroperitoneal lymph nodes, 143-144
      in trauma, 145-146
    advantages over conventional radiography, 127
    in aortic aneurysm and dissection, 88, 136, 137f
    approach in viewing scan, 128
    basic principles, 127-128
    of bone, 148
    of brain, 128-134
      brain scan compared with, 100-101

of chest, 134-138. *See also* Chest, CT of
with contrast
  in abdominal trauma, 145-146
  in head scan, 128
cost, 128
in fine-needle abdominal aspiration, 408, 408f, 409t
of head, 128-134
  in brain abscess, 133-134
  in brain tumor, 131-133, 132f
  in hydrocephalus, 134, 134f
  in intracranial vascular disease, 133, 133f
  in trauma, 128, 130-131, 130f, 131f
Hounsfield units for various body structures, 127, 127t
interventional procedures, 148-149
  biopsy, 148-149
  percutaneous drainage, 149
in kidney trauma, 173-174
of liver, liver scan compared with, 108
in lung nodule, 137
magnetic resonance imaging compared to, 424
in mediastinal mass, 136-137, 138f
metrizamide-enhanced, 146, 146f
of musculoskeletal system, 148
of pelvis, 144-146
  abscess, 145
  gallbladder, 140
  trauma, 145-146
radiation dose in, 127-128
in renal cell carcinoma, 173
in retroperitoneal lymphadenopathy, 88
single-photon-emission, 98
in soft-tissue tumors, 148
of spine, 146-147
ultrasound of pelvis compared with, 94
conventional, 6-7, 6f, 7f, 8f
  chest, 49-50, 49f
  of extremities, 39, 39f
  in facial trauma, 17f, 27
  in inflammatory and neoplastic disease of paranasal sinuses, 18f, 33
  nephrotomography with excretory urography, 245, 246f
positron-emission transaxial, 98
with radionuclide imaging, 98
of spine
  in cervical spine trauma, 22f, 33, 37-38
  in nontraumatic conditions, 24-27f, 38-39
Trachea, vascular ring compressing, 162-163
Transducers
  in blood pressure measurement, 380-381
  in photoplethysmography, 392
  in pressure wave measurements in cardiac catheterization, 330
Trauma
  abdominal, CT in, 145-146
  aortic pseudoaneurysm due to, 164, 164f
  of extremities. *See* Extremities, trauma
  head. *See* Head trauma
  minilaparoscopy in, 289-291, 289f
  in pelvis, 175
  to spine. *See under* Spine
Tuberculosis
  chest x-ray in, 45
  gallium lung scan in, 106

Ulcerative colitis, radiographic appearance, 235, 236f
Ultrasound, 59-94
  A mode, 59, 60f, 61

Ultrasound (Continued)
  of abdomen, 61, 63, 79-92
    adrenal glands, 85, 88f
    common bile duct, 79-81, 81f
    gallbladder, 79, 80f
    kidney, 84-85, 86-87f
    liver, 81-82, 82f
    needle puncture guidance by, 88, 91-92, 92f
    pancreas 82-83, 83f
    retroperitoneum, 85, 88, 90-91f
    spleen, 83-84, 84f
    testes, 85, 89f
  of aortic aneurysm, 88, 90f
  of breast, 69, 72-73f, 74
    mammography compared with, 69, 74
  of chest, 69, 72-73f, 74-75, 76-78f, 79. See also Echocardiography
    after mass discovered by xeromammography, 73f, 74
  difficulties in imaging, 63-65
  Doppler, 63, 382-388. See also Doppler ultrasound
    in carotid artery flow, 69, 70-71f
    duplex scanning, 69
  duplex scanning, 69, 70-71f
  in fine-needle abdominal aspiration, 408, 409t
  gray-scale imaging, 60f, 61
  of head, 65, 66f
    in craniotomy surgery, 65
    in infants, 65, 66f
  of heart. See Echocardiography
  historical developments in, 59
  of liver, liver scan compared with, 108
  M mode, 63
    in heart, 63
  mechanism of action, 59, 60f, 61
  of neck, 65-69, 67-68f, 70f
    carotid arteries, 69, 70-71f
    parathyroid, 68-69, 68f
    thyroid, 66-67, 67f
  in obstetrics, 61, 93f, 94
  of pelvis, 92-94, 93f
    CT compared with 94
    intravenous urography and barium enema compared with, 93-94
  real-time, 61, 62f, 63
    in gallbladder disease, 61
    linear array, 61, 62f, 63
    mechanical sector, 61, 62f, 63
    portability, 63
    resolution in, 63
Upper gastrointestinal series, 219, 222-227
  basics of interpretation, 224, 226
  diagnostic efficacy, 226-227
  multiphasic examination, 224
  single- versus double-contrast examination, 219, 222-223f, 224, 224f
    diagnostic efficacy, 226-227
  technical problems, 224
Ureter
  calculi, ureteropyeloscopy in removal, 244
  obstruction
    fine-needle aspiration cytology of, 401
    radionuclide imaging in, 110, 111f
  tumors, 244
Ureteropyeloscopy, 244
Urethra
  diverticulum, 252, 252f
  precaution in retrograde cystography, 249
  stricture, retrograde urethrography in, 250, 250f
  tear, 249
  trauma, retrograde urethrography in, 249-250
  voiding cystourethrography for, 251-252
Urethrography, retrograde, 249-250
  complications, 250
  indications, 249
  technique, 250
Urinary obstruction
  excretory urography in, 245
  radionuclide imaging in, 109, 110, 110f, 111f
  retrograde pyelography in, 248
  ultrasound in, 85, 86f
Urinary tract
  studies of, 243-254
    cystometrography, 252-254
    cystoscopy, 243-244
    excretory urography, 245-247
    retrograde cystography, 248-249
    retrograde pyelography, 247-248
    retrograde urethrography, 249-250
    ureteropyeloscopy, 244
    uroflow studies, 252, 253f
    voiding cystourethrography, 251-252
    vesicoureteral reflux, 251-252
Urinary tract infection, after retrograde pyelography, 248
Urine, uroflow studies, 252, 253f
Uroflow studies, 252, 253f
Urography
  excretory, 245, 246f, 247
    allergic reaction, 245, 247
    bladder appearance on, 248f
    complications, 245, 247
    contrast agent in, 245
    indications, 245
    interpretation, 245, 246-247f
    nephrotomography with, 245, 246f
    technique, 245
    in urinary obstruction, 245
  intravenous, ultrasound of pelvis compared with, 93-94

V wave
  pulmonary artery wedge pressure, 333
    in mitral regurgitation, 334, 338f
  right atrial pressure, 331, 331f
Vagal innervation, in acid-secretory testing, 371
Vagotomy
  Congo red test of efficacy, 373
  criteria for completeness of, 374-375
  2-deoxy-glucose testing, 375
  intraoperative gastric acid-secretory testing, 373-374
  pancreatic polypeptide testing, 375
  pH probes in stomach after, 373-374
  postoperative insulin test, 374
Valves, cardiac catheterization evaluation of, 340
Vascular disorders
  of colon, colonoscopy in, 277
  peripheral vascular disease, angiography in, 175-176, 178-179f
  radionuclide imaging, 123-124
  trauma, 175, 177f
    arteriovenous fistula in, 175, 176f
Vascular laboratory, 379-396
  blood pressure measurement
    direct, 380-382
    indirect, 379-380
  Doppler ultrasound, 382-388
  plethysmography
    air-filled, 389-390
    fluid-filled, 388-389
    impedance, 394-396

photo, 392-394
    strain-gauge, 390-392
Vascular malformations
    in brain, CT of, 133, 133f
    cerebral angiography in, 158, 159, 160f
Vascular resistance, cardiac catheterization in calculation of, 339-340
Vascular ring, aortic arch anomalies causing, 162-163
Vasculitis, cerebral arteries, 159
Vater, ampulla of, endoscopy of, 265
Veins, Doppler ultrasound studies of, 383
Venography
    impedance plethysmography compared with, 395
    inferior vena cava, 177-178
    of lower extremity, 177
        ascending, 177
        complications, 177
        descending, 177, 179f
    renal, 173
    superior vena cava, 177-178
Venous insufficiency
    photoplethysmography in, 392-394, 394f
    strain-gauge plethysmography in, 391-392
Venous thrombosis
    deep
        air-filled plethysmography in, 389, 390
        combination of diagnostic studies for, 395-396
        impedance plethysmography in, 394-396, 395f, 396f
        strain-gauge plethysmography in, 391, 392
        venography in, 177, 179f
    Doppler ultrasound in, 385
        diagnostic efficacy, 388
Ventilation, tests of, 301-305
Ventilation-perfusion scan, 104-106, 105f, 106f
    interpretation, 105
    procedure, 104-105
Ventricular abnormalities
    left ventricular hypertrophy, 315, 315f
    right ventricular hypertrophy, 315-317, 316f
Ventricular aneurysm, electrocardiogram in, 322
Ventricular arrhythmias, cardiac catheterization danger in, 328
Ventricular pressures, normal waveforms, 331-332, 332f, 333, 334f
Ventricular septum rupture, Swan-Ganz catheterization in, 347f
Ventriculoperitoneal shunt, radionuclide cisternography in evaluation of patency, 102, 102f

Vertebral angiography
    procedure, 156
    in vascular malformations, 159
Vertebral artery
    stenosis, 156
    subclavian steal phenomenon, 157
Vesicoureteral reflux, voiding cystourethrography for, 251-252
Vital capacity, forced, 301-302, 302f
Voiding cystourethrography, 251-252
Volvulus
    cecal, colonoscopy reduction, 278
    sigmoid, sigmoidoscopy in derotation of, 280

Weight, electrocardiogram related to, 312
Wolff-Parkinson-White syndrome, electrocardiogram in, 323f, 324
Wright respirometer, 302-303
Wrist trauma, radiography in, 33f, 34f, 41

X descent, 330, 331f
X-rays, 3-4. *See also* Radiation; Radiology; Radiography; *and under specific study*
    attenuation, 4
    Compton scattering, 4, 4f
    generation, 3-4, 3f
    image receptors of, 5
    interaction with matter, 4-5
        at atomic level, 4
        with object to be radiographed, 4
    photoelectric reaction, 4
    scattered radiation, 4-5, 5f
Xenon lung ventilation-perfusion test, 104-105, 307
Xeroradiography
    of breast, 6
    of extremities, 28f, 40
    image reception in, 6

Y descent, 331, 331f

Zenker's diverticulum
    endoscopy contraindication in, 267
    esophageal motility studies in, 367
Zollinger-Ellison syndrome
    acid-secretory testing in, 375
    gastrin-stimulation tests in, 371-372, 375
Zygomatic arch fracture, 16f